FOUNDATIONS OF ENVIRONMENTAL AND OCCUPATIONAL NEUROTOXICOLOGY

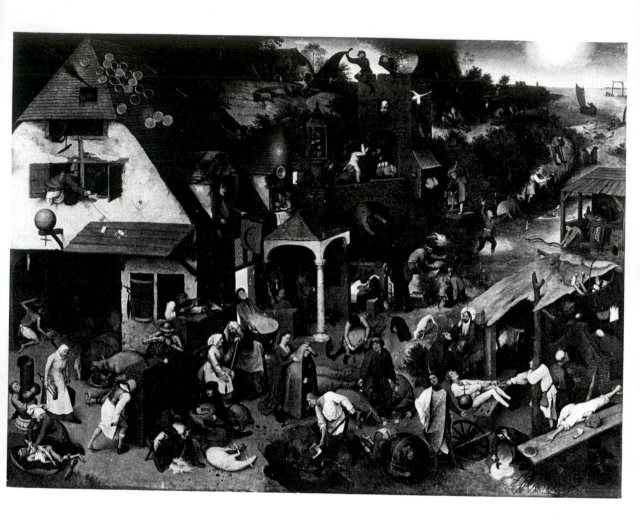

Pieter Bruegel, The Elder
The Netherlandish Proverbs, 1559

This painting illustrates the various occupations—and some of their hazards—of a medieval European village.

FOUNDATIONS OF ENVIRONMENTAL AND OCCUPATIONAL NEUROTOXICOLOGY

JOSÉ A. VALCIUKAS

WITH A NEW INTRODUCTION BY THE AUTHOR

TRANSACTION PUBLISHERS
NEW BRUNSWICK (U.S.A.) AND LONDON (U.K.)

Library of Congress Catalog Number: 2001057375
ISBN: 0-7658-0931-1
Printed in the United States of America

Library of Congress Cataloging-in-Publication Data

Valciukas, José A.
    Foundations of environmental and occupational neurotoxicology / José
A. Valciukas ; with a new introduction by the author.—Facsimile ed.
    p. cm.
Includes bibliographical references and index.
ISBN 0-7658-0931-1 (pbk. : alk. paper)
    1. Neurotoxicology. 2. Environmental toxicology. I. Title. [DNLM: 1.
Environmental Pollutants—toxicity. 2. Nervous System—drug effects.
    3. Occupational Diseases—chemically induced.]

RC347.5 .V35 2002
616.8'047—dc21   2001057375

To Alberto B. Bugeau, a born teacher and a good friend, from whom I am still learning after 32 years.

Contents

Introduction to the Transaction Edition

I wish to express thanks to Dr. Irving Louis Horowitz, chairman and editorial director of Transaction Publishers, Ms. Mary Curtis, president of Transaction Publishers, and Dr. Nathaniel J. Pallone, of Rutgers University's Center of Alcohol Studies, for their help in reissuing *Foundations of Environmental and Occupational Neurotoxicology*. I want thank Lauren Kittel for editing an earlier draft of this manuscript, and Michael Paley, assistant editor at Transaction Publishers, for help with the final version. I was saddened by the death of Dr. Sylvia Frank, who edited earlier versions of the present book.

*   *   *

This reissue of *Foundations of Environmental and Occupational Neurotoxicology* (*Foundations*) by Transaction Publishers occurs eleven years after the publication of the first edition of the book, in 1991, by Van Nostrand Reinhold. The book reflects my vision of a unique body of knowledge in which I was proficient during the mid-1980s, and that vision remains unchanged today. Given a free hand by Transaction to write a new introduction, I thought that an account of the personal context within which the book was written would be of interest for both those who already know my work and those who are reading it for the first time. I begin with a review of the circumstances that influenced my study and understanding of this discipline.

I was born in Argentina, finished my graduate education in the United States, and returned to Argentina after obtaining my Ph.D. (1970) in neuropsychology from the City University of New York (CUNY). I would eventually leave Argentina again to avoid the escalating civil war, and this decision was particularly influenced by an episode in which I almost lost my life as a result of a bombing of an American bank while I walking along Avenida 9 de Julio. The bank was there when I passed in front of it on my way to a sidewalk café on a lazy Sunday afternoon, and it was gone on the way home.

In 1975, while still in Argentina working as a member of the Carrera del Investigador Científico (Research Career of the National Council for Scientific and Technical Research), I won the Humboldt Fellowship from the Federal Republic of Germany. I relocated there in the winter of 1975-1976. After finishing up a two-month, total immersion course in German at the Goethe Institute in the small town of Murnau in Bavaria, I moved to Ulm (near Stuttgart). I was expected to continue my research on the topic of my doctoral dissertation—the visual-vestibular-cerebellar-oculomotor system—at the University of Ulm.

It was in Ulm, during my Sunday walks at the fortifications surrounding the old city, when I suddenly realized that I had been toying with three sets of keys. Looking back, the keys seemed to represent a kind of crossroads: There were the keys to my recently-purchased apartment in San Telmo, a neighborhood in Buenos Aires rich in history. There were the keys to my new apartment in Ulm, rented bare except for a bed and simple furniture. In 1976 Ulm was a kind of town where supermarkets—supplied by seasonal foodstuffs such as potatoes, carrots, onions, garlic, and the like—

closed at 6:00 PM, TV programming ended at 10:30 PM, and everybody was up at 5:00 AM. And there were the keys to the home of my friend Dyer Henke in St. Charles—a historical town a few miles from St. Louis, Missouri. My friend, now deceased, had been walking with me the day of the bombing episode in Buenos Aires. He gave me the keys to his house as a gesture of support in case I had the need to return to the United States in a hurry and without a job.

It was during that walk in early winter when I said to myself, "What do I do now? Do I remain in Germany where I can count on my personal safety and continue my professional career? Do I return to Argentina after 'normality' returns to the country?" In 1976, few knew that that year would mark the beginning of a horrific, full-fledged civil war in Argentina; even today nobody knows for sure how many people died during those events—perhaps as many as 20,000 according to some estimates. "Do I return to United States?" Although I had applied for a permanent residence in the United States, I still had not received the official documentation to immigrate legally to what was later to become my adopted country. There is a story about this, which I will tell you in a moment.

In the spring of 1976 I took a break from my work at Ulm and traveled once again to New York City. New York was dear to me because it was where I fulfilled my youthful dream of doing brain research. I first visited my dear friends Drs. Pedro and Tauba Pasik. Twelve years ago, and almost to the day, Drs. Pasik gave me a job as a research assistant at their laboratory of experimental neurology in the Department of Neurology at Mount Sinai Hospital (named the Mount Sinai School of Medicine in the 1960s), and they offered me a salary of $8,000 a year! I then asked my friends for advice about what to do after finishing my commitments with the Humboldt Foundation in Germany. Pedro Pasik said he had an idea: "Let me call somebody," he said. I overheard Dr. Pasik speaking to someone about an old student of his now living in Europe seeking a job in the United States. Dr. Pasik said that Dr.

Selikoff—whose name I had never heard before—would see me that morning.

Dr. Irving J. Selikoff (1915-1992) cut an impressive figure: he was very good-looking man who, during his pensive moments, reminded me of a Renaissance pope. He had suffered polio as a child and walked with difficulty. At first he would talk about certain topics with the enthusiasm of a young kid; in later years I saw a boss whose moods changed from manic excitement and wrath of biblical proportion to sadness, resignation, and depression. In spite of the fact that I perform psychological evaluations for a living, I cannot describe Dr. Selikoff's character: extraordinary people do not fit common molds. My interview with Dr. Selikoff was brief; he asked nothing about me. I later understood why: he was interested in "issues" more than "people," and many of us knew he could be a bad judge of people. That day he talked about something in which he appeared to be genuinely intrigued but, at the same time, gave the impression that, as a physician, he could not possibly know too much about the subject. He said that behavioral toxicology was an important research field and, would I be willing to create a unit devoted to that topic at the Environmental Sciences Laboratory? I left his office with my head spinning.

1976 was the 200th anniversary of the Independence of the United States, and New York was the place to be: in a few weeks New York's harbor would be abuzz with ships coming from all over the world; people would inundate New York eager to participate in the celebrations. Not me. Having accepted the invitation to spend some time in St. Charles with the friend who gave me the keys to his house, I spent the evening of the fourth of July of 1976 in the Ozark Mountains inside a camping tent. Although I was still intoxicated by the vivid memory of my brief conversation with Dr. Selikoff, I was not particularly thrilled by the thought of residing again in New York. However, there was no professional work for me in the mid-West at that time. After a brief stay in St. Charles, I returned to New York on my way back to Germany.

While in New York, I had a second interview with Dr. Selikoff. This time I was also interviewed by Dr. Ruth Lilis (now retired), whom I was later to admire as one of the most outstanding figures in occupational medicine in this country. My interview with Dr. Lilis obviously went well as I received an offer for a job at the Environmental Sciences Laboratory—in Dr Selikoff's words, "as soon as I was available from my commitments in Germany." I went back to Ulm and, soon after, received a notification to report to the American Embassy in Frankfurt for an interview with the Consul prior to my formal immigration to the United States. All the documentation had been sent to the American Embassy in Frankfurt from the American Embassy in Buenos Aires where I filed the application for immigration status about three years earlier.

I traveled from Ulm to Frankfurt and, once at American Embassy, a young neatly dressed black woman reviewed my documentation without having much eye contact with me. Everything was in order, except that what amounted to a "certification of good behavior" which I possessed had been issued by the FBI. The Embassy needed a formal statement from the New York City Police, as New York was the last city where I lived the longest. "But," I said, "I have a job waiting for me in New York! Could you not just accept the statement from the FBI, as it is, after all, more comprehensive than the one coming from the New York City Police?" The young lady was adamant—I had to write to New York and ask for a certificate of good behavior from the Police Department. Knowing the chaotic state in which New York was, I was almost certain that if I wrote to the Police Department in New York I would be waiting in Germany forever, and then I might not have even a job offer any longer. "Could I see the Consul, please?" I said. "I *am* the Consul!" the young lady snapped. There is an expression in Spanish— "Tierra, trágame" (may the earth open right under my feet, and may I be swallowed by it). I was confronted with my own prejudices and stereotyped expectations about people and positions. In 1976, black people in the United States were just gaining

equality in the placement of prominent positions, and it was only a few years earlier when women began burning their bras during demonstrations. The needed changes in my expectations came too suddenly, too late, and the damage was already done.

I called Dr. Selikoff in New York to explain why I would be delayed in Germany. It was one of the many lucky episodes of my life that one of his closest assistants, Mr. Sidney Sibel—also now deceased—used to work for the New York City Police Department. I waited in agony for several days in Wiesbaden, living in the house where my friend Dr. Maria Carmen Franck, with her husband and small children, lived. In my early twenties Dr. Franck was my mentor, and in *Foundations* I recognized her as someone who taught me that the process of learning the anatomy of the nervous system was fun. Back in 1963, at the time I was going to take the bus from Rosario to Buenos Aires to catch the plane that was to take me to New York, Dr. Franck ("Babby" to her friends") cut a lock of her hair and gave it to me as a present and as a wish of good luck. At the time of my stay with Dr. Franck, there were many Chileans in Wiesbaden and other cities in Germany; Chilean refugees visited the house where she and her husband lived. A form from the New York City Police indicating that there was no record of police apprehensions and/or involvement in criminal activities finally arrived, and it was time to say good-bye to my friends.

As I mention in *Foundations*, the first day at the Environmental Sciences Laboratory was educational. Dr. Selikoff called me early in the morning to tell me that I had to attend a lecture given by Dr. Charles Xintaras at the New York Academy of Sciences. Dr. Xintaras had edited a book entitled *Behavioral Toxicology* published in 1974; he is generally considered to be the father of the field in the United States. Soon after I recognized that if Dr. Selikoff liked you, he would call you incessantly to discuss ideas and projects. A few weeks after I reported to work he said to me: "José, during the course of your work here I will throw you balls; I do not expect for you to catch all of them, but I expect you to make something out of the ones you catch." Dr. Selikoff treated me like a prince; during the first weeks of my joining the Environmental Sciences Laboratory he arranged for an all-paid grand tour to visit the best American laboratories and the most recognizable experts in the field of behavioral toxicology so that, in his words, "I would have the opportunity to learn from the top and from the very best."

Not long after starting my new job, I checked my mailbox and noticed a small envelope that came from Germany; the envelope had black borders. I opened it, and there was a printed card written in German. I thought perhaps it was an announcement of a birthday or some event happening in Wiesbaden about which Babby would have wanted me to know. For more than ten years, Babby and I had corresponded, and we would send things to each other like clippings, fragments of poems, and pictures to remind ourselves that we were still good friends. It took me minutes to realize that the printed card was the notification of her death. Later on I learned that she died from lupus while in her early forties.

In the spring and summer of 1976 I knew very little about environmental sciences in general and occupational toxicology in particular. Now I realize that while I may have not known specific aspects of the field, I had a good training to absorb huge amounts of knowledge in a short period of time. (Dr. James Block—then a research psychologist who invited me to come to the Albert Einstein School of Medicine in 1963—used to say that "a Ph.D. is somebody who learns quickly"). Firstly, I had a good background in neuroanatomy and neurophysiology; at twenty-one I was a teaching assistant on the subject and—while still in Argentina—had explained the intricacies of the nervous system to people who sometimes doubled my age. From 1964 to 1970 I performed and published studies in experimental neurology with the Pasiks.

Secondly, I had a solid training in "classical" as well as in "modern" psychophysics. Classical psychophysics was taught at Queens College of the City University of New York (CUNY). During a midterm examination, Dr. William Battersby (now deceased) required his graduate students to plot from memory graphical representations of, for example, critical fusion frequencies as a function of retinal eccentricity. This was to illustrate the contribution of cones and rods in visual perception, a topic that went on to inspire my doctoral dissertation. Drs. Pasik and Dr. Battersby—who knew each other from the time they worked together under the direction of Dr. Morris B. Bender (no relation to Dr. Loretta Bender) at Bellevue Hospital in New York—built their own optical benches and many other pieces of experimental equipment. Both were much up to date in the recognition of the importance and the actual use of the then-emerging computer technology. In the later 1960s I already had a taste of the times to come: I collected data for my doctoral dissertation using a Digital (brand name) computer that had four kilobytes of memory!

I also had excellent training in "modern psychophysics." Late in the fall of 1971, Dr. Miguelina Guirao, a disciple of Dr. Stanley S. Stevens, the psychologist who proposed the "power law" to replace Fechner's "logarithmic law," returned to Harvard to finish papers left unwritten during her earlier stay at Dr. Stevens' lab. We flew together from Buenos Aires to New York. She went to Cambridge, and I stayed in New York with the Pasiks to finish my own papers left unwritten in late 1960s. Around Christmas time in 1971, Dr. Stevens died from a heart attack while skiing in Colorado. Among the many incredible things that happened to me during my life, I was invited to Harvard as a research associate by Dr. Guirao to help with her work because the future of Dr. Stevens' lab was uncertain. Once back in Argentina, Dr. Guirao and I wrote a comprehensive book in Spanish on the physiology and psychophysics of sensory systems, a book that is virtually unknown in the United States. My legitimate expectation to be recognized as the co-author of that book became subverted due to Argentina's brewing civil war when I fled the country late in 1975. Dr. Guirao never forgave me for leaving. I said that I would return, but I did not. In *Foundations*, published sixteen years after my departure from Argentina, I rescued, from memory, the knowledge that was pertinent to my own book; the knowledge was updated, as I had the opportunity to write my own book in New York, where I found multiple library resources. A friend of mine, some years after *Foundations* was published, gave me a copy of what was supposed to be my first book. I promised myself I would never write a book again unless I could do it all by myself.

"Classical," as well as "modern," psychophysics gave me the mathematical-statistical foundations of toxicology; psychophysics also left me distaste for scientific facts derived from ideal observers and college volunteers. Plotting "dose-response" relationships once a "threshold" value is exceeded requires the same mathematical-statistical strategies of those required for plotting "input-output" relationships in psychophysics. In industrial hygiene, threshold limit values (a redundancy) are the basis for regulation and control of exposures to chemical agents in the environment and the workplace; the numerical values of those thresholds are generally listed in tabular form for a large variety of chemicals. In psychophysics, threshold values depend upon many contributing factors and, as I mentioned early in the case of values for critical frequencies in various portions of the human retina, could require one's ability to read and interpret multidimensional graphs. Psychophysical functions in "classical" psychophysics rely on the notion of the "ideal" eye and the "ideal" ear, that is, the eye and the ear that nobody has. "Modern" psychophysics relies on the psychological characteristics of volunteers who, in most cases, happen to be highly educated Harvard students, or Swedish or Japanese citizens. My own experience in medical field studies of victims of environmental and/or occupational accidents contributed to my later long-lasting disgust for "scientific facts" that apply only to the privileged.

Thirdly, I had a good background in psychometrics and was familiar with most psychological tests that had been used to evaluate cognitive/motor functions and personality. In Argentina, I also was a teaching assistant in psychometrics and personality assessment, and saw and used tests that now are virtually unknown to most psychologists in the United States. However, I could not use psychometric tests in the manner I was taught to use them. Medical clinical surveys carried at the Environmental Sciences Laboratory imposed several space and time limitations in the administration of those tests. A medical survey is organized around the *medical* examination of people, the compilation of people's medical history, the review of their symptoms, and the collection of laboratory samples—including those routinely collected during a medical examination, such as blood and urine, but also fat, nails, hair, and others. A medical field survey of workers suspected to be exposed to asbestos—which I often joined because asbestos workers very often were not exposed to neurotoxic agents—included a number of lung function tests. Neuropsychological testing and electrophysiological determinations could never be administered due to the time allocated to the medical aspects of the field survey. In addition, I was not prepared—as few psychologists ever are—to administer psychological testing and carry out neurophysiological studies inside a union hall where I had to communicate with workers in Spanish, or on the lawn of a Canadian Indian reservation where I needed the help of people who could translate Mohawk into English for me.

"Necessity is the mother of invention," and there I was thinking about how I could compile a brief battery of psychological tests that I could administer within fifteen minutes during a medical field survey. The Block Design and the Digit-Symbol test of the Wechsler Scales of Adult Intelligence were easy to carry to the field, easy to administer particularly because most people found them credible, and during early trials, scores from these two tests gave magnificent bell-shaped distributions. I needed a test for screening global brain dysfunction, and I contemplated the possible adaptation of the Gottschalt figures, which turned out to be difficult for a hospital patient suffering from catastrophic brain damage, but not too challenging for a currently working blue-collar laborer. *Foundations* describes how I asked my colleagues who had children to bring children's books from which I could draw pictures of everyday objects anybody would recognize. I copied them on semitransparent paper, and then I selected ten of them and photocopied them one at a time, two at a time, three at a time, and so on until I got plates with a picture of ten superimposed outlines. Saturday and Sunday mornings at the lab, I made dozens of attempts to come up with the final four plates that would be used in numerous medical field surveys in which I participated. The plates were then copyrighted, and in a modest way I continued the tradition of my mentors by creating my own tools of work. The Embedded Figures Test was such a tool.

It was probably in the fall of that extraordinary year that was 1976 that I received my baptism of fire when I joined a team from the Environmental Sciences Laboratory in a medical survey of secondary lead smelter workers in Vernon, California. "Secondary" lead smelter workers are those who recycle old lead—most commonly from batteries—and retrieve the metal that is then sold in ingots. Not only did I administer psychological testing to ninety workers with the help of one assistant, but the night before the survey I made telephone calls to the home of workers who only spoke Spanish. I flew back to New York carrying the raw data on my plane seat like a precious cargo, and a few days later I began the process of entering the data via IBM punched cards. Inside a large, discarded suitcase, I carried the data from 103rd Street to 42nd Street in Manhattan where the CUNY computer center was located. In 1976, the screen of our "personal" IBM computer at the ESL measured about six by eight inches. Those were the years when your ability to creatively analyze your data depended on your aptitude to seek and maintain a friendly relationship with the head of the computer department, an individual who asserted his or her identity by becoming isolated from the rest of humanity by cathedral-quality, floor-to-ceiling glass panels.

A "group analysis" of the data was presented in February of 1977 at a lead conference sponsored by the Steel Workers of America, a branch of the U.S. AFL-CIO labor organization based in Washington, D.C. Blood lead levels were quite elevated and ninety workers exhibited a ranged of blood lead values ranging from very high to undetectable. Would those values correlate with psychological test results? The data were further analyzed at the Bell Laboratories in Murray Hill, New Jersey. My first encounter with staff members of the Bell Laboratories and my actual visit to their place of work is one of the most exhilarating experiences that I remember. Josef Eisinger and William E. Blumberg had recently patented the hematofluorometer (commonly called the "ZPP meter"), a piece of equipment that quantitatively measures lead effects on the human blood-forming system through the reflection of a drop of human blood excited with blue light. I did not have to help entering the data this time; the data were already entered in the computer when I arrived and were displayed on an unexpectedly unsophisticated X-Y plotter. A few hours later, we saw to our amazement that the age-corrected scores of psychological test scores belonging to secondary lead workers negatively correlated with ZPP levels (that is, as a group, the higher the ZPP value, the lower the score). These findings were important because they illustrated that workers currently employed and going about their daily duties showed subclinical effects induced by lead; the literature discussed cases of lead workers who were ill enough to be admitted into a hospital. These findings were soon to be published in *Science*. I had published many scientific papers before, and in later years would participate in many medical field surveys and publish many other papers, but none caused the excitement of such a highly-profiled contribution to a field virtually unknown to me only a few months ago.

As mentioned in *Foundations*, the idea of writing a book about the basis of environmental and occupational neurotoxicology came about when I myself was looking for such a book and I could not find it. However, as I try to remember events that happened twenty years ago, I realize that the book was conceived and written in bits and pieces since the early 1980s. In 1982 I published an article titled "Psychometric Techniques in Environmental Research" with Dr. Lilis; in the summary of this article the first sentence indicated that "behavioral changes may be the early and only manifestations of neurotoxicity." In 1984 I published a commentary in the a style of a "critique" titled "A Decade of Behavioral Toxicology." In the humanities, a "critique" belongs to a literary genre well known and highly appreciated; in the empirical sciences it still is often considered the work of someone who is showing sure signs of senility. In 1984 I wrote the first outline of *Foundations* in a manuscript sent for publication to the *International Archives of Occupational and Environmental Health* and titled "An Essay on Environmental and Occupational Neurotoxicology." An "essay" is also a format recognized in the humanities but frowned upon as old hat in the empirical sciences. The reviewer of my essay—it looked as if only one individual read the manuscript—considered it "interesting," but *Archives* rejected it for publication. "An Essay on Environmental and Occupational Neurotoxicology" is a condensed version of the book and was never published. In 1985 I contributed a paper to the World Health Organization (WHO) meeting in Copenhagen entitled "Control of Demographic Factors in the Analysis of Neurotoxicological Data" with the first-time-to-be-admitted-in-public confession that I wanted to show the Scandinavians the easy time they had with the analysis of data collected on workers who were 100 percent literate Caucasians. In 1985 Dr. Helena Hänninen, a pioneer in the use of psychometric testing in occupational neurotoxicology, invited me to Finland, her native country. I prepared two lectures for the trip: "The Myth of Objectivism: The Evolution of the State-of-the-Art in Environmental and Occupational Neurotoxicology" (again, very much in line with what a "critic" in the humanities would write), and another one on the "Art and Science of Designing Computer-Compatible Questionnaires." For reasons that I now do not recall, there was no time for me to de-

liver both lectures, and I gave my audience the choice of one over the other. My Finnish audience chose the topic on the design of computer-compatible questionnaires, then a novelty.

I was not sure if I could write *Foundations* by myself, but the prospect of editing a multi-authored book did not appeal to me very much. I also had a chip on my shoulder about the earlier book I co-authored but had to give up. *Foundations* was a more ambitious effort than the early book on the physiology and psychophysics of sensory systems, and I considered the possibility that the book might have to be a team effort. However, when I approached colleagues whose knowledge and experience I respected, they had to respond to their own sense of priorities: the publication of long-overdue scientific articles, writing or preparing annual reports for grant proposals, commitments to our Central Grant, lectures, depositions, family, travel, or yet another medical field survey. A book requires many months of planning, preparation, and actual writing. Few had the time to do it, so in the mid-1980s I decided to go on my own.

Dr. Selikoff, near the time of his retirement, gave me encouragement to write the book; at that time, he himself also needed help. Dr. Robert Schnitzer—a reputable scientist in his own right and a close collaborator of Dr. Selikoff at the time both worked in the treatment of tuberculosis with antibiotics, work that won Selikoff a Lasker Prize—was the managing editor of *Environmental Research*. Dr. Schnitzer was a man who, in his late eighties, openly expressed little tolerance for mediocrity; he was also experiencing the normal physical infirmities of advanced age. Dr. Selikoff founded both *Environmental Research* and *American Journal of Industrial Medicine*. He knew that I was writing a book and suggested to me—tongue-in-cheek, of course—that the weekly operations of *Environmental Research* would give me experience and inspiration.

Foundations was published in 1991, three years after I left the Environmental Sciences Laboratory; Dr. Selikoff died in 1992. The year 1988 was difficult. As anticipated by all of us who worked at the lab, Dr. Selikoff became emeritus and moved to an office at Mount Sinai on 98th Street. My earlier attempts to get funds for my own research—which would have allowed me not to depend on the Central Grant that gave life to the Environmental Sciences Laboratory and was the source of my salary—were unsuccessful. During all the years I was on the staff it was quite apparent that our type of human research based on medical field surveys was expensive and fiercely opposed by the industry. For example—possibly early in the 1980s—a grant proposal (written with Dr. Ruth Lilis) to evaluate residual neurotoxic effects of lead among lead battery manufacturing workers who were said to work under compliance with current recommended environmental thresholds for lead had to be explained and literally defended in front of more than a dozen of experts who, almost without exception, were paid professionals working for the industry. Another grant proposal for a study of whether long-term, low-level exposure to industrial solvents accelerated the process of cognitive "aging" among painters was also rejected. A prospective (follow-up) study of painter apprentices, who were at risk of exposure to industrial solvents, never came off the ground. I flew with Dr. Landrigan to San Diego, California to seek support from a labor union that had a school where such apprentices were trained; while in San Diego, I also made the first personal contacts for the publication of *Foundations*. Few days after returning from San Diego, Dr. Landrigan, the new director of the Environmental Sciences Laboratory, handed me the "pink slip," a very generous one, as I had an entire year to decide how I wanted to continue my professional career. An inner voice told me that if I wanted to continue my, by then, twelve-year career in the field of environmental and occupation health sciences, I had to finish the book.

From the summer of 1987 to the summer of 1988, I did nothing but write many papers that were due for publication and compile the first complete manuscript of *Foundations*, which probably amounted to a two-foot high pile including tables and illustrations. After many rejections, I eventually signed a contract with Van Nostrand Reinhold. At that time of signing the contract, I strongly believed that *Foundations* would have had a better exposure if I were still a member of the by then internationally prestigious Environmental Sciences Laboratory. Now I am not so sure: as I review the book more than a decade after its publication, it now looks like a document with a life of its own, and not needing any particular setting. If I remained at the Environmental Sciences Laboratory, and had not had a full year of a forced sabbatical, I think that I probably would never have had the uninterrupted time—so precious to a writer—to write the book. In 1988 I left Mount Sinai with the title of associate professor, and weeks later I began working as a senior forensic psychologist for the Supreme and Criminal Court in New York State. In 1991, the year of publication of the book, I received considerable media exposure as a result of my forensic work for the prosecution in the infamous case of New York State vs. Gonzalez, the man who set fire to the social club Happyland, where 87 people died, in what was then thought to be one of the worst tragedies in New York City. I visited the lab on the weekly basis, as I was still the managing director of *Environmental Research*. People who were in the inner circle watching the early dismantling of the Environmental Sciences Laboratory and the retirement of Dr. Selikoff appeared not to be happy about my *Foundations*. One close colleague of mine told me: "You have written so many articles about the subject, why do you have the need to write a book?"

Van Nostrand Reinhold won an award from the Association of American Publishers for "excellence in publishing in the medical field" (I do not have access to the actual words written on the plaque) for *Foundations*. Once the book was out, my publishers told me that the book would be used as a "model" for the publication of other books in the medical and technical fields. What happened afterwards is unclear to me, but the educated guess of many is that the book—created to be a scholarly textbook for a nonexistent discipline that I had envisioned—

became the victim of the realities of marketing. Van Nostrand went out of business and another company took over. I eventually received a letter from "the other company" stating that, because the book was not "performing well, *Foundations* would no longer be printed." The copyright reverted to me.

EPILOGUE

When Transaction approached me to publish a new edition of *Foundations,* the obvious question was posed as to whether or not I would update a book that was published more than a decade ago. Firstly, would I want to change the book's scope? The dictionary defines "scope" as the range covered by a subject; however, dictionary definitions are terse and they do not clarify whether a "subject" exists in and of itself or is created by an author or authors. There may be hundreds and even thousands of contributors to the field that I have called environmental and occupational neurotoxicology (E & O Neurotoxicology, hereafter), but the sum total of those contributions does not represent the scope of the field. The scope of *Foundations*, as I envisioned it, is a collection of scientific, technological, and humanistic knowledge that I think belongs together in this discipline. An earlier four-volume project that never materialized was titled *Environmental and Occupational Neurotoxicology: Science, Technology, Art, and Advocacy*, whose scope was wider than *Foundations*, but the material was most likely unpublishable. *Foundations* captured the essence of that earlier project in that it covered the idea of how a large number of professional disciplines—each one recognized in its own right—fit together in our understanding of how a number of natural and man-made chemical compounds affect our brain, mind, and behavior. Topics include existing knowledge about the neuropharmacological and toxicological action of those chemicals, their effects on specific areas of the nervous system, the consequences of those effects on the mind and behavior, the evaluation of confounders (that is, how one teases out the interpretation of effects that are most likely to be caused by those neurotoxic chemicals than by other factors), and the ethical dilemmas that we confront with the use and misuse of that knowledge, such as in the of neurotoxic agents of chemical warfare. The scope of E & O Neurotoxicology also covers its history, but it took a while to decide where to put it in the book. Those readers who have experienced first-hand the frustration of getting suggestions from professional editors might be amused to know that in previous versions of the book, I included the outline of its history *at the beginning*—following the classical format of introducing a discipline with its history—just to be told that few people would really be interested in knowing the history of a discipline that had yet to be properly reviewed. Then, in another version, when I placed the history *at the end*, I was told that the historical roots of the discipline that I envisioned was perhaps too interesting to be relegated to the back, with it looking like a mere appendix.

Secondly, the field of E & O Neurotoxicology is interdisciplinary, but would I want to rewrite *Foundations* from a neuropsychological perspective, which is, after all, the discipline on which I obtained my professional training? Professionals are encouraged to publish from their own training perspectives. The individual fresh from doing graduate work on molecular biology would advance his or her career by publishing reports and articles on his or her field; the graduate student in social psychology who performed a survey of Mexican lettuce pickers in California probably would publish his or her article in a behavioral sciences journal. However, the study of molecular changes of the brain of workers exposed to pesticides during lettuce collection is a valid topic of research in which the fields of molecular biology and behavioral sciences are brought together. One cannot think of such studies unless one stretches one's vision beyond the molds of established individual disciplines.

Professionalization almost always reduces the scope of a discipline; in E & O Neurotoxicology it breaks down the whole into parts, each reflecting a specific point of view: that of the neurologist, the psychiatrist, the neuropsychologist, the neuropharmacologist, the industrial hygienist, etc. In "The Myth of Objectivism," the lecture I prepared for my Finnish audience that I never delivered, I argued about the manner in which the acquisition of knowledge is sometimes effectively blocked by setting false state-of-the-art technologies which are only those emanating from a specific professional group. I once listened to a presentation in the late 1980s in which an industrial scientist argued that since CAT scanners were the "state-of-the-art" technology to determine if industrial solvents caused structural changes in the brains of workers, CAT scanning should therefore be the technology of choice to demonstrate the harmful effects, if any, of industrial solvents on the human brain. (The speaker was obviously not aware, from the structural point of view, that the brains of people afflicted with schizophrenia are not different from those of "normal people;" ten years later one will probably be expected to listen to the argument that positron emission tomography is the state-of-the-art technique to study the effect of solvents on people). Of course, that research will never be done, and perhaps should never be done; committed professionals who represent the interests of the industry may argue that since research has not performed up to standards, it is not contributory to our knowledge about neurotoxic affects of solvents in humans. However, there are good things to say about the professionalization of a discipline: it makes it easy to have an advanced knowledge of the audience one writes about because that audience is made up of the members of the writer's profession. The professionalization of a discipline also makes it easier to find a "market" for a book.

Would I think of rewriting *Foundations* so it could reach a different audience? Knowledge is not only targeted to those who already know, but also to those directly affected by or who could benefit from such knowledge. Knowledge of how natural substances and/or man-made chemical compounds affect the nervous system, mind, and behavior rarely reaches the individuals who are likely to be affected by them. Information is either lost or distorted vertically (that is, the transmission from people who know to people who do not know) or horizontally (that is, information that is shared among equals). Loss and distortion of information are sometimes the product of ignorance, and sometimes are intentional in order to meet explicit economic objectives (e.g., as in the industry's denial that nicotine in cigarettes is addictive). The problem of informing either the educated or the layman is compounded by our inability to change our minds or behavior in the presence of facts: we do not listen to facts; we deny facts to accommodate our own system of beliefs. Take AIDS, for example. The year 2001 marks a quarter of a century since the discovery of a pandemic that afflicts millions, has killed millions, and has affected many countries to the point that their economies and social institutions have been deeply shaken. However, many individuals still believe that AIDS is a "gay disease;" spokespeople for some countries tell us "they do not have the problem;" others claim that "HIV is not the cause of AIDS." Carbon monoxide is another example. People have been killed by carbon monoxide since humanity discovered how to preserve or make fire. However, I have yet to persuade the attendants who park my car in my garage to ask clients not to leave their cars running or "warm up" their cars while the vehicles are still parked in the windowless environment. I even remind the car attendants, people whom I know well and care for, that individuals commit suicide using carbon monoxide emanating from their car exhausts.

Ten years after the publication of this book, the field of E & O Neurotoxicology has gained wide recognition and has extended beyond its initial boundaries of acquiring knowledge about how the low-level, long-term exposure to certain chemical agents in the environment and the workplace affects mind and behavior. The field is stronger in its neuroanatomincal, neurochemical, neurophysiological, clinical, epidemiological, and statistical foundations. *Foun-*

dations was written at a time when HIV/AIDS was known only to a few, and I exuded optimism as I hoped that E & O Neurotoxicology would eventually help developing and developed countries minimize occupational neurotoxic illness through the processes of becoming aware of the issues, solving many methodological research problems, regulation, control, and enforcement of standards beyond "cost-effective" formulas. The book contains a plea for a better environment and workplace. *Foundations* was written to remind all of us of the need for a commitment and continuity of effort for a healthy environment and workplace. I hope that this reprint of the book will continue to remind us about that commitment.

José A. Valciukas
Ashland, New York

Preface

The subject of environmental and occupational neurotoxicology (referred to as E & O neurotoxicology throughout this book) has never before been viewed as a distinct body of knowledge. Perhaps, therefore, we need to justify the presentation of such knowledge and to examine the facts on which this corpus rests. Any illness affects our lives; many toxic agents produce disability and death. But neurotoxic agents in particular threaten the fabric of our lives in insidious ways. Neurotoxic agents, particularly those that affect brain functions, impair the very equipment we rely on for making decisions in our daily lives. To evaluate information, to make decisions, and to react in a consistent and reasonable manner to our perceptions of the world all are difficult enough; but it is of grave importance to know that the resource we rely upon—namely, the nervous system and the brain in particular—might be damaged by exposure to neurotoxic agents in the environment or the workplace.

The idea of writing this book occurred to me about 14 years ago when I myself was looking for such a book without success. I began collecting material, thinking I might fill the gap, but I soon realized the difficulty of the task. Clearly, the subject required that vast areas of knowledge be brought together—among them neuroanatomy, neurophysiology, neurochemistry, pharmacology, basic toxicology, clinical neurology, psychometry, mathematics, and statistics. In addition, one needed to be an historian, a sociologist, a political scientist, and sometimes an economist. The book I envisioned would draw together the various discrete disciplines which contribute to E & O neurotoxicology. For example:

- There are many excellent books of psychometrics and its foundations. However, none deals with how psychometric techniques are used for the evaluation of subclinical signs of neurotoxicology.
- There are many textbooks describing the foundations of basic electrophysiological procedures such as electroencephalography and electromyography. But the need to adhere to strict rules of statistical analysis when information from electrophysiological procedures are utilized is rarely mentioned.
- There are many lists of neurotoxic agents, but they include, indiscriminately, materials gleaned from in vitro and in vivo studies, studies performed in animal models, and clinical observations. The significance of the choice of model and experimental conditions for prevention of injury and for regulation and control of harmful substances in the environment and the workplace has yet to be satisfactorily discussed.

This book is not a compilation of my own research, which was the result of very specific needs that surfaced in the United States between the mid-1970s and the mid-1980s. Nor is the volume about the neurotoxicology of lead. Although I have made contributions to this field, I do not want to create the impression that lead is a paradigm for neurotoxicology as a whole. One familiar with the vast literature on lead research is not necessarily prepared to deal with the scientific and technical matters associated with other neurotoxic agents. Besides, so much has already been written about lead that one wonders how much knowledge is really needed to eradicate this environmental and occupational health problem. Lead has recently fired the imagination of scientists and writers as it did in the Middle Ages: a dozen or so books on lead have been published in the last decade alone.

In writing a book on neurotoxicology as it relates to environmental and occupational health, I wanted not only to present factual information, reviewing the pillars of our knowledge; I wanted to examine the thinking processes by which we link neurotoxic illness with environmental or occupational exposure to toxic agents. I also wanted to share with the reader matters that in my opinion are flaws, weaknesses, or uncertain areas in the field, with little or poor evidence or substantiation.

The possible confounders and how investigators deal with them also needed to be examined. The chapters on mass psychogenic illness and aging, for example, are cases in point. Several books have appeared since I began to work on this project, but none have dealt with the matters of confounders in the analysis and interpretation of human health data.

There were areas that had never been covered in textbooks before. I found, for example, that even the best informed of my colleagues knew little about the uses of neurotoxic agents during World War I. I felt that a chapter on the uses of neurotoxic agents in chemical warfare was essential.

The subjects of environmental and occupational health on the one hand and neurotoxicology on the other are each interesting in their own right. There are glamorous journalistic accounts of isolated aspects of the field and bone-dry technical material, and very little in between. Where I want to be is in the middle of these extremes. If readers find something here

worth pursuing further, they will find additional selected sources of information at the end of each chapter (though I make no claim to have read everything in every area). Professionals will benefit most from this book if they skip the chapters dealing with subject matter from their own field and read others with which they are less familiar.

This book is written for people who would like more knowledge of the biological, behavioral, and health sciences and those in any profession who would like to have an integrated view of this particular branch of the applied sciences. Safety and health coordinators and industrial hygienists, nurses, managers, and lawyers, for example, all might benefit from such a treatment. Another audience I would like to reach with this book is those individuals who contemplate midcareer adjustments from one field to another and perhaps lack the necessary background to make such a decision. I have therefore avoided technical language and jargon that would be understood only by certain members of any given profession but not by others. In these times of superspecialization, with each specialty often associated with its own obscure lingo, "translation" into a common vocabulary is often called for.

With this book I have tried to build bridges among disciplines and show that scientific knowledge is not "owned" by anybody and is derived from people trained in many different professional fields. Also, I have tried to give equal attention to the review of both the supposedly objective ("foolproof") techniques and the subjective ("fallible") nature of the scientific judgments that make the discovery and characterization of scientific facts possible.

THE ORGANIZATION OF THIS BOOK

The field of E & O neurotoxicology is an immense one that has been influenced by many people and circumstances over the years. In the Introduction to this volume I present the historical roots of this discipline and the several branches that have evolved from it in the past two decades, and recount some of the circumstances that gave rise to and shaped the issues we deal with today.

Part I of this book describes the labyrinths of the nervous system (generally considered the most complex organization of all living systems), how the various levels of biological structure can be viewed, and the techniques that are used to assess nervous function in humans.

Part II looks at the environment and the workplace, where people spend a significant part of their lives, to examine a vast array of naturally occurring and man-made chemical compounds that have a special affinity for man's nervous system. This section also examines current attempts to classify these substances.

Part III deals with the ways chemical compounds in the environment and the workplace are absorbed, distributed, and eliminated by the human body and how the excreted chemical compounds or their metabolites are used for biological monitoring of toxic substances in humans.

Part IV, the core of the book, describes how the search for possible toxic causation is conducted. This section explores the work of research laboratories to see how human health scientists organize their thoughts and strategies, how they apply the techniques that are available to ascertain human toxic dose and neurological or psychological outcome, and how they reach conclusions that given chemical compounds are or are not neurotoxic. How a health survey is organized and conducted and how the wealth of information that is generated from these surveys is preserved and updated in computer-based filing systems are also discussed.

Part V surveys the harvest of knowledge—sometimes abundant, sometimes meager—that has accumulated regarding the targets of neurotoxicity. Until recently, there was little impetus to much of this research because psychological functioning and behavior had not

been considered appropriate units of analysis. For example, it was readily accepted that the cerebellum—which controls balance and motor learning, among other things—was a target of neurotoxicity, but the notion that consciousness, perception, motor behavior, motivation and emotions, learning and memory, cognition, and personality might be targets was not. Yet, from a clinical point of view, behavioral alterations in nervous system functioning are easily recognizable by health professionals and laypeople alike. In the early 1970s the body of knowledge of environmental health sciences, toxicology, neuropsychology, and epidemiology was seen for the first time as a single corpus. It is only within that corpus that one can relate individual afflictions to environmental and occupational events.

Chapters 22 through 26 include descriptions of the basic functional organization of each sensory system, testing procedures available in the clinic and in the laboratory, and facts related to the effect of toxic agents on these systems.

There are merits and drawbacks in taking each sensory system one at a time. From a practical point of view, it is likely that the reader will profit more from an organization that reviews each individual sensory system separately. Furthermore, this organization serves to illustrate the fact that most of the studies have been conducted on the effects of toxic agents on two systems primarily—the somatosensory system and vision; thus, we know close to nothing about the toxic effects of neurotoxic agents on the chemical senses.

The disadvantage of reviewing each system separately is that the common features of the anatomy and physiology of all sensory systems is lost. For example, from an anatomic point of view, all sensory systems have a receptor (eg, skin receptors, hair cells, cones, and rods), bipolar cells, and relay nuclei. Despite the twists and turns that neural fibers undergo and the strange terminology that has accumulated over generations to describe these fascinating circuits, it is relatively easy to understand the basic functional organization of a sensory system. From the physiological point of view: all receptor cells generate an electrical potential (the generator potential) when activated by their specific stimuli; most of the time the receptor cells are directly linked to the afferent fibers of the bipolar cells (sometimes there is a synapse in between); all receptors use "labeled lines." All neural networks can perform a highly elaborate analysis of sensory information, a fact likely to be appreciated by students of the neurosciences and experimental psychology.

Those interested in the comparative study of the sensory systems might consult several of the excellent introductory sources, such as *Sensation and Perception: An Integrated Approach* (2nd ed), by Harvey R. Schiffman,[1] which provides emphasis on the human perspective, or *Neurobiology,* by Gordon M. Shepherd,[2] a delightful book that emphasizes animal behavior. For the advanced student, *Principles of Neural Science* (2nd ed), edited by Eric R. Kandel and James H. Schwartz,[3] is highly recommended.

Readers may notice the absence in this book of a chapter devoted to environmental and occupational toxic chemicals and pain. The reason is that there has been little human research in this area—I was unable to find a single comprehensive review devoted to this topic in the world literature.

Part VI presents some unresolved issues in environmental and occupational neurotoxicology in as balanced a manner as possible. It is difficult to group the various debates and

polarized opinions into a coherent, rational picture because the debates sometimes are scientific and sometimes not. Personal, philosophical, political, and scientific matters and national or cultural pride are important forces shaping environmental and occupational health sciences, a multidisciplinary and global activity. It would be naive to ignore these factors or to sweep them under the rug. But it is also dangerous to second-guess the motivation of people or to try to decipher why people think the way they do.

The following three issues fall into the category of "confounders" because sometimes it is difficult to decide whether we are seeing the effects of neurotoxic agents or something else. These issues have surfaced many times in national and international debates and published literature: the possible environmental causation of senile dementia (Chapter 32); whether what seems to be an environmental or occupational neurotoxically induced illness is in fact caused by chronic alcoholism, smoking, or other substance abuse (Chapter 33); and how and under what circumstances mass psychogenic illness can be separated from neurotoxin-induced illness (Chapter 34).

There are many other confounders. For example, there are many medical conditions—particularly neurological and psychiatric disorders—that may be wrongly interpreted as having an environmental or occupational origin. Conversely, there are definite environmental conditions that can produce neurological disorders. Failure to recognize these conditions may lead to human suffering and even death.

The following two issues can be classified as moral ones, revealing important aspects of human nature and society: the use of neurotoxic agents in chemical warfare (Chapter 35); and prevention of neurotoxic illness and our changing perception of "quality of life" (Chapter 36).

---

[1]Shiffman, HR (1982) *Sensation and Perception: An Integrated Approach, 2nd ed.* New York: John Wiley & Sons.

[2]Shepherd, GM (1983) *Neurobiology.* New York: Oxford University Press.

[3]Kandel, ER, and Schwartz, JH (eds) (1985) *Principles of Neural Science* (2nd ed). New York: Elsevier.

Acknowledgments

I sincerely feel that this book is the product of a team effort—a compilation of the knowledge and wisdom of people who touched my life and left a permanent imprint. I feel that I need to start by recognizing and honoring them: Dr. José Maria Gutierrez Marquez of the University of Litoral, Rosario, Argentina, from whom I learned anatomy and physiology of the nervous system in the late 1950s and who encouraged me to come to the United States for the first time; the late Dr. Maria Carmen Franck, who thought of the nervous system as something of beauty and something one ought to learn more about simply because it is fun to do so; Dr. Emma Spaney of Queens College of the City University of New York (CUNY) and Dr. José Olivio Jimenez from the Graduate Center of CUNY, both inspired teachers and scholars, who gave me extraordinary support during my difficult first years as a foreign student at the City University of New York; Drs. Pedro and Tauba Pasik, both Professors of Neurology at Mount Sinai School of Medicine, with whom I worked for my doctoral dissertation 20 years ago but who are best remembered as friends who followed my sometimes painful pilgrimage around the world, always giving me their love and support. Dr. Pedro Pasik, now Professor of Neurobiology, read and gave his critique on the introductory chapters dealing with the anatomy and physiology of the nervous system.

In 1976, Dr. Irving J. Selikoff of the Mount Sinai School of Medicine gave me a job at the Environmental Sciences Laboratory with the explicit objective of developing the field of behavioral toxicology for the laboratory under his direction; this was a field that he felt was of importance and about which—I now confess—I knew nothing. My first job assignment was to attend a lecture at the New York Academy of Sciences by Dr. Charles Xintaras, a lecturer who later became a good friend. It was Dr. Ruth Lilis, now at the Division of Environmental and Occupational Medicine, Mount Sinai School of Medicine, who thought I could do the job. Throughout the years we worked together, she was a constant source of inspiration. There are few people I truly admire; she is certainly one of them. Dr. Philip J. Landrigan, Director of the Division of Environmental and Occupational Medicine, Mount Sinai School of Medicine, gave me support during the transition years between Mount Sinai and my new career as a Senior Forensic Psychologist at the Criminal and Supreme Courts in New York City. Dr. Richard Rosner, Director of the Forensic Psychiatry Clinic for the Criminal and Supreme Courts, gave me support and encouragement to complete this book.

I thank Dr. Sylvia Frank, my original "language" editor, who, until recently, I thought would be the only one who would ever read this book from cover to cover. She kept me on a short leash not only from going astray on my knowledge of biochemical facts but in the logic and expression of my thoughts.

The following individuals read specific chapters and gave me their critiques: Mr. Fred Doby, who read several chapters during the preparation of the prospectus for the book but who, I am sure, prefers to be remembered as the one who helped me discover the therapeutic value of skiing while writing this book;

many of my students, colleagues, and close associates at Mount Sinai School of Medicine—Dr. Linda Glickman, Dr. Carla Campbell, Dr. Raymond Singer, Dr. Steven Solomon, Dr. Richard Letz, and Mrs. Annie Hernandez; Dr. Ken Anger, formerly at NIOSH in Cincinnati and now at the Oregon Occupational Health Center; Dr. Helena Hänninen, recently retired from the Occupational Health Institute in Helsinki, Finland; and Mr. Sheldon Samuels, who read the chapter dealing with the historical roots of our common discipline. Mr. Samuels also gave me financial and personal support during a critical phase of my professional career.

I thank the personnel of Levy Library, Mount Sinai Medical School—in particular Ms. Laura Lane DeVoe, Ms. Deborah Rogers, Ms. Jean Sullivant, and Ms. Harriet Meiss. Mrs. Marisse Burger, Assistant Editor of the *American Journal of Industrial Medicine,* took on the immense task of informing me of the latest developments in my field.

There were many individuals at Van Nostrand Reinhold who participated in the development and production of this book. My special thanks goes to Mark Licker and Judy Brief, for having faith in this project and providing support during all phases of the work.

I am particularly grateful also to Elizabeth Geller, whose outstanding editorial skills made me look a better writer than I really am.

I would like to thank Mr. Kenneth Casazza for providing free accommodation for two months at the K & J Campingrounds in the town of Ashland, New York during the final stages of production of this book. His generosity is greatly appreciated.

I was privileged to write the first draft of Chapter 36 while visiting the Astrophysical Observatory of Ampimpa, Province of Tucumán, Argentina, in 1985–1986. The privately owned observatory is located on top of a mountain, and the site for the scientific facility was donated by South American Indians who own the land. My ideas on priorities of health and disease as related to societal perception of quality of life originated there. To us, the creation of a privately owned astronomical laboratory in an area where tuberculosis is still endemic may seem an incongruity. But the inhabitants fully understand the mission of the research facility, and my impression is that the astronomical observatory, dominating the immense Calchaquíes Valley, is a secular symbol of their faith.

INTRODUCTION

The History of Environmental and Occupational Neurotoxicology

Environmental and occupational (E & O) neurotoxicology is a multidisciplinary science dealing with the study of chemical compounds found in the environment or the workplace that have deleterious effects on the nervous system and behavior of humans. These studies are sometimes simply aimed at identifying the presence of a harmful neurotoxic agent—eg, toluene as a causative agent in the outbreak of multitargeted neurological diseases among leather shoe manufacturers. However, the ultimate goal of E & O neurotoxicology is the understanding of the mechanisms of toxic action of such agents, with the aim of preventing illness and human suffering.

A redefinition of quality of life—which includes mental health and psychological factors in work practices as well as the subclinical manifestations of toxic illness—led to the creation of this discipline. The historical background leading to this definition is examined in this chapter.

Several fields converge in E & O neurotoxicology: neurosciences, neurotoxicology, toxicology, epidemiology and statistics, environmental and occupational health, and preventive medicine.

This chapter traces the evolution of this multidisciplinary field from Ramazzini, who created industrial medicine as we know it today, to the Industrial Revolution, to the social reforms of the 19th century and industrial hygiene in the United States at the turn of 20th century, and finally culminating in the Occupational Safety and Health Act (OSHA) of 1970 in the United States. Also described in this chapter are movements such as environmentalism and consumerism that help to highlight the important position this discipline maintains in the public eye.

HISTORICAL BACKGROUND

Historiographic Problems

Historiography is the science of writing history. One historiographic problem is the identification of sources from which a history—in this case, the history of E & O neurotoxicology—can be written.

This book deals with the foundations of our knowledge about neurotoxic "poisons" present in the environment or the workplace. The historical time span that needs to be accounted for is much shorter than that of naturally occurring toxins of plant and animal origin. It is only in the early 18th century that a well-documented interest in occupational diseases developed; the term "environmental medicine" was probably coined about two decades ago; the term "neurotoxicology" is equally young. The word "neurosciences" appeared in the early 1960s.

In attempting an historical account of occupational and environmental neurotoxicology some problems arise:

- The primary sources of information are scattered around the world, and the documents of historical interest are written in many languages including Chinese, Czech, Danish, English, Finnish, French, German, Italian, Japanese, Polish, Rumanian, Russian, Serbo-Croatian, Spanish, and Swedish. In some cases, when a scientist publishes an account of his or her work in English, extensive literature in other languages—in historiographic terms, the primary sources—already exist. In addition, the lack of an agreed-upon, universal scientific terminology creates even further communication problems.

- Occupational accidents and environmental disasters are often first seen as an internal problem in each country. In addition, in the past a strong sense of nationalism among scientists and public health workers around the world sometimes prevented the free exchange of information. After the explosion of a nuclear reactor in Chernobyl on April 26, 1986, Russia was forced to admit the tragedy only after elevated radiation levels were found in Sweden and Finland. It is therefore not surprising that accidents often never reach international scientific circles concerned with these matters.

- Many scientists who contributed to the earliest development of this discipline are still alive. This has its advantages and disadvantages. Among the advantages is the fact that we can still verify historical events by personal communication with the principal protagonists. Among the disadvantages is that we sometimes treat these people—who constantly review their own thoughts—as historical characters, as if their views were written in stone.

- The proliferation of chemical compounds and the scientific and technical reports associated with each one is staggering. Bransford (1984) has stated that "...throughout 1983, new chemical compounds were registered with the Chemical Abstracts Service division of the American Chemical Society at the rate of 70 per hour. Uses are found for 70,000 to 100,000 of these compounds. About 24,000 of them enter new products, such as dyes, plastics, paints and varnishes, preservatives and finishes." It is estimated that more than a fourth of the chemical compounds for which recommended standards exist—such as those published by the American Conference of Governmental Industrial Hygienists (ACGIH)—are neurotoxic (Anger and Johnson 1985).

- There is a lack of a comprehensive framework for historical analysis. The history of changing views in neurotoxicity has often been reviewed in terms of a single neurotoxic agent—lead. The danger of this historical approach is that lead is taken as a paradigm—a model for the study of other E & O neurotoxic illness and as a representative example of other toxic agents. However, lead is not a paradigm. To view lead as such is dangerous in that it inhibits the proliferation of knowledge of the effects of other neurotoxic agents that may be equally or even more dangerous.

- There is a general apathy for history as a subject matter. To paraphrase Thucidides, scientists tend to behave as though the most important things that ever happened in their field happened in their own lifetime.

More than an actual account of the history of occupational and environmental toxicology, the purpose of this chapter is to call attention to the need for beginning the collection of materials in such a manner that future professional historians of science can write a comprehensive account of the field.

An Overview of Sources

Much of the scientific reporting on environmental and/or occupational issues has been written by professional journalists. Some of the facts, trends, environmental catastrophes, and controversies about these events develop so quickly that scientists and scholars must depend on newspapers, television, and magazines intended for the general public as the first source of information. The depth and extent of knowledge of environmental sciences, the credibility of its protagonists, the hopes and frustrations of affected groups, and the mood of whole sections of the world where environmental and occupational exposure to neurotoxic agents has occurred are likely to be found in these sources rather than in scientific articles.

Many special-interest and general-interest magazines are excellent sources of historical information. For example, Rachel Carson's book *Silent Spring*—a leading document of 20th century environmentalism—was compiled from articles written for the magazine *The New Yorker,* and the tragedy of Bhopal was faithfully documented in *The New York Times.* Sometimes these so-called secondary sources overshadow scholarly accounts. Magazines such as *Scientific American* (particularly in its section "50 and 100 years ago"), *Environment, National and International Wildlife, Discover, Science '86* (the number changes as the year does; no longer in existence), *Science Digest* (no longer in existence), *The Sciences* (published by the New York Academy of Sciences), *The New Yorker, Time,* and *The New York Times* with its Tuesday "Science" section have each published remarkable articles on neurotoxic agents at one time or another.

Encyclopedias are sometimes good sources for a quick overview of fundamental scientific problems. For example, the *Encyclopaedia Brittanica* is an invaluable source of short biographical sketches of historical characters, accounts of massive poisoning, the history of specific aspects of forensic medicine, chemical warfare, regulation and control of toxic substances in the United States, Great Britain, and other countries of the world, and accounts of the discovery, manufacturing, distribution, and uses of individual toxic agents such as lead, mercury, and pesticides. *The Encyclopedia of Chemical Technology* is also a good source for this latter topic.

Some of this source material can be obtained through excellent computer-based information systems (TOXLINE, MEDLINE, etc). The Library of Congress and The National Library of Medicine have their own computer-based means of accessing documents related to the field of occupational and environmental health as well as the history of research for particular neurotoxic compounds. Almost without exception these systems have a cut-off year when they first began to store information in computer files. Thus, the search for historical sources needs to be done the old-fashioned way—ie, by consulting library cards or books containing photocopies of old library cards. The library of the New York Academy of Medicine has published numerous medical books of historical significance, including *Diseases of Workers* by Ramazzini (1713) published in 1964, a landmark book.

Restrictions, classifications, declassifications, and even destruction of documents by government agencies are at the present time creating a great deal of difficulty for professional historians. Hold (1983) has written an enlightening article on this subject. Some facts about the readiness for chemical warfare involving neurotoxic agents—nerve gas—in Europe during World War II were finally released to the general public in the early 1980s under the Freedom of Information Act.

From an historical point of view, the close association between knowledge and power must be recognized. Toxicology and politics have traveled hand in hand since antiquity.

Often, information has been (and still is) used or withheld for political purposes.

TOXICOLOGY

Toxicology literally means "the science of poisons." As a scientific discipline, toxicology is of relatively recent emergence in the last century. However, knowledge of the effects on humans of various minerals, plants, and animals has been available for centuries in many regions of the world, often by unrelated cultures. (For example, it has been thought that one of the reasons some ancient nomadic cultures in Europe settled down was the accidental discovery of beer brewing and the knowledge of beer's euphoric effects. For another example, South American Indians used the naturally occurring poison curare to kill animals for food for untold centuries before French scientists of the 18th century discovered its toxic and its beneficial medical properties as a local muscle relaxant.)

It is unfortunate that a modern, comprehensive world view account of this discipline has never been properly told. A contemporary book on the history of toxicology would indeed make fascinating reading. The origin, development, and modern trends in toxicology in general have been described in many scattered sources. But, as stated earlier, a comprehensive history of toxicology is still lacking. This is not surprising since, as Casarett and Bruce (1986) state, ". . . toxicology has evolved as a multidisciplinary field of study [and] definitions of toxicology often reflect the area of study from which the definition derives." [Those wishing to consult a brief, informative and interesting account of the field are directed to Casarett and Bruce's (1986) chapter "Origin and Scope of Toxicology." This source contains a brief history of toxicology. It includes toxicological aspects from antiquity, middle ages, the age of enlightenment, and modern times. Their references are guides to supplemental reading. These references are helpful to those who would like to pursue an in-depth study of the subject.]

The field of toxicology was not the particular domain of any one profession during antiquity and until the last century. At one time or another philosophers, physicians, pharmacists, drug dealers, professional poisoners, healers—including the vast pharmacological information known to Indians in North, Central, and South America—contributed to this knowledge. [*Kremer and Urdang's History of Pharmacy*, which is now in its fourth edition and was revised by Sonnedecker in 1976, is a good scholarly treatise on the subject. Written as a textbook for graduate students, it can be recommended as excellent reading. It contains numerous appendices, references, scholarly notes, bibliographic sources, and an enormous glossary of terms. La Wall (1927) is another important source.]

Since the middle 1970s toxicology as a discipline has rapidly blossomed. Two factors explain in part the rebirth of this interest: concern for the harmful effects of toxic agents in the environment and the workplace and drug abuse, which now has reached epidemic proportions.

Mateo José Buenaventura Orfila

Mateo José Buenaventura Orfila (1787–1853), a Spanish physician who worked in the French Court of Louis XVIII, is considered to be the father of modern experimental toxicology. Trained in both medicine and chemistry, he made numerous contributions to analytical procedures for the detection of poisons and wrote numerous treatises in toxicology and forensic medicine. It has been said that poisoning by arsenic, still popular at that time, declined significantly after Orfila described methods for its detection in the human body.

Orfila was born in Majorca in 1787, studied medicine in Valencia (Spain) and Barcelona, and compilations of the knowledge of his time. This included the chemistry of poisonous substances, work on practical chemistry, equipment design, pharmacological properties of poisons, pathological anatomy, signs and symptoms of toxic diseases, differential diagnosis, treatment, prevention, and forensic medicine. The fourth edition of *Traité de Toxicologie*, in two volumes, looks like a contemporary encyclopedia on the subject, except that Orfila's *Traité* is the work of a single person.

François Magendie (1783–1855), also an encyclopedist, is credited as being the founder of experimental toxicology (Brazier 1984, 1987). Magendie had different scholarly goals from those of Orfila. Orfila was preoccupied with the poisonous properties of household products, drugs, toxic agents at the workplace, and how this knowledge could be used in legal cases. Magendie was primarily interested in the value of poisonous agents as a research tool in pharmacology.

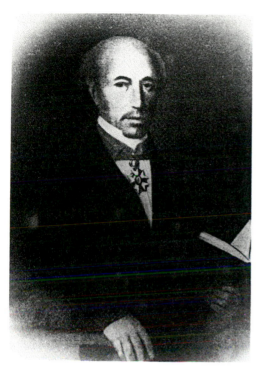

Mateo José Buenaventura Orfila (1787–1853). (From Instituto Fernando el Católico, Zaragoza, Spain, with permission.)

obtained a degree in Paris in 1811. In 1819 he was named professor in the Faculty of Medicine in Paris, where he was also professor of chemistry and dean of the faculty between 1831 and 1834. In 1816 he was appointed to the court of Louis XVIII, and then to the Royal Council of Public Instruction in 1834. He was the founder of the Orfila Museum of Comparative Anatomy. His works have been translated into English and German. Articles were published in 1953 on the occasion of the centennial of his death, but a comprehensive biography of Orfila in English is lacking. A biographical sketch is found in Beeson (1930); Loren Esteban (1961) has written a doctoral dissertation in Spanish on Orfila's life and work.

Orfila separated toxicology as a discipline from medicine and pharmacology. Both his *Directions for the Treatment of Persons Who Have Taken Poisons*, written in 1820, and later his *Traité de Toxicologie* (1843) are

OCCUPATIONAL MEDICINE

Health hazards associated with certain occupations have been recognized for many centuries (Goldwater 1936). Well-documented data support the view that in the Greco–Roman civilizations, physicians and writers knew about the dangers of specific trades and toxic agents. The earliest written reference to the poisonous effects of mercury and lead was made by Ulrich Ellenbog in 1472 in a brochure of eight pages. But it was the writings of Georg Agricola (1494–1555) and Theophrastus von Hohenheim (known as Paracelsus) (1493–1541) that firmly established the discipline of occupational medicine. (Occupational medicine is also known as industrial medicine.)

Bernardino Ramazzini

Bernardino Ramazzini (1633–1714) was the founder of industrial medicine as we know

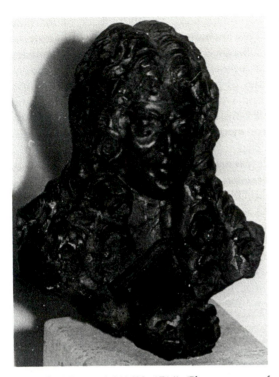

Bernardino Ramazzini (1633–1714). (Photo courtesy of Dr. Irving J. Selikoff.)

on the diseases of workers. These lectures formed the basis of his famous book: Diseases of Workers.

Ramazzini can also be considered the father of environmental medicine. He was interested both in climate per se and in the effects of atmospheric changes, humidity, and rain on human health. He occupies an important place in the history of meteorology that is often overshadowed by his recognized historical presence in occupational medicine.

it today. Ramazzini determined that a relationship exists between the worker's health and his occupation such that the worker's job could, under certain circumstances, be considered a disease-inducing agent. Citing Hippocrates on the importance of correctly questioning a patient on personal medical history, he added the question "What is his job?"

Born October 4, 1633 in the community of Carpi, a small town in the Modena region of Italy, Ramazzini went to Parma to pursue his medical education. Later, he went to Rome, where he worked with Antonio Maria de' Rosi from Ravenna, accompanying him on his patient visits. After contracting malaria, he was forced to resign his position and returned to Carpi. He married in 1665, and at the end of 1676 he and his family moved to Modena where he played an important role in the rebirth of this ancient Italian university. Ramazzini began his teaching career at the late age of 49. During the Modenese period (1682–1700), he taught physics and epidemiology and lectured

Ramazzini's fame spread internationally. In 1703, only a few years after his death, the second edition of *De Morbis Artificum Diatriba* was translated into English as *Diseases of Workers*. His book was extensively quoted and published in many editions around the world. The last edition was published in Leipzig in 1828, more than a century after Ramazzini's death.

Diseases of Workers is written in the florid style of Ramazzini's time. The author had no qualms about citing passages from Roman poets to illuminate an observation. The book contains both a compendium of diseases of selected trades and social groups and the practical foundations of occupational medicine. It makes numerous references to the effects of neurotoxic agents, particularly lead and mercury. In Chapter I, in which Ramazzini discusses the diseases of metal miners, his style of writing on two levels is apparent, as the following quote illustrates:

Various and manifold is the harvest of disease reaped by certain workers from the crafts and trades that they pursue; all the profit that they get is fatal injury to their health. That crop germinates mostly, I think, from two causes. The first and most potent is the harmful character of the materials that they handle, for these emit noxious vapors and very fine particles inimical to human beings and induce particular diseases; the second cause I ascribe to certain violent and irregular motions and unnatural postures of the body, by reason of which the natural structure of the vital machine is so impaired that serious diseases gradually develop therefrom. (Ramazzini 1713)

Bernardino Ramazzini influenced the philosophy and practice of this branch of medicine in many parts of the world. *Diseases of Workers* remained the most influential book on occupational medicine until the beginning of the 19th century. At that time, the Industrial Revolution led to the introduction of many new chemical compounds and the development of new work practices, forcing teachers and scholars to completely reorganize teaching handbooks.

The Industrial Revolution

"Industrial Revolution" is a term widely accepted to designate a period of complex events that changed England between 1760 and 1830, changes resulting from major historical breakthroughs that affected work practices:

- Changes in ownership of the means of production from the workers to the merchant.
- Large outlays of capital for the manufacture of new products and services.
- Division of labor: workers, until then artisans who knew every aspect of production, were assigned to specific aspects of the increasingly complex process of manufacturing products.
- Many great scientific discoveries and technical inventions that radically changed work practices.
- Discovery, characterization, and practical use of many new chemical compounds.

The Industrial Revolution was quickly exported to many other countries, which experienced similar social changes as a result.

The thrust of the Industrial Revolution created excesses and social injustices. There are bibliographic and literary sources, such as the works of Dickens (eg, *Hard Times,* written in 1854), that help to characterize the period:

It was a town of red brick, or of brick that would have been red if the smoke and ashes had allowed it; but as matters stood it was a town of unnatural red and black like the painted face of a savage. It was a town of machinery and tall chimneys, out of which interminable serpents of smoke trailed themself for ever and ever, and never got uncoiled. It had a black canal in it, and a river that ran purple with ill-smelling dye, and vast piles of buildings full of windows where there was rattling and a trembling all day long, and where the piston of the steam engine worked monotonously up and down, like the head of an elephant in a state of melancholy madness. It contained several large streets all very like one another, and many small streets still more like one another, inhabited by people equally like one another, who all went in and out at the same hours, with the same sound upon the same pavements, to do the same work, and to whom every day was the same as yesterday and tomorrow, and every year the counterpart of the last and the next. (Dickens, quoted in Hunter 1978, p. 93–94)

The Industrial Revolution, and the human health consequences it caused, were profoundly attacked. This resulted in the social reforms of the 19th century. These reforms attempted to regulate specific job practices such as child labor and abuses of apprenticeship and to improve working conditions for women. [Hunter's *The Disease of Occupations* (sixth edition, published in 1978) is one of the best sources for the changes in attitudes toward occupational health caused by the Industrial Revolution.]

This period of social change was followed by the Russian revolution of 1917, which left a distinctive mark on the philosophy and practice of industrial hygiene and medicine in many countries of the world, regardless of whether or not they subscribed to the communist credo.

Science was also affected by these historical changes. Historical writings are under constant revision, and sometimes—sadly to say—they are revised to accommodate contemporary social circumstances. Readers are alerted to these biases when consulting the sources compiled at the end of this chapter.

Alice Hamilton

Just as Ramazzini is considered to be the father of occupational medicine, Alice Hamilton (1869–1970) certainly was the mother of American occupational medicine. Fortunately, there is plenty of documentation relating to the life and work of this remarkable woman, including her biography and letters and several editions of her own handbook on occupational medicine.

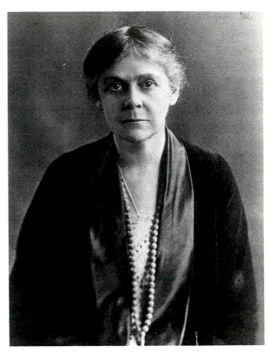

Alice Hamilton (1869–1970). (From The Schlesinger Library, Radcliffe College, with permission.)

Alice Hamilton was born in New York City on February 27, 1869. After receiving her medical degree from the University of Michigan in 1893, she continued her studies at Johns Hopkins University and in Germany. Between 1897 and 1905 she taught at the Northwestern University Medical School for Women.

She competed in a man's world. She was admitted to the faculty of Harvard University after she accepted three limitations: "She was not to enter Harvard Club, not to participate in the academic procession at Commencement, [and] not to expect the professional privilege of a quota of football tickets" (Curran 1970). She was an Assistant Professor at Harvard—a low academic position for a person of her reputation—between 1919 and 1935. She died in her cherished state of Connecticut on September 22, 1970, at the age of 101.

Dr. Hamilton entered the field of industrial medicine in 1910. Her first-hand observations of industrial diseases and her work, first in the state of Illinois and later for the federal government, led to the introduction of new hygiene practices and the passage of workers' compensation laws. She traveled extensively nationally and around the world, contacting the top occupational health leaders of her time. She was an acerbic critic of the ignorance and bad faith leading to the suffering and disease of workers.

Hamilton was noted for her passionate defense of workers' health. She vehemently fought the hypocrisy of managers and her own professional colleagues. Hamilton was an excellent and prolific writer; some examples taken from her 1943 book reveal her tongue-lashing style:

- "Another example used by the employer was alcoholism. The men were sick because they drank, and the employer did not need to prove it."
- "No hospital intern ever noted where the victim of plumbism [lead poisoning] had acquired the lead. Hospital history sheets noted carefully all the facts about tobacco, alcohol, and even coffee consumed by the leaded man."
- "Every article I wrote in those days, every speech I made, is full of pleading for the recognition of lead poisoning as a real and serious medical problem. It was easy to present figures demonstrating the contrast between lead work in the United States, under conditions of neglect and ignorance, and comparable work in England and Germany, under intelligent control."

CONSERVATION, ECOLOGY, AND THE ENVIRONMENT

In the United States, these three interrelated subjects form the basis of our present concern for the preservation of our environment and our interest in environmental influences on human health and behavior. Primitive people depended totally on nature. Their simple tools could do little to affect the immediate environment. The control of fire was perhaps the most damaging tool humans had that might produce profound changes in environment. Until the 18th century, nature was thought to be an endless supplier of humans' needs.

The mechanistic view of nature and the fusion of science and technology were the primary forces that led to the overexploitation of natural resources. Highsmith, in an undated article in *Encyclopedia Americana,* stated that the mechanistic view of nature "... may have contributed to the still prevalent conviction that parts of nature can be 'tinkered with' without regard to the whole— much as an automobile mechanic can adjust a carburetor without modifying the rest of the car." As early as the 13th century, though, Europeans had experienced the consequences of overexploitation of forests. Conservation was a social movement that began in the 19th century, built on the recognition that the delicate balance of nature could be profoundly upset by human activity.

In the 17th century, American colonists were granted power to control industries that might endanger public health and safety in the United States. Jared Eliot, George Washington, and Thomas Jefferson are representatives of the early conservation movement in America. However, the abundance of natural resources, the ease of acquiring land, and the limited population existing at the time were factors that drowned out early efforts in that direction. Late 19th century writers such as George P. Marsch alerted the public about excessive human actions that might adversely affect the physical condition of the globe. Theodore Roosevelt was the first conservationist president of the United States. In the United States, the National Park system is a major success in this area.

Rachel Carson's *Silent Spring*

The environmental movement gained momentum with the publication of the book *Silent Spring* (published in 1962). *The New York Times* called Rachel Carson's *Silent Spring* "... one of the most influential books of this century, helping to touch off an environmental revolution and changing the way the nation and much of the world looks at pesticides and pollutants generally."

Rachel Carson was born on May 27, 1907 in Springdale, Pennsylvania, where she attended school. She demonstrated her writing talents as a child, publishing fiction at an early age. In 1929

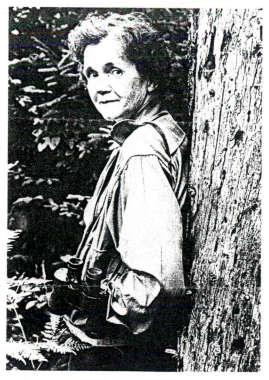

Rachel Carson (1907–1964). (Courtesy of the Rachel Carson Council.)

she received her Bachelor of Science degree from Pennsylvania College for Women, and in 1932 her Master of Arts degree in Zoology from Johns Hopkins University. Between 1936 and 1939 she had a permanent appointment as junior aquatic biologist at the Bureau of Fisheries. In 1941 she published Under the Sea Wind, *her first successful book. This was followed by two others that helped to establish her quality as a writer:* The Sea Around Us *and* The Edge of the Sea, *published in 1950 and 1955, respectively.* Silent Spring *appeared in 1962 after a three-part condensation in* The New Yorker. *The chemical industry soon mounted a personal and scientific attack on her, even before* Silent Spring *was published. Velsical Chemical Corporation, a large manufacturer of pesticides, tried to intimidate the publisher into withdrawing the book by threatening a lawsuit over "inaccuracies" in the description of their products. Carson died in Silver Springs, Maryland on April 14, 1964.*

To a large extent, Rachel Carson succeeded in her message because of her powerful writing style. Some literary critics place her in the same category as Thoreau. "A Fable for Tomorrow," the introductory chapter to *Silent Spring,* is only two pages long, but it is written in such rich literary style that it "grabs even the casual peruser" (Gardner 1983).

There was once a town in the heart of America where all life seemed to live in harmony with its surroundings. The town lay in the midst of a checkerboard of prosperous farms, with fields of grain and hillsides of orchards where, in spring, white clouds of bloom drifted above green fields. In autumn, oak and maple and birch set up a blaze of color that flamed and flickered across a backdrop of pines. The foxes barked in the hills and deer silently crossed the fields, half hidden in the mists of the fall mornings. . . . Then a strange blight crept over the area and everything began to change. Some evil spell had settled on the community: mysterious maladies swept the flocks of chickens; the cattle and sheep sickened and died. Everywhere was a shadow of death. The farmers spoke of much illness among their families. In the town the doctors had become more and more puzzled by new kinds of sickness appearing among their patients. . . . There was a strange stillness. The birds, for example—where had they gone? (Carson 1962)

Environmental Disasters Involving Neurotoxic Agents

A series of industrial environmental disasters involving neurotoxic agents has caused an increased awareness of the dangers of environmental pollution.

Japan, which experienced the horrors of the nuclear bombing of Hiroshima and Nagasaki, was again hit hard in 1953 and 1960 with outbreaks of methylmercury poisoning, which occurred in Minamata Bay and the District of Niigata. The source of exposure was mercury-contaminated fish. Profound mental retardation was reported among children born from intoxicated mothers. A new disease—Minamata disease—was named associated with this tragedy (Takeuchi 1977). Until these episodes, methylmercury had not been considered an environmental health problem.

From the middle 1950s to the early 1970s several fungicide-related epidemics occurred in Iraq, West Pakistan, and Guatemala; they all involved the ingestion of bread prepared from fungicide-treated seeds. In Iraq between 1971 and 1972, 6530 individuals were affected. This outbreak is considered the worst non-war-related environmental disaster ever.

Environmental accidents widely publicized in the mass media have also occurred in the United States. In 1973, an accident of catastrophic proportions took place in the United States, in Michigan. It involved the accidental contamination of polybrominated biphenyls (PBBs) in the food chain. A fire retardant was accidentally mixed with farm animals' feed. Eggs, meat, and milk products became contaminated (Kay 1977).

Numerous other less-known industrial accidents have occurred in the United States. Many involved workers who handled or were in close contact with toxic agents. Schaumburg and Spencer (1980) have reviewed industrial accidents involving acrylamide (a monomer), chlordecone and leptofos (both pesticides), DMAPN (a catalyst used in the production of polyurethane foam), lead, *n*-hexane and methyl-*n*-butyl ketone (both solvents), manganese, organomercury, and organotin.

The environmentalists' passionate message is based on these human tragedies. In the 1970s, when public concern about environmental issues reached its peak, there was a marked increase in research on environmental problems. But rhetoric, the prediction of imminent doom first in mass media and then in books, hurt the environmental movement severely. The 1980s experienced a decline in personnel and resources for environmental research.

Environmental medicine and epidemiology—to be discussed below—are two disciplines that have become strongly related. The latter was a firmly established discipline that, about a generation ago, joined forces with those who were studying environmental and occupational health problems.

EPIDEMIOLOGY

"Epidemiology is the study of the distribution and determinants of health-related states and events in populations, and the application of this study to the control of health problems" (Last 1986). The word "epidemiology" derives from "epidemics," meaning, in Greek, "upon the people." Epidemiology is the scientific study of epidemics of infectious agents, and, in recent years, noninfectious agents as well. Occupational health problems, such as the study of the effects of toxic agents on nervous system functions, are a recent addition to its domain.

Epidemiology deals with two broad categories of problems: mortality—the study of death and its causes—and morbidity—the study of illness and its causes. The study of chronic illness caused by the presence of neurotoxic agents in the environment and the workplace falls into the latter category.

The epidemiological method is a systematic way of planning, executing, analyzing, and interpreting results derived from the study of large groups of people. Of particular importance in environmental and occupational toxicology are methods for determining the causes of neurotoxic diseases. The topics of epidemiological methodology relevant to this field are the identification of individuals at risk, the study design, sources of error of measurement, and screening. Some elements of the epidemiological method, such as sampling, overlap with the field of statistics.

ENVIRONMENTAL MEDICINE

Irving J. Selikoff

Occupational health is a subdivision of environmental medicine. As stated above, the founder of modern occupational medicine—Bernardino Ramazzini—was interested in research on environmental matters as well as occupational health problems. Dr. Irving J. Selikoff (1915–), professor emeritus and director of the Environmental Sciences Laboratory at Mount Sinai Medical School in New York City, is the leader of environmental medicine as we know it today. Selikoff is a towering figure in modern science, having made contributions to medicine, epidemiology, and regulation and control of toxic substances in the environment and in public health. He is often called "the Ramazzini of our times."

Irving J. Selikoff was born in New York City on January 15, 1915. He obtained his Bachelor of Science degree at Columbia University in 1935 and his Medical degree at the Royal College of Scotland in 1941. He is a member of the American Board of Preventive Medicine and many other medical and scientific societies. After his crowning achievements for the treatment of tuberculosis by means of isonizide, for which he was awarded the Lasker Award in 1955, he began a second career as an occupational physician devoted to the carcinogenic properties of asbestos.

He founded the Environmental Sciences Laboratory in 1961 and gathered around him top scientists in the field. He founded the journal Environmental Research *in 1967 and* American Journal of Industrial Medicine *in 1980. An honorary degree awarded by Tufts University in 1979 marks the first time an honorary doctoral degree was ever awarded in environmental medicine. Selikoff has been consulted by legislators and managers of leading industrial and labor organizations in matters of legislation regarding environmental and occupational health problems. He is considered to be one of the most politically influential people of our times (*National Journal *1985).*

Selikoff influenced very deeply the field of occupational and environmental neurotoxicology. First, he guided those in the field along the philosophical lines already developed for other toxic substances—eg, that the toxic effects of environmental and occupational neurotoxic agents in humans are best understood when studied in humans. Second, during the period of his directorship at Mount Sinai's Environmental Sciences Laboratory in New York City, he organized medical field surveys of neurotoxic agents—asbestos, lead, polybrominated biphenyls (PBBs), polychlorinated biphenyls (PCBs), industrial solvents, pesticides, etc. Third, he created an enthusiastic atmosphere encouraging the development of new ideas, techniques, and cooperative efforts between institutions. At this writing, Dr. Selikoff continues his epidemiological studies on asbestos and his commitment to public health preventive medicine.

CONSUMERISM

Traditionally, it had been felt that physicians and scientists from academia and industry were the only ones capable of understanding how environmental and occupational problems affect people. The voices of "common people" had rarely been heard. In the middle 1960s, however, the consumer movement changed all that. Occupational and environmental physicians have discovered that the victims of occupational health problems and those affected by environmental disasters are the first sources of medical information. Consumerism has deeply influenced the manner in which we perceive our work and environment.

Consumerism is a movement seeking increased control of information on goods and services consumed by individuals. In preindustrial economies, the relationship between producers and consumers was regulated by the principle of *caveat emptor* ("let the buyer beware"). This principle fails in industrial economies where the buyer is manipulated through advertisements or, because of lack of information, is forced to trust the safety of products or services.

Although laws protecting the consumer have existed for many years, the consumer movement achieved prominence through the efforts of Ralph Nader. His book *Unsafe at any Speed,* published in 1965, marked the beginning of this movement. Consumerism led to drastic changes in practices regarding the dissemination and witholding of information in the best interest of the individual. The right to know and labeling of harmful products are an example of the former; confidentiality of information, the latter. The movement has influenced areas of quality and safety of products and services, pricing practices, selling and credit, informed consent, advertisement claims, etc.

As a result of consumer pressure, scientists developed a keener awareness that "applied research" was not always research for the common good. People began to ask sharper and sharper questions. For example, it is no longer possible for a responsible scientist to say, "No evidence has linked occupational exposure to solvents and a deterioration in mental performance." Now someone will ask, "Do we know that for sure, or do you say that because the experiments that might help to answer such questions have never been performed in humans?" "No evidence" is an expression that has been ambiguously applied both to the case of many experiments having proven no association between exposures and diseases and to the plain lack of information on a subject. In the past, this kind of questioning posed by the public to scientists or political leaders was unheard of. For a long time, it was successfully argued that the nature of the work performed by scientists could not be judged by the general public. Thus, the issue of the ethical implications of research can be viewed as a product of consumerism. In this view, science is not a suprahuman activity, and scientists are not above the law.

PSYCHOLOGY

Environmental and occupational neurotoxicologists use the tools of neuropsychologists and clinical neurophysiologists in the assessment of nervous system deficits suspected to be caused by toxic agents. Until these professionals joined hands with epidemiologists and toxicologists, human data were largely confined to subjective symptoms and signs obtained during the neurological examination. Psychologists introduced the concept of "subclinical neurotoxic signs," an extension of "minimal brain damage," a term that has been overused and is now largely abandoned.

Psychology is a discipline that studies mind and behavior. It was born in Germany in the middle of the last century, and was aimed at the study of human and animal behavior. The method of human psychology was originally introspection, a look into oneself, where psychologists studied subjective phenomena.

At the beginning of this century (circa 1910) the thought took hold that in order to be on sure footing, psychology needed to be based on something everybody could observe. Behavior could be observed; the inner workings of other people's minds could not. The works of the Russian physiologists Bechterev and Pavlov reached the shores of the United States, and their English translations in the 1930s left an indelible mark on psychology. John B. Watson, the founder of behaviorism in the United States, long searching for the scientific basis of psychology, argued that unconditioned reflexes—reflexes one is born with—and conditioned reflexes—learned responses—are all one needed to know in order to predict behavior.

Psychology has been fragmented into dozens of branches, not all of them equally influential in E & O neurotoxicology. Approaches, concepts, and techniques that are now part of the body of E & O neurotoxicology come from at least six branches of psychology—namely, behavioral psychology, individual differences, occupational psychology, environmental psychology, neuropsychology, and social psychology.

Behavioral Psychology. Behavorial psychology is a branch of psychology that considers behavior the object of its study. The language created by Bechterev and Pavlov and greatly enriched in the 1930s by B. F. Skinner (1904–1990), a leading Harvard psychologist, described behavior in terms of observable stimuli and observable responses. Subjective phenomena had no place in Skinner's system because they could not be studied scientifically. Although attempts were made, the language of Skinner could not be successfully translated to human neurotoxicology. One of the main reasons human neurotoxicologists working with human beings in problems of environmental and occupational health and neurotoxicologists conducting research in laboratory animals on basic mechanisms of toxic action cannot communicate is the lack of a common language.

In addition, vast territories of essential psychological research that did not fit Skinner's system were ignored. For example, since the time Skinner wrote his doctoral dissertation at Harvard, he argued that a knowledge of the physiology of the nervous system was unnecessary in order to predict behavior. When the works of Russian physiologists working on the control of air quality by means of objective methods became known in the United States, the process of intellectual assimilation into Skinner's phraseology continued. The conclusions of the Russian physiologists were immediately translated into Skinner's mold, but the physiology was left out. In early studies of behavioral pharmacology, a drug was often used to prove the theoretical point that drugs can be a "discriminative stimulus" affecting behavior in a predictable manner.

Individual Differences. Also known as *differential psychology,* this is an applied branch of psychology that studies differences in skills and abilities among people. Because the measurement of these abilities requires special equipment—such as that utilized in the determination of reaction time, motor coordination, visual perception, auditory localization, etc—differential psychology and experimental (laboratory) psychology provided, in the 1960s, the early armamentarium for the study of neurotoxic effects under laboratory conditions. The application of differential psychology is now called *human factors engineering.* In Europe it is called *ergonomics.*

Occupational Psychology. Occupational psychology utilizes the instruments of the human factors engineer for the selection of the right worker for a given job. It, too, has changed its name, and is now being called *industrial and organizational (I & O) psychology* to accommodate a society that increasingly relies on services more than the production of goods. I & O psychologists work in close cooperation with management. Occupational and I & O psychologists have contributed little to our understanding of how neurotoxic agents act at the workplace.

The historical views of psychologists on occupation and cognitive functions are exemplified by the words of Woodworth, a psychologist who taught at Columbia University. Woodworth, like many leaders in the field, was an encyclopedist: he knew probably everything worth knowing in his field. However, the possibility that neurotoxic agents could cause deteriorations in cognitive function was not even suspected by psychologists at the time. If it was, the academic philosophy was that these problems were the territory of applied psychologists and not the concern of research-oriented pure scientists. This view still permeates research performed in this branch of psychology. Woodworth (1921) wrote:

> Occupations which demand much mental activity, provided they are well paid, attract individuals of high intelligence. So we should expect, and the expectation is partially supported by facts. The tests of recruits in the Army showed that, on the average, professional men ranked highest, bookkeepers and clerks rather high, mechanics fairly well, and other occupations in order, with unskilled laborers at the bottom. Such was the *average* result, but it was equally noticeable that the *spread* of intelligence, for almost every occupation, was very wide. Some professional men, for instance, did not rank high, and some laborers did rank high, and the most intelligent of the laborers surpassed the least intelligent of the professional men.
>
> A man's occupation cannot be the cause of his high or low intelligence, since the adult intelligence level of the individual is usually reached and established before he enters on his occupation. Rather intelligence level is a factor in his selection of an occupation.

Many of the correlations between toxic exposures and neuropsychological performance are still misunderstood because of this rigid conception of natural job selection, that is, that one job is best suited to our natural talents. Neurotoxic agents are thought to be associated with neuropsychological performance when a dose–response relationship between indicators of exposure and absorption can be demonstrated. In many studies, levels of skills and occupation are taken as possible confounders.

Neuropsychology. Neuropsychology is a branch of psychology specializing in the effect of brain lesions on behavior. It became a specialization of psychology in the early 1960s. By then, after some initial struggle, clinical psychology had become a discipline accepted within medicine, particularly within psychiatry. But, as the complexities of the brain began to unravel as a result of the birth of the neurosciences, which evolved at about the same time, it became apparent that the classical training of psychologists was inadequate to assess psychological dysfunction produced by brain lesions. At that time, only traumatic and degenerative causes were prominently studied. It is only as recently as the early 1980s that neuropsychologists have gained an insight into behavioral consequences of neurotoxic exposures. To this author's knowledge, there are still no formal courses on human behavioral toxicology or human neurotoxicology either at the undergraduate or at the graduate level in the United States.

Environmental Psychology. The objective of environmental psychology is the study of the effects of physical settings and architectural designs on the mental health of individuals. The term appeared in literature in the late 1950s. It was first intended to bring attention to numerous perceptual experiments in humans under laboratory conditions in which the environment was shown to play an important role in the determination of behavior. It has since become an applied discipline thanks to the effort of Dr. Harold Proshansky and his colleagues at the City University of New York.

Social Psychology. Social psychology is the study of humans conceived of as part of a group. It is closely related to sociology, in which the group—not the individual—is the subject matter of inquiry. Social psychologists made an unexpected entry into the field in the middle 1980s, and some significant contributions have already resulted. They proposed a wider perspective within which neurotoxic agents need to be studied. For example, a child is indeed poisoned by lead, but the socioeconomic status of the parents is an important determinant of these exposures as well. Besides, social psychologists accustomed to studying complex phenomena come to the field with impressive credentials in the

use of imaginative models yet to be discovered by classically trained toxicologists and epidemiologists.

THE BIRTH OF BEHAVIORAL TOXICOLOGY

Behavioral toxicology is the study of toxic agents on behavior and the use of behavioral methods for the monitoring of toxic substances in the environment and the workplace. The discipline existed in Europe without a name as early as 1930. But it was not formally recognized there or in the United States until the late 1950s or early 1960s.

One can view the birth of behavioral toxicology as occurring within a wide framework of social changes, particularly changing views in occupational health, or as a novel approach in toxicological evaluation. The views are not necessarily contradictory.

In the former (wider) view, behavioral toxicology was born when, as a result of more than 200 years of social change, the concept of the quality of life changed. Quality of life standards changed from a fatalistic, unchallenged—even accepted—view that death may result from one's job to the successful plea that both physical and psychological factors in work practices should be taken into consideration. Labor organizations played an important role in the improvement of working conditions in the United States. It can be argued that the message of behavioral toxicology was recognized at least as promptly by American leaders in the field of occupational health as by the scientists who studied the neurotoxic effects of chemical agents and drugs. Dr. Helena Hänninen (1985) from Finland and Mr. Sheldon Samuels (1986) from the AFL-CIO in the United States, for example, seem to think that the birth of behavioral toxicology occurred in the context of social changes.

But not all agree with this interpretation. Dr. Kenneth Anger (1985), formerly at the National Institute of Occupational Safety and Health and now at the Oregon Health Sciences University at Portland, credits the newly acquired knowledge of specific toxic agents—notably carbon monoxide and carbon disulfide—as having prompted research on these subjects.

Dr. Rodney R. Beard of the Department of Community and Preventive Medicine, Stanford University, raised the intriguing possibility that behavioral toxicology was introduced to the United States as a result of national prestige. After the realization that Russia had stricter environmental standards for air pollutants and that behavioral methods were used to establish these standards, many U.S. scientists began adapting the behavioral approach. (In the Soviet Union electrophysiological techniques were—and still are—favored; in the United States the well-established techniques of experimental psychology began to be utilized.) Beard wrote in 1974:

> Interest in behavioral toxicology in the United States began in the later part of the 1950s, principally because we learned that the Russians were setting more stringent standards than us for air quality in industry. . . . There were cries of outrage at the thought that anyone should be so brash as to think they could be better than us. It was learned that the exacting Russian standards, some of them over ten times as strict as ours, were based on what seemed to be peculiar ideas, such as the protection from odors—not only noxious odors, but any odors, and protection from physiological responses—not only from pathological responses, but from any responses at all. Finally, it was said that some standards were based on studies done by 'Pavlovian methods.'

None of us who were concerned about industrial health appeared to be aware that the study of the influence of toxic agents upon the behavior of animals was already well established in the United States. Such work had gone on for years in the pharmacology laboratories. When the first volume of *Annual Reviews of Pharmacology* was published in 1960, it had a long report by Dews and Morse on Behavioral Pharmacology. However, nothing had yet been done with any of the industrial solvents or other industrial materials. Only drugs had

been tested by this technique, which showed such great promises of useful applications.

Behavioral toxicology in the United States was finally firmly established as a result of three converging influences. The first of these was the knowledge of the human work involving psychological and electrophysiological methods in Europe, particularly Russia and Finland.

Germany had dominated many branches of sciences and medicine until World War II. Alice Hamilton, for example, did not consider her training complete until she visited Germany and many other European centers of learning early in this century. She spoke very highly of trends in industrial medicine in that country. For example, it is difficult to grasp the devastating effects that carbon disulfide caused among workers in the last century without consulting Lauderheimer's Die Schwefelkohlenstoffvergiftung der Gummiarbeiter *(published in 1899). At that time, many Eastern European scientists, and even the Japanese, published their works in German.*

After World War II the use of German language in scientific circles fell into disrepute. An intriguing possibility that deserves further research is that many (including the Russians) knew many of the sources written in German but were not expected to quote them. In the United States German sources were almost certainly not consulted.

The other converging influences were the branching out of psychopharmacologists—originally trained in research with animal models—into areas of industrial toxicology, and passage of the Occupational Safety and Health Act (OSHA) of 1970.

It is difficult—and unwise—to pinpoint any historical figure in particular who can be said to be the founder of behavioral toxicology. However, the pioneering work of Hänninen has been recognized worldwide. In 1985 she wrote an autobiographical account of how she entered the field:

> During my first ten years at the Institute [of Occupational Health, Helsinki, Finland] most

of the patients who were sent to a psychologist were not the ones with an occupational disease but those with various psychological problems, psychiatric symptoms, or psychosomatic diseases. Dealing with these kinds of problems corresponded with my education as a clinical psychologist. However, in this particular setting I learned to extend my clinical interview from childhood experiences and marital problems of the patients to their occupational experiences, and to evaluate the possible relationships of the latter to their psychological problems. In that I learned much about the importance of work to mental health.

Occasionally patients with a suspected occupational disease due to some neurotoxic agent . . . were also sent for psychological assessment. They presented me with both a problem and a challenge. In fact, nobody could advise me exactly what to look for, except for the traditional differentiation between organic and psychogenic disturbances.

In an early publication from the Institute of Occupational Health in Helsinki, those clinical activities were described by Hänninen and Lindström under the term "toxicopsychology." But that term never caught on in American circles.

As stated earlier, Hänninen was one of the first to apply psychometric techniques to the evaluation of neurotoxicity in humans. Her early publications on the subject date back to the early 1960s. But other articles on sensory physiology as a basis for air quality standards, for example, were available in English as early as 1962 (Ryazanov 1962).

The Occupational Safety and Health Act of 1970

In the United States, behavioral toxicology received an important endorsement by the Occupational Safety and Health Act of 1970. The United States has passed many occupational safety and health laws regulating specific sectors of the workforce; however, this Act was the most comprehensive of these. The spirit of the law is clearly stated:

The Congress finds that personal injuries and illnesses arising out of work situations impose a substantial burden upon, and are a hindrance to, interstate commerce in terms of lost production, wage loss, medical expenses, and disability compensation payments.

The Congress declares it to be its purpose and policy, through the exercise of its powers to regulate commerce among the several States and with foreign nations and to provide for the general welfare, to assure so far as possible every working man and woman in the Nation safe and healthful working conditions and to preserve our human resources.

This law was the first to mention that research on psychological problems at the workplace is needed. The section on research and related activities (Section 20a) reads:

The Secretary of Health, Education, and Welfare, after consultation with the Secretary and with other appropriate Federal departments or agencies, shall conduct (directly or by grants and contracts) research, experiments, and demonstrations relating to occupational safety and health, including psychological factors involved, and relating to innovative methods, techniques, and approaches for dealing with occupational safety and health problems.

Behavioral toxicology became known in the United States thanks to the publication of two multiauthored books in 1974, one by Xintaras, Johnson, and DeGroot and the other by Weiss and Laties. However, since the subject matter grows in different countries at different times, scientific articles in various languages on the value of behavioral methods for the evaluation of the effect of neurotoxic agents in the environment and the workplace are continuing to appear in the scientific literature.

CONCLUSIONS

Environmental and occupational neurotoxicology is a multidisciplinary science dealing with the study of chemical compounds found in the environment and the workplace that cause harmful effects on the nervous system of humans. The field is the core at which neuropsychology, toxicology, and epidemiology and statistics converge. The human neurotoxicologist studies the toxic effects of environmental and occupational agents within the framework of toxicology and with tools from computer sciences, epidemiology, and statistics.

Morally, environmental and occupational neurotoxicology responded to a redefinition of the concept of "quality of life," a definition that guarantees a safe place in which to live and a healthy place in which to work. Thus, the discipline is closely linked to the ideals of the environmental movement, ecology, consumerism, labor organizations, and the people's right to know.

REFERENCES

Anger, WK (1985) Overview of NIOSH neurobehavioral testing/research. *Neurobehav Toxicol Teratol* 7:289–290.

Anger, WK and Johnson, BJ (1985) Chemicals affecting behavior. In *Neurotoxicity of Industrial and Commercial Chemicals, Vol 1,* JL O'Donoghue (ed) pp 51–148. Boca Raton, FL: CRC Press.

Beard, RR (1974) Early developments of behavioral toxicology in the United States. In *Behavioral Toxicology: Early Detection of Occupational Hazards,* C Xintaras, BL Johnson, and I De Groot (eds) pp. 427–431. Washington, DC: US Department of Health, Education and Welfare, Public Health Service, Center for Disease Control, National Institute for Occupational Safety and Health.

Beeson, BB (1930) Orfila, pioneer toxicologist. *Ann Med Hist* 2:68–70.

Bransford, JS (1984) Proliferation of new chemical increasing need for data bases. *Occup Health Safety* 4:32–35.

Brazier, MAB (1984) *A History of Neurophysiology in the 17th and 18th Centuries: From Concept to Experiment.* New York: Raven Press.

Brazier, MAB (1987) *A History of Neurophysiology in the 19th Century.* New York: Raven Press.

Carson, R (1962) *Silent Spring.* Greenwich, CT: Fawcett Publications.

Casarett, LJ and Bruce, MC (1986) Origins and scope of toxicology. In *Toxicology: The Basic Science of Poisons,* 3rd ed, CD Klaasen, MO Amdur, and J Doull (eds) pp. 3–10. New York: Macmillan.

Curran, JA (1970) *Founders of Harvard School of Public Health, with Bibliographic Notes.* New York: Josiah Macy Jr Foundation.

Dews, PB and Morse, WH (1961) Behavioral pharmacology. In *Annual Review of Pharmacology,* WC Cutting, RH Dreibach, and HW Elliott (eds) pp. 145–174. Palo Alto, CA: Annual Reviews.

Gardner, CB (1983) *Rachel Carson.* New York: Frederik Ungar.

Goldwater, LJ (1936) From Hippocrates to Ramazzini: Early history of industrial medicine. *Ann Med Hist* 8:27.

Hamilton, A (1943) *Exploring the Dangerous Trades.* Boston: Little, Brown.

Hänninen, H (1985) Twenty-five years of behavioral toxicology within occupation medicine: A personal account. *Am J Ind Med* 7:19–30.

Highsmith, RM (undated) History of conservation. In *Encyclopedia Americana,* pp. 635–637.

Hold, C (1983) Historians deplore classification rules. *Science* 222:1215–1218.

Hunter, D (1978) *The Disease of Occupations,* 6th ed. London: The English University Press.

Kay, K (1977) Polybrominated biphenyls (PBB), environmental contamination in Michigan 1973–1976. *Environ Res* 13:64–93.

Last, JM (1986) *Maxcy-Rosenau Public Health and Preventive Medicine,* 12th ed. Norwalk, CT: Appleton-Century-Crofts.

Laudenheimer, R (1899) *Die Schwefelkohlenstoffvergiftung der Gummiarbeiter.* Leipzig: Veit & Co.

La Wall, CH (1927) *The Curious Lore of Drugs and Medicines (Four Thousand Years of Pharmacy).* Garden City, NJ: Garden City Publishing.

Lorén Esteban, S (1961) *Mateo José Buenaventura Orfila: Estudio Crítico-Biográfico de su Obra e Influencia.* Zaragoza: Institución "Fernando el Católico" de la Excel Diputación Provincial de Zaragoza.

Nader, R (1965) *Unsafe at Any Speed: The Designed-In Dangers of the American Automobile.* New York: Grossman.

Orfila, MJB (1820) *Directions for the Treatment of Persons Who Have Taken Poisons, and Those in State of Apparent Death; Together with the Means of Detecting Poisons and Adulterations in Wine; Also of Detecting Real from Apparent Death* [Translated from the French by RH Black]. London: Longman, Hurst, Ress, Orne, and Brown.

Orfila, MJB (1943) *Traité de Toxicologie,* 4th ed. Paris: Fortin.

Ramazzini, B (1713) *De Morbis Artificum Diatriba* (translated as *Diseases of Workers). New* York: New York Academy of Medicine.

Ryazanov, VA (1962) Sensory physiology as basis for air quality standards: The approach used in the Soviet Union. *Arch Environ Health* 5:480–494.

Samuels, SW (1986) *The Environment of the Workplace and Human Values*. New York: Alan R Liss.

Schaumburg, HH and Spencer, OS (1980), Selected outbreak of neurotoxic disease. In *Experimental and Clinical Neurotoxicology,* OS Spencer and HH Schaumburg (eds) pp. 883–889. Baltimore: Williams & Wilkins.

Sonnedecker, G (1976) *Kremer and Urdang's History of Pharmacy,* 4th ed. Philadelphia: JB Lippincott.

Takeuchi, T (1977) Neuropathology of Minamata disease in Kumamoto: Especially at the chronic stage. In *Neurotoxicology,* L Roizin, H Shiraki, and N Grcevic (eds) p. 235. New York: Raven Press.

Weiss, B and Laties, VG (eds) (1974) *Behavioral Toxicology*. New York: Plenum Press.

Woodworth, RS (1921) *Psychology*. New York: Henry Holt.

Xintaras, C, Johnson, BL, and DeGroot, I (eds) (1974) *Behavioral Toxicology, Early Detection of Occupational Hazards*. Washington, DC: US Department of Health, Education and Welfare, Public Health Center for Disease Control, National Institute for Occupational Safety and Health.

SUGGESTED READINGS

Adams, F (trans) (1939) *The Genuine Works of Hippocrates*. Baltimore: Williams & Wilkins.

Agricola, G (1556) *De Re Metallica* (translated 1950 by HC Hoover and LH Hoover). New York: Dover Publications.

Alluisi, EA (1975) Optimum uses of psychobiological, sensorimotor, and performance measurement strategies. *Hum Fact* 17(4):309–320.

Amstrong, RD, Leach, LJ, Belluscio, PR, et al. (1963) Behavioral changes in the pigeon following inhalation for mercury vapor. *Am Ind Hyg Assoc J* 24:366–375.

Anonymous (1968) *British Journal of Industrial Medicine:* The first 25 years. *Br J Ind Med* 25:1–3.

Ashford, NA (1976) *Crisis in the Workplace*. Cambridge, MA: MIT Press.

Aub, JC, Fairhall, LT, Minot, AS, et al. (1926) *Lead Poisoning*. Baltimore: Williams & Wilkins.

Bakir, F, Damluji, SF, Amin-Zaki, L, et al. (1973) Methylmercury poisoning in Iraq: An inter-university report. *Science* 181:230–241.

Barners, HE (1963) *A History of Historical Writing,* 2nd ed. New York: Dover Publications.

Barnhart, CL, Steinmetz, S, and Barnhart, RK (1973) *The Barnhart Dictionary of New English since 1963*. Bronxville, NY: Barnhart/Harper & Row.

Beritic, T (1989) Spinal origin of human lead neuropathy: This paper marks the 150th anniversary of the Paralysie de Plomb ou Saturnine by L. Tanquerel des Planches. *Am J Ind Med* 15:643–656.

Berman, A (ed) (1966) *Pharmacological Historiography, Proceedings of a Colloquium Sponsored by the American Institute of the History of Pharmacy on the Occasion of the Institute's 25th Anniversary*. Madison, WI: American Institute of the History of Pharmacy.

Bernal, JD (1971) *Science in History, Vol 2, The Scientific and Industrial Revolutions*. Cambridge, MA: The MIT Press.

Bernard, C (1857) *Leçons sur les Effets des Substances Toxiques et Médicamenteuses*. Paris: J Balliere et Fils.

Bignami, G (1976) Behavioral pharmacology and toxicology. *Annu Rev Pharmacol Toxicol* 16:329–366.

Blackman, DE and Sanger, DJ (1978) *Contemporary Research in Behavioral Pharmacology*. New York: Plenum Press.

Blackmon, LR (1967) *A Bio-Bibliography of Rachel Carson (1907–1964)*. Washington, CD: Catholic University of America, Master of Science Dissertation.

Boakes, R (1984) *From Darwin to Behaviourism: Psychology and the Minds of Animals*. New York: Cambridge University Press.

Boring, EG (1950) *A History of Experimental Psychology*. New York: Appleton-Century-Crofts.

Borkin, J (1978) *The Crime and Punishment of IG Farben*. New York: The Free Press.

Brimblecombe, P (1987) *The Big Smoke: A History of Air Pollution in London since Medieval Times*. London: Methuen.

Brodeur, P (1974) *Expendable Americans*. New York: Viking Press.

Brook, P (1972) *The House of Life: Rachel Carson at Work with Selection of her Writings, Published and Unpublished*. Boston: Houghton Mifflin.

Brooks, C and Cranefield, P (1959) *The Historical Development of Physiological Thought*. New York: Hafner.

Brown Travis, C, McLean, BE, and Ribar, C (eds) (1989) *Environmental Toxins: Psychological, Behavioral and Sociocultural Aspects, 1973–1990*. Washington, DC: American Psychological Association.

Buess, H (1962) The beginnings of industrial medicine in England. *Br J Med* 19:297–302.

Buess, H (1967) Ueber den Beitrag deutscher Aertze zur Arbeitmedizin des 19 Jahrhunderts. In *Der Artz und der Kranke,* W Artelt (ed) pp. 166–178. Stuttgart.

Burnham, D (1984) Facts? Let them eat docudrama. *The New York Times* June 4.

Burnham, D (1984) Computers worry historians. *The New York Times* August 26.

Burnham, D (1984) Censorship accords signed by thousands, study shows. *The New York Times* June 14.

Caldwell, AE (1970) *Origins of Psychopharmacology: From CPZ to LSD.* Springfield, IL: Charles C Thomas.

Campbell, WA (1971) *The Chemical Industry.* London: Longman.

Cantarow, A, and Trumper, M (1944) *Lead Poisoning.* Baltimore: Williams & Wilkins.

Carlton, DE (1983) *Behavioral Pharmacology.* New York: WH Freeman.

Carone, PA, Kieffer, SN, Yolles, SF (eds) (1984) *History of Mental Health in Industry: The Last Hundred Years.* New York: Human Sciences Press.

Carter, LJ (1973) Environmentalists seek new victory in a frustrating war. *Science* 181:143.

Carter, LJ (1976) Michigan's PBB incident: Chemical mix-up leads to disaster. *Science* 192:240–243.

Cartwright, FF (1972) *Disease and History.* London: Rupert Hart-Davis.

Chalupa, B, Synkova, J, and Sevcik, M (1960) The assessment of electroencephalographic changes and memory disturbances in acute intoxications with industrial poisons. *Br J Ind Med* 16:238–241.

Chen, KK (1969) *The American Society for Pharmacology and Experimental Therapeutics.* Washington, DC: Judd and Detweiler.

Chyzer, BA (1908) *Uber die in ungarischen Tonwarengewerbe vorkommenden Bleivergifungen.* Jena, GDR: Fischer.

Clarke, KK (1969) *The Apothecary in Eighteen-Century Williamsburg: Being an Account of His Medical and Chirugical Services, as Well as of His Trade Practices as a Chemist.* Williamsburg: Colonial.

Chen, E (1979) *PBB: An American Tragedy.* Englewood Cliffs, NJ: Prentice Hall.

Clarke, R (1968) *We All Fall Down: The Prospect of Biological and Chemical Warfare.* London: Allen Lane, Pinguin Press.

Clendening, L (ed) (1942) *Source Book of Medical History.* New York: Dover Publications.

Cohen, A and Margolis B (1973) Initial psychological research related to the occupational safety and health act of 1970. *Am Psychol* 28:600.

Comstock, EG (1978) Morbidity due to non-poisoning. *J Occup Med* 20:755–758.

Corn, JK (1978) Historical aspects of industrial hygiene: I. Changing attitudes toward occupational health. *Am Ind Hyg Assoc J* 39:695–699.

Corsi, P and Weindling, P (1983) *Information Sources in the History of Science and Medicine.* London: Butterworth Scientific.

Daumas, M (1979) *A History of Technology and Invention: Progress through the Ages.* New York: Crown Publishers.

David, A (1986) In memoriam: Professor Jaroslav Teisinger, MD. *Am J Ind Medicine,* 9:495–496.

de Boor, W (1956) *Pharmakopsychologie und Psychopathologie.* Berlin: Springer-Verlag.

Déjérine-Klumpke J (1889) *Des Polynévrites en Général et des Paralysies et Atrophies Saturnines en Particulier.* Paris: F Alcan.

Dibner, B (1958) *Agricola on Metals.* Norwalk, CT: Burndy Library.

Di Pietro, P (1983) *Bernandino Ramazzini (Carpi of Modena 1633–Padua 1714) on the CCCL anniversary of his birth, Archives of the Collegium Ramazzini, Vol 1, Proceedings of the First International Symposium on the Celebration of the 350th Anniversary of the birth of Bernardino Ramazzini.* Carpi, Italy: Collegium Ramazzini.

D'Itri, PA and D'Itri, FM (1977) *Mercury Contamination: A Human Tragedy.* New York: John Wiley & Sons.

Doull, J, Klaassen, CD, and Amdur, MO (1983) *Casarett and Doull's Toxicology: The Basic Science of Poisons,* 3rd ed. New York: Macmillan.

Duffy, J (1990) *The Sanitarians: A History of American Public Health.* Urbana, IL: University of Illinois Press.

Ekel, GJ (1974) Use of conditioned reflex methods in Soviet behavioral toxicology research. In *Behavioral Toxicology: Early Detection of Occupational Hazards,* C Xintaras, BL Johnson, and I De Groot (eds). pp. 432–440. Washington: DC: US Department of Health, Education and Welfare, Public Health Service, Center for Disease Control, National Institute for Occupational Safety and Health.

Ekel, GJ and Teichner, WH (1976) *An Analysis and Critique of Behavioral Toxicology in the USSR.* Cincinnati: US Department of Health, Education and Welfare, Centers for Disease Control, National Institute for Occupational Safety and Health, Division of Biomedical and Behavioral Sciences. DEW (NIOSH) publication No. 77-160.

Erb, W (1874): Ein Fall von Bleilähmung. *Arch Psychol (Frankf)* 5:445–446.

Felton, JS (1976) 200 years of occupational medicine in the US. *J Occup Med* 28:809.

Freindly, J (1984) Journalism schools are long on students, short in respect. *The New York Times* June 3.

Fries, GF (1985) The PBB episode in Michigan: An overall appraisal. *CRC Crit Rev Toxicol* 16(2):105–156.

Gamberale, F (1975) Behavioral toxicology: A new field of job health research. *Ambio* 4:43–46.

Garrison, FH (1929) *An Introduction to the History of Medicine, with Medical Chronology, Suggestions for Study, and Bibliographic Data.* Philadelphia: WB Saunders.

Gilfillan, SC (1965) Lead poisoning and the fall of Rome. *J Occup Med* 7:53–60.

Goldberg, ME, Haun, C, and Smyth, HF (1962) Toxicologic implication of altered behavior induced by an industrial vapor. *Toxicol Appl Pharmacol* 4:148–164.

Goldberg, ME, Johnson, HE, Pozzani, UC, et al. (1964) Effect of repeated inhalation of vapors of industrial solvents on animal behavior. I. Evaluation of nine solvent vapors on pole-climbing performance in rats. *Am Ind Hyg Assoc J* 25:369–375.

Goldwater, LJ (1936) From Hippocrates to Ramazzini: Early history of industrial medicine. *Ann Med Hist* 8:27.

Goldwater, LJ (1946) *Mercury: A History of Quicksilver.* New York: New York Press.

Goodman Gilman, A, Goodman LS, and Gilman, A (1980) *Goodman and Gilman's The Pharmacological Basis of Therapeutics,* 6th ed. New York: Macmillan.

Grandjean, E, Münchinger, T, Tirrian, V, et al. (1955) Investigations into the effects of exposure to trichloroethylene in mechanical engineering. *Br J Ind Med* 12:131–142.

Greenwood, M (1932) *Epidemiology, Historical and Experimental.* Baltimore: Johns Hopkins University Press.

Griffenhagen, GB (1957) *Tools of the Apothecary.* Washington, DC: American Pharmacological Association.

Grun, B (1963) *The Timetables of History: A Horizontal Linkage of People and Events.* New York: Touchstone/Simon and Schuster.

Grund, W (1968) *Toxicologie und Arbeitsmedizin.* Berlin: VER Verlag Volk und Gesundheit.

Guthrie, DA (1946) *A History of Medicine.* Philadelphia: JB Lippincott.

Gutierrez Fernández, F (1975) *Magendie, Fundador de la Toxicolgía Experimental.* Barcelona: Gráficas Diamante.

Haber, LF (1958) *The Chemical Industry during the Nineteenth Century.* Oxford: Clarendon Press.

Hall, G (1984) Franz Koelsch: Pioniers des medizinichen Arbeitsschutzes. *Arbeit Soc Prev Med* 19:218–222.

Hamilton, A (1925) *Industrial Poisons in the United States.* New York: Macmillan.

Hamilton, A (1984) Forty years in the poisonous trades. *Am J Ind Hyg* 9(1):5–17.

Hänninen, H (1964) Psychische symtome bei schwefelkohlenstroffvergiftung. *Excerpta Med* 62:894–897.

Hänninen, H and Lindström, K (1976) *Behavioral Test Battery for Toxicopsychological Studies used at the Institute of Occupational Health in Helsinki.* Helsinki: Institute of Occupational Health.

Hardy, HL (1983) *Challenging Man-Made Disease: The Memoirs of Harriet L Hardy.* New York: Praeger.

Harvey, JA (1971) *Behavioral Analysis of Drug Action.* Glenview, IL: Scott, Foresman.

Haublein, H-G (1959) Aus der Geschichte des Arbeitergesundheitsschutzes in Deutschland. In H-G Haublein and Kersten (eds), pp. 7–36. *Der Artz im Betribs-Gesundheitsshutz,* Berlin: VEB Verlag Volk und Gesuntheit.

Hawkins, TR (1987) A history in progress: NIEHS, the first 20 years (1966–1986). *Environ Health Perspect* 75:7–10.

Hayes, AW, Schnell, R, and Miya, TS (eds) (1983) *Developments in the Science and Practice of Toxicology.* Amsterdam: North Holland Elsevier.

Haynes, W (1945) *This Chemical Age.* New York: Alfred A Knopf.

Holmstead, B and Lilihestrand, G (eds) (1963) *Readings in Pharmacology.* Oxford: Pergamon Press.

Hordern, A (1968) Psychopharmacology: Some historical considerations. In *Psychopharmacology: Dimensions and Perspectives,* CRB Joyce (ed) pp. 95–148. London: Tavistock.

International Labour Office (1983) *Encyclopedia of Occupational Health and Safety,* 3rd ed. Geneva: ILO.

Ittelson, WI, Proshansky, HM, Rivlin, LG, et al. (1974) *An Introduction to Environmental Psychology.* New York: Holt, Rinehart and Winston.

Iverson, SD and Iverson, LL (1975) *Behavioral Pharmacology.* New York: Oxford University Press.

Jaffe, B (1976) *Crucibles: The Story of Chemistry from Ancient Alchemy to Nuclear Fission,* 4th rev ed. New York: Dover Publication.

Joravsky, D (1989) *Russian Psychology: A Critical History.* Cambridge, MA: Basil Blackwell.

Judkins, BM (1986) *We Offer Ourselves as Evidence: Toward Workers' Control of Occupational Health.* Wesport, CT: Greenwood.

Karbe, K-H (1973) Der Stand of Arbeitsmedizin in Deutschland im Jahrzeit der burgerlichen Revolution. *Deutsch Gesundheit* 9:423–426.

Kehoe, RA (1962) Cummings memorial lecture: Education and training in industrial hygiene. *Am Ind Hyg Assoc J* 23:175–180.

Kelman, S (1981) *Regulating America, Regulating Sweden: A Comparative Study of Occupational Safety and Health Policy.* Cambridge, MA: MIT Press.

Kingsland, SE (1985) *Modeling Nature: Episodes in the History of Population Ecology.* Chicago: University of Chicago Press.

Kovacks, G (1968) The history of industrial psychiatry. *Can Psychiatr Assoc J* 13:93–94.

Kuratsune, M, Yoshimura, T, Matsuzaka, J, et al. (1971) Yusho, a poisoning caused by rice oil contaminated with polychlorinated biphenyls. *Publ Health Rep* 86:1083–1091.

Kuratsune, M, Yoshimura, T, Matsuzaka, J, et al. (1972) Epidemiologic study on Yusho, a poisoning caused by ingestion of rice oil contaminated with a commercial brand of polychlorinated biphenyls. *Environ Health Perspect* 1:119–128.

Kirk-Othmer Encyclopedia of Chemical Technology, 3rd ed (1978–1984). New York: Wiley–Interscience.

Lacy, A (1988) Rachel Carson's legacy. *The New York Times* March 10.

Lain Entralgo, P (1963) *Historia de la Medicina Moderna y Contemporánea*. Barcelona: Científica-Médica.

Lain Entralgo, P (1971) *Historia Universal de la Medicina*. Barcelona: Salvat.

Lal, H (1977) *Discriminative Stimulus Properties of Drugs*. New York: Plenum Press.

Landrigan, PJ (1985) Academic occupational health and environmental medicine: Current directions. *Bull NY Acad Med* 61(10):901–916.

Laties, VG (1979) IV Zavadskii and the beginnings of behavioral pharmacology: An historical note and translation. *J Exp Anal Behav* 32:463–472.

Laties, VG (1986) Lessons from the history of behavioral pharmacology. In *Advances in Behavioral Pharmacology, Vol. 5, Developmental Behavioral Pharmacology*. Hillsdale, NJ: Lawrence Erlbaum Associates.

Lee, DK (1970) The National Institute of Environmental Health Sciences. *Am Ind Hyg Assoc J* 31:637–640.

Lee, WR (1964) Robert Baker: The first doctor in the factory department, Part 1, 1803–1858. *Br J Ind Med* 21:85–93.

Lee, WR (1964) Robert Baker: The first doctor in the factory department, Part II, 1858 onwards. *Br J Ind Med* 21:167–179.

Lee, WR (1968) The history of the statutory control of mercury poisoning in Great Britain. *Br J Ind Med* 25:52–62.

Lee, WR (1972) Emergence of occupational medicine in Victorian times. *Br J Ind Med* 30:118–124.

Legge, RT (1920) *Industrial Diseases and Industrial Poisons*. New York: T Nelson.

Legge, TR (1936) The history of industrial medicine and occupational diseases. *Ind Med* 5:300–314, 371–377, 420–430, 513–517, 569–576, 633–638.

Legge, T (1934) *Industrial Maladies*. London: Oxford University Press.

Legge, T and Goadby, KW (1912) *Lead Poisoning and Lead Absorption*. London: Arnold.

Leicester, HM (1956) *The Historical Background of Chemistry*. New York: Dover Publications.

Levy, BS and Wegman, DH (1983) *Occupational Health: Recognizing and Preventing Work-Related Disease*. Boston: Little, Brown.

Lilienfeld, AM (1976) *Foundations of Epidemiology*. New York: Oxford University Press.

Lipton, MA, DiMascio, A, and Killam, KF (1978) *Psychopharmacology: A Generation of Progress*. New York: Raven Press.

Long, PO (ed) (1985) *Science and Technology in Medieval Society*. New York: The New York Academy of Sciences.

Macht, DI (1928) *The Holy Incense: A Botanical, Pharmacological, Psychological, and Archeological Appreciation of the Bible*. Baltimore: Waverly Press.

Magnudson, HJ, Fassett, DW, Gerade, HW, et al. (1964) Industrial toxicology in the Soviet Union: Theoretical and applied. *Am Ind Hyg Assoc J* 25:185–197.

Malan, RM (1963) Occupational health in Eastern Europe. *Br J Ind Med* 20:154–164.

Maurisen, JPS (1981) History of mercury and mercurialism. *NY State J Med* 81:1902–1909.

Mayers, MR (1958) Alice Hamilton, MD. *Am Ind Hyg Assoc J* 19:449–452.

McCarry, C (1971) *Citizen Nader*. New York: New American Library.

McCord, CP (1953) Lead and lead poisoning in early America: Benjamin Franklin and lead poisoning. *Ind Med Surg* 22:393–399.

McCord, CP (1954) Lead and lead poisoning in early America: The lead pipe period. *Ind Med Surg* 23:27–31.

McEwen, FL and Stephenson, GR (1979) *The Use and Significance of Pesticides in the Environment*. New York: John Wiley & Sons.

McIntosh, RP (1985) *The Background of Ecology: Concept and Theory*. New York: Cambridge University Press.

Meek, WJ (1954) *The Gentle Art of Poisoning: Medico-Historical Papers*. Madison, WI: University of Wisconsin Press.

Meillère, JPG (1903) *La Saturnisme: Etude Historique, Physiologique, Clinique, and Prophylactique*. Paris: O Doin.

Möbius, PJ (1886) Ueber einige ungewöhnliche Fälle von Bleilähmung. *Z Nervenheilk* 1:6–13.

Morgan, JP and Tullos, TC (1976) *The Jake Walk Blues: A toxicological tragedy mirrored in American popular music. *Ann Intern Med* 85(6):804–808.

Mouson, RR (1980) *Occupational Epidemiology*. Boca Raton, FL: CRC Press.

Musson, AE and Robinson, E (1969) *Science and Technology in the Industrial Revolution*. New York: Gordon and Breach.

Nash, RF (1989) *The Rights of Nature: A History of Environmental Ethics*. Madison, WI: University of Wisconsin Press.

National Journal (1986) 150 who made a difference. June 14, No. 24.

The New York Times (1986) Silent Spring led to safer pesticides, but use is up. April 21, p. A14.

Niedringhaus Davis, L (1984) *The Corporate Alchemists: Profit Takers and Problem Makers in the Chemical Industry*. New York: William Morrow.

Niyogi, SK (1980) Historical development of forensic toxicology in America up to 1978. *Am J Forens Med Pathol* 1:249–264.

Northrup, HR (1978) *The Impact of OSHA: A Study of the Effects of the Occupational and Safety Act on Three Key Industries, Aerospace, Chemicals and Textiles*. Philadelphia: Industrial Research Unit.

Nriagu, JO (1983) *Lead and Lead Poisoning in Antiquity*. New York: John Wiley & Sons.

Oliver, T (1914) *Lead Poisoning: From the Industrial, Medical, and Social Points of View.* London: HK Lewis.

Olmsted, JMD (1944) *François Magendie: Pioneer in Experimental Physiology and Scientific Medicine in XIX France.* New York: Schuman.

Oppenheim, H (1885) Zur pathologischen Anatomie der Bleilähmung. *Arch Psychol (Frankf)* 16:476–495.

Pachter, HM (1961) *Paracelsus: Magic into Science.* New York: Collier.

Pauli, JM (1984) The origin and basis of threshold limit values. *Am J Ind Med* 5:227–238.

Peterson, I (1986) Study of effects of agent orange on veterans is stalled in dispute. *The New York Times,* May 19, p. A1.

Poling, A (1986) *A Primer of Human Behavioral Pharmacology.* New York: Plenum Press.

Proctor, RW and Weeks, DJ (1990) *The Goal of BF Skinner and Behavioral Analysis.* New York: Springer-Verlag.

Proshansky, HM, Ittelson, WH and Rivlin, LG (eds) (1970) *Environmental Psychology: Man and His Physical Setting.* New York: Holt, Rinehart & Winston.

Reekie, D and Weber, MW (1979) *Profits, Politics, and Drugs.* London: Macmillan.

Remak, E (1876) Zur Pathogenese der Bleilähmungen. *Arch Psychol (Frankf)* 6:1–56.

Rom, WN (Ed) (1983) *Environmental and Occupational Medicine.* Boston: Little, Brown.

Roosevelt, N (1970) *Conservation: Now or Never.* New York: Dodd, Mead.

Rose, ME (1971) The doctor in the industrial revolution. *Brit J Ind Med* 28:22–26.

Rosen, G (1968) *A History of Public Health.* New York: MD Publications.

Ruffin, JB (1963) Functional testing for behavioral toxicology: A missing dimension in experimental environmental toxicology. *J Occup Med* 5(3):117–121.

Schertz, RG and Robertson, WO (1978) The history of poison control centers in the United States. *Clin Toxicol* 12(3):291–296.

Schilling, RSF (1979) Donald Hunter: The first editor of the *British Journal of Industrial Medicine. Br J Ind Med* 36:242–243.

Seiden, LS and Dykstra, LA (1977) *Psychopharmacology: A Biochemical and Behavioral Approach.* New York: Van Nostrand Reinhold.

Shabecoff, P (1982) EPA chief assailed on lead violation. *The New York Times* April 13.

Shabecoff, P (1982) Environmentalists come of age. *The New York Times* October 13.

Shabecoff, P (1984) Cleaning up the EPA vocabulary. *The New York Times* June 13.

Shabecoff, P (1985) Environmental movement is facing changes. *The New York Times* April 4.

Sheail, J (1987) *Seventy-Five Years in Ecology: The Brit-*ish Ecological Society. Palo Alto, CA: Blackwell Scientific.

Shuster, L (ed) (1962) *Readings in Pharmacology.* Boston: Little, Brown.

Smith, CS (ed) (1968) *Sources for the History of the Science of Steel.* Cambridge, MA: MIT Press.

Srivastava, G (1954) *History of Indian Pharmacy.* Calcutta: Pindars.

Stillman, JM (1920) *Theophrastus Bombastus von Hohenheim, Called Paracelsus: His Personality and Influence as Physician, Chemist and Reformer.* Chicago: Open Court Publishing.

Stoddart, AM (1911) *The Life of Paracelsus: Theophrastus von Hohenheim.* London: John Murray.

Stoerring, GE (1936) Gedachnisverlust durch Gassevergiftung, ein Mensch ohne Zeitgedächtnis. *Arch f.d. ges. Psychol* 95:436–511.

Takeuchi, T, Eto, N, and Eto, K (1979) Neuropathology of childhood cases of methylmercury poisoning (Minamata disease) with prolonged symptoms, with particular reference to the decortication syndrome. *Neurotoxicology* 1:1–20.

Teisinger, J (1939) Periferni neuritidy z povolani. *Cas lek ces* 33:1–8.

Tanquerel des Planches, L (1839) *Traité des Maladies de Plomb ou Saturnines.* Paris: Ferra.

Teleky, L (1923) Die Streckerschwäche als Symptom der Bleiaufnahme und Bleivergiftung. *Klin Wochenschr* 2:876–908.

Teleky, L (1924) Die Symptome der Bleivergiftung, ihre Bedeutung für Frühdiagnose und Diagnose. *Munch Med Wochenschr* 71:266–269.

Tekely, L (1935) Klinik und Begutachtung der Bleivergiftung. *Schweiz Med Wochenschr* 65:229–234.

Teleky, L (1951) Industrial hygiene in West Germany. *Ind Hyg Q* 12:23–82.

Teleky, L (1953) *Gewerbliche Vergiftungen.* Berlin: Springer Verlag.

Theophilus (1100?) *On Divers Art: The Foremost Medieval Treatise on Painting, Glassmaking and Metalwork* [translated from the Latin with introduction and notes by John G Hawthorne and Cyril S Smith]. New York: Dover.

Thomas, L (1986) *The Lasker Awards: Four Decades of Scientific Medical Progress.* New York: Raven Press.

Thompson, CJS (1931) *Poisons and Poisoners, with Historical Accounts of Some Famous Mysteries in Ancient and Modern Times.* London: H Shaylor.

Thompson, T and Schuster, CR (1968) *Behavioral Pharmacology.* Englewood Cliffs, NJ: Prentice-Hall.

US Department of Health, Education, and Welfare (1977) *Human Health and the Environment, Some Research Needs, Chapter 13, Behavioral Toxicology,* pp. 329–350. Washington, DC: NIEHS.

US Department of Labor (1976) *Brief History of the American Labor Movement.* Washington, DC: Superintendent of Documents, US Government Printing Office.

Valciukas, JA (1984) A decade of behavioral toxicology: Impressions of a NIOSH/WHO workshop in Cincinnati, May 1983. *Am J Ind Med* 5:405–406.

Valciukas, JA (1984) Kodo zuroku: A Japanese *De Re Metalica. Am J Ind Med* 6:397–398.

Valciukas, JA (1985) The role of the psychologist in occupational neurotoxicology: A propos of Huszco et al's "Psychology and Organized Labor" *Am Psychol* 40:1053–1054.

Valciukas, JA (1985) Pioneers in occupational neurotoxicology. *Am J Ind Med* 78:1.

Valciukas, JA and Lilis, R (1980) Psychometric techniques in environmental research. *Env Res* 21:275–297.

Valentin, M (1978) *Travail des Hommes et Savants Oubliés: Histoire de la Medicine du Travail, de la Securité, et de l'Ergonomie.* Paris: Docis.

Vigliani, EC (1950) Clinical observations on carbon disulfide intoxication in Italy. *Industr Med Surg* 19:240–242.

Waitt, AH (1942) *Gas Warfare: The Chemical Weapon, Its Use, and Protection against It.* New York: Duel, Sloan, and Peter.

Waldron, HA (1973) Lead poisoning in the ancient world. *Med Hist* 17:391–399.

Wedeen, RP (1989) Were the hatters of New Jersey mad? *Am J Ind Med* 16:225–233.

Weiss, B (1983) Behavioral toxicology and environmental health science. *Am Psychol* 1174–1187.

Whiteside, T (1979) *The Pendulum and the Toxic Cloud: The Course of Dioxin Contamination.* New Haven: Yale University Press.

Whorton, JC (1974) *Before "Silent Spring": Pesticides and Public Health in Pre-DDT America.* Lawrenceville, NJ: Princeton University Press.

Wiener, PP (ed) (1974) *Dictionary of the History of Ideas: Studies of Selected Pivotal Ideas.* New York: Charles Scribner's Sons.

Wilson, R (1987) A visit to Chernobyl. *Science* 236:1636–1640.

Winslow, CEA (1952) *Man and Epidemics.* Princeton, NJ: Princeton University Press.

Woodwell, GM (1984) Broken eggshells: The miracle of DDT was short-lived, but it helped launch the environmental movement. *Science* 84:115–117.

Woolley, DE (1984) A perspective of lead poisoning in antiquity and the present. *Neurotoxicology* 5(3):353–362.

Wright, W (1922) A clinical study of fur cutters and felt-hat workers. *J Ind Hyg* 4:296–304.

Xintaras, C (1964) *Application of the Technique of Evoked Response to Industrial Toxicology.* Doctoral Thesis, University of Cincinnati, Cincinnati.

Part I

Fundamentals and Techniques

1

Main Components of the Nervous System

Knowledge of the main components of the nervous system is generally recognized as being essential for an understanding of the gross neuropsychological manifestations of neurotoxic illness, the rationale for the use of specific techniques for the assessment of nervous system functions, and the understanding of pharmacological mechanisms of neurotoxic action.

One of the most basic approaches in the understanding of nervous system function is to differentiate control of voluntary muscles and viscera and to determine whether central and/or peripheral structures are involved. The nervous system may be divided into two major compartments: the somatic and the visceral nervous system. The *somatic nervous system* innervates and controls voluntary (skeletal) muscles. These include, for example, the neural pathways that convey sensory information of limb position—even when the eyes are closed—and the neural pathways that carry voluntary motor commands for arm, finger, or toe movement. The *visceral nervous system* controls internal organs that are not normally under the influence of voluntary control, such as changes in the rate of the heartbeat, the dilation and constriction of blood vessels, the dilation and constriction of the pupils, etc.

Environmental and occupational toxic agents often have multiple neural targets. For example, lead is a poison the chronic toxic effects of which are known to include the gastrointestinal system, neuromuscular pathways, central nervous system, blood-forming system, kidneys, and others. For reasons that are not yet completely understood, lead sometimes has a preferential effect on the somatic nervous system, as in the "lead palsy" observed in severe forms of occupational lead poisoning. This form of paralysis is thought to be the result of the effect of lead on the nerve cells, nerves, and neurochemical events controlling muscles of the upper and lower limbs and hand. But lead also can cause alterations in the gastrointestinal system and the visceral portion of the nervous system, such as in the case of "lead colic" observed in advanced stages of intoxication. Somatic and visceral signs of lead poisoning can occur separately or in combination.

Figure 1.1 illustrates another important division of the nervous system: central and peripheral. The *central nervous system* includes the bulk of nervous tissue—the spinal cord, brainstem, cerebellum, and cerebrum. They are called "central" because all derive from the *neuraxis*, an early structure in the nervous system's embryonic development. Most of the

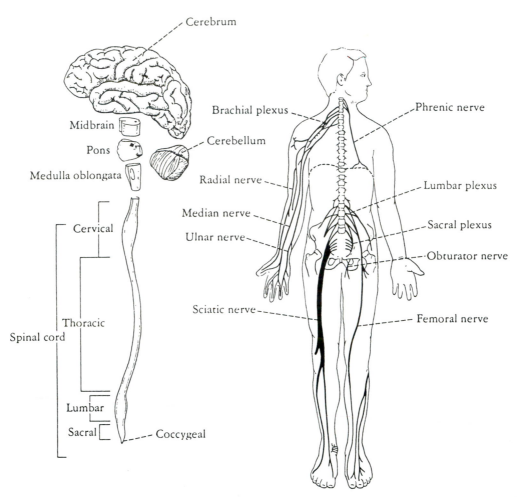

Fig. 1.1. Left: The main components of the central nervous system. Right: The peripheral nervous system, excluding the cranial nerves. (From Snell 1980.)

central nervous system is protected by a bony structure comprised of the vertebral column and the cranium. All neural tissue located outside the neuraxis is referred to as the *peripheral nervous system.*

Somatic and visceral portions of the nervous system are related to their peripheral and central components; thus, many permutations are possible. For example:

- Peripheral nerves from the spinal cord send messages to move somatic voluntary muscles, resulting in movement.
- The cerebral cortex, a central structure, also controls somatic voluntary muscles.
- Peripheral autonomic nerves that are part

of the visceral system control internal visceral organs such as heart, lungs, and endocrine glands.
- Central structures such as the hypothalamus also control visceral organs.

Toxic-induced paralysis can result from the effect of a neurotoxic agent on either the central or peripheral nervous system or, most frequently, both. For example, on the one hand, in severe cases of lead poisoning, there is motor paralysis presumably caused by the effect of lead on motor neurons of the spinal cord and the nerves that transmit motor messages. On the other hand, the flaccid paralysis produced by some organophosphorus pesticides results from the interference of the toxic agent with the neurotransmitter at the neuromuscular junction, that is, where the nerve interfaces with muscle.

The recognition of this difference in the cause of the paralysis is essential for the proper diagnosis, treatment, and rehabilitation of victims of neurotoxic diseases. For example, nerves in the peripheral nervous system can recover after traumatic injury or toxic damage. Central neural structures are in general more often permanently damaged; function is recovered only when other areas of the nervous system take over the functions previously performed by the damaged structures.

THE CENTRAL NERVOUS SYSTEM

The Spinal Cord

The spinal cord is a whitish structure situated within the vertebral canal that extends from the foramen magnum—a large opening at the base of the skull—to the lower level of the first lumbar vertebra (Fig. 1.2). The spinal cord, which is approximately cylindrical in shape, is artificially divided into four portions: cervical, thoracic, lumbar, and sacral-coccyxeal. Figure 1.3 is a cross-sectional view of its main components and protective membranes, called the *meninges* (the dura mater, the arachnoid, and the pia mater).

The anatomic configuration of the spinal cord varies as one progresses from the caudal *(Latin for tail) to the* cervical *(Latin for neck) portion of the spinal cord. Consistently, in animals and humans, structures located on the back are called* dorsal, *whereas those on the front are called* ventral. *This terminology allows anatomists to use the same terms for the description of the nervous system of both animals and humans. The need for making these comparisons is essential when animals are used as models of human neurotoxic illnesses.*

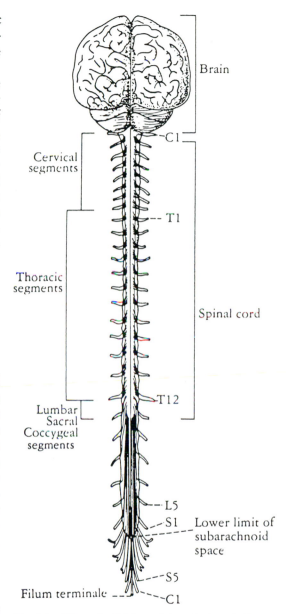

Fig. 1.2. The main divisions of the spinal cord. (From Snell 1980.)

The most prominent features of the spinal cord are the *gray matter*, appearing in cross sections as a centrally located butterfly-shaped region containing the cell bodies of nerve cells called *neurons*, and the *white matter*, wrapped around the gray matter, containing the myelin-covered fibers of the neurons called *axons*. "Gray matter" is an ancient term that

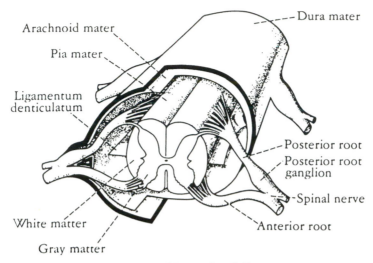

Arachnoid mater

Pia mater

Ligamentum
denticulatum

Dura mater

Posterior root

Posterior root
ganglion

Spinal nerve

Anterior root

White matter

Gray matter

Fig. 1.3.   A cross-sectional view of the spinal cord. (From
Snell 1980.)

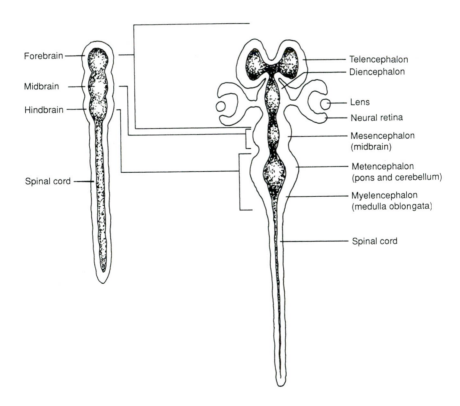

Forebrain

Midbrain

Hindbrain

Spinal cord

Telencephalon
Diencephalon

Lens
Neural retina

Mesencephalon
(midbrain)

Metencephalon
(pons and cerebellum)

Myelencephalon
(medulla oblongata)

Spinal cord

Fig. 1.4.   Major components of the developing brain at
4 weeks (left) and at 6 weeks (right) of development.
(Adapted from Kandel and Schwartz 1985.)

designates the portion of the brain containing the bodies of nerve cells. "White matter" is the gross appearance of nerve fibers. Both terms were in use even before nerve cells and fibers could be observed under the light microscope. Their names derive from the appearance of nerve cells and their fibers seen as a collection of elements. Additional features of the spinal cord are described below as the anatomic organization of the spinal nerves is described.

The Brain

The brain lies in the cranial cavity, a continuation of the vertebral canal protected by the meninges. The brain is divided into three major components; in ascending order—that is, from the caudal to the cervical portion of the nervous system—they are the **hindbrain** (also called the rhombencephalon), the **midbrain** (the mescencephalon), and the **forebrain** (the prosencephalon). These components are easily identified in the developing brain (Fig. 1.4). As the nervous system continues its development, the hindbrain is further subdivided into the medulla oblongata and the pons and cerebellum; the midbrain continues to be identified as such; and the forebrain is subdivided into the diencephalon and the telencephalon or cerebrum.

The Hindbrain. The three major components of the hindbrain that need to be recognized are the medulla oblongata, the pons, and the cerebellum. (See Figs. 1.5 and 1.6.)

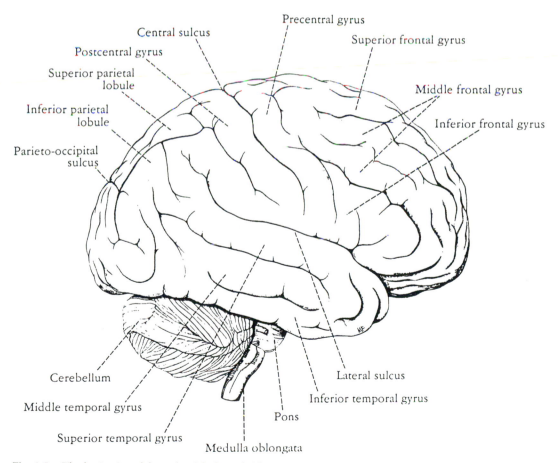

Fig. 1.5. The brain viewed from the right lateral side. (From Snell 1980.)

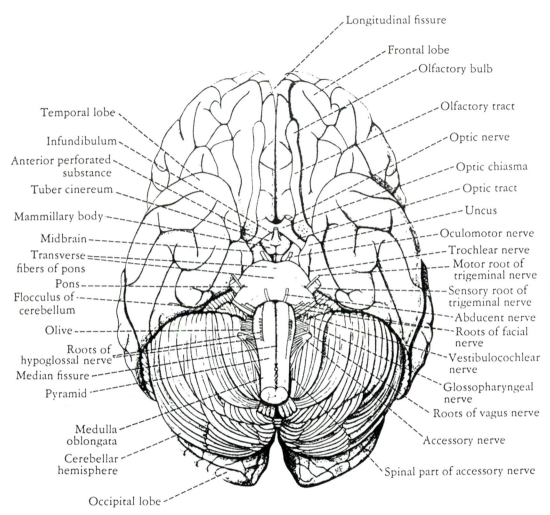

Temporal lobe

Infundibulum

Anterior perforated
substance

Tuber cinereum

Mammillary body

Midbrain

Transverse
fibers of pons

Pons

Flocculus of
cerebellum

Olive

Roots of
hypoglossal nerve

Median fissure

Pyramid

Medulla
oblongata

Cerebellar
hemisphere

Occipital lobe

Longitudinal fissure

Frontal lobe

Olfactory bulb

Olfactory tract

Optic nerve

Optic chiasma

Optic tract

Uncus

Oculomotor nerve

Trochlear nerve

Motor root of
trigeminal nerve

Sensory root of
trigeminal nerve

Abducent nerve

Roots of facial
nerve

Vestibulocochlear
nerve

Glossopharyngeal
nerve

Roots of vagus nerve

Accessory nerve

Spinal part of accessory nerve

Fig. 1.6. The brain viewed from below. (From Snell 1980.)

The *medulla oblongata,* a cone-shaped structure, is delimited by the spinal cord below and the pons above. The medulla oblongata contains neural structures that control heart rate and breathing, sometimes the targets of neurotoxic agents and drugs causing death.

The *pons* ("bridge") derives its name from the large number of fibers traversing its anterior aspect en route to the cerebellar hemispheres. It is located between the medulla oblongata and the midbrain.

The *cerebellum*—Latin for "little brain"— forms a wedge between the brainstem and the lower portion of the brain's occipital lobe.

It consists of a median portion called the vermis and two laterally placed hemispheres. It is characteristically corrugated in appearance, and, when compared in various vertebrates, its features have remained remarkably constant throughout animal evolution. In contrast, other brain structures, particularly the cerebral cortex, vary markedly from "lower" to "higher" organisms, achieving their greatest complexity in humans.

The cerebellum receives sensory information and sends motor messages essential for motor coordination. The cerebellum is responsible (among other numerous functions) for programming the execution of fine movements. This programming or scheduling requires the accurate timing of sensory inputs and motor responses. The cerebellum is often the target of numerous neurotoxic agents, eg, alcoholic beverages, many industrial solvents, and lead.

The Midbrain. The midbrain is a narrow part of the brain connecting the hindbrain to the forebrain. The structures that need to be identified in the midbrain are the cerebral aqueduct, the tectum, the cerebral peduncles, the substantia nigra, and the red nucleus.

The *cerebral aqueduct* is a channel that connects the third and fourth ventricles; the *cerebrospinal fluid* (CSF) flows through this opening. In Chapter 9, on absorption, distribution, and elimination of toxins, and Chapter 20, dealing with effects of neurotoxic agents on the developing brain, the roles of the CSF and of the blood–brain barrier as a selective protective mechanism are examined. The cerebral aqueduct is a landmark feature of the midbrain that helps to identify such other anatomic features as the tectum and the cerebral peduncles.

The *tectum* is a part of the midbrain lying dorsal to the cerebral aqueduct. Four surface swellings are the most prominent features of the tectum: the two *superior* and the two *inferior colliculi*. As will be seen in later chapters in this volume, the superior colliculi participate in visual and oculomotor functions, whereas the inferior colliculi are part of the auditory system.

The *cerebral peduncles* lie dorsal to the cerebral aqueduct and are formed by fibers that connect the cortex with lower levels of the brainstem and spinal cord. The *substantia nigra* ("black substance") is a paired nucleus formed in part by a band of pigmented nerve cells. The *red nuclei* are a pair of ovoid masses of cells also receiving their name from their color.

The Forebrain. In the adult brain, the *diencephalon* ("between brain") is completely hidden from view. The major features that

need to be recognized in the diencephalon are the thalamus and the hypothalamus.

"Thalamus" means "inner room." The thalami are a pair of egg-shaped masses of gray matter lying on either side of the third ventricle, forming the upper part of its vertical walls. Thalamic nuclei are named with two—sometimes three—words. The first word indicates the group to which the particular nucleus belongs; the second word indicates the nucleus within the group. The groups are named roughly after their anatomic placement within the thalamus: anterior, medial, lateral, ventral, intralaminar, midline, and reticular. Examples of some of the nuclei to be encountered in later chapters are the lateral geniculate body (LGB), the medial geniculate body (MGB), and the reticular (R). The collection of thalamic nuclei provide five main functions:

1. Sensory information to primary areas of the cerebral cortex.
2. Information about ongoing movement to motor areas of the cerebral cortex.
3. Information on the activity of the limbic system to areas of the cerebral cortex related to this system.
4. Information on intrathalamic activity to association areas of the cerebral cortex.
5. Information on brainstem reticular formation activity to widespread areas of the cerebral cortex.

The name *hypothalamus* means literally "under the thalamus." It forms the base of the third ventricle, an important reference point for the imaging of the brain. The hypothalamus is a complex, minute neural structure responsible for many aspects of behavior such as drives, motivation, and emotion. It is the link between the nervous and the neuroendocrine system, to be reviewed below. The pituitary gland is linked by neurons to the hypothalamic nuclei. It is well established that the hypothalamic nerve cells perform many neurosecretory functions. The hypothalamus is linked with many other major regions of the brain, including the rhinencephalon—the primitive cortex originally associated with olfaction—and the limbic system, including the hippocampus.

The *cerebrum* is the largest component of the brain, consisting of two cerebral hemispheres connected by a mass of white matter called the *corpus callosum*. The *cerebral cortex* is the surface layer of each cerebral hemisphere. Deep sulci, or grooves, serve as reference points to separate important anatomic regions: the central and the lateral sulci (Fig. 1.5). The *frontal lobe* lies in front of the central sulcus. The *parietal lobe* begins at the back of the central sulcus and lies next to the *occipital lobe*. The latter occupies the posterior portion of the brain. The *temporal lobe* begins well inside the folding of the lateral sulcus and extends into the ventral aspects of the brain hemispheres.

Two important components of the cerebrum are reviewed here: the basal ganglia and the limbic system. Additional features and systems of the cerebrum are reviewed later in the discussion of specific targets of toxic action.

The *basal ganglia* are nuclei of nerve cells—not ganglia (clumps of nerve cells) as their name implies—located toward the center of the brain. They are easily recognized during a gross morphological examination of the human brain. The most important nuclei of this group are the *caudate nucleus,* the *putamen,* and the *globus pallidus,* known collectively as *corpus striatum.* From the functional point of view, this system includes the substantia nigra and the subthalamic nucleus, which anatomically is part of the diencephalon.

The basal ganglia comprise major centers of the extrapyramidal motor system. (The pyramidal system, to which the term is contrasted, is described below.) The *extrapyramidal system* is selectively affected by many neurotoxic agents (eg, manganese). In the past two decades, important discoveries have been made concerning the role these nuclei play in several neural degenerative diseases (eg, Parkinson's disease, Huntington's chorea).

The *limbic system* is comprised of convoluted neural structures branching out in many directions, particularly with the hypothalamus. The *amygdala* and the *hippocampus* are easily recognizable limbic structures; others, such as the septal nuclei, less so. The limbic system is involved in the control of emotional expression. The hippocampus is believed to be a structure where many memory processes occur.

THE PERIPHERAL NERVOUS SYSTEM

The peripheral nervous system is the portion of the nervous system that includes motor, sensory, and autonomic neurons located outside the central nervous system. The term describes the anatomic distribution of this system, but functionally it is artificial. The bodies of peripheral motor fibers, for example, are located within the central nervous system. In experimental, clinical, and epidemiological neurotoxicology, the term "peripheral nervous system" describes a system that is selectively vulnerable to the effects of toxic agents and that is able to regenerate.

The Spinal Nerves

It was mentioned earlier that the most prominent features of the spinal cord are the gray matter, containing the cell bodies of the neurons, and the white matter, containing the myelinated axons of the neurons. The ventral and dorsal roots are where the peripheral nerves enter and leave the spinal cord along its length.

The ventral region of the spinal cord's gray matter contains nerve cells that regulate motor function; the middle region of the thoraxic spinal cord is associated with autonomic functions. The dorsal portion receives sensory information from the spinal nerves (Fig. 1.7). Adjoining vertebrae contain openings to allow root fibers forming the spinal nerves to leave the spinal canal. There are 31 pairs of spinal nerves, which are named according to the region of the vertebral column with which they are associated: eight cervical, 12 thoracic, five lumbar, five sacral, and one coccygeal. A *metamere* is a region of the body innervated by a spinal nerve (Fig. 1.8). By carefully examining the motor and sensory functions of metameres, neurologists can infer the location of lesions where damage occurs.

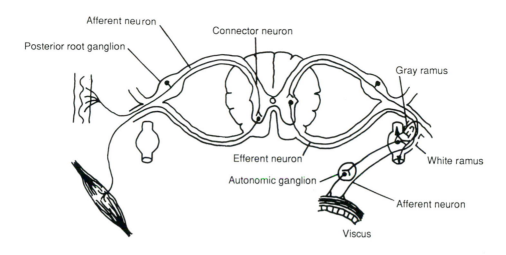

Fig. 1.7. Cross-section of the spinal cord, showing the functional organization of a single spinal nerve. (Adapted from Snell 1980.)

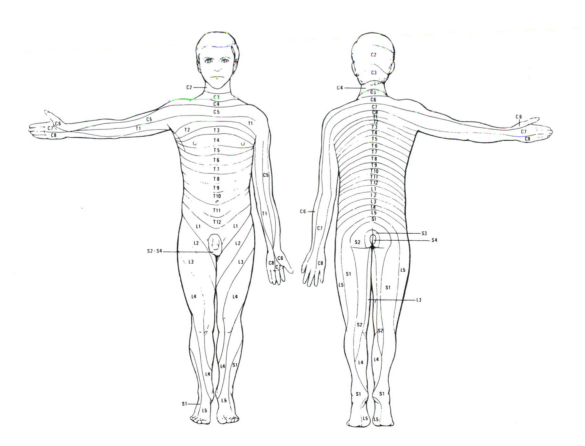

Fig. 1.8. The segmental distribution of the spinal nerves (the metamerae). C, cervical; T, thoracic; L, lumbar; S, sacral. (From Kandel and Schwartz 1985.)

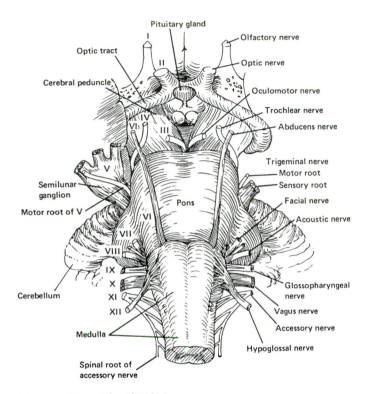

Fig. 1.9. The cranial nerves. (From Chusid 1982.)

Table 1.1. List of the Cranial Nerves and Their Functions

Number	Name	Function
I	Olfactory	Sensory input from olfactory receptors
II	Optic	Sensory input from retinal ganglion cells
III	Oculomotor	Motor output to four of six extraocular eye muscles
IV	Trochlear	Motor output to superior oblique eye muscle
V	Trigeminal	Main sensory input from the face
		Motor output to the jaw muscles
VI	Abducens	Motor output to posterior rectus eye muscle
VII	Facial	Main motor output to muscles of the face
		Sensory input from some taste buds (chorda tympani nerve)
VIII	Acoustic	Sensory input from the inner ear and the vestibular organ
IX	Glossopharyngeal	Sensory input from some taste buds and the carotid body
		Motor output to muscles of throat, larynx, and salivary glands
X	Vagus	Main parasympathetic motor output to muscles of heart, lungs, and gut
		Motor output to muscles of pharynx
		Sensory input from some taste buds
XI	Accessory	Motor output to sternocleidomastoid and trapezius muscles
XII	Hypoglossal	Motor output to the tongue musles

Adapted from Romer and Parsons (1977) and Brodal (1981) in Shepherd (1987).

The Cranial Nerves

"*Brainstem*" is a comprehensive term that designates the region of the nervous system that includes the medulla, the pons, and the midbrain. The brainstem is a continuation of the spinal cord upward and forward (ventrally). It is in this region that most of the cranial nerves make their exits and entrances (Fig. 1.9). There are 12 pairs of cranial nerves; Table 1.1 describes the name and main function of each pair. Cranial nerves are reviewed further in Chapter 3 in the discussion of the details of the clinical neurological examination and in Part V, where motor and sensory systems are described as targets of neurotoxic agents.

THE AUTONOMIC NERVOUS SYSTEM

The autonomic nervous system (controlling involuntary funtions) has two main components: the sympathetic and the parasympathetic nervous system (Fig. 1.10). These are peripheral aspects of the autonomic nervous system. The sympathetic nerves controlling visceral activity arise from the thoracic and lumbar portions of the spinal cord; parasympathetic nerves arise from the brainstem and the sacral portion of the spinal cord.

Both the sympathetic and the parasympathetic nerves have ganglia between the neural fiber that leaves the spinal cord and the effector (the gland or muscle—such as the heart—that responds to the nerve impulse). The positions of these ganglia differ for the sympathetic and the parasympathetic system. In the sympathetic system, the ganglia are located near the spinal cord; in the parasympathetic system, they are located close to the organs they control. The organization of the sympathetic nerves is well illustrated in Fig. 1.10, right side.(But the significance of this differential placement is not clear.) The autonomic nervous system also has central components; the hypothalamus is the site where many autonomic functions are integrated.

The main role of the autonomic nervous system is to regulate the activity of smooth muscles, the heart, glands in the digestive canal, sweat glands, and adrenal and other endocrine glands. The role of the autonomic functions in the preservation of the body's internal environment is reviewed further in Chapter 28, dealing with the effects of neurotoxic agents on motivation and emotion.

THE NEUROENDOCRINE SYSTEM

Hormones have generally been considered to be chemical messengers that are released from cells into the bloodstream to exert their action on target cells some distance away. Until recently, hormones were distinguished from neurotransmitters, to be reviewed in the next chapter dealing with the neurobiology of neurotoxic diseases. The latter are chemical messengers released from neurons onto a synapse between the nerve terminals and another neuron or an effector, that is, muscle or gland. With the discovery that classical neurotransmitters such as dopamine could act as hormones, the distinction between neurotransmitters and hormones became less and less clear. Thus, based on purely anatomic considerations, hormones derived from nerve cells may be called *neurohormones*. But, from a functional point of view, as shall be seen in the next chapter, the nervous system can be thought of as a truly neurosecretory system.

The hypothalamus controls endocrine functions through a link with the pituitary gland (also called the hypophysis). Until the middle 1950s the endocrine glands were viewed as a separate system governed by the pituitary gland, often called the "master gland." At that time, a neurovascular hypothesis was advanced that established the functional role of the hypothalamic–hypophyseal factors in the control of endocrine function. In this view, the endocrine hypothalamus provides the final common neuroendocrine pathway in the control of the

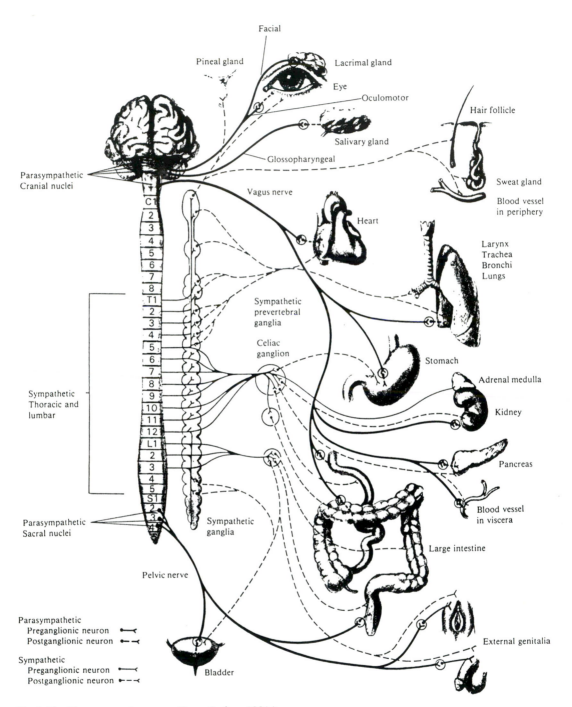

Fig. 1.10. The autonomic system. (From Carlson 1981.)

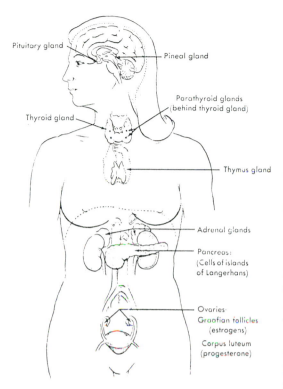

Pituitary gland

Pineal gland

Parathyroid glands
(behind thyroid gland)

Thyroid gland

Thymus gland

Adrenal glands

Pancreas:
(Cells of islands
of Langerhans)

Ovaries·
Graafian follicles
(estrogens)

Corpus luteum
(progesterone)

Fig. 1.11. The major components of the neuroendocrine system in the female human. (Reproduced by permission from Anthony, Catherine Parker, and Thibodeau, Gary A.: Textbook of Anatomy and Physiology, ed. 12, St. Louis, 1987, Times Mirror Mosby College Publishing.)

tal work deals with the effects of neurotoxic agents on the immune system via the neuroendocrine system. However, the body of information is so meager—and sometimes so controversial—that it does not merit a review at this time. Consequently, the functional organization of the neuroendocrine system is not further discussed in this book.

CONCLUSIONS

Information on basic neural processes is constantly evolving. Even basic notions of neuroanatomy change as new techniques make it possible to understand how portions of this immensely complex system are related to each other. Neurosciences, a discipline that has evolved since the 1950s, has revolutionized our views of the brain and its function.

Neurotoxicology is also a rapidly evolving discipline. But oddly, human and animal experimentation on the effects of neurotoxic agents has often not kept pace with the most recent developments in the neurosciences. Thus, old and new models of brain functions coexist in the clinical and experimental neurotoxicological literature. The reader has to be very critical about stated or implied models of brain functions underlying research reports, particularly in human neurotoxicology.

endocrine system (Fig. 1.11). It has now been firmly established that the endocrine system is itself regulated by the central nervous system as well as the endocrine inputs. Thus, the term "neuroendocrinology" is an adequate term to describe the discipline that studies the reciprocal integrated roles of the nervous and the endocrine systems in the control of physiological processes.

Based on animal experimentation, environmental and occupational toxic agents are suspected to play a role in the human neuroendocrine system. Most recent experimen-

REFERENCES

Anthony, CO and Thibodeau, GA (1987) *Textbook of Anatomy and Physiology* (12th ed). St. Louis: Times Mirror/Mosby College Publishing.

Brodal, P (1981) *Neurological Anatomy in Relation to Clinical Medicine* (3rd ed). New York: Oxford University Press.

Carlson, NR (1981) *Physiology of Behavior.* Boston: Allyn and Bacon.

Chusid, JG (1982) *Correlative Neuroanatomy and Functional Neurology.* Los Altos, CA.: Lange Medical Publications.

Kandel, ER and Schwartz, JH (eds)(1985) *Principles of Neural Science* (2nd ed). New York: Elsevier.

Romer, AS and Parsons, TS (1977) *The Vertebrate Body*. Philadelphia: Saunders.

Shepherd, GM (1987) *Neurobiology* (2nd ed). New York: Oxford University Press.

Snell, RS (1986) *Clinical Neuroanatomy for Medical Students* (2nd ed). Boston: Little, Brown.

SUGGESTED READINGS

Adelman, G (ed) (1987) *Encyclopedia of Neuroscience*. Boston: Birkhäuser.

Blalock, JE and Bost, KL (eds) (1988) *Neuroimmunoendocrinology*. Basel: Karger.

Carpenter, MB and Sutin, J (1983) *Human Neuroanatomy* (8th ed). Baltimore: Williams & Wilkins.

Freir, S (ed) (1989) *The Neuroendocrine–Immune Network*. Boca Raton, FL: CRC Press.

Gazzaniga, MS (1989) Organization of the human brain. *Science* 245:947–952.

Hadley, ME (1984) *Endocrinology*. Englewood Cliffs, NJ: Prentice-Hall.

Harris, GW (1955) *Neural Control of the Pituitary Gland*. London: Edward Arnold Ltd.

Johnson, RH, Lambie, DG, and Spalding, JMK (1984) *Neurocardiology: The Interrelationships between Dysfunction in the Nervous System and Cardiovascular System*. London: WB Saunders.

Krieger, DT and Hughes, JC (eds) (1980) *Neuroendocrinology*. Sunderland, MA: Sinauer Associates Inc.

Meltzer, HY (ed) (1987) *Psychopharmacology: The Third Generation of Progress*. New York: Raven Press.

Narahashi, T and Chambers, JE (eds) (1989) *Insecticide Action: From Molecule to Organism*. New York: Plenum.

Nauta, WJH (1986) *Fundamental Neuroanatomy*. New York: WH Freeman.

Plomin, R, DeFries, JC, and McClearn, GE (1980) *Behavioral Genetics: A Primer*. San Francisco, CA: WH Freeman.

Riedere, P, Kopp, N, and Pearson, J (1990) *An Introduction to Neurotransmission in Health and Disease*. New York: Oxford University Press.

Shepherd, GM (ed) (1990) *The Synaptic Organization of the Brain*. New York: Oxford University Press.

Siegel, GJ, Agranoff, BW, Albers, RW and Molinoff, PB (eds) (1989) *Basic Neurochemistry: Molecular, Cellular and Medical Aspects* (4th ed). New York: Raven Press.

Thibodeau, GA and Anthony, CP (1988) *Structure and Function of the Body* (8th ed). St. Louis: Times Mirror/Mosby College Publishing.

Thomas, JA, Korach, KS, and McLachlan, JA (eds) (1985) *Endocrine Toxicology*. New York: Raven Press.

Walsh, TJ, and Emerich, EF (1988) The hippocampus as a common target of neurotoxic agents. *Toxicology* 49:137–140.

2

The Neurobiology of Neurotoxic Disease

The soft warm living substance of the brain and nervous system stands in stark contrast to the rigid metal and plastic hardware of a modern day computer, but at the fundamental level there are clear similarities between these two apparently disparate organizational systems and, of course, one is a product of the other. Not only are the nerve cell units (neurones) self-repairing and self-wiring under the grand design built into our genes, but they can also promote, amplify, block, inhibit, or attenuate the micro-electric signals which are passed on to them and through them, and thereby give rise to signaling patterns of myriad complexity between networks of cerebral neurons, and this provides the physical substrate of mind (Bradford 1987).

The understanding of neurotoxic diseases has changed substantially as new approaches have been developed. There has been a progression from the characterization of gross morphological changes that occur in the nervous system as a result of neurotoxic illness to the study of cellular mechanisms of toxicity and, finally, to the search for the molecular basis of toxicity. These approaches coexist, and all three contribute essential information for the evaluation of the effects of neurotoxic agents in humans.

CHANGING VIEWS OF NEUROTOXIC ILLNESS

Since the Greeks, science has attempted to explain complex phenomena in terms of elemental processes. Neuroscience, a modern discipline that emerged in the 1950s for the multidisciplinary study of nervous system function and behavior, is no exception to this tendency. For a brief review of the early and current evolution of the neurosciences see Gross (1987) and many other related references in *Encyclopedia of Neurosciences* (Adelman 1987). Table 2.1 is a comparative chart of the range of physical dimensions covered by each approach. The following are noteworthy: brain structures are measured in centimeters and millimeters; cell structures are measured in micrometers, millionths of a meter; and physicochemical processes that occur within neurons, in nanometers, 1000ths of a micrometer, and even smaller units.

The Gross Morphological Approach

Neurology is a division of medicine specializing in the diagnosis and treatment of diseases of the nervous system. Classical neurology attempted to understand behavioral

Table 2.1. Various Levels of Biological Structure

Dimension	Field	Structures	Method
0.1 mm (100 μm) and larger	Anatomy	Organs	Eye and simple lenses
100 μm to 10 μm	Histology	Tissues ⎫	Various types of light
10 μm to 0.2 μm (200 nm)	Cytology	Cells, bacteria ⎭	microscopes, x-ray microscopy
200 nm to 1 nm	Submicroscopic morphology Ultrastructure	Cell components, viruses	Polarization microscopy, electron microscopy
Smaller than 1 nm	Molecular and atomic structure	Arrangement of atoms	X-ray diffraction

Table 1.1 from *Cell and Molecular Biology* by EDP DeRobertis and EMF DeRobertis, copyright © 1980 by Saunders College Publishing, a division of Holt, Rinehart and Winston, Inc., reprinted by permission of the publisher.

or psychological changes in terms of gross morphological alterations in brain structure, and this basic approach has not changed much over the years. Then and now, motor paralysis is explained by damage to neurons, nerves, and/or muscles; partial loss of vision by specific lesions of visual pathways; speech disturbances unrelated to sound-producing devices such as the the larynx or the mouth by damage to cortical centers mediating speech. In clinical neurology, morphological and neuropathological methods are still fundamental to the understanding of mechanisms of toxic injury. A document on principles and methods used for the assessment of neurotoxicity published by the World Health Organization (1986) states:

> The information derived from morphological studies is highly relevant to the interpretation of biochemical, neurophysiological, and behavioral data. Structural changes have always been the firm foundation on which analysis of clinical neurological disease has been based. Both diagnosis and prognosis depend heavily on previous neuropathological experience for their accuracy. Moreover, treatment of neurological disease can only be satisfactorily planned by using the knowledge gained from experimental and morphological studies that have provided an understanding of the pattern by which neural cells are affected.

From the gross morphological point of view, neurological diseases are grouped as trau-matic, vascular, neoplastic, genetic, degenerative, infectious, and toxic-metabolic. Among the latter, two large classes are recognized: those neurological diseases resulting from the effect of naturally occurring neurotoxins and those resulting from man-made drugs and chemical compounds released in the environment or the workplace.

Virchow (1821–1902) is the founder of modern pathology. Neuropathology is one branch of the theoretical and empirical science Virchow envisioned. Clinical neuropathology is a case-oriented method of investigation based on naked-eye observation of neurological disturbances in humans and the search for an explanation of these changes in terms of morphological changes occurring in neural tissues. Experimental neuropathology is a branch of the neurosciences that tries to understand the mechanisms of neural diseases by reproducing its major features in animal models.

Many anatomic and histological techniques are employed in forensic neuropathology to determine the causes of illness and death, particularly if they are criminally caused. At the moment of death, important neurochemical processes are profoundly distorted in a few seconds, and all electrical activity ceases. What is left for a neuropathologist to observe are structural changes such as edema or tissue degeneration. The nerve tissue also undergoes drastic biochemical changes after its removal during biopsy. Some of these changes can be arrested by means of well-known histological procedures, eg, dropping the sample into liquid nitrogen, whose temperature is −200°C (about −400°F).

Clinical, forensic, and experimental neuropathologists know the manner in which nerve tissue may be removed from living or dead organisms. Among Virchow's contributions is the detailed description of how different human organs need to be removed from the body to facilitate their study. Tissues need to be processed before neurons can be seen under the light or electron microscope. Good histology and neuropathology handbooks contain literally hundreds of combinations of fixation and staining procedures that allow clinical and experimental researchers to see particular details of nervous tissue organization. The WHO (1986) document mentioned above reviews some of these techniques.

Literally, a *neuropathy* is any disease of the nervous system. But "neuropathy" is a term rarely used by itself. A peripheral neuropathy is, for example, any disease affecting the peripheral nervous system. A polyneuropathy—an alteration of multiple neural sites—is largely confined to the peripheral nervous system as well. The understanding of toxin-induced neuropathies requires the integration of several sources of data:

- The results of biochemical laboratory tests (eg, blood, cerebrospinal fluid, urine).
- The results of laboratory tests performed to detect levels of neurotoxic exposure and absorption in urine, blood, various secretions, nails, hair, etc.
- Imaging of the nervous tissue.
- Nerve or muscle biopsy whenever possible or indicated.
- A postmortem analysis of nervous tissue and other organs.
- In certain cases there may be also an attempt to reproduce neurotoxic syndromes in experimental animals under controlled laboratory conditions.

Classical neuropathological descriptions of neurotoxic diseases contain several important distinctions essential for the understanding of the mechanisms of neurotoxic illnesses. One of them is whether changes in gross morphological examination of the brain tissue are the direct or indirect effect of a given toxic agent. Chronic alcoholism, for example, may be associated with a profound psychosis (Korsakoff's psychosis). Until a generation ago, these neuropsychological alterations were thought to be caused by alcohol itself. Later, it was realized that the psychosis is primarily caused by malnutrition, as individuals who suffer from chronic alcoholism usually do not eat properly.

When neuropathologists describe *cerebral edema*, a swelling of brain tissue often associated with acute neurotoxic poisoning, the details of the description include how herniation of the brain occurs and the mechanical forces that push the brain tissue around the complex labyrinth of cavities engulfed in an unyielding skull. Sometimes a quantitative determination of the extent of cerebral edema is possible. The ratio of skull capacity to brain volume and the brain's water content and specific gravity are calculated by empirical formulas handed down through several generations of pathologists.

The description of the devastating effects of *anoxia* (lack of oxygen) constitutes another example of the classical neuropathological approach. Lack of oxygen to brain tissue can result from three major situations:

1. Damage to nervous tissue may be caused by primary lack of oxygen, labeled *anoxic anoxia,* low oxygen in the external environment. An example of this type of anoxia is the brain damage suffered by mountain climbers who lose their oxygen supply at high altitude where low oxygen pressure prevails.
2. The blood vessels may fail to bring oxygen to the brain (*ischemic anoxia*), as in certain cases of atherosclerosis or blockage of blood vessels.
3. Because of altered metabolic processes, nerve cells may receive an inadequate supply of oxygen in the blood (*cytotoxic anoxia*). This is the mechanism by which cyanide produces death, by interfering with the red blood cell's capacity to bind and transport oxygen.

The Cellular Approach

Santiago Ramón y Cajal (1852–1934), a Spanish neuroanatomist, is considered the founding father of the cellular approach in neurobiology.

In his writings, Virchow uses the term "cellular pathology," but in fact he describes pathological changes in tissues, not cells. During Virchow's time the neuron had not yet been discovered. Ramón y Cajal demonstrated for the first time that nervous tissue is not a network of cells but follows the general rules of the cellular doctrine proposed in 1839 by Mathias Jacob Schleiden (1804–1881) and Theodor Schwann (1810–1992). The cellular doctrine stated that the cell is the basic unit of all living tissue.

For some time it was thought that the cellular doctrine did not apply to nervous tissue. Using a silver-based staining technique proposed by the Italian anatomist Camillo Golgi (1843–1926), with whom Ramón y Cajal later shared the Nobel prize in Medicine and Physiology in 1906, Ramón y Cajal demonstrated the cellular nature of all nerve tissue. During the course of his long life, Ramón y Cajal made immense contributions to the field of comparative neuroanatomy.

Ramón y Cajal's contributions to modern neuroscience are many, but among his most remarkable feats was his series of predictions on the physiological properties of neurons based only on observations of their structure. This is not unlike someone being able to explain how a previously unseen type of computer works by just looking at its circuitry. Among these observations were that conduction of the nervous impulse occurs from cell body to axon and that neurons are separated from each other by gaps, later called "synapses," a term coined by Sherrington (1857–1952), an English physiologist.

Since Ramón y Cajal's time, neuroanatomists have observed, drawn, and photographed nerve cells, showing hundreds of different shapes. After a long period of time extending roughly from 1870 to 1920, a tax-onomy of cells emerged. What stimulated the development of the cellular approach in neurobiology—and many years later in neurotoxicology—was, among other factors, the availability of a vast array of neural tissue fixation and staining procedures. A critical reviewer of the classical literature on toxic-induced cellular changes needs to know the assets and limitations of these technical procedures. Radiolabeling techniques available today, for example, have revolutionized the manner in which basic research and neuropathological investigations are conducted. The classification of neurotoxic agents by Spencer and Schaumburg reviewed in Chapter 8 of this volume is an example of the cellular approach in neurotoxicology.

The Molecular Approach

Historically, the level of biological analysis has proceeded from the description of organs to tissues to cells. Cell neurobiology is an important discipline within the neurosciences. About 30 years ago the chemical (molecular) events underlying the neuron's transmission of the action potential began to be understood, as well as how the synthesis and release of many neurotransmitters at the neural synapse occurred. The discipline of *molecular neurobiology* thus emerged.

The molecular approach in toxicology is one seeking the understanding of mechanisms of toxicity in terms of biochemical processes at the molecular level. It has both theoretical and practical consequences. From a purely theoretical point of view, this approach has contributed to the understanding of several fundamental neural processes:

- The chemical structure of the genetic material present in the nerve cell nucleus.
- The types of proteins generated by messenger, transfer, and ribosomal RNA.
- The structure and distribution of molecular layers of membranes, the gateway for entrance of specific ions into the neuron.

- The number and types of molecules contained in synaptic vesicles.
- The very small electrical potentials generated by the release of neurotransmitters into synapses.
- The pharmacological characteristics of the targets of neurotransmitters.

The most powerful asset of molecular neuroscience is, however, the attempt to explain and manipulate nervous system function and, ultimately, behavior by means of physicochemical and pharmacological processes. From a practical point of view, molecular neuroscience has contributed to the development of large varieties of therapeutic drugs. Antipsychotic drugs, for example, have changed our view of the nature of psychiatric diseases and the way we manage them. Diazepam, a mood modifier generally known under the trade name Valium, is one of the most used drugs today.

It is almost certain that in the near future the molecular approach will force us to make sharper characterizations of the observations typical of the gross morphological and even the cellular era of scientific research. For example, the distinction between "organic" and "functional" diseases—a distinction that has divided disciplines such as neurology on the one hand and psychiatry and psychology on the other—will probably have to be abandoned because the distinction is so general that it adds little information about the nature of a neurological disorder.

THE FUNCTIONAL ORGANIZATION OF THE NERVOUS SYSTEM AT THE CELLULAR AND MOLECULAR LEVEL

Nerve cells are the functional units of the nervous system. The nervous system is believed to have ten thousand million such cells. There are two types of nerve cells, *neurons* and *glia,* the glia being present in greater proportions than neurons.

The Neuron

Figure 2.1 is an idealized diagram of a neuron with its three most important structural features: the cell body, the dendrites, and the axon. The *dendrites* are finely branched processes near the cell body of a neuron. The dendrites receive excitatory or inhibitory effects via neurotransmitters. The *cytoplasm* is the content of the cell body in which the *organelles,* including the cell nucleus and other inclusions, are found (Fig. 2.2). The nucleus contains the cell's chromatin, the genetic material. The *axon hillock* is the portion of the cell body that gives origin to the axon. The *terminal boutons* are the terminal points of the axon. The terminal boutons contain the presynaptic membranes from which neurotransmitters are released into the synaptic cleft.

Organelle is also a term that sometimes designates a complex structure such as the Golgi apparatus as well as relatively simpler ones such as secretory granules and synaptic vesicles. Determining how these organelles act in health and in disease is one of the most active areas of research today in neurobiology. Only those organelles the reader is likely to encounter in original papers and other documents describing neurotoxicological research at the molecular level are dealt with here.

The nucleus of the nerve cell is atypical compared with that of other living cells in that although it contains the genetic material deoxyribonucleic acid (DNA), this material is not involved in the process of cell division. After reaching maturity, nerve cells do not divide (an exception to this rule are the neurons of the olfactory epithelium). The nucleus contains the *nucleolus,* rich in ribonucleic acid (RNA). The DNA contains information for directing the synthesis of *messenger RNA* (mRNA). mRNA moves from the nucleus to the cell's cytoplasm, where it carries messages, with the aid of *transfer RNA* (tRNA) and *ribosomal RNA* (rRNA), for the synthesis of protein. Three types of proteins have been identified: cytosolic protein, which form

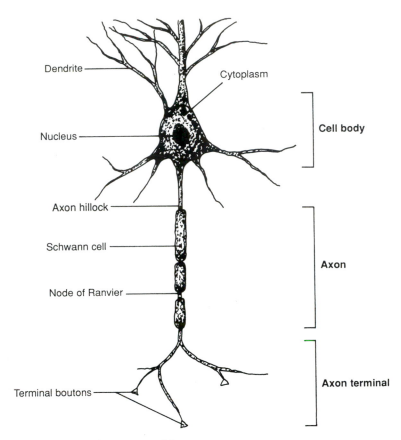

Fig. 2.1. The anatomy of the neuron.

the fibrillar elements of the nerve cell; mitochondrial proteins, which attach themselves to the mitochondria, organelles inside the cell that generate energy for cell activity and proteins that form membranes and secretory products.

In the cell body, the endoplasmic reticulum, the Golgi apparatus, the mitochondria, and the lysosome are the most prominent anatomic features. The endoplasmic reticulum suffers marked changes during neuronal degeneration. A rough or smooth endoplasmic reticulum has been identified on the basis of the presence or absence of ribosomes, complex organelles where protein synthesis takes place, attached to its surface.

The *Golgi apparatus* is a biochemically important station where proteins generated by ribosomes are transformed into cell membranes and secretory material. The latter include secretory substances in synaptic vesicles. The *mitochondria* are the power-generating stations of the cell. They generate ATP (adenosine triphosphate), a molecule that is essential for the process of energy transfer and utilization. The *lysosome,* also found in the cytoplasm of the nerve cell, is widely described as the digestive system of the nerve cell. It contains highly destructive enzymes. Exogenous material captured by phagocytic vacuoles are fused with the lysosomes. Lysosomes also form autophagic vacuoles and act as scavengers within the nerve cell. Neurons are now conceived of as modified secretory cells. Secretory granules accumulating in the Golgi apparatus are the precursors of *synaptic vesicles,* which store neurotransmitter substances, the chemical messengers between nerve cells.

The fibrillar elements form the skeleton of

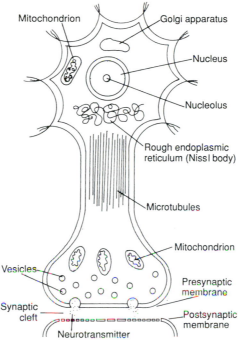

Mitochondrion

Golgi apparatus

Nucleus

Nucleolus

Rough endoplasmic
reticulum (Nissl body)

Microtubules

Mitochondrion

Vesicles

Presynaptic
membrane

Synaptic
cleft

Postsynaptic
membrane

Neurotransmitter

Fig. 2.2.   The organelles.

the neuron and participate in the trophic function of the neuron, acting as vehicles of transmission. Axonal transport can be anterograde (cell body to axon terminal) and retrograde (axon terminal to cell body) (Fig. 2.3). From the thickest to the thinnest, three types of fibrillar elements are recognized: *microtubules, neurofilaments,* and *microfilaments.*

Glial Cells

In contrast to nerve cells, glial cells do not, by themselves, carry electrical messages. There are two types of glial cells, the *macroglia* and the *microglia.* The macroglia include at least three types of cells: astrocytes, oligodendrocytes, and ependymal cells. Microglial cells are primarily scavenger cells, removing de-

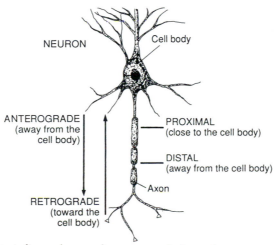

NEURON

Cell body

ANTEROGRADE
(away from the
cell body)

PROXIMAL
(close to the cell body)

DISTAL
(away from the cell body)

Axon

RETROGRADE
(toward the
cell body)

Fig. 2.3.   Terms to indicate places and movement relative to the neuron.

bris after neural damage or infection has occurred.

The glial cells also have distinctive microscopic and ultramicroscopic features. Glial cells physically support neurons, but a number of physiological properties are also now beginning to be understood. Among the most important neuron–glial interactions are the glial cell's role in providing the neurons with nutrients, removing fragments of neurons after their death, and, most importantly, contributing to the process of chemical communication.

Glial cells, in sharp contrast with neurons, can divide and thus can reproduce themselves. Tumors of the nervous system, for example, result from an abnormal reproduction of glial cells.

Myelin

What appears in the macroscopic observation of neural tissue as "gray matter" and "white matter" has a microscopic and biochemical counterpart. Microscopically, the gray matter contains the neuronal cell bodies, whereas the white matter is the tissue comprised of neural fibers or axons. The "white" appearance is caused by a sheath, composed of a fatty substance called myelin, covering those fibers. The myelin of the peripheral nerves originates from the membrane of the *Schwann cell,* which wraps around the axon. The myelin of fibers in the central nervous system is provided by the membranes of the *oligodendrocytes* (a variety of glial cells). Oligodendrocytes usually myelinate several axons, whereas the Schwann cell is associated with only one axon. Discontinuities of the myelin sheath, designated *nodes of Ranvier,* exist between continuous Schwann cells or oligodendrocytes. It is estimated that in the longest central motor pathway, up to 2000 Schwann cells form the myelin cover. Myelin facilitates the propagation of the action potential, as described below.

The myelin may be a specific target of neurotoxic agents. A morphological classification of neurotoxic substances describes characteristic neuropathological changes of the myelin as *myelinopathies.*

Trophic Function of the Neuron

The normal functions of the neuron include protein synthesis, axonal transport, generation and conduction of the action potential, synaptic transmission, and formation and maintenance of the myelin. Some of the basic trophic functions (ie, those having to do with the transport of nutrients) of the neuron were described as early as the 19th century by sectioning the axons (axotomy). Among the processes uncovered, one of the most important is *Wallerian degeneration,* named after Waller, the English physiologist who described it. Before reviewing the normal functions of the neuron, it is essential to review the features of Wallerian degeneration. This provides a good opportunity to describe well-known changes in organelles as a result of either traumatic or toxic damage. Parenthetically, the terms used to describe Wallerian degeneration produced by traumatic axotomy are the same ones used to describe changes resulting from neurotoxic agents.

At the cellular level, neuropathological changes resulting from toxic damage to neural tissue are far more complex that those occurring as a result of traumatic damage. It is only recently that changes in neurons affected by neurotoxic agents have been observed. Figure 2.3 (right side) describes the concepts of proximal and distal. *Proximal* (near the cell body) and *distal* (away from the cell body) refer to a given place within the neuron, taking the cell body as a reference point. Figure 2.3 (left side) illustrates the concept of anterograde and retrograde, terms referring to displacement of elements within the neuron. *Anterograde* refers to the movement of elements from the cell body to the distal portion of the neuron. *Retrograde* refers to the movement of elements from the distal portion of the neuron toward the cell body.

Twenty-four hours after transection (cutting) of the axon, the most distinctive feature to be seen is swelling of the proximal and distal stumps, the original site of mechanical trauma. Swelling results from accumulation of fluids and membranous elements on both sides of the site of injury. These changes are not unlike those observed in a rain-flooded two-way road with vehicles stopped on both sides of the flooded area. In this analogy, stalled vehicles are the swelling. Swelling on both sides of the injury site were the first indications neuroscientists had that the trophic function of the neuron is bidirectional, ie, that the movement of nutrients can occur in both an anterograde (Fig. 2.4) and a retro grade fashion.

After a few days, regeneration of the en-

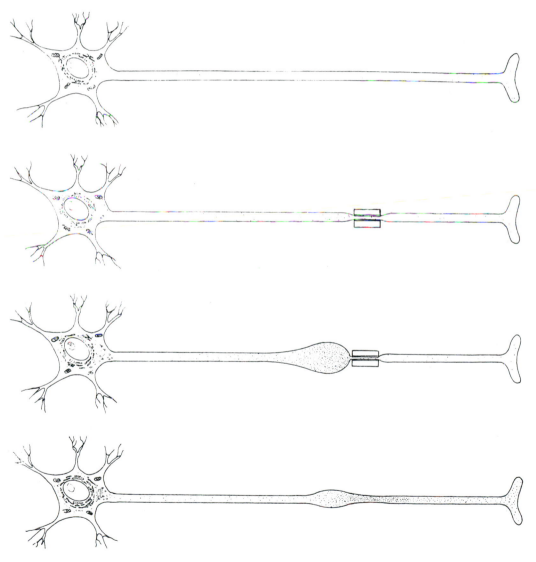

Fig. 2.4. Axoplasmatic flow toward the distal portion of the nerve fiber, as demonstrated by constriction of a nerve fiber. (From Ottoson 1983.)

sheathed axons, ie, those covered with myelin, occurs. Sprouts grow from the proximal stump, moving at the rate of 1 to 3 mm per day. Under favorable conditions, sprouts reach the distal stump. When renervation—joining of the stumps—is completed, the basic features of normal transmission are reestablished.

The cell body of the injured neuron undergoes profound structural changes known since the light microscope was the only observational instrument available—eg, disintegration of the *Nissl substance*. (Nissl substance is another name for the rough endoplasmic reticulum.) A description of ultrastructural changes in protein synthesis and axonal transport is now possible through the use of radiolabeling and ultramicroscopic techniques.

Microscopic and ultramicroscopic events of Wallerian degeneration, a pathological process, give insights into what neurons do under normal circumstances. Such normal functions as protein synthesis, axonal transport, the generation and conduction of action potentials, synaptic transmission, and the maintenance and formation of the myelin are reviewed here. For readers not familiar with the enormous body of knowledge now accumulated in the neurosciences, it needs to be stated that each of these topics is itself the subject of many highly specialized books.

If molecular neurobiology is said to be a young discipline, the neurobiology of the neurotoxic processes is still in its infancy. True, the molecular basis of action of many neurotoxins and pharmacological agents is well understood. But with some notable exception—eg, lead, methylmercury, acrylamide—the molecular basis of toxicity of the vast majority of environmental neurotoxic agents is unknown. That is why, instead of describing the molecular neurobiology of a select group of occupational and environmental neurotoxic agents, we still are forced to refer to the comparatively abundant strategies and examples from classical neuropharmacology or the science of modern drug manufacture.

Synthesis and Transport of Membranes and Secretory Proteins

As stated above, neurons are now considered as modified secretory cells. Following the description of Schwartz (1985), the synthesis and distribution of proteins are described as undergoing four phases: synthesis, assembly, and export; translocation; maturation and release; and recycling. After their manufacture, membrane and neurosecretory proteins are finally assembled in the Golgi apparatus. Membranes and neurosecretory proteins are exported from the Golgi apparatus by an anterograde axonal transport either at a fast rate, approximately 400 mm per day, or slowly, 0.3 to 3 mm per day. Fibrillar elements such as microtubules, neurofilaments, and microfilaments are thought to provide the support for this translocation of organelles, but the details of how this occurs are still not clear. The journey may, for certain neurons with particularly long axons, take several days. The synaptic vesicles eventually reach their final destination at the axonal terminal. There, synaptic vesicles achieve "maturation" and are ready for release.

Transient Signals

Neurochemical processes involving ions (charged particles) of sodium, potassium, calcium, and chloride result in three types of transient signals: the generator potential, the action potential, and the synaptic potential.

The *generator potential* is characteristic of receptors and thus is also known as the receptor potential. The main characteristic of this electrical potential is that its magnitude is proportional to the specific sensory stimulus for that particular receptor; it is a graded potential. Receptor potentials have been recorded in all specialized sensory systems. For example, when the intensity of light stimulating a single retinal photoreceptor increases, the magnitude of the generator potential increases. Similarly, the generator potential of a Pacinian corpuscle—a receptor located in the skin and associated with the sensation of touch and vibration—varies in proportion to the mechanical pressure exercised on the single receptor.

Generator potentials can be depolarizing and excitatory and hyperpolarizing and inhibitory. This means that if the receptor has the ability to reduce the normal voltage of the axon membrane, that membrane is "prepared" for firing. On the other hand, if the receptor increases the axon membrane's voltage, its threshold for firing is increased, and therefore it is "unprepared" for firing. Synaptic potentials, described below, have identical depolarizing (excitatory) or hyperpolarizing (inhibitory) properties.

The *action potential* results from depolarization of the resting membrane potential. The resting membrane potential (about -60 mV) results from an inbalance of ion charges in both sides of the cell membrane. The action potential is triggered when the generator potential achieves firing threshold. A key characteristic of the action potential is that it transmits signals in an all-or-none fashion. Neurons transmit electrical signals by modulating the frequency of discharges. The more vigorous stretching of a single muscle spindle, a receptor inside the muscles, the greater is the frequency of the discharge measured at the axon level.

A power function relates the intensity of the specific sensory stimulus to the rate of firing of single cells. This means that if the logarithm of the rate of firing of single neurons is plotted against the logarithm of the magnitude of specific sensory stimuli (eg, light, sound, mechanical pressure) a straight line is obtained. Sensations—subjective events that are almost certainly the expression of basic neurophysiological processes occurring at the receptor level—are also related to the magnitude of their stimulus by a power function. Thus, neurophysiologists tend to interpret this well-established stimulus–response relationship at the receptor level (the power function) as the explanation of why, at the psycholog-

ical level, the magnitude of the sensation is related to the power of its stimulus too. This assumption has been confirmed by studies in humans in which the activity of individual nerve fibers of the limb's somatic sensory system and subjective impressions have both been recorded.

The *synaptic potential* is the potential generated in the neuron adjacent to a synapse (postsynaptic neuron) as a result of a chemical transmitter interacting with the chemical receptor of the neighboring neuron.

Those unfamiliar with the neurophysiological literature need to be alerted to the fact that the term "receptor" has at least two meanings. First, it applies to single units responsible for sensory transduction, eg, light into a generator potential. Second, "receptor" also means the chemical target of a chemical substance, drug neurotransmitter, etc—eg, nicotinic and muscarinic receptors—described below.

Synaptic potential, like generator potentials, are graded. Their magnitude is proportional to the amount of chemical neurotransmitter(s) to which the postsynaptic neurons are sensitive. The postsynaptic receptors can, like generator potentials, be depolarizing (excitatory) or hyperpolarizing (inhibitory). Figure 2.5 is an illustration of how signals are temporally related to each other.

Synaptic Transmission

As stated earlier, one of Ramón y Cajal's major contributions to our understanding of brain morphology was the proposal that the neuron is the basic unit of the nervous system. Earlier, it was thought that the nervous system was an uninterrupted network of cells and fibers. The Spanish neuroanatomist reasoned that gaps must exist between neurons: the synapses.

Discussion of the general features of synaptic transmission requires description of the details of the axon terminal, the synaptic ves-

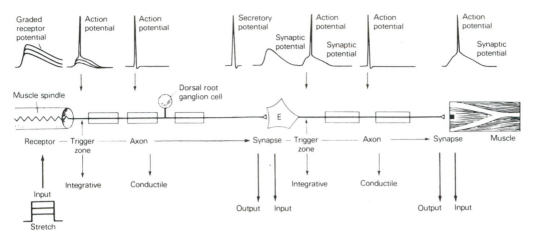

Fig. 2.5. Temporal relationships between transient signals. (From Kandel and Schwartz 1985.)

icles, the presynaptic membrane, the synaptic cleft, a brief introduction to what neurotransmitters do, and a description of the postsynaptic membrane with its receptors. (See Fig. 2.2, bottom, for illustration of general synaptic organization.)

The *axon terminal* is literally where the neuron ends at the tip of its axon. It is an irregularly shaped structure measuring between 1 and 5 μm. The axon terminal may contain mitochondria, a sign of high metabolic activity. The axon terminal is delineated by its membrane; many physical and neurochemical processes of neurotransmission occur at the presynaptic portion of this membrane.

The *synaptic vesicles*, transported via the axon, reach the axon terminal in their fullest stage of "maturation." Synaptic transmission occurs as a result of vesicles bursting open, releasing neurotransmitter substances into the synaptic cleft. Each of these events (bursting of vesicles) is associated with a minuscule electrical discharge called *"miniature end-plate potentials"* (MEPP). Neurotransmitters reach the membrane of an adjacent neuron, the postsynaptic neuron, where receptors for these specific neurotransmitters are located. Neurotransmitters also reach effectors (muscle and glands). The space between the presynaptic neuron and the effector is called the *neuroeffector junction.*

At one time, it was believed that synaptic transmission was an electrical process. An electrical charge generated at the presynaptic membrane was thought to jump across the synapse, reaching the membrane of the postsynaptic neuron. As basic neurochemical and electrophysiological mechanisms began to be better understood, synaptic transmission became recognized as a chemical process, the most important stages of this process being synthesis, transport, release, and fate of the neurotransmitter. However, under some circumstances electrical transmission indeed occurs without the aid of neurotransmitters. Such electrical synapses are called *gap junctions.*

Neurotransmitters and Their Receptors

A *neurotransmitter* is a chemical substance that, when released from axon terminals by the action potential, stimulates or inhibits adjacent neurons or effector organs such as muscle and glands. Known neurotransmitters and their neural pathways have been intensively studied, and new ones are constantly being discovered (Table 2.2). In fact, the most active areas of research concern the chemical characterization of neurotransmitters, how neurotransmitters are synthesized, released, and terminated, where in the nervous system they are disturbed, and how the key stages of synaptic function can be modified by drug or neurotoxic agent action.

Table 2.2. Neurotransmitters, Putative Neurotransmitters, and Neuroactive Peptides

System	Compound
Amino acidergic	γ-Aminobutyrate (GABA)
	Aspartate
	Glutamate
	Glycine
	Taurine
Cholinergic	Acetylcholine
Histaminergic	Histamine
Monoaminergic	Epinephrine
	Dopamine
	Norepinephrine
	Serotonin
	Tryptamine
Peptidergic	Angiotensin
	Bombesin family (2 members)
	Bradykinin
	Calcitonin gene-related peptide (CGRP)
	Carnosine
	*Caerulein
	Cholecystokinin family (5 members)
	Corticotropin
	Corticotropin-releasing hormone (CRF)
	Dynorphin family (5 members)
	*Eledoisin
	Endorphin family (2)
	Enkephalin family (2)
	Gastrin family (2 members)
	Luteinizing-hormone-releasing-hormone (LHRH)
	Melatonin
	Motilin
	Neurokinins (2 peptides)
	Neuromedin family (4 members)
	Neuropeptide K
	Neuropeptide Y
	Neurotensin
	Oxytocin
	Peptide Histidine Isoleucine (PHI)
	*Physalaemin
	Sleep-inducing peptides (4 peptides)
	Somatostatin
	Substance K
	Substance P
	Thyroid hormone-releasing hormone (TRH)
	Vasoactive intestinal peptide (VIP)
	Vasopressin
Purinergic	Adenosine
	ADP
	AMP
	ATP

From Bradford (1987), p. 554.
*Found mainly in lower vertebrates.

Some neurological and psychiatric disorders are now understood to be caused by chemical changes in neurotransmission—eg, myasthenia gravis, Parkinson's disease, certain forms of affective disorders such as depression, severe distortion of thought processes such as in schizophrenia, and Alzheimer's disease. Although excellent isolated reports on the effect of several environmental and occupational neurotoxic agents on neurotransmission have been published, the body of knowledge is meager compared with that existing for neuropsychiatric diseases. Pharmacological studies of manufactured drugs require an understanding of how drugs affect neurotransmission. Drug manufacture and neurotransmission research are thus intimately related. The changing views of drug action have been lucidly summarized by Feldman and Quenzer (1984).

A review of the cellular targets of toxicity and particularly of neurotransmission is necessary. Acetylcholine (ACh), a fairly well characterized neurotransmitter, is used as an illustration.

NEUROTOXIC AGENTS AND NEUROTRANSMISSION

The effects of neurotoxic agents on neurotransmission are characterized by the site in the nervous system where they act, their chemical receptors, the time course of their effects, whether neurotoxic agents facilitate, block, or inhibit neurotransmission, or whether neurotoxic agents alter the termination or removal of the neurotransmitter's pharmacological action.

One of the first questions investigators ask themselves is where a given neurotransmitter is found in the nervous system. Acetylcholine (ACh), for example, is the main transmitter of the autonomic system, in both its sympathetic and parasympathetic components. Neurotransmitters that mimic the effect on the sympathetic division of the autonomic system are called *sympathomimetics,* whereas those that affect the parasympathetic division

are called *parasympathomimetics.* Acetylcholine is found in sympathetic and parasympathetic synapses.

Acetylcholine is also found in neuromuscular and neurosecretory junctions. Both the central and peripheral nervous systems have widely distributed cholinergic synapses (ACh when used as an adjective is called "cholinergic"). A neural mapping of the cholinergic distribution of ACh has been reconstructed. Some of these mappings have actually been seen briefly in vivo by means of imaging techniques.

It is also important to describe the receptors for specific neurotransmitters, their pharmacological properties, and whether their activation will result in excitation or inhibition. Acetylcholine, for example, is known to have at least two types of receptors: *nicotinic* and *muscarinic.* The first is called "nicotinic" because it is activated by nicotine, the alkaloid found in tobacco leaves. The second is called "muscarinic" because it is activated by muscarine, another alkaloid found in certain mushrooms. Both nicotinic and muscarinic receptors can be either excitatory or inhibitory. By now, the excitatory or inhibitory properties of cholinergic receptors—receptors sensitive to the chemical effects of ACh—in brain structures and body organs have been well characterized.

The time course of pharmacological effects of the neurotransmitter on its specific receptors has also been studied. Nicotinic receptors react very quickly to the presence of ACh; ACh produces a rapid depolarization of the postsynaptic membrane where the receptor is located. Muscarinic receptors, on the other hand, are comparatively slower. On the basis of these observed differences in time course, nicotinic receptors are thought to be involved in the rapid conduction of information across synapses.

There are neurotoxins or drugs that mimic the effects of neurotransmitters on their receptors. An *agonistic* substance is one that acts on a receptor, showing pharmacological properties similar to its specific neurotransmitter. Nicotine is thus an agonist for the nicotinic receptor. Another example is apomorphine. Apomorphine, an emetic obtained by treating morphine with strong acids, has the same effects as dopamine on dopamine receptors. Apomorphine is thus a dopamine agonist.

Investigators also look for *antagonists,* substances that create a chemical bond with the receptor, preventing the action of agonist substances. Historically, professional poisoners worth their salt were expected to know the antagonists or antidotes—a term now in disuse—of all poisons. Antagonists are also called receptor blockers. For example, curare, a naturally occurring drug in certain plants that kills by paralyzing skeletal muscles, is an antagonist of nicotinic receptors. Atropine, a powerful autonomic drug derived from *Atropa belladonna,* is an antagonist of muscarinic receptors.

There are also substances that block the synthesis of neurotransmitters. Acetylcholine is synthesized by linking acetyl coenzyme A (acetyl CoA) and choline. Hemicholinium, a synthetic compound, interferes with the synthesis of ACh and, as a result, is called an ACh synthesis blocker. Other substances, such as the venom of the black widow spider, accelerate the release of the neurotransmitter into the synaptic cleft. These substances are called ACh depletors. Still others prevent the release of an already mature neurotransmitter. Botulinus toxin, produced by a bacterium, prevents the synaptic vesicles from releasing ACh into the synaptic cleft. Botulinus toxin is, then, an ACh release blocker.

Reuptake is an essential mechanism for termination of many transmitters. Still other transmitters have enzymes involved in their removal or the termination of their pharmacological action. For acetylcholine, a key enzyme is cholinesterase, which removes acetylcholine after its action. Substances that inhibit the action of cholinesterase are referred to as anticholinesterase agents. Organophosphate pesticides and some extremely lethal neurotoxic agents used in chemical warfare ("nerve gas") are anticholinesterase agents.

Current knowledge of receptors for other neurotransmitters, their agonists and antagonists, synthesis blockers, depletors, release blockers, and substances that inhibit the termination of neurotransmitter action or its uptake are reviewed by Cooper et al. (1986), Goodman Gilman et al. (1985), and Feldman and Quenzer (1984). The latter is particularly informative in reviewing techniques, the investigator's thinking process, historical false leads, and current uncertainties.

CONCLUSION

The difficulties experienced by neuroscientists in linking known processes that occur at the molecular level in the neuron with events at the cellular level that in turn may explain how normal and pathological neuropsychological changes occur are clearly stated in the following:

> . . . (A)t the molecular level, an explanation of the action of a drug is often possible; at the cellular level, an explanation is sometimes possible, but at a behavioral level, our ignorance is abysmal (Cooper et al. 1986).

REFERENCES

Adelman G (1987) *Encyclopedia of Neurosciences.* Boston: Birkhäuser.

Bradford, HF (1987) Neurotransmitters and neuromodulators. In *The Oxford Companion to the Mind,* RL Gregory (ed), p. 550. New York: Oxford University Press.

Cooper, JR, Bloom, FE, and Roth, RT (1986) *The Biochemical Basis of Neuropharmacology* (5th ed). New York: Oxford University Press.

De Robertis, EDP and De Robertis, EMF (1980) *Cell and Molecular Biology* (7th ed). Philadelphia: Saunders College.

Feldman, RS and Quenzer, LD (1984) *Fundamentals of Neuropsychopharmacology.* Sunderland, MA: Sinauer Associates.

Goodman Gilman, A, Goodman, LS, and Gilman, A (1985) *Goodman and Gilman's the.Pharmacological Basis of Therapeutics* (7th ed). New York: Macmillan.

Gross, CG (1987) Early history of neurosciences. In *Encyclopedia of Neurosciences,* G Adelman (ed), pp. 843–846. Boston: Birkhäuser.

Kandel, ER and Schwartz, HJH (eds) (1985) *Principles of Neural Science* (2nd ed). New York: Elsevier.

Ottoson, D (1983) *Physiology of the Nervous System.* New York: Oxford University Press.

Schwartz, JH (1985) Synthesis and distribution of neuronal protein. In *Principles of Neural Science* (2nd ed), pp. 37–57. New York: Elsevier.

World Health Organization (1986) *Principles and Methods for the Assessment of Neurotoxicity Associated with Exposure to Chemicals, Environmental Health Criteria 60,* Geneva: WHO.

SUGGESTED READINGS

Agrawal, AK, Squibb, RE, and Bondy, SC (1981) The effects of acrylamide treatment upon the dopamine receptor. *Toxicol Appl Pharmacol* 58:89–99.

Agrawal, DK, Misra, D, Agarwal, et al. (1982) Influence of sex hormones on parathion toxicity in rats: Antiacetylcholinesterase activity of parathion and paraoxon in plasma, erythrocytes, and the brain. *J Toxicol Environ Health* 9:451–459.

Aldridge, WM, Clothier, B, Forshaw, P, et al. (1978) The effect of DDT and pyrethroids cismetrin and decamethrin on the acetylcholine and cyclic nucleotide content of rat brain. *Biochem Pharmacol* 27:1703–1706.

Ali, SF, Hong, JS, Wilson, WE, et al. (1982) Subchronic dietary exposure of rats to chlordecone (kepone) modified levels of hypothalamic beta-endorphins. *Neurotoxicology* 3:119–124.

Ames, RG, Brown, SK, Mengle, DC et al. (1989) Cholinesterase activity and depression among California agricultural pesticide applicators. *Am J Ind Med* 15:143–150.

Bainave, RJ and Cage, PW (1973) The inhibitory effect of manganese on transmitter release at the neuromuscular junction of the toad. *Br J Pharmacol* 47:339–352.

Bancroft, JD and Stevens, A (1977) *Theory and Practice of Histological Techniques.* New York: Churchill Livingstone.

Barker, JL and Mckelvy, JF (eds) (1983) *Current Methods in Cellular Neurobiology: Electrophysiological and Optical Recording Techniques,* Vol. 3. New York: John Wiley & Sons.

Bartholini, G, Lloyd, KG, and Morselli, PL (1986) *GABA and Mood Disorders.* New York: Raven Press.

Bondy, SC, Harrington, ML, Anderson, C, et al. (1979) Low concentration of an organic lead compound alters transport and release of putative neurotransmitters. *Toxicol Lett* 3:35–41.

Bondy, SC, Tilson, HA, and Agrawal, AK (1981) Neurotransmitter receptors in brains of acrylamide-treated rats. II. Effects of extended exposure to acrylamide. *Pharmacol Biochem Behav* 14:533–537.

Bonilla, E (1980) L-Tyrosine hydroxylase activity in the rat brain after chronic administration of manganese chloride. *Neurobehav Toxicol* 2:37–41.

Bradford, HF (1986) *Chemical Neurobiology: An Introduction to Neurochemistry.* New York: WH Freeman.

Brown, SK, Ames, RG, and Mengle, DC (1989) Occupational illness from cholinesterase-inhibiting pesticides among agricultural workers applicators in California, 1982–1985. *Arch Environ Health* 44(1):34–39.

Bull, RJ, and Luthenhoff, SD (1975) Changes in the metabolic responses of brain tissue to stimulation, in vitro, produced by in vivo administration of methylmercury. *Neuropharmacology* 14:351–359.

Chang, L (1977) Neurotoxic effects of mercury: A review. *Environ Res* 14:329–373.

Cooper, GP and Manalis, RS (1983) Influence of heavy metals on synaptic transmission: A review. *Neurotoxicology* 4(49):669–684.

Cooper, GP, Suszkiw, JB, and Manalis, RS (1984) Presynaptic effects of heavy metals. In *Cellular and Molecular Toxicology,* T Narahashi (ed) pp. 1–21. New York: Raven Press.

Damstra, T (1978) Environmental chemicals and nervous system dysfunction. *Yale J Biol Med* 51:457–468.

Damstra, T and Bondy, SC (1980) The current status and future of biochemical assays for neurotoxicity. In *Experimental and Clinical Neurotoxicology,* PS Spencer and HH Schaumburg (eds) pp. 820–833. Baltimore: Williams & Wilkins.

Damstra, T and Bondy, SC (1982) Neurochemical approaches to the detection of neurotoxicity. In *Nervous System Toxicity,* CL Mitchell (ed) pp. 349–373. New York: Raven Press.

Diemer, NH (1982) Quantitative morphological studies of neuropathological changes. *CRC Crit Rev Toxicol* 10(1):215–263.

Emson, PC (1983) *Chemical Neuroanatomy.* New York: Raven Press.

Gottlieb, DI (1988) GABAergic neurons. *Sci Am* 258(2):82–89.

Holtzman, D, Herman, MM, Shen Hsu, J, et al. (1980) The pathogenesis of lead encephalopathy: Effects of lead carbonate feeding on morphology, lead contents, and mitochondrial respiration of immature and adult rats. *Virchows Arch [Pathol Anat]* 387:147–168.

Hrdina, PD and Singhal, RL (1981) *Neuroendocrine Regulations and Altered Behavior.* New York: Plenum Press.

Jasper, HH and Sourkes, TL (1983) Nobel laureates in neuroscience: 1904–1981. *Annu Rev Neurosci* 6:1–42.

Jonsson, G (1980) Chemical neurotoxins as denervation tools in neurobiology. *Annu Rev Neurosci* 3:169–187.

Kandel, E (1982) The origins of modern neuroscience. *Annu Rev Neurosci* 5:299–303.

Kimelberg, HK and Norenberg, MD (1989) Astrocytes. *Sci Am* 260(4):66–76.

Lampert, PW and Schochet, S (1968) Demyelination and remyelination in lead neuropathy: Electron microscopic studies. *J Neuropathol Exp Neurol* 27:527–545.

Mardsden, CA (1984) *Measurement of Neurotransmitter Release in Vivo*. New York: John Wiley & Sons.

Myers, RR, Powell, HC, Shapiro, H, et al. (1980) Changes in endoneurial fluid pressure, permeability and peripheral nerve ultrastructure in experimental lead neuropathy. *Ann Neurol* 8(4):392–401.

Nathan, P (1988) *The Nervous System* (3rd ed). New York: Oxford University Press.

Norton, S (1978) Is behavior or morphology a more sensitive indicator of central nervous system toxicity? *Environ Health Perspect* 26:21–27.

Patterson, PH (1978) Environmental determination of autonomic neurotransmitter function. *Annu Rev Neurosci* 1:1–17.

Pentschew, A and Garro, F (1976) Lead encephalo-myelopathy of the suckling rat and its implications on the porthyrinopathic nervous disease. *Acta Neuropathol (Berl)* 6:266–278.

Poduslo, JF, Low, PA, Windebank, AJ, et al. (1982) Altered blood nerve barrier in experimental lead neuropathy assessed by changes in endoneurial albumin concentration, *J Neurosci* 2(10):1507–1514.

Powell, HC, Myers, RR, and Lampert, PW (1980) Edema in neurotoxic injury. In *Experimental and Clinical Neurotoxicology*, PS Spencer and HH Schaumburg (eds) pp. 118–138. Baltimore: Williams & Wilkins.

Ramón y Cajal, S (1937) *Recollections of My Life*. Cambridge, MA: The MIT Press.

Ramsay, RB, Krigman, MR, and Morell, P (1980) Developmental studies of the uptake of choline, GABA, and dopamine by crude synaptosomal preparations after in vivo and in vitro lead treatment. *Brain Res* 187:383–387.

Reichardt, LF and Kelly, RB (1983) A molecular description of nerve terminal function. *Annu Rev Biochem* 52:871–926.

Schrier, BK (1982) Nervous system culture as toxicologic test system. In *Nervous System Toxicity*, CL Mitchell (ed) pp. 337–348. New York: Raven Press.

Segarra, JM (1970) Histological and histochemical staining methods: A selection. In *Neuropathology: Methods and Diagnosis*, CG Tedeschi (ed) pp. 233–269. Boston: Little, Brown.

Shepherd, GM (1987) *Neurobiology* (2nd ed). New York: Oxford University Press.

Siegel, GJ, Agranoff, B, Albers, RW, et al. (eds) (1988) *Basic Neurochemistry* (4th ed). New York: Raven Press.

Silbergeld, DK (1983) Localization of metals: Issues of importance to neurotoxicology of lead. *Neurotoxicology* 4(3):193–200.

Silbergeld, EK (1984) Mitochondrial mechanisms of lead neurotoxicity. In *Cellular and Molecular Neurotoxicology*, T Narahashi (ed) pp. 153–164. New York: Raven Press.

Silbergeld, EK, Hruska, R, Miller, L. et al. (1980) Effect of lead in vivo and in vitro on GABAergic neurochemistry. *J Neurochem* 34(6):1712–1718.

Silbergeld, EK, Miller, LP, Kennedy, S, et al. (1979) Lead, GABA, and seizures: Effects of subencephalopathic lead exposure on seizure sensitivity and gabaergic function. *Environ Res* 19:371–382.

Smith, RS and Bisby, MA (eds) (1987). *Axonal Transport*. New York: Alan R. Liss.

Snyder, SH (1984) Drug and neurotransmitter receptors in the brain. *Science* 224:22–31.

Spencer, PS and Bischoff, MC (1982) Contemporary neuropathological methods in toxicology. In *Nervous System Toxicity*, CL Mitchell (ed) pp. 259–275. New York: Raven Press.

Spencer, PS and Schaumburg, HH (eds) (1980) *Experimental and Clinical Neurotoxicology*. Baltimore: William & Wilkins.

Spencer, PS, Schaumburg, HH, Raleigh, RL, et al. (1975) Nervous system degeneration produced by the industrial solvent methyl *n*-butyl ketone. *Arch Neurol* 32:219–222.

Shellengerber, MK (1984) Effects of early lead exposure on neurotransmitter systems in the brain: A review with commentary. *Neurotoxicology* 5(3):177–212.

Shankland, DL (1982) Neurotoxic action of chlorinated hydrocarbon insecticides. *Neurobehav Toxicol Teratol* 4:805–811.

Takeuchi, T, Eto, N, and Eto, K (1979) Neuropathology of childhood cases of methylmercury poisoning (Minamata disease) with prolonged symptoms with particular reference to the decortication syndrome. *Neurotoxicology* 1:1–20.

Thomas JA, Korach, KS, and McLachlan, JA (1985) *Endocrine Toxicity*. New York: Raven Press.

Tilson, HA and Sparber, SB (eds) (1987) *Neurotoxicants and Neurobiological Function*. New York: Wiley-Interscience.

Virchow, R (1986) Post-mortem examinations and the position of pathology among biological studies. Methuchen, NJ: Scarecrow Reprint Corporation [originally published in 1873].

Wilson, WE (1982) Dopamine-sensitive adenulate cyclase in activation by organolead compounds. *Neurotoxicology* 3:100–107.

Wince, LC, Donovan, CA, and Azzaro AJ (1980) Alterations in the biochemical properties of central dopamine synapses following chronic postnatal $PbCO_3$ exposure. *J Pharmacol Exp Ther* 214:642–650.

Wu, Y-Q, Wang, J-D, Chen, J-S et al. (1989) Occupational risk of decreased plasma cholinesterase among pesticide production workers in Taiwan. *Am J Ind Med* 16:659–666.

Yamamura, HI, Enna, SJ, and Kuhar, MJ (1981) *Neurotransmitter Receptor Binding*. New York: Raven Press.

3

The Clinical Neurological Examination

The clinical neurological examination is the systematic study of signs and symptoms associated with the normal or abnormal function of the nervous system through observation and probes. In the clinic, a physician makes a judgment of the possible causes (etiology) of abnormal signs and symptoms. Only physicians trained in neurology perform this kind of examination.

The clinical neuropsychological examination, reviewed primarily in Chapter 4, is a comprehensive evaluation of the functional status of an individual known or suspected to suffer from nervous system damage. In the United States, psychologists trained in neuropsychology perform this examination.

In epidemiological surveys, information derived from the systematic clinical examination of a large number of individuals affected by neurotoxic agents is sometimes the only data available. Surveys designed to ascertain the prevalence and causes of neurological diseases may or may not include psychometric, electrophysiological, or imaging procedures, but they almost always include a systematic study of neurological signs and symptoms.

The book *Pictorial Manual of Neurologic Tests: A Guide to the Performance and Interpretation of the Neurological Examination*

(Van Allen and Rodnitzky 1981) is a good source regarding how the neurological examination is conducted and the rationale behind the different probes.

THE EXAMINATION

The neurological examination is carried out in somewhat different manners depending on the context within which the study is conducted. In the clinic, the neurological examination is typically carried out by a single physician and includes the patient's medical history, the physical (neurological) examination, and a review of neurological signs and symptoms. In epidemiological surveys, these three components of the examination are sometimes the responsibility of three different teams of professionals.

The reason for splitting the components of the neurological examination among several professionals is to avoid bias. Epidemiological surveys are often conducted under pressure. Immediately after an environmental accident has occurred, for example, a community may request that all at potential risk be examined. Some may argue that should a physician know where the individual was placed at the moment of the explosion of a chem-

ical plant, for example, recording of signs and symptoms may be biased. Seasoned physicians resent the view that their clinical judgment can be easily influenced by the wealth of information available at the time of an environmental or occupational tragedy. During an environmental health emergency when human lives are at stake, matters of epidemiological design sometimes need to be necessarily overlooked. Yet, during litigation, the "design" and "bias" of epidemiological surveys are often under attack.

Decision Trees in the Neurological Evaluation

Neurologists perform three types of evaluations. In the *symptomatic examination* they observe symptoms and signs of a disease. In the *anatomic examination* they ascertain the probable portions of the nervous system affected. The *diagnosis* is a statement of the type of possible causes of neurological illness. In medicine, the cause of a disease is called its etiology.

The physical examination consists of a series of probes performed in a systematic manner. The probes are based on the principle of branching—ie, if condition A exists then probe X, otherwise probe Y. This is the reason why in medical field surveys it is so difficult to design a computer-compatible questionnaire for data obtained when performing a physical examination. In poorly designed survey questionnaires, the logic to which neurologists adhere during the course of a physical examination is often obscure if not misleading.

The neurological examination is aimed at examining broad areas of nervous system function. But if and when anomalies are suspected or detected, neurologists probe as much as necessary. From the neurologist's point of view, psychometric and neurophysiological techniques (discussed in Chapters 4 and 5) are ancillary techniques that may help to resolve uncertainties of diagnoses raised during the course of the clinical examination.

When neurologists examine a person suspected of being affected by environmental or occupational exposure to a neurotoxic agent,

they rule out other neurological conditions such as traumatic, degenerative, vascular, metabolic, or infectious diseases. This is called the *differential diagnosis* of an illness. Juntunen and Haltia (1982) have described the decision tree that neurologists follow from the suspicion of a neurotoxic syndrome to its diagnosis (Fig. 3.1).

Observation of the Patient's Physical Appearance

As the examiner walks toward the patient to greet him or her for the first time, the examiner performs the first evaluation, that of the patient's physical appearance. Long years of experience, intuition, and sharp observational skills help to collect qualitative data of this nature. Changes in the subject's physical appearance are likely to occur in chronic conditions. For example, facial expression and posture characteristics of the aged may be observed in young people. Unusual skin conditions, unkempt and dirty clothing, tics, and abnormal gestures or body movements are all important data that the alert clinician takes into consideration. The observation—usually recorded in written notes—concentrates on conditions that are clearly not the function of economic factors or personal inclinations. Changes in fashions and cultural norms are, of course, important factors to be considered in making an evaluation of the physical appearance of a patient seen in the clinic or the participant in a medical field survey.

Very little effort has been made to standardize this phase of the clinical examination or the epidemiological survey dealing with physical appearance. On certain occasions, a picture or a film of the patient is made to illustrate points relative to his or her physical appearance. These are valuable to document the time course of either the onset of the disease or its recovery. The examiner requests permission from the patient or the immediate family to obtain pictures or films. In addition, the examiner is aware of issues of confidentiality of information when this information

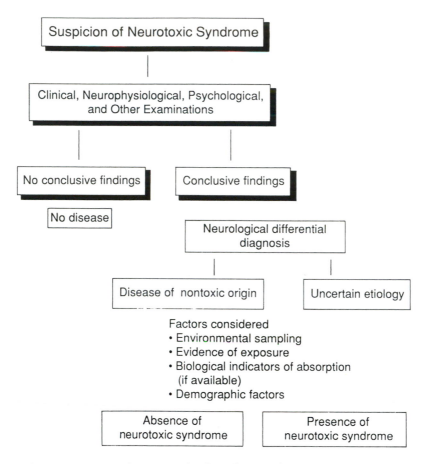

Fig. 3.1. Juntunen's decision tree for the evaluation of neurotoxic diseases. (From Juntunen and Haltia 1982.)

is planned to be presented in public, particularly if the patient can be clearly identified by the photograph. A worker, for example, may rightly fear that a picture obtained in the privacy of an office may reach management, thus jeopardizing his or her job.

The Medical and Occupational History

A detailed family and medical history includes data on hospitalization(s) and reason(s) for hospitalization, present or past: cardiovascular, gastrointestinal, genitourinary, skin, blood, ear, nose and throat conditions, nervous system, musculoskeletal, metabolic diseases, cancer, etc. A history of accidents is also usually recorded. The medical history also includes past and present use of medication, alcohol intake, tobacco use, and recreational drug use. Finally, it also includes family history to assess hereditary, degenerative, deficiency, and possible metabolic diseases. Chapter 13 (Surveys) contains an example of a computer-compatible form used to obtain information on the medical history of a survey participant.

An occupational history is recorded in order to ascertain activities and probable exposures in previous and present work. The significance of the use of occupational history for the evaluation of possible toxic exposures is discussed in more detail in Chapter 11. During medicoepidemiological surveys the occupational history is sometimes recorded by professional interviewers. This is to optimize the time of the examining physician, time that is generally at a premium, or to control bias that may arise should the physicians become familiar with subjects' occupational exposures.

The Probes

A probe is different from a test. A *probe* is the examination of the status of the nervous system of an individual with the naked eye or by use of very simple equipment. For example, a simple and effective probe of color vision consists of asking the patient in the clinic to identify all pieces that are red from a collection of pieces of wool in a basket. However, the examiner knows that someone with alterations in color perception can discriminate color on the basis of the brightness of objects. Thus, this simple probe may not suffice when the examinee is a worker who badly needs to depend on an accurate detection of color. In such a case, the examiner may request a formal test of color perception.

As a rule, a *test* is a probe that has been standardized on the basis of a statistically representative number of functionally normal people satisfying various criteria of test development. (The meaning of a psychological test is discussed in Chapter 4, Psychometric Techniques.) The types of probes performed are intimately linked to the understanding professionals have of the gross morphological organization of the nervous system. For example, when necessary, a professional familiar with tests and procedures to investigate eye movements will request the performance of a test for otolith functions (ie, the normal presence of rotary components of the eye) as recorded by means of electrophysiological procedures, as the head is oriented in different spatial positions. Another with long experience in the examination of the minimally brain-impaired will include probes that, from the outside, seem close to psychometric testing. An example of this is to ask the patient to hand draw in the clinic to uncover subtle changes in the patient's vis-

ual field. (In a drawing of a clock, sometimes patients with visual field defects do not draw significant areas of the clock.)

Neurologists consider the following probes essential in the course of a routine neurological examination:

- Gait and posture
- Cranial nerves
- Motor examination
- Tendon reflexes
- Sensory evaluation.

Gait and Posture.   In the maintenance of the upright posture and walking, a substantial portion of the nervous system is brought into action. Examination of the posture and gait provides important clues to the status of the nervous and musculoskeletal systems, general health, and sometimes mental status.

The *gait examination* includes the observation of presence of arm swing, the ability to perform rapid turning without losing balance, and the ability to walk on toes and heels. Tandem walking, in which the patient is asked to walk heel to toe down a line on the floor, is a very sensitive test for general motor coordination. Tandem walking reduces the base for maintaining balance, demanding greater ability to compensate for changes in posture as walking proceeds. It is a widely used test for assessing overt signs of alcohol intoxication.

Gait abnormalities may result from a variety of conditions. Foot drop and high stepping are seen in some neuropathies characterized by axonopathies, neurological diseases affecting the axons of neurons. Slapping and unsteady gait are associated with dysfunction of the spinal cord's dorsal column (where peripheral sensory fibers enter the spinal cord). Abnormal walk and clumsiness often result from exposure to neurotoxic agents such as metals (manganese, mercury), solvents (carbon disulfide, methyl *n*-butyl ketone, *n*-hexane), monomers (acrylamide), pesticides (DDT, kepone), and gases (ethylene chloride). Some gait anomalies such as those derived from solvent exposure may be erroneously interpreted as drunkenness by plant managers and fellow workers.

The *posture examination* is the observation of the patient in standing position with feet slightly separated and with feet together. The posture examination often includes the *Romberg test* (Fig. 3.2A) in which the patient stands with feet together with eyes closed or open and the examiner takes notes of balance and tendency to fall on one side. In the *sensitized Romberg test* (Fig. 3.2B), performed when the results of the Romberg tests are ambiguous, the heel of one foot touches the toe of the other along a line.

Pathological alterations in the striatum, a component of the basal ganglia system, may be associated with bizarre jerky movements accompanied by flinging of the arms and facial grimacing. In the initial phases of the disorder, the patient sometimes hides the abnormal movements by pretending they are intentional, for example, by fixing his necktie or combing his hair with his hands.

Cranial Nerves.   This includes the examination of the sensory organs, muscles, and functions that depend on the functional integrity of the cranial nerves as described in Chapter 1. Traditionally, cranial nerves are designated by Roman numerals. The examination is performed seriatim from nerves I to XII.

The examination of the olfactory nerve (I) is performed with the patient's eyes closed, testing one nostril at a time. Aromatic substances such as vanilla bean, coffee, tobacco, peppermint, etc. are adequate. But the use of odoriferous compounds diluted in alcohol may produce misleading findings. For example: Alcohol, an irritant, can be detected through the stimulation of the trigeminal nerve (V) even after olfactory nerves are severed; and chronic occupational exposure to solvents may be associated with severe impairment of olfactory functions.

Four probes are used to evaluate the optic nerve (II): fundoscopy, visual acuity, visual fields, and color perception.

A

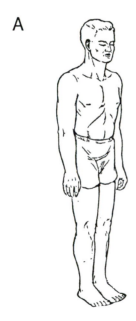

B

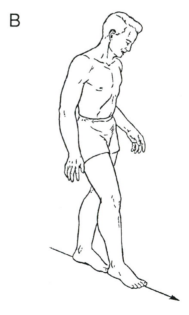

Fig. 3.2.   The Romberg test. (From *Pictorial Manual of Neurologic Tests: A Guide to the Performance and Interpretation of the Neurological Examination* (2nd ed), by MW Van Allen and RL Rodnitzky © 1981 by Yearbook Medical Publishers, Inc., Chicago, IL.

Fundoscopy is the examination of the fundus of the eye, where the surface of the retina can be seen. The fundoscopic evaluation is made by means of an optical instrument called the *opthalmoscope*. The optic papilla is where neural fibers originating in the retina gather to become the optic nerve. It is an oval area crossed by small blood vessels and devoid of visual receptors. Changes in blood vessel appearance and coloration are in some cases indicative of atherosclerosis. Edema of the papilla is associated with an increase in intracranial pressure, sometimes indicative of tumors.

Visual acuity is the ability to detect, resolve, and perceive fine detail of a visual display. The evaluation of visual acuity is essential for the interpretation of the findings of tests involving vision. Most of the psychometric tests described in Chapter 4 are relatively insensitive to changes in visual acuity. Nonetheless, when in doubt, the examiner uses simple probes—such as requesting the examinee to read written material of different sizes—to make a quick evaluation of this important confounder. Many factors account for a reduction in visual acuity. Some are changes in the transparency of the optical media of the eye, such as corneal lacerations or cataracts (opacity of the intraocular lens). Some others result from damage to the neural pathways involved in visual perception.

Our *visual field* is everything we can see around us with both eyes without moving the head. Changes in the visual fields make it possible to localize the site of neural lesions in the visual pathway. Once they leave the retina, the visual fibers that form the optic nerve preserve a topological integrity—ie, their positions with respect to each other—despite twists and turns of the nerve bundles. A simple test of the visual field is performed in the clinic with one's fingers and sometimes with the aid of colored pencils. But the characterization and extent of *scotomas*—loss of vision in specific regions of the visual field—is detected by visual field testing.

Assessment of *color perception* is possible by use of simple tests. Some of them are plates with letters and numbers shaped by arranging circles of different colors; others involve color sorting. However, as indicated above, the clinician is aware of the significance of brightness in perception of color.

Examining the III nerve usually means observing pupil size, reaction to light, and the action of some extraocular muscles allowing the elevation of the eyelids. The pupil dilates as the radial muscles of the iris contract; conversely, the pupil has a pinpoint appearance as the sphincter muscle of the iris contracts. These muscles are under the control of the autonomic nervous system. Neurotoxic agents affecting autonomic functions are likely to produce pupillary alterations. Certain organochlorinated pesticides such as DDT cause the pupil to dilate; pupillary changes are also associated with drug abuse.

The presence of dilated pupils is a common cause of *photophobia*, an exaggerated sensitivity to light. It is a common practice to observe the kind of glasses the subject carries even if he or she does not use them during the course of examination. Heavily tinted glasses are sometimes an indication of photophobia. (But children and teenagers sometimes use heavily tinted glasses to imitate entertainment idols.)

Failure to open the eye (dropped lid or *ptosis*) may be caused by lesions of the III nerve.

To evaluate the extraocular muscles innervated by the III, IV, and VI nerves, the examiner asks the patient to move his or her eyes about in a horizontal and vertical plane. Limitations of eye movement and double vision can thus be noted.

Nystagmus—repetitive movement of the eyes—has fast and slow phases. By convention, the direction of the nystagmus is designated by the direction of the fast phase. Nystagmus may be elicited normally by stimulation of the vestibular organs, such as when the ears are irrigated with cold or warm water (caloric nystagmus). Nystagmus on lateral monocular fixation is present in approximately 25% of the general population; nystagmus on lateral binocular fixation is a sign of neurological dysfunction. The presence of nystagmus is associated with alterations of neural pathways of the vestibulocerebellar–oculomotor system. Acute and chronic exposure to neurotoxic agents such as alcohol and solvents may produce gross alterations in eye movements that can be observed by the naked eye. Others, such as the subtle alterations caused by lead and mercury, require the use of oculographic methods for their detection.

Pinpricks and touch over the face are used to assess the functional integrity of two overlapping sensory systems whose information is carried by unmyelinated (pain) and myelinated (touch) fibers. These two are carried by the sensory branch of the V nerve, the trigeminal nerve. The corneal reflex is tested by touching each cornea with a wisp of cotton.

Examination of the symmetry of facial movements is performed to evaluate the VII nerves controlling facial muscles. These nerves are tested by observing and touching the muscles of the face as the patient closes his or her jaw tightly and moves the mandible from side to side. The anterior two-thirds of the tongue is innervated by the sensory branch of the VII nerve carrying taste sensations.

Hearing can be severely affected by ototoxic drugs such as the antibiotic streptomycin. Deafness often occurred after the early massive use of antibiotics to treat tuberculosis. Although isolated cases have been reported, hearing is rarely affected by neurotoxic agents in the workplace. Noise-induced hearing damage, quite prevalent in many worksites, may be a more likely explanation of hearing impairment. In the clinic, the noise produced by rubbing the index finger against the thumb can be used as an effective stimulus. Some patients need audiometric testing for their sensitivity to a wide range of frequencies, generally from 125 to 30,000 Hz.

The functions of the IX–X nerves are assessed by an examiner's careful observation of speech—particularly slurred speech, the presence of gag reflex, and the ability to swallow.

The XI nerve innervates the muscles that control the symmetry of shoulder muscles and rotation of the head, whereas XII controls the movement of the tongue. The examiner assesses the functional integrity of this nerve by observing midline presence of atrophy or abnormal tongue movements.

Motor Examination.   The motor examination is directed at the evaluation of muscle tone, motor strength, and motor coordination. Chapter 27 presents a more detailed review of motor disturbances caused by neurotoxic agents.

Some neurological conditions are characterized by neuromuscular disorders such as the presence of atrophy (muscle degeneration), fasciculation (involuntary twitches of the muscles), tone-resistance to passive movement, and tremor. Evaluation of atrophy and fasciculation sometimes calls for testing of individual muscles. Often, electrophysiological procedures—particularly electromyography and nerve conduction velocity determinations—aid the diagnosis. The examiner ascertains whether metabolic or structural lesions are located in the ventral horn of the spinal cord, the ventral root, or the peripheral motor nerve.

Evaluation of muscle tone and resistance to passive movement can lead to the diagnosis of either spasticity or rigidity. *Spasticity* is characterized by a "clasp-knife" resistance; the resistance increases as the examiner continues to apply force. *Rigidity* is a sort of "lead-pipe" resistance characterized by uniformly increased resistance throughout the range of motion. Spasticity often results from lesions of the "upper motor neuron" systems.

In general, an "upper motor neuron" is located in the nervous system at higher levels than the spinal cord. As is shown in Chapter 27, experimental work in laboratory animals seems to contradict early simplistic views on the causes of spasticity. In general, lesions and toxic agents affecting the "lower motor neuron," those of the spinal cord and its motor nerves, are associated with weakness, flaccidity, muscle atrophy, and fasciculation.

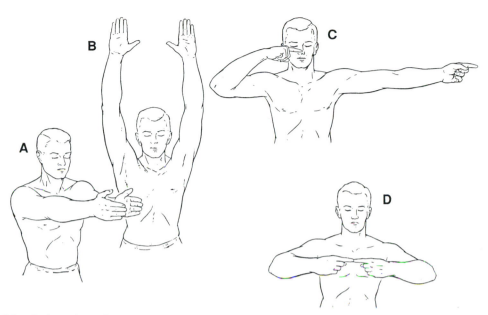

Fig. 3.3. Probes of coordination of arms and hands. (From *Pictorial Manual of Neurologic Tests: A Guide to the Performance and Interpretation of the Neu-* *rological Examination* (2nd ed), by MW Van Allen and RL Rodnitzky © 1981 by Yearbook Medical Publishers, Inc., Chicago, IL.)

Tremor is the involuntary periodic oscillation of a body member. Three categories of tremor are recognized: resting tremor, intentional tremor, and postural tremor. *Resting tremor*, as its name indicates, is present at rest. It is exaggerated when limbs are relaxed and lessens during the execution of a voluntary movement. It is often of basal ganglia origin. Resting tremor needs to be differentiated from *physiological tremor,* a normal oscillation of body parts between 8 to 13 Hz. *Intentional tremor* is manifested when one attempts to perform a movement at will (volitional movement). It is a sign of cerebellar disease. A maneuver to elicit intentional tremor is to ask the patient to touch his or her nose with the index finger of one hand. *Postural tremor* is observed with the part of the body maintaining a posture, such as holding the hands outstretched. It diminishes when the limbs are relaxed, reappearing as soon as movement begins. Neurotoxin-induced tremors tend to be symmetrical, such as those induced by mercury, DDT, acrylamide, etc. Asymmetric resting tremor is more likely to be consistent with fairly localized neural lesions.

Motor coordination results from the integration of sensory input and motor outputs. One important set of cues is brought by *muscle sense* or *kinesthesia.* Figure 3.3 (A and B) shows typical neurological tests to evaluate *proprioception,* the ability to recognize the position of limbs in space. In A the man is asked to place his arms in front of him with his eyes closed. In B, he is asked to elevate one arm—for example, the left— and then position the right arm at the same height. Figure 3.3 (C and D) reveals simple tests of motor coordination performed under clinical conditions. In C the man is being asked to touch his nose alternately with the index finger of his right and left hand with eyes closed. In D the man is asked to touch his two index fingers with eyes closed.

Motor coordination is a learned sequence of motor acts, such as those involved in buttoning one's shirts or tying one's shoes. The cerebellum is the main neural structure involved in the scheduling and appropriate sequencing of motor acts including motor learning. The timing of these learned sensory and motor cues is easily disrupted as a result of a large variety of neurotoxic chemical agents. That is why motor coordination probes have long been used in the quick assessment of intoxicated persons, such as the assessment performed by police officers who need to ascertain possible alcohol intoxication among car drivers.

Reflex Examination.   The reflex examination consists of the testing of deep tendon and superficial cutaneous reflexes. Deep tendon reflexes are elicited by tapping the tendon of major muscles with a soft rubber percussion hammer. The reflex activity of the biceps, triceps, quadriceps, and gastrocnemius is thus examined. American neurologists use the convention of designating the magnitude of reflex action with a scale ranging from zero to four. "Zero" indicates the absence of reflex activity, whereas "four" is a gross exaggeration of the response, often accompanied by several beats of clonus (a rhythmic muscle contraction evoked by and sustained during muscle stretch).

The clinical interpretation of findings is always challenging. The absence of these reflexes may be associated with alterations at many different levels of the nervous system, including the integrity of receptors within muscles. The exaggeration of reflexes is often part of spasticity, a syndrome caused by alterations in upper motor neurons, neurons located at higher levels than the spinal cord.

The *Babinski response*, a cutaneous reflex, is an abnormal neurological sign consisting of the extension of the great toe and fanning of the other toes as a result of striking the most lateral portion of the sole with a sharp object such as a key or a safety pin. Normally, there is no flexion of all toes as a result of this type of sensory stimulation. The Babinski sign is normal in babies; its disappearance is a measure of the progressive myelinization of the nervous system. In the adult, the Babinski response is found with lesions of the corticospinal tract.

Sensory Evaluation.   The sensations of pain, cold, and warmth on the one hand and of touch and mechanical vibration on the other

are mediated by the somatosensory system (described in detail in Chapter 23). Sensations of pain and temperature are conducted by thin, unmyelinated fibers, whereas touch and vibration are mediated by thick, myelinated fibers. Thus, in lesions affecting the dorsal column of the spinal cord, sensations of touch and vibration disappear or are greatly diminished, whereas pain and temperature sensations remain unchanged. The mapping of body sites where sensations are altered or have disappeared or a dissociation pattern of sensation (ie, one type of sensation is lost while the other remains) appears allows the probable localization of lesions.

Autonomic Nervous System

The evaluation of autonomic nervous function is part of a thorough neurological examination. This includes questions and probes regarding frequency of urination, changes in regularity and frequency of heart beat, amount of urinary output, presence of diarrhea or constipation, impotence, sudden reduction in blood pressure leading to fainting, lacrimation, changes in pupil diameter, and dryness of mouth and skin, among others. When necessary a physician may require the performance of specific tests of autonomic system function—eg, sweating tests, special electrocardiographic tests.

Neurotoxic agents of occupational origin known to cause autonomic system defects in acute or chronic doses include DDT, lead, arsenic, the large majority of industrial solvents, dimethylaminopropionitrile (DMAPN)—used in the manufacture of polyurethane foams—and many others. Most of these effects are presumed to be of central nervous system origin since peripheral neuropathies involving the autonomic system are uncommon. Table 3.1 lists signs and symptoms of autonomic system failure.

The differential diagnosis between occupational and *iatrogenic toxicopathies* (caused by medical treatment) is essential. Many medications have been specifically developed

Table 3.1. Symptoms and Signs of Autonomic Failure

System	Symptom	Sign
Cardiovascular	Dizziness	Orthostatic hypotension
	Vertigo	Supine hypertension
	Syncope	
	Fatigue	
Gastrointestinal	Dysphagia	Altered swallowing
	Distention	Hypomotility
	Constipation	Hypermotility
	Diarrhea	
	Abdominal pain	
Genitourinary	Urinary urgency, frequency, and incontinence	Altered sacral reflexes
	Fecal incontinence	Sphincter dysfunction
	Impotence	
Temperature regulation	Flushing	Altered sweating or skin temperature
	Hyperhidrosis	
	Anhidrosis	Abnormal sweat test
	Heat intolerance	Hyperpyrexia
Exocrine glands	Irritated eyes	Changes in lacrimation or salivation
	Tearing	
	Dry/moist mouth	
General/diffuse	Diplopia	Extraocular palsy
	Night blindness	Horner's syndrome
	Nasal stuffiness	Boggy mucosa

From Hamill (1987).

to act on the autonomic system—eg, cardiovascular drugs. Whenever the effects of environmental and occupational toxic agents are studied, the possible effect of these medications should, of course, be ruled out. Among these are widely prescribed tranquilizers, antidepressants, antihypertensive medications, particularly the so-called β blockers, and medications prescribed to regulate cardiac rhythm such as perhexylene.

Substance abuse and alcoholism are the third major sources of substances that can produce autonomic effects. The addictive nature of many neurotoxic drugs is explained in part by the critical, sometimes long-lasting, alterations in metabolic pathways. It is now suspected that some abused substances have a synergistic effect with neurotoxic agents of occupational origin—eg, exposure to industrial solvents and alcohol use together can increase the toxic effect.

Neurotoxins of plant and animal origin often produce marked autonomic effects that are sometimes fatal. Well known are the autonomic effects of the bite of the black widow spider and the cobra, the sting of the scorpion, and toxins released by bacteria such as those that cause botulism and tetanus, as well as mushroom poisoning (*Amanita muscaria*).

EXAMINATION OF MENTAL STATUS

Examination of mental status consists of observations of the subject's behavior and simple probes to evaluate nervous system function. Sometimes, a physician has to perform this evaluation very quickly and under unusual circumstances. An example is the teenager who has attempted suicide by ingestion of an insecticide. Another example is the examination of a large group of workers affected by the sudden release of a neurotoxic chemical in the environment.

The actual clinical neuropsychological examination is aimed at the evaluation of level of consciousness, attention and concentration, prevailing mood, memory, language, constructional abilities, and cognitive functions. The clinical evaluation of these basic dimensions is directed to the ascertainment of whether they are within normal limits or an expression of brain disease, that is, whether an underlying structural or toxic-metabolic change in the nervous system can be demonstrated. The limits that supposedly separate normality from neurological disorders (resulting from organic factors) or psychiatric diseases (often called "functional diseases") are not as distinct as once thought.

Throughout the remainder of this chapter the main emphasis is on the examination performed on people who experience readily observable conditions suspected to be associated with the intake of neurotoxic agents.

Evaluation of Level of Consciousness

This is designed to determine where a subject is placed in a continuum ranging from a reasonable state of alertness to deep coma. Specific terms used for key stages within this range are *alertness*, *lethargy*, *stupor*, and *coma*. In Chapter 21 the relationship of levels of consciousness with the sleep–wake cycle is explored in detail.

In clinical neurotoxicology one can observe acute episodes of poisoning, such as from carbon monoxide, where the stage of consciousness progresses from confusion to coma and death in a few minutes. Thus, the determination of level of conciousness is of fundamental importance. The adequate evaluation of almost all other dimensions of mental functioning depends on whether the clinician can talk to an alert, cooperative individual or has to rely on the information given by a relative or friend of a comatose patient in an emergency room.

The level of alertness can also be evaluated by simple tests that can be applied at the bedside. In one, the patient is requested to count numbers from 1 to 10 and then from 10 backwards. It is possible to make the test more difficult by asking the patient to serially subtract sevens from 100 (eg, 100, 93, 86, 79, and so on). There are numerous simple paper-and-pencil tests that can be used on relatively healthy or mildly impaired individuals.

Attention

This is aimed at ascertaining the subject's ability to focus his or her mind on specific external or internal stimuli at will or on command. At bedside, the clinician is interested in whether the patient is "tuned" to the environment, reacting to what is personally meaningful. But many factors affect a person's interest in his or her surroundings. Age and education are important—for example, an aging person may be fascinated by the sight of a pigeon picking seeds in a park, a scene not likely to impress a busy business person.

Concentration is related to attention. *Concentration* is the ability to maintain the focus of personally meaningful stimuli for an appropriate period of time. Inability to concentrate, exemplified in the remark "my mind wanders," may be a common symptom of clinical significance. *Distractibility* refers to the ease with which stimuli may disrupt the focusing of one's attention. Extreme polarization of attention is easy to understand in a musician who, for example, during a particularly creative period of a day, goes without eating or drinking for many hours.

The Prevailing Mood

Affect is the pattern of observable behaviors that is the expression of a subjectively experienced emotional state. Common examples of affect are euphoria, anger, and sadness. Affect is variable over time, in response to changing emotional states, whereas mood refers to a pervasive and sustained emotion. A range of affect may be described as "broad" (normal), "restricted" (constricted), "blunted," or "flat."

Depression is a common mood disorder encountered in some stages of neurotoxic illness. (Depression is sometimes *the* most common neuropsychiatric symptom in community-based surveys, particularly among the aged.) Depression may be associated with a cloudiness of consciousness, which might be the reason a subject does not perform well during the administration of psychometric tests. Apathy, sudden or slow changes in mood, or elation states not resulting from any particular personal event, feelings of being "high," and inappropriate laughter all are examples of moods with clinical significance that need to be taken into account in evaluating a patient.

There are standardized questionnaires for the assessment of chronic emotional states. The Profile of Mood States, described in Chapter 28, has been developed for a detailed probe of prevailing feelings. It can be used both in the clinical examination of people affected by neurotoxic agents and in epidemiological studies of groups exposed to such agents.

Learning and Memory

Clinical examinations performed in the context of environmental and occupational neurotoxicology cover the entire life span, from the possible deleterious effects of some neurotoxic agents *in utero* through the possible role of other toxic agents in the early onset of senility. Evaluation of learning and memory, therefore, is targeted to different life stages. A pediatrician or a child neuropsychologist is well trained in the recognition of the various maturational stages of the nervous system. In the child, learning of a large variety of motor and verbal skills is only possible when the nervous system achieves a certain level of maturity.

The evaluation of learning in the adult is very limited when conducted at the bedside. An uncooperative, apathetic patient often gives a distorted picture of his or her mental status. Since learning is so dependent on consciousness, motivation, and moods, the information provided by a patient's relative may be more appropriate in evaluating alterations in learning and memory.

There are many psychometric tests of learning developed in experimental psychology, such as paired associated learning or learning lists of numbers. These have been applied in epidemiological studies on the effects of neurotoxic agents. There is no consensus on the usefulness of these tests in the clinic. Computer-based testing procedures such as the ability to learn a series of numbers have been described for the study of learning in the adult (Chapter 29).

Memory disturbances are often found in many clinical descriptions of the effects of neurotoxic agents at the workplace. Office filing technology and computer jargon permeate the description of this important mental process. Memory is described as a process involving "registering," "storing," and "recalling" information and motor acts.

A scientist or a health professional is interested in knowing the subject's "recall" capacity for visual, auditory, and motor skills in three arbitrary time spans: immediate, recent, and remote. "Immediate" recall, sometimes called *short-term memory*, refers to the ability to recall a meaningful event that has occurred in the past few minutes. Subjects may leave a pot boiling on the stove for hours, or put water into the pot but not remember moments afterward what they meant to do. In extreme cases, such as those suffering from Alzheimer's disease, relatives are forced to remove the knobs of the stoves of people living alone to avoid such dangerous actions. "Numbers recall" during a clinical examination may or may not capture these extreme examples of disturbances of "immediate" or "recent" memory. Examiners cannot always put together whether significant failure in a test of immediate recall is in fact caused by alterations in concentration, mood, or lack of interest rather than by "recall" capacity.

Alterations in memory can be very profound, even leading to total memory loss, called *amnesia*. But most often memory defects are subtle; the inability to remember where one's favorite tools have been placed and missing highway exits while driving in familiar environments are examples. Forensic professionals are very aware of the presence of "amnesia" among malingerers (persons feigning illness to avoid responsibility or claim monetary "compensation").

Tests of short-term memory are available—eg, the Benton Visual Retention test, which has been used in both epidemiological and clinical studies.

Language

Language is an acquired skill in the use of body-generated signs for communication purposes. It encompasess both the signs and the set of usage rules the individual learns in a given culture. *Speech* refers specifically to the communication process carried out by sounds generated by the phonatory (speech-producing) system and registered by auditory, muscle, and skin receptors. The written language is a valuable source for the evaluation of communication, personality, and even motor disorders (eg, revealing hand tremor).

The clinical evaluation of language and speech is difficult because of the diversity of theories on the nature and neural control of speech. The clinician needs to be familiar with classical speech syndromes in making a differential diagnosis (eg, is it a neurotoxin-induced language defect or aphasia?). *Aphasia* is the inability to communicate. An extensive vocabulary exists to describe the large variety of aphasic syndromes. An important controversy currently exists regarding the classification and labeling of many speech disorders, particularly their localizing value, ie, where the neural lesion is located. The evaluation of language and speech in clinical neurotox-

icology still needs to be developed to its fullest capacity. Language and speech are underrepresented in the clinical literature on the neurotoxicity of occupational and environmental agents.

Clinical neurotoxicologists pay close attention to a large variety of motor and sensory mechanisms and demographic factors such as native language, age, education, and ethnic background in the interpretation of their findings. Slurred speech, for example, caused by acute ingestion of alcoholic beverages is an easily observable phenomenon. But reading difficulties caused by lead absorption in children need to be scrutinized further. Readily available labels such as *alexia* (loss of reading ability), *dyslexia* (difficulties in learning to read), *agraphia* (difficulties in writing), and *disprosody* (alterations in speech intonation) can be misleading and may inhibit further observations of unique patterns of speech disorders caused by neurotoxic agents. It is universally recommended that restraint be exerted in the use of these terms in favor of explicit descriptions of the language deficit whenever health professionals need to use them.

Thus far, there are no language or speech tests that have been proposed for the evaluation of subclinical manifestations of neurotoxic illness, subtle signs of dysfunction that precede actual illness or clinically recognizable disease.

Constructional Abilities

Subtle qualitative features of mental status are seen when subjects are asked to do things, such as to reproduce pictures or to assemble simple puzzles. Subjects challenged with such tasks have to plan a solution in their minds and then execute the steps toward the solution of the problem. Defects may be present in the perception of the task, in the planning of the task, or in its execution. That is why tests to assess constructional abilities are sometimes called "visuomotor" tests. There are numerous psychometric tests specifically developed to assess constructional abilities. The Block Design test described in the next chapter, for example, is widely used in both clinical and epidemiological studies of large groups of toxin-exposed individuals. In this test the subject duplicates geometric patterns with cubes.

There are many other tests aimed at the assessment of subclinical changes in constructional ability: reproduction of drawings, drawings on command, a large collection of object assembly tests, puzzles, etc.

Cognitive Functions

Despite a concerted research effort to understand the nature of intelligence, this highest order of cognitive function remains elusive. Is the vast array of primary mental functions considered evidence of intelligent behavior primarily inherited or acquired through education? This question has not been answered; the pendulum swings in both directions and the controversy is heated up at least once in each generation of scholars [see Gould (1981) for a lucid review of this problem].

When evaluating neurotoxin-induced disease, some clinicians rely on simple probes or tools to evaluate "intelligence." For example, a child neuropsychologist will ask a 9-year-old boy to perform simple arithmetic calculations, will ask information about his name and the name of his dog, and will ask him to recite a sentence or repeat numbers or assemble a puzzle, such as the figure of a person. In evaluating children, the amount of detail in the drawing of a person and how the parts of the body are linked give a good measure of cognitive functioning. However, often a clinical neurologist will need the help of a trained child neuropsychologist in the evaluation of difficult cases where neuropsychiatric signs are observed. Some health professionals use the total battery or fragments of well-standardized intelligence scales such as Wechsler's (described in Chapter 4).

Review of Symptoms and Signs

Universal lists of neurological symptoms and signs that could be used by untrained technicians to evaluate people suspected of having been exposed to neurotoxic agents have been proposed from time to time. One such checklist (Johnson 1987) is the following, in which subjects are asked to refer to the past month in recognizing the following symptoms:

Increasing Fatigue
Lightheadedness or Dizziness
Difficulty Concentrating
Confusion or Disorientation
Difficulty Remembering
Difficulty Remembering Noticed by
    Friends or Relatives
Need Notes to Remember Things
Difficulties in Understanding Written
    Material
Irritability Without a Reason
Depression Without a Reason
Heart Palpitation Without Exertion
Sleep Disturbances
Decreased Sexual Desire
Difficulty Maintaining an Erection
Difficulty With Balance or Coordination
Presence of Cramps in Legs
Loss of Muscle Strength in Legs or Feet
Loss of Muscle Strength in Arms or Hands
Decreased Grip Strength
Persistent Numbness, Tingling, or Pins-
    and-Needles Sensation in Fingers
Persistent Numbness, Tingling, or Pins-
    and-Needles Sensation in Toes
Headaches
Frequent Headaches at Work
Frequent Headaches Outside Work
Nausea for No Apparent Reason
Problems with Vision
Difficulty Driving Home from Work
Skin Rashes
Skin Excessively Dry or Cracked
Perspiration for No Apparent Reason
Unusual Taste in the Mouth
Frequent Stomach Pain
Changes in Bowel Habit, Cramps, or
    Constipation
Problems with Urination
Difficulty Breathing

Although such a list is of limited and questionable value when no other sources of information are available, readers under such circumstances are cautioned that no chemical, pharmacological, or medical knowledge supports the validity of such a list. Certain clusters of signs and symptoms are appropriate for the evaluation of a number of neurotoxic agents, but life-threatening conditions such as snake poisoning or poisoning with chemical products in the household could be overlooked.

Only physicians trained in toxicology can make the differential diagnosis between occupational (or environmental) diseases and medical conditions that might have other causes. Table 3.2 is a partial list of nonoccupational conditions that may mimic neurotoxic illness.

TERMS

Environmental and occupational neurotoxicology is a discipline that brings together the efforts of many health professionals, each contributing his or her field's own language. Many controversies on the proper use of terms have arisen and faded away over the past century. Presently, international efforts are being made to develop a unifying classification of neurotoxic signs, symptoms, and diseases that result from exposure to agents in the environment and the workplace. In the United States, the American Psychiatric Association (1987) published the *Diagnostic and Statistical Manual of Mental Disorders* (revised third edition) (DSM-III-R). But the DSM-III-R contains scant information on the large number of psychological and neuropsychiatric disorders caused by toxic chemicals other than by prescription or recreational drug abuse. The following deals with definitions of terms used in this chapter and later on throughout this volume.

To begin with a definition of one of the most common terms, a *sign* is an observable manifestation of disease (eg, hyperreflexia). In the neurotoxicological literature, the term *symptom* is sometimes used interchangeably with sign. Symptom often means a subjective complaint, eg, irritability, headache, depression. A *syndrome* is a set of signs and symptoms, eg, acute toxic encephalopathy.

Signs, symptoms, and syndromes develop over time. Clinical neurotoxicologists need to study the evolution of syndromes over time, also known as the time course or the natural history of the disease. Some syndromes develop in a matter of minutes or less (eg, loss of consciousness because of carbon monoxide poisoning); others may take a few days (eg, motor palsy from lead poisoning and the notorious delayed neurotoxicity of nerve agents used in chemical warfare).

Short-time toxic effects are called *acute*. In the vast majority of cases, acute neurotoxic effects imply that they are reversible after neurotoxic exposure ceases. Minutes, hours, or days after cessation of the neurotoxic exposure, individuals may return to their base line of neuropsychological functioning (as is the case, for example, with exposure to trichlorethylene). Symptoms, signs, and syndromes that develop or persist over long periods of time are called *chronic*. Chronic sometimes but not always implies "irreversible," meaning that permanent damage to the nervous system has occurred. However, this is an oversimplified statement because the limit of the nervous system's recovery power is largely unknown. An example of a chronic syndrome is the severe neuropathy produced by toluene sniffing.

There are other important terms. *Subclinical* refers to neurotoxic effects experienced by the affected individual but leading to no major condition requiring medical attention. Whether repeated exposure to neurotoxic agents at the workplace or in living environments produces subclinical effects leading to permanent damage to the nervous system is

Table 3.2.   Nonoccupational Neurological Conditions Mimicking Neurotoxic Illnesses

Acute encephalopathies	Myelopathies
Hepatic	B_{12} vitamin deficiency
Uremic	Drug-induced (eg, clioquinol)
Alcohol withdrawal	Demyelinating diseases
Electrolyte disturbance	Tabes dorsalis
Endocrinopathies	Indolent neoplasms
Viral encephalopathies	Lathyrism
Pharmaceutical agents	Hereditary spastic paraparesis
Anoxia	Cervical spondylosis
Postanoxia	Cranial neuropathies
Hypoglycemia	Systemic sclerosis
Chronic encephalopathies	Chronic meningitis
Multiinfarct dementia	Trigeminal neuropathies
Diffuse angiopathies	Bell's palsy
Alzheimer's disease	Diabetic neuropathy
Pharmacological agents	Miller–Fisher syndrome
(eg, bromism)	Myasthenia gravis
Wernicke–Korsakoff syndrome	Botulism
B_{12} vitamin deficiency	Indolent neoplasm and hematomas
Endocrinopathy	Syphilis
Neurosyphilis	Aneurysm
Chronical subdural hematomas	Optic neuropathies
Indolent neoplasms	Demyelinating diseases
Remote effects of neoplasms	Syphilis
Viral encephalopathies (eg, AIDS)	Drug-induced
Ataxias	Nutritional
Spinocerebellar degenerations	Chronic meningitis
Indolent neoplasms and hematomas	Hereditary diseases (eg, Leber's optic atrophy)
Remote effects of neoplasms	Indolent neoplasms
Vertebrobasilar insufficiency syndrome	Peripheral neuropathy
Alcoholic cerebellar degeneration	Diabetes
Demyelinating disease	Guillain–Barré syndrome
Extrapyramidal movement disorders	Vascular neuropathies
and tremors	Drug-induced
Wilson's disease	Nutritional (alcohol)
Huntington's disease	Hereditary neuropathies
Postanoxia encephalopathy	Disproteinemia
Dystonia musculorums deformans	Remote effects of malignancy
Idiopathic Parkinson's disease	Muscle weakness other than neuropathy
Drug-related dyskinesias	Polymyositosis
Essential tremor	Myasthenia gravis
Demyelinating diseases	Hypokalemia
Anxiety	Tick paralysis
Indolent neoplasms	Alcohol myopathy

Adapted from Johnson (1987).

now an active area of investigation. Subclinical refers to neurotoxic effects that cannot be observed during the course of the clinical examination either by the naked eye or by means of simple probes; thus, subclinical is a matter of "degree."

Another term, .*preclinical*, refers to neurotoxic effects that may lead to metabolic changes, behavioral effects, subjective symptoms, or neurological or psychiatric signs or symptoms leading to the impression that if exposure to neurotoxic agents were to continue, these exposures might eventually lead to a full-blown neurological or psychiatric disorder; thus, "preclinical" is a matter of time.

The concept of subclinical or preclinical manifestations of neurotoxic illness is not widely accepted. On one hand, it is obvious that if we were able to detect something that we predict will happen, that information is useful for disease prevention. On the other, there are experts who disagree on whether the search for subclinical or preclinical manifestations of neurotoxic illness that do not bother the patient is worth pursuing.

There are also disagreements about the classification of major neuropsychiatric disorders caused by acute or chronic exposure to neurotoxic agents in the workplace. A neuropsychiatric impairment that, in the judgment of a clinician who has all relevant data, has been induced by a neurotoxic agent is called a *toxic encephalopathy* or *toxic encephalosis*. Many reserve the term neuropathy for disorders of the peripheral nervous system. Thus, exposure to certain pesticides may produce a toxic peripheral neuropathy.

Another disagreement in terminology is the designation of a disease or illness as functional or organic. A *functional disorder* is considered by some to be the expression of changes in nervous system function—eg, the inability of neurotransmitters to act on target cells. The term "functional" means that no structural damage to the nervous system can be demonstrated, either in experimental laboratory animals or at postmortem examination. The term *organic disorder* implies an observable change in some anatomic portion of the nervous system structure caused by trauma, the burst of a major blood vessel (stroke), or a disorder caused by a neurotoxic agent.

The distinction between functional and organic is often found in the clinical literature dealing with toxic neuropathies. However, neuroscientists who work on the neural basis of behavior are not likely to use these terms. Major advances have been made in our understanding of the neurochemical basis of behavior, and new technologies are now available to help clinicians in ascertaining the etiology (the causes) of neural disorders.

One of the most heated debates surrounds the definition of *dementia*. Dementia is a profound breakdown in mental functioning. Most clinicians use the term dementia to characterize a mental deterioration that has an organic origin—eg, the long-term practice of boxing leading to brain trauma—or is the sequel of an unknown neuropathological process, eg, senile dementia. There exists a lively controversy on whether the term dementia can also be applied to describe the profound neuropsychological changes resulting from chronic exposure to toxic agents in the environment or workplace. An example of this is the term proposed by some investigators as the "painter's syndrome," where a profound deterioration of mental functions resembling dementia may be demonstrated. For a review of this problem see Waldron (1986).

REFERENCES

American Psychiatric Association (1987) *Diagnostic and Statistical Manual of Mental Disorders* (3rd ed. rev.) Washington, DC: APA.

Gould, SJ (1981) *The Mismeasure of Man.* New York: WW Norton.

Hamill, RW (1987) Autonomic dysfunction: Clinical disorders and pathophysiological mechanisms. In *Encyclopedia of Neuroscience,* G. Adelman (ed) p. 94. Boston: Birhhäuser.

Johnson, BL (ed)(1987) *Prevention of Neurotoxic Illness in Working Populations.* New York: John Wiley & Sons.

Juntunen, J (1982) Alcoholism in occupational neurology: Diagnosed difficulties with special reference to the neurological syndromes caused by exposure to organic solvents. *Acta Neurol Scand (Suppl)* 92:89–108.

Van Allen, MW and Rodnitzky, RL (1981) *Pictorial Manual of Neurological Tests: A Guide to the Performance and Interpretation of the Neurological Examination.* Chicago: Year Book Medical Publishers.

Waldron, HA (1986) Solvents and the brain (Editorial). *Br J Ind Med* 43:73–74.

SUGGESTED READINGS

Aaserud, O, Hommeren, OJ, Tvedt, B et al. (1990) Carbon disulfide exposure and neurotoxic sequelae among viscose rayon workers. *Am J Ind Med* 18:25–37.

Acres, J and Gray, J (1978) Paralytic shellfish poisoning. *Can Med Assoc* 119:1195–1197.

Arlien-Søborg, P (1984) Chronic toxic encephalopathy in house painters. *Acta Neurol Scand [Suppl]* 99:105–113.

Arlien-Søborg, P, Henricksen, L. Gade, A, et al. (1982) Cerebral flow in chronic toxic encephalopathy in house painters exposed to organic solvents. *Acta Neurol Scand* 66(1):34–41.

Asbury, AK and Johnson, PC (1978) *Pathology of Peripheral Nerve.* Philadelphia: WB Saunders.

Bagnis, R, Kuberski, T, and Laugier, S (1979) Clinical observations of 3,009 cases of ciguatera (fish poisoning) in the South Pacific. *Am J Trop Med Hyg* 28:1067–1073.

Baker, EL. White, RF, and Murawski, BJ (1985) Clinical evaluation of neurobehavioral effects of occupational exposure to organic solvents and lead. *Int J Ment Health* 14(3):135–158.

Bakir, F, Damluji, SF, Amin-Zaki, L, et al. (1973) Methylmercury poisoning in Iraq: An inter-university report. *Science* 181:230–241.

Bannister, R (ed) (1989) *Autonomic Failure* (2nd ed). New York: Oxford University Press.

Baraitser, M (1990) *The Genetics of Neurological Disorders* (2nd ed). New York: Oxford University Press.

Beritik, T (1984) Lead neuropathy. *CRC Crit Rev Toxicol* 12(2):149–213.

Bickerstaff, ED and Spilane, JA (1989) *Neurological Examination in Clinical Practice* (5th ed). Boca Raton, FL: CRC Press.

Blackburn, AB (1983) Review of the effects of agent orange: A psychiatric perspective on the controversy. *Mil Med* 148(4):333–340.

Braceland, FJ (1942) Mental symptoms following carbon disulfide absorption and intoxication. *Ann Int Med* 16:246–261.

Bowers, MB, Goodman, EM, and Sim, VM (1964) Some behavioral changes in man following anticholinesterase administration. *J Nerv Ment Dis* 138:383–389.

Buxton, PH and Hayward, M (1967) Polyneuritis cranialis associated with industrial trichloroethylene exposure. *J Neurol Neurosurg Psychiarty* 30:511.

Byers, RK and Lord, E (1943) Late effects of lead poisoning on mental development. *Am J Dis Child* 66:471–494.

Campbell, RJ (1989) *Psychiatric Dictionary* (6th ed). New York: Oxford University Press.

Chapel, J and Husain, A (1978) The neuropsychiatric aspects of carbon monoxide poisoning. *Psychiatr Opin* 15(3):33–37.

Cherniak, MG (1986) Organophosphorus esters and polyneuropathy. *Ann Int Med* 104:264–266.

Clark, G (1971) Organophosphate pesticide and behavior: A review. *Aero Med* 42:735–740.

Collins, RT (1961) *A Manual of Neurology and Psychiatry in Occupational Medicine.* New York: Grune & Stratton.

Damasio, H and Damasio, AR (1989) *Lesion Analysis in Neuropsychology.* New York: Oxford University Press.

de la Burde, B and Choate, MS, Jr (1972) Does asymptomatic lead exposure in children have latent sequelae? *Pediatrics* 8:1088–1091.

de la Burde, B and Choate, MS, Jr (1975) Early asymptomatic lead exposure development at school age. *Pediatrics* 8:638–642.

DeJong, RN (1967) *The Neurologic Examination.* New York: Harper & Row.

DelCastillo, J (1970) The influence of language upon symptomatology in foreign-born patients. *Am J Psychiatry* 127:242–244.

Dille, JR and Smith, PW (1964) Central nervous system effects of chronic exposure to organophosphate insecticides. *Aero Med* 35:475–478.

Dreisbach, RH (1980) *Handbook of Poisoning: Prevention, Diagnosis, and Treatment.* Los Altos, CA: Lange Medical Publications.

Dyck, PJ, Thomas, PK, and Lambert, EH (eds) (1975) *Peripheral Neuropathy.* Philadelphia: WB Saunders.

Ecobichon, DJ and Joy, RM (1982) *Pesticides and Neurological Diseases.* Boca Raton, FL: CRC Press.

Edgerton, RB and Karno, M (1971) Mexican-American bilingualism and the perception of mental illness. *Arch Gen Psychiatry* 24:286–290.

Ekenbäck, K, Hulting, J, Persson, H, et al. (1985) Unusual neurological symptoms in a case of severe crotaloid envenomation. *J Toxicol* 23:357–364.

Feldman, RG (1982) Central and peripheral nervous system effects of metals: A survey. *Acta Neurol Scand [Suppl]* 92:143–166.

Feldman, RG (1982) Neurological picture of lead poisoning. *Acta Neurol Scand [Suppl]* 92:185–199.

Feldman, RG (1982) Neurological manifestations of

mercury intoxication. *Acta Neurol Scand [Suppl]* 92:201–209.

Fengsheng, H (1985) Occupational toxic neuropathies: An update. *Scand J Work Environ Health* 11:321–330.

Flodin, U, Edling, C, and Axelson, O (1984) Clinical studies of psychoorganic syndromes among workers with exposure to solvents. *Am J Indust Med* 5:287–295.

Folstein, MF, Folstein, SE, and McHugh, PH (1975) "Mini-mental state": A practical method for grading the cognitive state of patients for the clinician. *J Psychiatr Res* 12:189.

Gade, A, Mortenson, EL, and Bruhn, P (1988) Chronic painter's syndrome: A reanalysis of psychological test data in a group of diagnosed cases, based on comparisons with matched controls. *Acta Neurol Scand* 77:293–306.

Gardner, H (1975) *The Shattered Mind: The Person After Brain Damage*. New York: Vintage Press.

Gazzaniga, MS and Ledoux, JE (1978) *The Integrated Mind*. New York: Plenum Press.

Gershon, S and Shaw, FH (1961) Psychiatric sequelae of chronic exposure to organophosphorus insecticides. *Lancet* 1:1371–1374.

Goodwin, DM (1989) *A Dictionary of Neuropsychology*. New York: Springer-Verlag.

Grinker, RR (1926) Parkinsonism following carbon monoxide poisoning. *J Nerv Ment Dis* 64:18–28.

Hagstadius, S, Ørbaek, P, Risberg, J, et al. (1989) Regional cerebral blood flow at the time of diagnosis of chronic toxic encephalopathy induced by organic solvent exposure and after cessation of exposure. *Scand J Work Environ Health* 15(2):130–135.

Hartman, DE (1987) Neuropsychological toxicology: Identification and assessment of neurotoxic syndromes. *Arch Clin Neuropsychol* 2(1):45–65.

Heilman, KM and Valenstein, E (eds) (1985) *Clinical Neuropsychology* (2nd ed). New York: Oxford University Press.

Horan, JM, Kurt, TL, Landrigan, P, et al. (1985) Neurologic dysfunction from exposure to 2-+-butyl-azo-2-hydroxy-5-methylhexane (BHMH): A new occupational neuropathy. *Am J Public Health* 75:513–517.

Joseph, R (1990) *Neuropsychology, Neuropsychiatry, and Behavioral Neurology*. New York: Plenum Press.

Juntunen, J (ed)(1982) Occupational neurology. *Acta Neurol Scand [Suppl]* 92:1–218.

Juntunen, J (1984) Organic solvent intoxication in occupational neurology. *Acta Neurol Scand [Suppl]* 98:105–120.

Juntunen, J and Haltia, M (1982) Polyneuropathies in occupational neurology: Pathogenic and clinical aspects. *Acta Neurol Scand (Suppl)* 92:59–73.

Juntunen, J, Matikainen, E, Anti-Poika, M, et al. (1985) Nervous system effects of long-term occupational exposure to toluene. *Acta Neurol Scand* 72(5):512–517.

Karmo, M. (1966) The enigma of ethnicity in a psychiatric clinic. *Arch Gen Psychiatry* 14:516–520.

Knave, B, Mindus, P, and Struwe, G (1979) Neurasthenic symptoms in workers occupationally exposed to jet fuel. *Acta Psychiatr Scand* 60(1):39–49.

Kolb, B and Whishaw, IQ (1985) *Fundamentals of Human Neuropsychology* (2nd ed). New York: WH Freeman.

Larsen, F and Leira, HL (1988) Organic brain syndrome and long-term exposure to toluene: A clinical, psychiatric study of vocationally active printing workers. *J Occup Med* 30(1):875–878.

Leestma, JE and Kikpatrick, JP (1987) *Forensic Neuropathology*. New York: Raven Press.

LeQuesne, PM (1981) Toxic substances and the nervous system: The role of clinical observation. *J Neurol Neurosurg Psychiatry* 44:1.

Levine, SP, Cavender, GD, Langolff, GD et al. (1982) Elemental mercury exposure: Peripheral neurotoxicity. *Br J Ind Med* 39:136–139.

Levinson, D (1987) *A Guide to the Clinical Interview*. Philadelphia: WB Saunders.

Lewin, R (1985) Parkinson's disease: An environmental cause? *Science* 229:257–258.

Lilis, R, Fishbein, A, Eisinger, J, et al. (1977) Prevalence of lead disease among secondary lead smelter workers and biological indicators of exposure. *Environ Res* 14:255–285.

Lilis, R, Valciukas, JA, Malkin, J, et al. (1985) Effects of low-level lead and arsenic exposure on copper smelter workers. *Arch Environ Health* 40:38–47.

Littorin, ME, Fehling, C, Attewell, RG, et al. (1988) Focal epilepsy and exposure to organic solvents: A case reference study. *J Occup Med* 30(10):805–808.

Maghazaji, HI (1974) Psychiatric aspects of methylmercury poisoning. *J Neurol Neurosurg Psychiatry* 37(8):954–958.

Mancuso, TF and Locke, BZ (1972) Carbon disulfide as a cause of suicide. *J Occup Med* 14:595–606.

Martin, JB and Reichlin, S (1987) *Clinical Neuroendocrinology* (2nd ed). Philadelphia: FA Davis.

Mathers, LH (1985) *The Peripheral Nervous System: Structure, Function and Clinical Correlations*. Menlo Park, CA: Addison-Wesley.

Matikainen, E and Juntunen, J (1984) Autonomic dysfunction in toxic states: Alcohol and solvents. *Acta Neurol Scand [Suppl]* 98:130–133.

Min, SK (1986) A brain syndrome associated with delayed neuropsychiatric sequelae following acute carbon monoxide intoxication. *Acta Psychiatr Scand* 73(1):80–86.

Morgan, JP (1982) The Jamaica ginger paralysis. *JAMA* 248:1864–1867.

Morton, WE and Caron, GA (1989) Encephalopathy:

An uncommon manifestation of workplace arsenic poisoning. *Am J Ind Med* 15:1–5.

Nishida, H and Yamada H (1984) A case report of cerebellar ataxia due to the use of lacker thinner. *Kyushu Neuropsychiatry* 30(1):55–61.

Ochoa, J (1980) Criteria for the assessment of polyneuropathy. In *Experimental and Clinical Neurotoxicology,* PS Spencer and HH Schaumburg (eds) pp 681–707. Baltimore: Williams & Wilkins.

Olson, WH, Brumback, RA, Gascon, G, et al. (1989) *Handbook of Symptom-Oriented Neurology.* Boca Raton, FL: CRC Press.

Perl, TM, Bédard, T, Kosatsky, T, et al. (1990) An outbreak of toxic encephalopathy caused by eating mussels contaminated with domoic acid. *N Engl J Med* 322(25):1775–1780.

Potvin, AR and Tourtellotte, WW (1985) *Quantitative Examination of Neurologic Functions.* Boca Raton, FL: CRC Press.

Rustan, H and Hamdi, T (1974) Methylmercury poisoning in Iraq: A neurological study. *Brain* 97:499–510.

Savage, EP, Keefe, TJ, Mounce, LM, et al. (1988) Chronic neurological sequelae of acute organophosphate pesticide poisoning. *Arch Environ Health* 43:38–45.

Shiffman, HR (1982) *Sensation and Perception: An Integrated Approach* (2nd ed). New York: John Wiley & Sons.

Spencer, PS and Schaumburg, HH (eds) (1980) *Experimental and Clinical Neurotoxicology.* Baltimore: Williams & Wilkins.

Spencer, PS and Schaumburg, HH (1985) Organic solvent neurotoxicity: Facts and research needs. *Scand J Work Environ Health* 11 (Suppl 1):53–60.

Sterman, AB, and Schaumburg, HH (1980) The neurological examination. In *Experimental and Clinical Neurotoxicology,* PS Spencer and HH Schamburg (eds) pp 675–680. Baltimore: Williams & Wilkins.

Strub, RL and Black FW (1985) *The Mental Status Examination in Neurology* (2nd ed). Philadelphia: FA Davis.

Tabershaw, IR and Cooper, WC (1966) Sequelae of acute organic phosphate poisoning. *J Occup Med* 8:5–20.

Tariot, PN (1983) Delirium resulting from methylene chloride exposure: Case report. *J Clinic Psychiatry* 44(9):340–342.

Taylor, JR, Selhorst, JB, Houff, SA, et al. (1978) Chlordecone intoxication in man. *Neurology* 28:626–630.

Teitelbaum, JS, Zatorre, RJ, Carpenter, S, et al. (1990) Neurologic sequelae of domoic acid intoxication due to the ingestion of contaminated mussels. *N Engl J Med* 322(25):1781–1787.

Thomas, PK (1980) The peripheral nervous system as a target for toxic substances. In *Experimental and Clinical Neurotoxicology,* PS Spencer and HH Schaumburg (eds) pp 35–47. Baltimore: Williams & Wilkins.

Torvik, A, Lindboe, CF, and Rogde, S (1982) Brain lesions in alcoholics: A neuropathological study with clinical correlations. *J Neurol Sci* 56:233–248.

US Department of Health, Education and Welfare (1977) Occupational diseases: A guide to their recognition (rev ed). Washington, DC: Superintendent of Documents, US Printing Office.

Valciukas, JA, Lilis, R, Wolff, MS, et al. (1978) Comparative neurobehavioral study of a polybrominated-biphenyl exposed population in Michigan and a nonexposed group in Wisconsin. *Environ Health Perspect* 23:199–210.

Valciukas, JA, Lilis, R, Singer, R, et al. (1985) Neurobehavioral changes among shipyard painters exposed to solvents. *Arch Environ Health* 40:47–52.

Victor, M, Adams, RD, and Collins, GH (1989) *The Wernicke-Korsakoff Syndrome and Related Neurologic Disorders Due to Alcoholism and Malnutrition* (2nd ed). Philadelphia, PA: FA Davis.

Vigliani, EC (1954) Carbon disulfide poisoning in viscose rayon factories. *Br J Ind Med* 11:235–244.

Vinkin, PJ and Bruyn, GW (eds) (1979) *Handbook of Clinical Neurology,* Vols 36 and 37. Amsterdam: North Holland.

Whorton, MD and Obrinsky, DL (1983) Persistence of symptoms after mild to moderate acute organophosphate poisoning among 19 farm field workers. *J Toxicol Environ Health* 11:347–354.

World Health Organization (1985) *Chronic Effects of Organic Solvents on the Central Nervous System and Diagnostic Criteria.* Copenhagen: WHO.

Wright, W (1922) A clinical study of fur cutters and felt-hat workers. *J Ind Hyg* 4:296–304.

4

Psychometric Techniques

It has been known from clinical studies that environmental and occupational neurotoxic agents could sometimes produce profound changes in behavior and neuropsychological functioning. With the introduction of psychometric techniques to assess those changes, it became possible to assess the effects of these agents in a quantitative manner that later made it possible to establish dose–response relationships between exposures and neuropsychological function.

BACKGROUND

The term "psychometric" means, literally, measurement of the mind. A *psychometric test* is a task or a set of tasks given under standard conditions designed to assess some aspects of a person's knowledge, skill, or personality. In environmental and occupational neurotoxicology, psychometric tests are administered to evaluate manifestations of nervous system dysfunction that are suspected to result from exposure to toxic agents.

Psychometry was born early in the 19th century in response to two challenges: the objective definition of mental retardation and the identification of school children with special education needs. Alfred Binet (1857–1911) is credited with being the first to develop a battery of psychometric tests for measuring mental age. The concept of intelligence quotient (IQ) was proposed by William Stern (1871–1938). During World War I, Army Tests were developed for recruitment of American soldiers. Many of the psychometric tests used today in human neurotoxicology, eg, the Digit Symbol test, now part of the Wechsler Intelligence Scale, can be traced to army tests assembled hastily during that period. For some excellent accounts of the history of psychometric testing, see Boring (1950).

The concept that individuals should meet specific challenges successfully in order to qualify for admission to certain circles of a social organization is found in most world cultures. In ancient China, civil employees were chosen on the basis of tough examinations; leaders among American Indians were selected, and retained their positions, on the basis of their proven bravery; in many cultures in Africa, adolescents have to demonstrate their hunting abilities before being admitted to adulthood.

It is generally acknowledged that the Finnish psychologist Helena Hänninen was the first to administer psychometric tests for the evaluation of the effects of toxic agents on the nervous system among workers exposed to potentially harmful agents. Naked-eye evaluation of the clinical symptoms of occupational neurotoxicity has a much longer history, dating back to Ramazzini (1633–1714) and Hamilton (1869–1970).

A psychometric test is both a task used in the clinic and a research tool. As a task in the clinic, it represents a challenge to the individual being tested. For example, some tests measure how quickly one can react to the presence of a light; others measure how accurately one can reproduce from memory geometric figures just presented; still others measure how steady one's hands are in a task requiring hand–eye coordination. As a research tool, psychometric techniques allow the quantitative assessment of psychological and/or behavioral changes caused by previously unsuspected neurotoxic agents.

The Standardization of Tests

In psychology, *test standardization* is a technical word that means the process in which the validity, reliability, sensitivity, and specificity of a given test are shown. However, there are many variations in meaning of the word "standard" even in the behavioral sciences. "Standard" may mean that the test or tests are widely known (eg, standard tests were used for the evaluation of . . .), that they have been used in a given fashion (eg, psychometric procedures were used in a standardized fashion), etc. (A further discussion of the variation in meaning of the word "standard" is found below in this chapter.)

The technical process of test standardization is a lengthy one. Briefly, the following definitions apply.

A test is *valid* if it measures the function that the test developer claims it measures, eg, reaction time, recent memory, motor coordination. In practice, validation of a test often consists of performing a study on how the test scores of the new test correlate with the scores of an old, well-established psychometric test. Expert ratings of people's behavior or performance are sometimes used as a source in the validation of a test. In environmental and occupational neurotoxicology this requirement is sometimes difficult to fulfill. Psychometric tests are used to assess subclinical manifestations of toxic illness, manifestations not readily observable by the clinician during the course of a neurological examination against which a test may be validated.

A test is *reliable* if it measures consistently what it is expected to measure. In the process of ascertaining how reliable a test is, a test developer employs statistical techniques to determine the internal consistency of a test—whether all the items of the test measure the same attribute—and the ability of the test to produce the same results when used over time.

A test is *sensitive* if it is able to pick up a neuropsychological dysfunction in individuals known from other sources to be suffering from such dysfunction. The Block Design test, for example, is a very sensitive test for detecting brain dysfunction and a large variety of mental disorders.

A test is *specific* if it is able to identify nonneurologically affected individuals who, from an independent source, are known to be healthy. **No psychometric test has ever been claimed by reputable professionals to be specific either for any neurological or psychiatric dysfunction or for any neurotoxic chemical agent or drug.**

It should be emphasized here that the process of standardization applies to any data-acquisition technique—electrophysiological methods (Chapter 5), imaging techniques for the visualization of the live brain (Chapter 6), checklists, personal inventories, sampling devices for assessment of environmental exposures among workers (Chapter 11), chemical analytical techniques for the detection of specific chemical compounds, some of which are known to be toxic (not covered in this book), biochemical markers of neurological and psychiatric dysfunctions (Chapter 9), clinical protocols of signs and symptoms of neurological or psychiatric diseases (Chapter 13), reproductive questionnaires (Chapter 14), markers of early aging (Chapter 32), and objective indicators of alcohol or drug abuse

(Chapter 33). Parenthetically, psychologists, often criticized for dealing with a "soft" discipline, are the ones who have made the most valuable contributions to the field of technique standardization.

Foundations of Psychometric Tests

What do psychometric tests measure? The answer to this question depends on, among other things, theoretical postures and the professional background and training of the neurotoxicologists who happen to use them. For some, a test such as the Block Design test (to be described below) measures visual organization; for others, it is a measure of a fundamental psychological process called cognition. In the Russian tradition evolved from the work of Sechenov (1829–1905), Bekhterev (1857–1927), and Pavlov (1849–1936), a psychometric test measures higher central nervous system functions. Wechsler, who incorporated the earlier Knox cubes—the basis for the Block Design test—into his widely used test battery, considers the scores in the Block Design test to be a measure of intelligence.

"Visual organization," "cognition," "higher central nervous system function," and "intelligence" are abstractions. In the technical literature, they are called constructs. A *construct* is something that is postulated as underlying nervous system function—therefore explaining how human behavior and/or thinking occurs—that cannot be directly measured. Constructs often are useful as labels that allow communication among professionals of the same as well as different disciplines. However, constructs should never be considered "real" entities. For an enlightening discussion of the use and misuse of constructs in science see Gould (1981).

With the advent of both the philosophical school of operationism and the psychological school of behaviorism, the latter represented by the work of B. F. Skinner (1904–1990) of Harvard University, labels describing mental functions began to be discarded. Operationism is a school of thought developed in the United States around 1927 as a result of the writings of P. W. Bridgman (1882–1961). This school maintains that scientific truths should be understood in terms of the operations scientists perform to obtain their data.

According to the operationism school of thought it is not necessary to state anything about what these tests measure. We know that psychometric tests can discriminate between subjects affected by neurotoxic agents and individuals not so exposed; ie, they are reliable and sensitive. In the absence of any overt picture of neurotoxic poisoning, psychometric test scores correlate with biological indicators of neurotoxic absorption; ie, they are valid and reliable. But we often cannot say why this is true. Behaviorism, as a psychological school of thought, was born in this philosophical environment.

The Use of Psychometric Tests

Psychometric tests are used in different contexts: as monitoring devices for the early detection of neuropsychological dysfunction among people exposed to environmental or occupational toxic agents, as part of a comprehensive clinical evaluation of individuals poisoned by neurotoxic agents, and as research tools. In order to know what psychometric tests do and their significance in environmental and occupational neurotoxicology, these three contexts have to be clearly distinguished.

Psychometric procedures are used as screening procedures in the study of environmental disasters or occupational accidents. The context is generally a medical field survey. The selection of the proper screening battery is guided by the neurotoxic agent(s) involved (when known) and the time and facilities available. In most of these studies, group results are reported. A screening battery is not comprehensive enough to make a clinical evaluation of the status of an individual who has, for example, collapsed after carbon monoxide inhalation. But data obtained from medical field surveys provide important indications as to whether there is reason for concern. Additionally, more comprehensive studies may be recommended on the basis of data obtained from medical field surveys.

A medical field survey, discussed in detail in Chapter 13, can be quite hectic. Except for blood and urine tests that are performed immediately after the subject has registered, subjects complete the various laboratory tests and examinations in no particular order. The purpose of the various tests has already been explained to the subject at the time of registration.

The question most frequently asked about the screening battery by subjects taking the test is whether this is a "test of intelligence." The answer to the question is obviously a courteous "No." One can add: "We would like to test the speed of your reactions to several tests of performance. These are not pass-or-fail tests: we would just like to know how much you can do."

Under field conditions, errors are committed by examiners much more frequently than under clinical conditions. Thus, scoring of the tests is not attempted during the field survey, where the goal is quality and completeness of the data collected.

A comprehensive battery of psychometric tests can also be used in clinical settings, eg, a hospital or private practice. Clinical psychologists are trained in the use of psychometric procedures for the evaluation of intelligence, personality disorders, evidence of brain damage, developmental problems in children, etc. Forensic psychologists are employed by the courts as consultants in assessing defendants in various phases of legal proceedings, such as competence to stand trials, prepleading investigation, suspected malingering, presentence evaluation, etc. Most recently, psychologists have acted as expert witnesses in courts in cases of suspected intoxication at the workplace. In the United States, the evaluation of preclinical or subclinical effects of neurotoxic agents in the environment or the workplace has only recently been called to the attention of professionals working in various fields. (The role of different professionals in such assessment is discussed in more detail in Chapter 38.)

In addition, psychometric tests are used as a research tool. For example, a new test can be proposed for the evaluation of a known neurotoxic agent for which a single test or a battery of psychometric tests has already been proposed, eg, the assessment of the neurotoxicity of organic mercury. Usually, the motivation for the development of new psychometric tests is to speed up the process of test administration while obtaining comparable results. As another example, a neurotoxic agent about which little is known in humans may be recognized as an environmental or occupational problem. On the basis of what is known from in vitro experiments with neural tissue exposed to neurotoxic agents, from animal models, and from pathological findings in a number of patients exposed, for example, to polybrominated biphenyls, health researchers may propose a psychometric battery designed to study the neurotoxic effects of exposure to these chemical compounds. As a result of these studies, some psychometric tests may be proven to be sensitive to the effects of neurotoxic agents, and others not.

What follows is a review of single psychometric tests, comprehensive batteries for adults and children, and tests that have been used for clinical and research purposes. Because there are thousands of tests already published and hundreds more added every year, the selection has been guided by the following criteria: (1) the tests have been used in human neurotoxicological studies, preferably by several investigators around the world, and (2) their sensitivity, validity, and reliability have been demonstrated.

REPRESENTATIVE TESTS

Classification of psychometric tests is difficult and is the subject of continuing controversy. Such classifications are generally based on constructs. For example, a test for the assessment of moods, such as the Profile of Mood States (POMS), does not mean that we know what moods are. As stated above, "mood" is a construct, a label attached to an unobservable phenomenon.

In spite of these limitations, environmental and occupational neurotoxicologists around the world seem to agree that the following "constructs" should be tapped in a core battery for screening purposes: measures of speed, motor coordination, visual integration, cognitive functions, measures of memory, evaluation of prevailing moods, and tests of verbal abilities.

Measures of Speed

Reaction time tests are among the oldest research tools in psychological research, and for several generations reaction timers have mirrored prevailing technologies in physical appearance. They were first built based on picturesque clock-type mechanisms. Then, electrical and electronic reaction timers became available. With the advent of personal computers it was almost inevitable that computer-based reaction timers would be developed. A large variety of computer games use the principles of reaction time measurement as their foundation. Although there have been numerous attempts to unify the physical characteristics of reaction timers, because their construction is so linked to the latest available technology, reaction-timer prototypes rapidly become obsolete in each generation.

Reaction time can be measured in response to simple stimuli (simple reaction time) or to a complex pattern of changing configuration, such as those of flight simulators or of computer games (complex reaction time). Some investigators use reaction time as the only test for screening purposes (Gamberale 1985).

Reaction timers have a distinct advantage over most other performance tests proposed for screening purposes. Most people, regardless of their background, age, and education, find them credible and appropriate for neu-

rotoxicological evaluation. Some have heard or read about the effect of alcohol on reaction time, and therefore, they accept that reaction time can be used for the evaluation of the effects of neurotoxic agents. Some other tests, such as those for the evaluation of personality, are not so easily accepted, as their use is often considered an invasion of privacy.

Scoring procedures for reaction time tests are not simple. In general, however, the shorter the reaction time—measured in milliseconds—the "better" the score. Each individual has his or her own statistical distribution of measures of reaction time. The distribution of, let's say, 20 samples of measures of John Doe's reaction time may or may not be statistically "normal." For all subjects, whether to take the shortest time value, the mean, the median or a given quartile is always an issue. Guidelines for the use of appropriate statistics have yet to be developed.

Motor Coordination

Tests of motor coordination have been incorporated in many short batteries developed for screening purposes. "Motor coordination" is a construct that is applied to different abilities as disparate as driving a car or threading a needle. The most common tests of motor steadiness are the Santa Ana Dexterity test and the grooved pegboard test.

The *Santa Ana Dexterity test* consists of a metal board in which four rows of square holes are cut (Fig. 4.1). Square plastic pegs having a cylindrical head with a black semicircle and a matching white semicircle are fitted to the holes. The subject has to lift and rotate each peg 180 degrees. Scores are based on the number of pegs turned in 30 seconds. The test is performed first with the preferred hand, then with the other hand, and finally with both hands. The test is not commercially available, but several laboratories around the world have obtained copies furnished by Dr. Helena Hänninen (Hänninen and Lindström 1976).

The Santa Ana Dexterity test has known

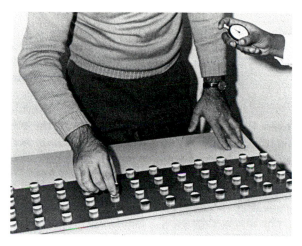

Fig. 4.1. The Santa Ana Dexterity test. (Test provided by Dr. Helena Hänninen, Institute for Occupational Health, Helsinki, Finland.)

shortcomings when its use is attempted in medical field surveys. In this situation, where as a rule 30 to 60 subjects a day need to be tested, the requirement of placing all the pegs back into the original position three times is a heavy burden for those administering the test. Under clinical conditions, on the other hand, Hänninen and her collaborators find this test to be a sensitive indicator for the study of the neurotoxicity of lead (Hänninen et al. 1978).

There are several other types of motor coordination and dexterity tests. Some were developed for the purpose of personnel selection. In a typical example, as in the *grooved pegboard dexterity test,* subjects are instructed to insert key-shaped pieces of metal into grooved metal holes. Holes are cut in such a manner that the subject has to rotate the metal piece in several positions to match the grooves cut in the metal sheet. Subjects are instructed to perform the task with both the preferred and the other hand. The score is the time in seconds that the subject takes to complete the task.

Two additional tests of motor steadiness or motor coordination have been proposed for an ideal screening battery of psychometric tests: the Mira y Lopez test and finger tapping. In the *Mira y Lopez test* subjects are

required to draw straight and zigzag lines and staircases with both hands. The task must be accomplished with and without visual guidance. Hänninen and Lindström (1976) have used this text extensively and have provided a scoring procedure. However, the scoring is cumbersome and time-consuming. It is best suited for a medical setting rather than for screening. The test itself was created by a Brazilian and is well known in Latin America in Spanish and in Europe in its German translation. It is hardly known in the United States except for those familiar with the work of Hänninen and Lindström (1976).

Finger tapping is a test comprising many well-known batteries of tests for assessment of brain damage (Reitan and Davidson 1974). The commercially available device for finger tapping is clumsy and requires considerable effort to strike the key. The box containing the key is not attached to a firm base, and either the subject or the test administrator has to hold the box to prevent its tumbling. Some subjects develop strategies for tapping. They tap, letting the finger vibrate over the key, thus developing extremely fast rates. Poorly motivated and noncompetitive subjects tap at very low rates. A computer-based version of the test overcoming these limitations has been developed by Richard Letz at the Mount Sinai School of Medicine in New York City, and is available through the Neurobehavioral Examination System (NES).

Visual Integration

In the *Bender–Gestalt test* (BGT), the individual undergoing evaluation is shown nine printed cards with geometric designs of various levels of complexity. He or she is instructed to copy these figures one by one as well as possible on a single page. There is no time limit in this test. The test is very brief and nonverbal. In drawing the figures, the person undergoing evaluation needs to rely on perceptual and motor abilities that are sometimes disrupted by brain damage (called "organicity" in the literature dealing with this test). Since the BGT was published in the late 1930s, this test has become an instrument of choice for psychologists who need to make a quick evaluation of suspected brain damage.

There have been many procedures for scoring test results. The one described by Lacks (1984), who also has provided an excellent review of the background of the BGT, relies on behavioral observations during the execution of the test plus items checked in a scoring checklist. Among the behavioral observations are signs of fatigue, insufficient attention to the stimuli, extremely rapid and careless execution of the drawings, dissatisfaction expressed for poorly executed drawing or attempts to correct errors, poor motor coordination or hand tremor, and apparent difficulty in seeing the figures. Features of the drawing included in the checklist are rotation, overlapping difficulties, simplification, fragmentation, retrogression (drawing showing characteristics of a younger age than the subject), collision tendency among the figures, closure difficulties, angular difficulties, and wrong relative sizes among patterns. The number and qualitative features of these behavioral observations and errors are used to conclude that the defendant does or does not exhibit signs of "organicity."

Cognitive Functions

The three tests reviewed first are the core of the author's own screening battery of psychometric testing (Valciukas and Lilis 1980). In their development, we relied on the concept of "apical behavior" described in Chapter 20. In short, the core battery of tests has to tap fundamental nervous system function without which other mental functions cannot be executed. "Apical behavior" is a construct—"the apex of behavior" is its highest manifestation. Apical behavior is synonymous with "higher-order central nervous system function" prevalent in Russian terminology.

In our studies of several groups of workers exposed to neurotoxic agents and controls, we have used the Block Design test (BD) from the Wechsler Intelligence Scale (WIS), the Digit Symbol test (DS), also from WIS, and the Embedded Figures test (EF). The Block Design test (Fig. 4.2) is widely used in the evaluation of neurotoxic agents. The test provides a quick and objective measure of the subject's ability to "perceive spatial relations." Extensive literature exists on the rationale underlying the use of this test in normal and in brain-damaged individuals (Matarazzo 1972). The examinee is presented with cubes having two red sides, two white sides, and two sides drawn from red and white triangles joined at the hypotenuse. The task involves arranging the cubes in such a way that the top surface of four (or nine) cubes reproduces a design displayed by the test administrator. In the first six trials, only four cubes are used, and the designs are relatively simple. In the last four trials (three, in the newest version of the Wechsler), nine cubes are used, and the designs are more complex. The score is based on the number of patterns correctly duplicated as well as the speed with which the task is accomplished. Figure 4.3 shows the correct reproduction of a pattern and some common mistakes in reproduction.

It is unfortunate that in recent revisions of the test no effort has been made to improve

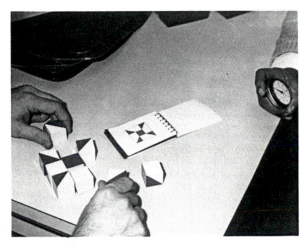

Fig. 4.2. The Block Design test. (The Psychological Corporation, New York.)

the scoring procedures. The procedure for scoring the first six designs can be easily memorized; the last four additional designs require that score norms be constantly present. Moreover, the population of the United States has aged considerably since the Knox cubes, later transformed into the Block Design test, were proposed as a psychometric tool. Many normal aged persons in their 70s cannot complete the last designs in less than 3 minutes, but they do complete it if one gives them enough time to finish the task. No scores are provided for these cases; in the available norms they are considered "failures." In ad-

ministering the test, if one sees that the subject is working in a rational, planned fashion, one needs to wait up to 4 minutes or more before withdrawing the pattern. We have extended the scales downward, and if subjects finish the task, they get at least one point.

The *Digit Symbol test* (Fig. 4.4) assesses the subject's ability to manipulate symbols according to a code. Because of its simplicity and sensitivity, this test is one of the most important components in batteries of tests used to assess neurological deficits. The subject is given a list in which digits from 1 to

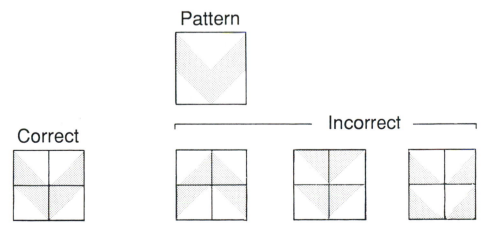

Fig. 4.3. Correct and incorrect reproduction of a pattern in the Block Design test.

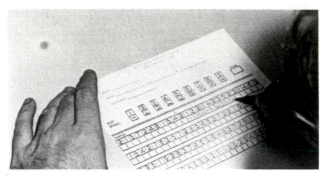

Fig. 4.4. The Digit Symbol test. (The Psychological Corporation, New York.)

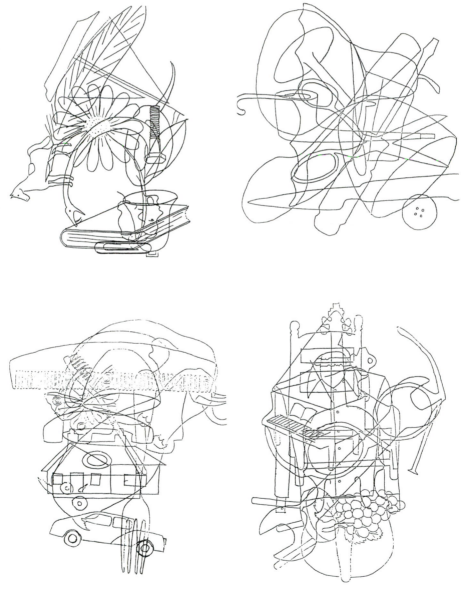

Fig. 4.5. Four plates used in the Embedded Figures test. (Copyright by Dr. José A. Valciukas, as appearing in Valciukas and Singer 1982; reproduced by permission of Academic Press.)

9 are associated with symbols and are given a form containing blank spaces next to a list of random digits. Subjects are instructed to fill the blanks with the symbols that correspond to each number. In a computer-based version of the test, the codes are reversed; the subjects are presented with the symbols and have to fill in the digits. The computer-based version makes the test more "cognitive" by removing the motor component present in the paper-and-pencil version of the test. Additional information on this test can be found in Matarazzo (1972).

The *Embedded Figures test* (Fig. 4.5) is an adult adaptation of figures used in the perception of overlapping and embedded figures by children of different ages (Ghent 1956). It measures the ability to distinguish figures from a background, an essential perceptual phenomenon extensively studied by psychologists of the Gestalt school. The subject is shown four sets of 10 superimposed outline drawings of common objects and is required to identify as many as possible. Further description of this test is found in Valciukas and Singer (1982).

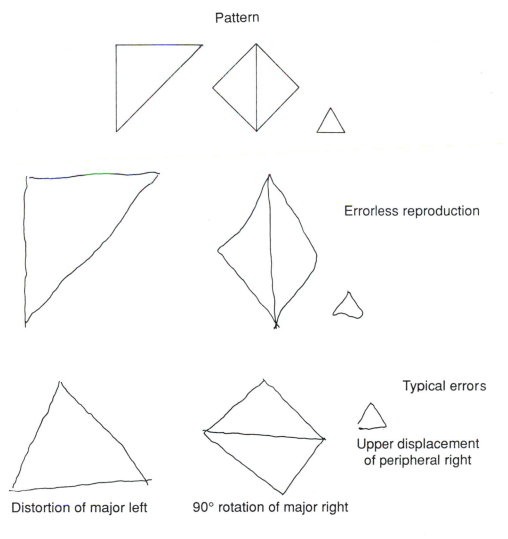

Pattern

Errorless reproduction

Typical errors

Upper displacement of peripheral right

Distortion of major left   90° rotation of major right

Fig. 4.6. Reproduction of a plate from the Benton Visual Retention test.

Measures of Memory

The *Benton Visual Retention test* (BVRT) (Fig. 4.6) is a clinical and research instrument used to assess visual perception and, in particular, visual memory. This test, or variations of it, has been recommended for the assessment of brain dysfunction caused by neurotoxic agents (Johnson 1987). The subject is shown 10 designs of increasing complexity, each for 10 seconds; this is followed by the immediate reproduction, from memory, of the designs by the subject. Both the number of correct reproductions and the error scores are used to assess the functional status of the subject's visual memory. Although norms for certain populations are available in the literature, norms for blue-collar workers need to be developed because age and education are important factors to be considered in the interpretation of the results. The commercially available set gives little information on validity and reliability studies. The test taps multiple domains including concentration, attention, and visuomotor coordination. Thus, in the clinic, the test gives a good deal of information not provided by other psychometric tests. Persons who are suspected of being unable to draw should be tested at the end of the session by having them reproduce the plates by direct copying.

Assessment of Moods

For the quick assessment of basic moods and quick follow-ups, particularly after accidents where absorption of a neurotoxic agent has occurred, the use of the *Profile of Mood States* (POMS), or inventories similar to it, has been recommended for the core battery of tests for neurotoxicological evaluation (Johnson 1987). The inventory is presented as 65 five-point adjective rating scales comprising six mood or affective states. Examples of these moods or states are Tension–Anxiety (T), Depression–Dejection (D), and Anger–Hostility (A). The instructions are simple: "Below is a list of words that describe feelings people have. Please read each one carefully. Then, fill in ONE space under the answer to the right that best describes HOW YOU HAVE BEEN FEELING DURING THE PAST WEEK INCLUDING TODAY." The numbers refer to the following descriptive phrases: 0, not at all; 1, a little; 2, moderately; 3, quite a bit; and 4, extremely.

The test is commercially available, and there are several companies offering services to read, score, and even interpret the score sheets. If the test is administered via a microcomputer, a trained technician is necessary for its administration, and a clinical psychologist with special training in neurotoxicology is needed for the interpretation of the results. The POMS has some drawbacks. Some of the adjectives describing moods are ordinarily not used in everyday language (example: peeved, muddled), and they may not be understood by individuals with limited education.

Tests of Verbal Abilities

The measurement of language and speech has a prominent place in the neuropsychological evaluation of patients suffering from brain damage. Although tests of verbal abilities have been proposed by investigators who work with relatively homogeneous linguistic groups (Hänninen and Lindström 1976), when used in heterogeneous groups, such as those existing in large cities, they are heavily dependent on command of language and culture. For a discussion of the use of language-dependent tests, see Anastasi (1982).

There are numerous tests for the evaluation of speech, language, and verbal abilities. Some of them, such as the *Peabody Picture Vocabulary test* (Dunn 1965), require that the subject match a spoken word to a picture. In tests of word fluency, subjects are required to say in 60 seconds all the words they can think of starting with F, S, P, or T. Because of the need to evaluate learning difficulties in the child, an extensive collection of tests of verbal abilities exists for this age group.

COMPREHENSIVE BATTERIES FOR THE ADULT

A number of batteries have been developed for individual assessment of the adult; this chapter also contains descriptions of batteries for infants and children. In the majority of cases these comprehensive batteries are administered in private offices or clinical settings. At the time of this writing, there are large-scale studies among veterans of the Vietnam War exposed to agent orange in which comprehensive batteries are used for epidemiological research, but results have not yet become available. Three widely used instruments are the Minnesota Multiphasic Personality Inventory (MMPI), the Wechsler Scale for the Measurement of Adult Intelligence (WAIS), and the Halstead–Reitan battery for neuropsychological assessment. There are numerous other batteries of tests developed for specific purposes (Buros 1974, 1975a, b, 1978). For a critical evaluation of such tests, consult Anastasi (1982). In the most recent protocols for the assessment of disability, a licensed test administrator should be able to document observational data as well.

Readers should be alerted to the fact that almost anybody can develop a test and obtain a copyright or patent. Many are commercially available and have received "endorsements" but have never been critically evaluated in peer-reviewed journals. Test-publishing companies often actively seek authors who want to publish their tests. Even college textbooks, which sometimes describe a given psychometric test extensively, escape critical scrutiny.

The *Minnesota Multiphasic Personality Inventory* (MMPI) was developed in 1937 (Hathaway and McKinley 1942). In Hathaway's obituary in *The New York Times* (1984), the MMPI was described as being ". . . the most widely used psychological test in the world." To date there have been over 5000 publications of the MMPI, and it has been translated into most major languages.

The MMPI consists of 550 affirmative statements to which the examinee gives the response "True," "False," or "Cannot say." In the individual form of the test, the statements are printed on separate cards, which the respondents sort into the three categories. Examples of the statements are: "I do not tire quickly"; "Most people will use somewhat unfair means to gain profit or an advantage rather than lose it."

A revised copy of the MMPI (the MMPI-2) became available in August, 1989. The University of Minnesota Press added some scales and deleted questions from the early version that were found to be offensive. Like its predecessor, the MMPI-2 asks true–false questions about feelings, symptoms, attitudes, and beliefs. The MMPI-2 sample includes 2600 people from Minneapolis, Cleveland, San Diego, Seattle, Norfolk, VA, Philadelphia, and Chapel Hill, NC and from the surrounding rural areas. The percentage of minorities represents that of the 1980 US Census. In revising the test, its publishers initially hoped to develop a shorter test. Length was found to be an inconvenience in the early version. This was not possible, and in fact the MMPI-2 ended up with an additional scale. However, the test items have been reordered in such a manner that if a subject answers the first 370 items the test administrator can still score the basic scales.

As a result of a factor-analytical analysis the individual items are classified on "clinical scales" such as Hypochondriasis (Hs), Depression (D), or Hysteria (H). The test is now available for automatic computer interpretation (Lachar 1983). However, it is strongly recommended that a clinical psychologist with specific training in neurotoxicology be in charge of the ultimate interpretation of the results. Further information about the MMPI appears with great frequency in many sources; a good guide to the immense literature is found in Anastasi (1982).

The *Wechsler Appraisal of Adult Intelligence* was created by David Wechsler (1896–1981). In the words of Matarazzo (1981), ". . . probably the work of no other psychologist, including Freud or Pavlov, has so directly impinged upon the lives of so many people." Wechsler is known for three major contributions to the field of psychometry: (1) the development of the test that bears his name; (2) the substitution of a deviation quotient for Binet's and Stern's concept of mental age that related raw score to chronological age—the intellectual quotient or IQ (In the computation of the deviation quotient, a group of the subject's age is taken as a reference for the appraisal of intelligence); and (3) the clinical testing of multilingual populations. Part of Wechsler's career took place at the Bellevue Hospital in New York City, where he was exposed to many different ethnic groups.

Wechsler's battery is not only a test of intelligence but also is a comprehensive assessment of psychological profiles. The battery can be used for the evaluation of brain damage and various psychiatric disorders. It consists of 11 subsets: information, vocabulary, picture completion, picture arrangement, similarities, digit span, object assembly, arithmetic reasoning, comprehension, digit symbols, and block design. Many subsets of Wechsler's battery have been used extensively in neurotoxicological research. Many professionals tend to discard those items that are heavily dependent on cultural and language factors, such as general information and vocabulary subsets. Some of the tasks may look silly for many healthy adults—eg, the assembly of a puzzle consisting of a human body and another of a human hand. However, these puzzles are very difficult to complete for brain-damaged individuals.

The *Halstead–Reitan battery* is one of the most widely used tests for the assessment of brain damage (Halstead 1947; Reitan and Davison 1974). The set consists of the following tests: categories, critical frequency fusion (CFF), tactile performance, rhythm, speech sound perception, finger tapping, and time sense. Some clinical psychologists add to this core set the trail-making test and an aphasia and agnosia test. It is generally recommended that the Wechsler Bellevue Intelligence Scale I or the Wechsler Adult Intelligence Scale and the MMPI-2 be administered along with the Halstead–Reitan battery. Thus defined, the complete administration of the Halstead–Reitan battery takes between 6 and 8 hours.

The *Luria–Nebraska battery* is based on research performed by Luria (1966, 1973). Luria and Majovski (1977) have provided an excellent review of the context within which the battery evolved. The battery consists of 269 items representing 11 basic nervous system functions: motor, rhythm, tactile, visual, receptive speech, expressive speech, writing, reading, arithmetic, memory, and intellectual process. The effort to standardize the content, administration, and scoring of this essentially qualitative battery has occurred only recently, so its full impact on current neurotoxicological and clinical thinking has yet to be evaluated.

The biggest advantage of the Luria–Nebraska battery over its most obvious competitor, Halstead–Reitan, is that it takes about $2\frac{1}{2}$ hours to administer. Flexible use of test items is possible, since they are considered as "units." Most batteries are built on the concept of "subtests," such as the Wechsler and the Halstead–Reitan. It is claimed that the "units" in the Luria–Nebraska test can be added or subtracted without altering the essential nature of the test. No such claim has been made on "subtests" of the other two well-known batteries.

The batteries discussed above—Wechsler, Halstead–Reitan, and Luria–Nebraska—provide an important arsenal for neurotoxicological evaluation. Thus far, the use of these batteries has been aimed at the important problem of recognizing early signs of brain damage. One school of thought would use certain responses to these tests as an indication of localization of brain dysfunction, although with the advent of nervous system imaging techniques (discussed in Chapter 6) suspected anomalies of structure and function can now be seen directly. The role of these batteries, however, in the assessment of disability and compensation is undeniable.

It is hoped that as the field of clinical and

experimental neurotoxicology continues to develop, we will see more and more applications of these batteries for the assessment of neurotoxic effects. A good introduction to the features of batteries of tests in nontechnical language is found in Green (1981).

COMPREHENSIVE BATTERIES FOR CHILDREN

Psychometric techniques have been used in babies and children in behavioral teratology or pediatric neurotoxicology. The purpose of this research is to determine whether a child's physical and cognitive development has been affected by neurotoxic exposure at home, in the immediate environment, or in utero. Some of these techniques have been in existence since the 1940s. The most widely known are herein reviewed. Those interested in a more comprehensive description of their uses are directed to Anastasi (1982), from which test publishers can be reached.

Developmental Scales

The recognition that the behavior of infants and children undergoes developmental stages can be traced to the important work by Gesell and Amatruda (1947). In the newest version of the *Gesell developmental schedules,* five behavioral patterns are assessed: adaptive, gross motor, fine motor, language, and personal–social. The battery can be used from the age of 4 weeks to 5 years. It relies on the examiner's observational skills plus some information supplied by the child's parents; high interobserver reliability can be reached after adequate training in its use. This scale, and others to be described below, are more appropriate to supplement medical examinations in clinical settings. In fact, because the tests are dependent on the availability of trained personnel and time, they have not, as a rule, been used in neurotoxicological research.

The *Bayley Scales for Infant Development*

were developed by Bayley and co-workers for a longitudinal study: the Berkeley Growth Study. The battery can be used for assessing development of children between 2 months and $2\frac{1}{2}$ years of age. Three groups of tests are provided: a mental scale, a motor scale, and an infant behavior record. The size of the standardization sample is impressive: it was selected to be representative of the United States population in terms of residence, geographical regions of the country, and demographic characteristics of parents and children.

The *McCarthy Scale of Children's Ability* is meant to be used for children between the ages of $2\frac{1}{2}$ and $8\frac{1}{2}$ years. It consists of six subscales: verbal, perceptual–performance, quantitative, general cognitive, memory, and motor. The standardization is based on 1032 cases, a sample that includes approximately 100 children at each of the 10 selected age levels.

There are other scales based on Piaget's theories of the child's mental development. But in the opinion of Anastasi (1982), an authority on psychometric testing, "all such scales are in experimental form" and "few are commercially available."

Tests of Intelligence

Tests of intelligence that have been used for the assessment of neurotoxic agents on child mental development include the Wechsler Preschool and Primary Scale of Intelligence (WPPSI) and the Wechsler Intelligence Scale for Children (WISC-R). The WPPSI includes 11 subtests only 10 of which are used to calculate IQs. The subtests are grouped into a Verbal, a Performance Scale, and a Full Scale, from which three different measures of IQ are calculated. The administration of the subtests is alternated to maintain the children's interest and cooperation.

The *Wechsler Preschool and Primary Scale of Intelligence* was standardized on a national sample of 1200 children: 100 boys and 100 girls in each 6-month age group from 4 to 6½ years. The sample was stratified against the 1960 US Census data with reference to geographic region, urban–rural residence, proportion of whites and nonwhites, and father's occupational level. Raw scores on each subtest were converted to a normalized standard score with a mean of 10 and a standard deviation of 3. The scaled scores on the Verbal, Performance, and Full-Scale IQ were then converted to an IQ with a mean of 100 and a standard deviation of 15.

The *Wechsler Intelligence Scale for Children,* revised edition 1974 (WISC-R), consists of 12 subtests. Two of these subtests are used only as alternates or as supplementary tests. The subtests are grouped into a Verbal and Performance Scale. The Verbal Scale includes information, similarities, arithmetic, vocabulary, and comprehension. The Performance Scale includes picture completion, picture arrangement, block design, object assembly, and coding (or mazes). The raw scores of each subtest are converted into a standard score within the child's own age group. Tables of such standardized scores are provided for every 4-month interval between the ages of 6 and 16 years. The scores of the subtest scales are expressed in relation to a mean of 10 and a standard deviation of 3. The subtest scores are added and converted into an Intelligence Quotient (IQ) with a mean value of 100 and a standard deviation of 15. Verbal, Performance, and Full IQ can be computed in a similar fashion. The standardization of the WISC-R included 100 boys and 100 girls at each year of age from 6½ through 16½ years, totaling 2200 cases. The WISC-R was stratified on the basis of the 1970 US Census with respect to geographic regions, urban–rural residence, occupation of head of household, and race (white versus nonwhite).

ADMINISTRATION OF COMPREHENSIVE BATTERIES

Tests described in the previous section should ideally be administered by a psychologist.

(Psychology is a licensed profession in the United States as well as in many other countries.)

Scoring Procedures

The scoring procedure of a screening battery encompasses two phases: (1) the scoring procedures of each test according to the rules the test developer(s) proposed for it, and (2) some elementary statistical procedures by which individuals are classified as being "above normal limits," "within normal limits," or "below normal limits." The first phase is described in Fig. 4.7 in a simplified manner. The second requires additional explanation.

A screening battery is used for research or monitoring purposes. When biological indicators of neurotoxin exposure such as blood lead levels (or lead absorption as zinc protoporphyrin) are available, a dose–response relationship between psychometric test scores and these biological indicators sometimes can be established (to be discussed in detail in Chapter 19).

In epidemiological research, the analysis of dose–response relationships is always based on group data. As a rule, a screening battery does not provide information about the status of an individual subject's nervous system

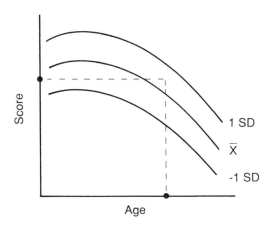

Fig. 4.7. Outline of the principle of test scoring. $\overline{X}$, median; SD, standard deviation.

functioning. But a screening battery can uncover individuals with neurological or psychiatric disorders, individuals who in the opinion of the test administrator require further evaluation.

Thus, the question of whether there is a potential neurotoxic effect from exposure to neurotoxic agents is both formulated and answered in statistical terms. That is why neurotoxicologists involved in the use of a screening battery in epidemiological surveys must develop a strategy for test score analysis even before going into the field. Among the most commonly used strategies are the classification of individuals as being "within 2 standard deviations of the mean" (if the distribution of scores is normal, which is rarely the case), "above or below the median" (for scores that are not normally distributed), or "falling within the first quartile" (or other percentile measure).

Scoring Procedures for Individual Subjects. All batteries discussed above share a common feature: they have been developed to assess personality characteristics, cognitive levels of functioning, and indications of brain damage in **single individuals**. The appearance and performance of the single subject—a patient suspected of being affected by a neurotoxic agent(s)—are compared with group data of individuals sharing similar characteristics, such as gender, age, and education.

Some of the scoring rules and test interpretations have been so highly developed that, as stated earlier, the individual's performance in some of these batteries—eg, the MMPI-2—can be "interpreted" by a programmed computer. Others contain recommendations for computing indices among specific sets of tests, such as contrasting language-dependent test scores with performance test scores in the Wechsler's battery. However, a clinical report resulting from the examination of a single individual does not contain merely a numerical profile. In most cases, a clinical report written by trained psychologists includes many observations and examples that

can be significant for the assessment of neurotoxicity but are not necessarily part of the test.

As has been well demonstrated by pioneers in the field of clinical toxicology, such as Hänninen and her mentor Hamilton, it is possible to perform good research while performing a clinical evaluation aimed at assessing the health status of an individual. A careful description of a series of case reports has been the basis of many well-documented neurotoxic effects. Under these circumstances, the clinical investigator is free to choose any test that seems appropriate for the assessment of his or her patient. Dr. Morris B. Bender (1905–1983), one of the world's leading neurologists, used to invent simple tests during the examination of his patients.

The freedom that is needed for the deep insight of a sometimes subtle psychopathological process certainly cannot be achieved by the use of a fixed clinical protocol. But epidemiologists and regulatory agencies need quantitative data on which to base their recommendations. The creative process that is constantly needed to keep science fresh and the requirement of quantitative data to make science useful often occur in different arenas.

Scoring and Interpretation Procedure for Group Data. Individual psychometric testing and, more recently, neuropsychological and neurotoxicological evaluation have solid statistical, neurophysiological, and toxicological bases. Individuals who administer these tests are specifically trained in the administration, scoring, and interpretation of test results. Part of this education consists of following highly structured guidelines for scoring, consulting atlases, case reports, and, most importantly, working for a period of time with someone very familiar with all required phases.

However, there are no similar guidelines on how to interpret group data obtained from comprehensive test batteries. Chapter 17 contains a detailed review of this topic.

Consensus on the Use of Psychometric Techniques in Neurotoxic Illness Prevention

Since the middle 1980s numerous attempts have been made to achieve an international consensus on a core of psychometric techniques useful for screening and prevention purposes (Valciukas 1984). These efforts are mentioned here because health experts who worked with psychometric techniques appeared to have been the first to recognize the need for such an international consensus. However, as can be seen in the contents of the most recent publications, since that time, animal models and clinical, pathological, electrophysiological, and imaging techniques have been added in international meetings on consensus. Only the most significant can be briefly reviewed here: *Principles and Methods for the Assessment of Neurotoxicity Associated with Exposure to Chemicals* published by the World Health Organization in Geneva in 1986 and *Prevention of Neurotoxic Illness in Working Populations* edited by Johnson in 1987.

Principles and Methods is a document intended to "aid in the design and assessment of studies concerned with exploring the association between exposures to chemicals and the development of adverse neurobehavioral effects." Although the WHO emphasizes animals as "systems" and "models," the book was written as an attempt to provide an overview of the principles of neurobehavioral assessment and to identify methods that have been successfully applied to the study of neurotoxicity in the past. The meeting grew out of a meeting held in Moscow in 1983 and strongly reflects the view of eastern European countries at the time. The book is organized into five sections: general principles, neurobehavioral methods, neurophysiological methods, morphological methods, and biochemical and neuroendocrinological methods.

Prevention of Neurotoxic Illness is divided into three sections: literature review, consensus and recommended methods, and strategies for prevention. The first section (literature review) provides the rationale for clinical, experimental, and epidemiological studies in assessing worker exposure to neurotoxic chemicals. This section summarizes a wide range of clinical reports, epidemiological investigations, and experimental studies. Also discussed in this section is the field application of research findings in the early detection and prevention of neurotoxic diseases. International guidelines for use and testing of human subjects in research studies are discussed, particularly ethical principles and participants' rights.

The second section (consensus and recommended methods) describes epidemiological, clinical, neurobehavioral, and neurophysiological methods used in early detection. Specific needs and purposes are identified, and test batteries for these contexts are recommended. Table 4.1 is a summary of such recommendations.

The third section addresses critical issues and additional methodologies such as hygienic standards, industrial hygiene practices, engineering controls, work practices, and material substitutions.

At this writing, an update of such consensus from a joint meeting by the National Institute of Occupational Health (NIOSH) and the Pan American Health Organization (PAHO) that took place in Washington, 1989 is soon due to appear (WK Anger, personal communication). From time to time, consensus documents have been unavoidably dominated by professionals who work in various branches of the environmental and occupational health sciences and who understandably attempt to have their disciplines achieve as much recognition as possible. The role of the professions and the context of research are discussed in Chapter 38.

EXPERIMENTAL PSYCHOMETRIC TESTS

We are currently witnessing the first attempt to standardize a multiple-purpose battery of

Table 4.1. Recommended Battery of Psychometric Tests for Evaluation of Neurotoxic Illness

Functional Domain	Core Tests	Additional Tests	Tests to be Developed Later
Motor speed		Finger tapping	Two-plate tapping
Motor steadiness	Aiming (Pursuit Aiming II)	Flanagan Coordination	Mira Tremometer with spectral analysis Body sway Tracking
Attention/response speed	Simple reaction time	Choice reaction time Simple reaction time (British Applied Psychology Unit)	Series of reaction time tasks with increasing complexity
Perceptual–motor speed	Digit Symbol (WAIS-R)*	Bourdon–Wiersma Neisser Letter Search Identical numbers	
Manual dexterity	Santa Ana (Helsinki version)	Minnesota Rate of Manipulation Test—Turning Subtest Purdue Pegboard Lafayette Pegboard Test	Mirror drawing Other psychomotor tests
Visual perception/memory	Benton Visual Retention	Benton Visual Reproduction Visual retention (WMS†) Block design (WAIS-R) Symmetric drawing	Embedded Figures Raven's Progressive Matrices Figure classification Picture completion (WAIS-R)
Auditory memory	Digit span (WAIS, WMS)	Logical memory (WMS) Associative learning (WMS) Serial digit	Tests for various aspects of memory Various memory span tests Memory tests with delayed recall Tests for auditory and semantic processing
Verbal abilities		Similarities (WAIS-R) Stroop Color-Naming Test	Verbal comprehension tests Word knowledge tests Word fluency tests
Attention/vigilance		PASAT (Paced Auditory Serial Attention Test) Continuous performance test	Other tests for attention or vigilance Time-sharing tasks
Affect	POMS (Profile of Mood States)	EPI (Eysenck Personality Inventory, version B) Taylor Manifest Anxiety Scale	Psychiatric ratings

*Wechsler Adult Intelligence Scale—Revised.
†Wechsler Memory Scale.
(Johnson 1987.)

psychometric tests for the assessment of brain damage induced by neurotoxic agents. Because, as indicated above, "standardization" has several meanings, it is important to review them in this section devoted to recommendations for test developers. "Standardization" means "uniformity of procedure" (Anastasi 1982). For example, test administrators in the United States, Australia, Colombia, and Finland use the same battery of tests, scoring procedures, and their own norms established under certain fixed conditions. "Standardization" also refers to the process of test development by which the author(s) of the test establishes the validity, reliability, and sensitivity of the test as a clinical or research tool. Cronbach (1984) uses the term with this connotation.

A review of the various phases of test standardization is beyond the scope of the present volume. Many sources cover this topic (Anastasi 1982; Cronbach 1984).

Guidelines for Psychometric Test Developers

The following are current guidelines for test developers compiled from various sources (Lezak 1976; Osmon 1983; Johnson 1987):

- Rationale and research base
- Degree of challenge for the subject or patient
- Cost
- Accessibility to instrumentation and supporting documentation
- Preparation for administration requirements
- Facility requirements
- Ruggedness and portability
- Ease of administration
- Credibility
- Professional requirements and special training for test administration
- Total time requirement
- Ease of scoring
- Data generation (quantitative and qualitative)

- Ease of interpretation
- Comprehensiveness and degree of redundancy with other tests
- Sensitivity to demographic factors, such as ethnic background, language, and culture.

Rationale and research base. A test can be developed in a variety of contexts. Some are empirical; they seem to work and have been in service for years. Examples are the Rorschach test, which, in spite of continuous use since it was proposed in the early 1920s, has been rated consistently as a poor psychometric tool (Anastasi 1982). Others have been developed in the context of neuropsychological research and have a fairly good rationale and research support.

As the field of environmental and occupational (E & O) neurotoxicology continues to develop, new tests for the assessment of central nervous system function or the functional status of specific target areas of the nervous system are welcome. Adaptations of older tests are also useful. For example: The Block Design, essentially a puzzle, is said to have been known by the Chinese thousands of years ago. The documentation of the Block Design per se or as a subset of Wechsler's battery for the assessment of child and adult intelligence is enormous. In most cases, computer-based testing procedures are an adaptation of familiar psychometric tests.

As a rule of thumb, a new test should never be "tried out" under field conditions. One should be thoroughly familiar with the test and possible sources of problems in one's home clinical setting, private office, or research laboratory before using it under field conditions. Many new tests have failed not only in E & O neurotoxicology but in many other branches of applied psychology. Failures are, as a rule, not reported in the literature. Many failures happen when the proponent of the test is not present in the field to make quick adjustments when necessary. If an experimental test does not live up to its expectations, not only is the credibility of the investigator at stake, but the overall medical field survey is jeopardized.

Degree of challenge for the subject or patient. A psychometric test should be a challenging task. Ideally, one would like to develop a test that could be administered to a patient admitted to the hospital with a stroke, to a blue-collar worker who is healthy enough to be able to perform normal daily activities, and to someone who claims—in court—to have suffered from environmental neurotoxic exposure. But this goal is difficult to achieve. Most of the tests developed for neurologically impaired individuals are not difficult enough for a worker examined in a medical survey. He/she finds them "silly." There are other problems as well.

If one were to ask who the Vice President of the United States is to a worker—a common question from clinical neurological or psychiatric examinations to determine whether the subject is well oriented in time or is aware of his/her environment—the question and the answer to that question will be known to most of those participating in the survey, and both the question and the answer will be passed along to everybody waiting to be examined at the testing booth. On the other hand, a computer testing procedure may be challenging enough for the relatively healthy worker but become a formidable task for someone experiencing the aftereffects of acute neurotoxic poisoning.

Cost. Project directors are, as a rule, budget conscious. Tests for neurotoxicological assessment that represent a significant percentage of the budget of a total research effort or medical field survey are not likely to be welcomed no matter how good they are. For this reason, paper-and-pencil tests are often favored.

Accessibility to instrumentation and supporting documentation. Several tests that have been proposed as the core of a battery of tests are not commonly available in the United States. As indicated above, the Santa Ana Dexterity test has been used extensively in Finland for the assessment of the neurotoxicity of various agents, but this test has poor

documentation and is not even mentioned in American textbooks dealing with psychometric tests.

Test developers must provide thorough clinical information on tests (eg, blueprints and circuitry) in case repair work is necessary. Ideally, computer-based procedures should provide the programs that generate the stimuli and, most importantly, the quantification of responses. If this is not possible because of copyrights or patents, test developers have to assure the user of such procedures which tests have been performed for the sake of quality control. Unfortunately, this topic has not been discussed as often as it should be.

Preparation for administration requirements. The need for reasonable preparation is rarely mentioned in current recommendations for a battery of tests assessing neurotoxicological effects. An instrument that is too complicated or that requires several hours (or even days and weeks) of preparation prior to its actual administration is definitely an inconvenience.

The Benton Visual Retention (BVR) test is highly regarded and in fact is recommended in the NIOSH/WHO core battery (Johnson 1987). For the examination of 300 individuals, 3000 pieces of white paper are required. For one who is involved in data management (see Chapter 14), each piece should contain the identification member of the individual and must have the number of the plate the subject attempted to copy. In the BVR tests, labels fulfill the additional requirement of providing the position of each piece of blank paper when subjects, patients, or defendants draw the memorized pattern.

The system or device should be easily understood by the test administrator. He or she should be able to repair or replace the system in case of breakdown. Ideally, no specially trained technicians or engineers should be required during the actual administration of the tests. Most laboratories cannot pay an engineer to accompany a neurotoxicologist to a medical field survey to be sure that everything works according to plan. Backups should be available for parts that can be easily lost, stolen, or broken.

Facility requirements. In Chapter 13 the circumstances under which a medical field survey is performed are described. In our experience, most local people who help to set up the site where the medical examination will take place are very cooperative in providing requirements needed for several testing sessions. However, note that tests of attention, concentration, or verbal comprehension and vigilance tasks requiring a silent room are unrealistic for conditions existing during medical field surveys. The booth where psychometric tests are administered is usually nothing but a table, two chairs, and a desk lamp in a small space delimited by hanging white sheets stapled to hanging ropes. Most paper-and-pencil tests can, however, be performed under such conditions.

Ruggedness and portability. Tests should be made from sturdy materials that will tolerate the unexpected conditions found in large or small hospitals unfamiliar to testing personnel. The rule of thumb is that the total instrumentation and the test results should be carryable by one person of average strength aboard an airplane.

Ease of administration. The test instructions should be clearly understood by subjects: they should be brief and to the point. But workers should not be treated as patients. At times, a professional accustomed to the examination of severely brain-damaged people or people affected by psychiatric disorders must adjust quickly to the fact that most people examined in a field survey are "normal," some coming to the testing site with their own cars, some traveling several hundred miles through several states. Before testing begins, defendants examined in the course of "toxic torts" require special instructions regarding the type and scope of information collected and issues of confidentiality.

Credibility. Even for individuals not involved in litigations, why the test is administered should be explained to the subject; this is now required by law. One must never assume that the subject understands what one is trying to do, even though psychological tests have been around for many years and most people have encountered them at some point in their lives. The context and purpose of the investigation—as understood by the subject—is of paramount importance in the acceptance of psychometric tests. The Digit Symbol test is readily accepted by most subjects even though a measure of mild exhaustion is often observed at the time the task is completed among subjects performing the test. A personality inventory is less readily accepted; as indicated above, some consider such inventories an invasion of privacy. However, a detailed questionnaire on stressful events, strain, sources of support, plus a personal inventory is readily accepted. The credibility of the test is important for additional factors. If even one out of eight tests comprising a psychometric battery is rejected by subjects, it is likely that the rest of the tests will not be accepted either. During the performance of medical field surveys, rumors may spread among examinees, and the booth where psychometric testing is performed will be avoided.

Professional requirements and special training for test administration. A good rule to follow is that the test administrator should not require that a task be performed that he or she is unwilling or unable to perform. During the developmental phase of the test, the test developer must have the test administered to himself/herself by someone else in order to grasp the potential problems and to solve them as required. Sometimes there are subjects with special needs (eg, the elderly, those with multilingual backgrounds) who require the intervention of an experienced test administrator.

A group of technical personnel is usually necessary in order to examine, let's say, 100 persons per day. At times, persons who help to administer the test must be found locally and trained in a matter of hours. Although it is desirable that tests be administered by highly qualified professionals, there are times when such professionals are not available. A highly efficient team can nevertheless be created with the help of alert and dedicated people.

Total time requirement. Some of the most comprehensive batteries of psychometric tests—such as the Halstead–Reitan—require several hours to be administered. In addition, scoring, interpretation, and writing the report and the conclusions can take many additional hours for each subject. These time allocations are unrealistic under medical field survey conditions. In medical field examinations, the collection of laboratory specimens and special tests may take 5 to 6 hours per subject. Under ideal circumstances, and particularly when the assessment of a potentially neurotoxicological problem is involved, the survey director may allow 1½ hours per person at the most for all psychometric testing.

Ease of scoring. As any experienced psychometrist knows, test scoring can sometimes be the most time-consuming part of the test. The time it takes to score some tests used—and even recommended—for the assessment of neurotoxicity is unrealistically long (an example is, the Benton Visual Retention test). Even the widely used Block Design test does not have easy-to-memorize scoring rules. The Digit Symbol test is one of the easiest, particularly when the commercially available scoring plate is used.

Data generation. Many psychometricians now favor computer-compatible forms containing the "menu" of all possible responses. Item analysis, an essential aspect of test development, is greatly facilitated by the use of these forms. Some experienced researchers feed data directly into personal computers. The file structure of these computer-based procedures should be known and understood by other people collaborating on the project, particularly the data manager, before decisions on the mode of data retrieval are made.

Ease of interpretation. Psychometric tests play an important role in differential diagnosis. By means of quantitative and qualitative analysis of results, it is sometimes possible to ascertain the nature of the brain lesion (eg, diffuse versus localized). But at the pre-

sent time, psychometric techniques are playing a relatively minor role in this type of assessment. During the past four decades there have been many advances in the detection of brain lesions. Imaging techniques allow us to "see" the living brain (Chapter 6). Therefore, the issue of using results of psychometric tests for the localization of brain lesions is now less crucial.

Rather, the role of psychometric tests is important in two fundamental aspects: assessment of preclinical or subclinical manifestations of neurotoxic effects and assessment of rehabilitation potential. The assessment of manifestations of behavior too subtle to be detected during the course of a routine clinical examination is what gave rise to the discipline of behavioral toxicology. In addition, the patient, his/her family, and health care team all need to know the time course of rehabilitation after neurotoxic exposure has ended. Moreover, psychometric testing is often recommended for purposes of deciding on compensation. Much more research is needed on the use of psychometric techniques in assessing rehabilitation potential.

Comprehensiveness and redundancy. Ideally, a psychometric test should be able to tap every basic dimension of mind and behavior: a battery of tests should be comprehensive. Even today, proposed batteries are difficult to suit everybody's professional needs. A comprehensive battery that is good for the assessment of brain trauma is not necessarily good for the assessment of the sequelae of neurotoxic poisoning; a test good for the clinic is not necessarily the best for forensic purposes where malingering is suspected. More importantly, there is still no universal agreement on what the basic dimensions of human behavior are.

Redundancy of tests, an unwanted feature, is often encountered in attempts to develop comprehensive batteries. Two (or more) tests should not be administered if they measure the same construct. An exception to this rule is the unusual circumstance when the results of one test are in doubt and additional information is sought. Redundancy of individual test items, as found in the scales of the MMPI-2, is, of course, a highly valuable feature of the test itself.

Avoiding redundancy is relatively easy. There are many statistical tools to show that two or more tests tap essentially the same brain function—technically, the same "construct." This is shown when the results of two psychometric tests are highly correlated or may become apparent as a result of factor analysis (Chapter 19).

With testing time always at a premium when one performs a comprehensive battery of psychometric tests, an examiner would like to eliminate tests that are redundant. But when one is administering a short, screening-type battery of tests with, let us say, the sole objective being assessment of cognitive function, redundancy is an asset (Valciukas and Lilis 1980). A high correlation among tests is, in the latter case, a good check of the presence of possible spurious effects—eg, low performance in the first test because of anxiety.

Other desirable features. The features identified below vary in importance according to the experience and context in which the researcher or clinician performs his/her activities. (This discussion is restricted to those that apply to the area of E & O neurotoxicology). Tests that depend heavily on language should be avoided. In multilingual America, especially in cosmopolitan areas like New York, test results obtained from a bilingual or multilingual person cannot be evaluated alongside results from a subject whose native language is English. This problem is recognized in the psychological literature but has not been properly discussed in neurotoxicological research. (The problem of language is further discussed below as an issue associated with the testing of linguistic minorities.) Tests should not be biased against any racial or cultural minority; such a bias might appear in a test developed by a representative of a leading cultural, ethnic, or linguistic majority who may have been blind (or careless) about test characteristics not easily recognized by these minorities.

COMPUTER-BASED TESTING PROCEDURES

Since the late 1970s, computer-based testing procedures have been developed for the assessment of neurotoxicity under clinical, laboratory, and field conditions. The author is unaware of applications of computer-based testing procedures for forensic purposes.

One of the earliest computer-based tests, developed in 1979, is the Behavioral Test Battery for Health Hazard Evaluation developed by Evelyn Williams of the Department of Psychology, New Mexico State University. It consists of subtests designed to measure psychological processes related to decision making, attention, motor performance, perceptual efficiency, memory span, scanning rate, and cognitive processing. The norms provided were based on 61 college-age individuals, 28 females and 33 males.

Except for the use of this unusual group as "norms," this was a very sophisticated battery even by today's standards. There is no quarrel in using college students as part of test development; the problem arises when these "norms" are referenced in studies of the effects of neurotoxic agents in the general population or among blue-collar workers. The description of the battery's features is available as a report to the National Institute for Occupational Safety and Health (Williams 1979).

Current Computer-Assisted Systems

The most widely known recent computer-based tests are the ones developed by Eckerman and his collaborators (1985) and Baker and Letz (Baker et al. 1985). Eckerman's system, called APPLETOX, was a joint project by the Department of Psychology of the University of North Carolina and the Health Effects Research Laboratory—Neurotoxicology Division of the United States Environmental Protection Agency. One of the most interesting features of this project was that, since its inception, the project's developmental status (including self-critiques) had always been available to those interested in the subject. The following is the series of tasks listed in their status report of May, 1983:

1. Keypress training.
2. Visual duration threshold with masking.
3. Simple auditory reaction time.
4. Choice auditory reaction time.
5. Choice visual reaction time with distracters.
6. Color block names.
7. Classification of letters as normal or reversed.
8. Switching attention: position/number/color.
9. "Fuzzy set" classification: cups and bowls.
10. Memory scanning for digits.
11. Forward digit span on touch telephone.
12. Learning supraspan digit strings on telephone.
13. "Simon sez" span of location sequences.
14. Continuous recognition of common words.
15. Keeping track of categories.
16. Keeping track of locations.
17. Recent chronological memory.

Implementation was contemplated for the following:

18. Testing vibratory threshold with signal detection approach.
19. Hand-with-ball judgment or up/down/front/back mannequin.
20. Physical/nominal picture matching.
21. Tone pattern recognition.
22. Continuous recognition of pictures.
23. Motor assessment: wrist movement accuracy, rate, memory, tremor, strength, and reflex sensation.

The APPLETOX (Eckerman et al. 1985) was expected to be a brief screening battery consisting of tests aimed at the detection of sensory, cognitive, and motor impairments.

Information on the development of this battery was available through a mailing list. The documentation contained information about the planned tasks and reactions to criticisms. In the latest documentation available (May, 1983), the project remained a good exercise in experimental psychology. However, to my knowledge, the authors did not test human subjects affected by neurotoxic chemicals in the environment or the workplace.

In 1985, Richard Letz, at Mount Sinai Medical Center, and collaborators published validation studies of their version of a computer-based neurobehavioral system for occupational and environmental epidemiology developed at the Harvard School of Public Health (Baker et al. 1985). The system is designed for an IBM personal computer or compatibles. In their most recent publication the battery consisted of the following tasks:

1. Symbol–digit.
2. Hand–eye coordination.
3. Simple reaction time.
4. Continuous performance.
5. Digit span.
6. Paired associated learning.
7. Paired associated recall.
8. Visual retention.
9. Pattern memory.
10. Memory scanning.
11. Vocabulary.
12. Mood scales.
13. Pattern recognition.

One of the distinctive features of this computer-based system is the background of its developers. Well grounded in the problems of assessment of occupational and environmental neurotoxicology, the authors tested their battery on workers exposed to organic solvents as they were developing the system.

Many other systems have been created to meet special needs such as testing the neurologically impaired. Some of these systems could be potentially useful for the assessment of highly trained personnel such as those in charge of cleaning up waste dumps. Contrary to the claims of many, computer-based systems automatically select and eliminate a large group of uneducated or unsophisticated workers or victims of environmental accidents.

Computer-based testing procedures are brief, good under conditions of continuously changing technical support staff, and comprehensive.

Indeed, as a data-collection device, systems available today do allow the rapid collection of data. However, the need to know a computer language such as advanced BASIC or machine language and to work for hours, if not days, to make the slightest modification in the fixed program is rarely mentioned. As occurs in the development of any custom-made software, one is permanently dependent on the programmer for the execution of changes. The computer programmer may have his or her own views as to how the test should be developed or corrected.

Computer-based testing procedures guarantee that the testing is performed—sometimes by a technician—under uniform circumstances. However, it is the general consensus that no one who is not professionally qualified to perform psychological testing should try to administer psychometric tests.

Many of the computer-based procedures are said to cover large segments of basic dimensions of neuropsychological functioning. This is hardly the case, for essential dimensions such as constructional abilities (as assessed in the Block Design) are entirely missed by computer-based testing procedures. At times, the instrumentation seems to take precedence over the real problems of health hazard evaluation or assessment of neurotoxicity. On many occasions, particularly in the evaluation of accidental exposure to little-known neurotoxic agents, one has literally to design simple tests on the spot.

An Update on Computer-Assisted Systems

Computers have been used not only for data acquisition but for evaluation as well. That is, the interpretation of test results is generated via a computer. In an editorial published in 1983 in the journal *Science,* Matarazzo— an authority on psychometric testing—raised important issues regarding the indiscriminate use of computer-based testing procedures and computer-generated test interpretations. "Since the results of psychological tests can affect decisions concerning employment, the handling of handicapped . . . , and diagnostic functions such as estimating deficits associated with brain damage, the quality of these tests is a legitimate matter for general concern." Such tests have a ". . . spurious appearance of objectivity and infallibility as a halo effect from the computer." Lastly, Matarazzo rightly stated that "Psychological testing carried out by a console is no more synonymous with psychological assessment than is the printout from a laboratory computer synonymous with professional assessment in clinical medicine" (Matarazzo 1983).

Since their inception, computer-based testing procedures have created lively debate. In a reply to Matarazzo's editorial, Green (1983) states that ". . . a paper-and-pencil test does not lose its power when it migrates to a computer." This may be so for the United States, where computers are readily available. However, many recent environmental and occupational accidents in countries other than the United States have taught us that our world is not confined to the limits of the continental United States. It is often forgotten that in most countries of the world, a computer is still an exotic commodity. Green stated that ". . . the appearance of infallability is closely related to the appearance of precision of numerical test scores, a problem that predates the computer."

ISSUES RELATED TO PSYCHOMETRIC TESTING

An investigator prepared to use psychometric tests for the evaluation of neurotoxic effects must be aware of other issues surrounding psychometric testing. Such matters as informed consent, truth in testing, privacy of information, bias in testing, psychometric testing and the individual's ethnic background, and psychometric testing among linguistic minorities are reviewed.

Informed Consent

Historically, the need for informed consent developed as a result of abuses by researchers (such as in the testing of subjects with drugs whose long-term effects were unknown at the time, or using prison inmates with syphilis to ascertain the time course of the disease). It is only in the past decade that proof of compliance with ethical standards has been required in research protocols from institutions seeking local, state, or federal funding. Many prestigious private funding organizations also request adherence to ethical standards.

Truth in Testing

This issue may not be apparent to someone not familiar with the details of psychological testing. Truth in testing literally means that one should do what one tells the subject one is going to do.

The following is a fairly good example of what to tell a subject about why psychometric tests are used in a particular field survey: "I will measure the speed of your reactions in several tests; when we come back to the lab, we will compare the results of your tests with other people working under different conditions." The explanation can be extended: "As you know, we are here to study whether people have been affected by substance X. What we do is measure whether high levels of substance X are or have been present here; then, we will compare your results as a group with levels of substance X to see whether there is any association." Further: "An association between the results of several people and levels of substance X will indicate to us that you—as a group—are affected by substance X. Remember, this is a group study; to determine whether you as a person are currently affected requires a more extensive evaluation of all the data we have gathered about you."

The following was an actual statement of someone guiding a local official through the different testing stations during the course of a medical field survey: "This is a place where people play with cubes and other things." Obviously, this is an example of a poor explanation. We instruct our technical personnel who have been trained locally to call a senior member of the team when an examinee asks for additional information about the purposes of the tests.

Many would disagree with the idea of a full disclosure of the true purpose of the test. Epidemiologists argue that by giving so much detail, one may introduce information biases. (Malingering and information bias are discussed in Chapter 12.) The grounds for objection are that by informing the subject about the purpose of the test, one may create a bias: the subject will try to perform badly to show that he/she is affected by substance X. This fear in most medical surveys is unfounded. Most subjects in medical field surveys try to do their best even when they are seriously handicapped. A healthy subject is invariably motivated by the challenge provided by most tasks. Moreover, he/she knows that one does not know the levels of biological indicators of exposure (ie, blood lead levels, urinary levels of mercury) at the moment of testing; one only collects specimens (blood, urine, hair, etc). Sometimes, the laboratory analysis of these specimens takes months to complete.

However, when people are examined in the context of toxic torts, the prior information they have before the forensic evaluation may be voluminous. A lawyer acting as a counsel to the defendant may, at the time of testing, have read as much about the offending toxic substances as the test administrator himself or herself. Before testing, the counsel has in many cases already explained to the defendant the purposes of the tests. Supposedly unsophisticated blue-collar workers sometimes come to the clinic with a highly organized file of clippings telling all about the signs and symptoms they are suffering, information that has been collected by several members of the family.

Privacy of Information and Examinee's Right of Access to Records

This issue deals with when and to whom the information gathered about a subject is available. The researcher needs to guarantee that a subject's name and any part of his/her personal data will not be disclosed without permission. In certain states, violation of this rule—if substantiated—is enough reason for a professional to have serious problems with his/her professional license. In New York State, if a visitor to a drug and alcohol rehabilitation center reveals the name of anyone other than the one he/she is visiting, this revelation may lead to a fine of $500.

In certain medical field surveys, workers may come to the testing site on their own time or on weekends because management will not authorize these examinations. Disclosure of the list of participants is thus feared by the examinees. At the Mount Sinai School of Medicine, we have been able to perform extensive examinations among thousands of workers in the past because we were able to keep our promise of privacy of information.

However, this information should be disclosed to the subject if he/she so requests. At times information is needed when the data from a particular study are requested for legal evaluation in court or simply when the subject needs to discuss his/her health status with a private physician. A medical field survey is usually followed by a rather comprehensive medical report sent to the subject and his/her private physician if required. Obviously, the subject is free to share the medical information with the company physician. Historically, these "subject-centered" policies have grown out of the fact that many companies do not inform their employees of test results.

Thus far we have referred to the scientist's direct obligations toward the individual research subject. But scientific concepts can and have been used for wider, political purposes. A notorious example of the social consequences of scientific research involved the interpretation of data of whites and blacks in tests of intelligence. Gould (1981) has written an admirable book on the "scientific" proofs of racism. Additional information on the subject is found in Bersoff (1981).

Bias in Testing

A psychometric test should be constructed in such a manner that its contents, administration procedures, and the analysis of its results do not give better chances to one group than another. If farmers were to develop a test of practical information on farm living and practices, most city dwellers who never lived on a farm would certainly fail: the test would be unfair to city dwellers. A comprehensive review of bias in testing is found in Cole (1981). Messik (1980) has written a comprehensive technical article on test validity and the ethics of assessment.

There are many types of test bias. The two most important ones directly affecting psychometric testing for neurotoxicological evaluation are cultural bias and linguistic bias. These are discussed below.

Psychometric Testing and Ethnic Background.
In many standardized psychometric tests, blacks score consistently lower than whites. Is this "proof" that blacks are intellectually inferior to whites? There are few topics in science associated with so many publications defending one or the other position. Let us examine how this issue affects E & O neurotoxicology.

The original developers of "behavioral toxicology" were Scandinavians. We are told that they do not have racial or ethnic minority problems in their countries since their populations are considered genetically and culturally homogeneous. As a result of such ideal testing circumstances, the issue of how to analyze neurotoxicological information in the presence of cultural and racial confounders was never addressed in the first publications on the subject.

Consider the following situation. As a group, blacks score lower than whites in certain psychometric tests. Let us assume that we compare two groups. Group A contains 30% blacks and group B 45% blacks. If we use a psychometric test for which blacks score lower than whites, we would conclude that group B scored significantly lower than A. If group B happens to be the study group—the group known to be exposed to neurotoxic agents—then most probably one would conclude that agent X is adversely affecting group B. The fact is that agent X probably has nothing to do with the difference in test results: we have not been careful enough in the selection of tests and have underestimated the importance of a good research design. That is why group differences should never be taken by themselves as a basis for a judgment of neurotoxicity.

When one analyzes the contribution of demographic confounding factors such as race in judgments of neurotoxicity, subtle factors may be overlooked. Unfortunately, job discrimination is still with us in ways surprising even to the most aware investigators. Blacks are sometimes assigned dirtier jobs than whites. As a result, biological indicators of neurotoxic exposure or absorption may be observed in greater proportion among blacks than whites. Without a careful examination of occupational histories, we may conclude that blacks are "more sensitive" to neurotoxic exposure than whites.

These issues have received little attention in neurotoxicological research. Chapter 18 contains a discussion of procedures for controlling for ethnicity. The social context of testing has been discussed by Gordon and Terrell (1981).

Psychometric Testing among Linguistic Minorities.   We conclude this chapter with an examination of the second most important source of bias in psychometric testing applied to neurotoxicological research: language. A psychometric test used for the assessment of neurotoxic effects should be fair to those whose native language is not English. More generally, a clinician or experimental neurotoxicologist should be aware of the role of bilingualism (or multilingualism) in the interpretation of test results.

Native language should also be taken into consideration in the interpretation of test results derived from linguistically heterogeneous groups. Whenever possible, the groups should be "stratified" (see Chapter 18) by language. The potential effects of language can also be analyzed in the context of a multiregression model (Chapter 18). The importance of this factor has been recognized in a meeting of the NIOSH/WHO, where experts from various parts of the world met to develop a unified core battery for neurotoxicological assessment (Johnson 1987). An examination of biases in testing linguistic minorities is found in Olmedo (1981).

CONCLUSIONS

A psychometric test is a standardized procedure to assess basic dimensions of human mind and behavior. Many psychometric tests originally developed for education and clinical psychology have been adapted for the assessment of toxin-induced neurological impairment. They have been shown to be valid, sensitive, and reliable techniques for the assessment of such changes. But they are not specific. A trained neuropsychologist needs to interpret the findings obtained by means of these procedures.

Additionally, the judgment of neurotoxicity is not based on findings derived from isolated cases only. Sometimes even group differences in psychometric test results are not incontrovertible proof that the differences can be explained by the exposure to a neurotoxic agent(s). The strongest case is based on a demonstrable relationship between measures of performance and measures of exposure and absorption.

REFERENCES

Anastasi, A (1982) *Psychological Testing* (5th ed). New York: Macmillan.

Baker, EL, Letz RE, Fidler, AT, et al. (1985) A computer based neurobehavioral evaluation system for occupational and environmental epidemiology: Methodology and validation studies. *Neurobehav Toxicol Teratol* 7:369–377.

Bersoff, DN (1981) Testing and the law. *Am Psychol* 36(10):1047–1056.

Boring, EG (1950) *A History of Experimental Psychology.* New York: Appleton-Century-Crofts.

Buros, OK (ed) (1974) *Tests in Print II.* Lincoln: University of Nebraska, Buros Institute of Mental Measurement.

Buros, OK (ed) (1975a) *Intelligence Tests and Reviews.* Lincoln: University of Nebraska, Buros Institute of Mental Measurement.

Buros, OK (ed) (1975b) *Personality Tests and Reviews II.* Lincoln: University of Nebraska, Buros Institute of Mental Measurement.

Buros, OK (ed) (1978) *The Eighth Mental Measurement Yearbook.* Lincoln: University of Nebraska, Buros Institute of Mental Measurement.

Cole, NS (1981) Bias in testing. *Am Psychol* 36(10):1067–1077.

Cronbach, LJ (1984) *Essentials of Psychological Testing* (4th ed). New York: Harper & Row.

Dunn, LM (1965) *Expanded Manual for the Peabody Picture Vocabulary Test.* Minneapolis: American Guidance Service.

Eckerman, DA, Caroll, JB, Foree, D, et al. (1985) An approach to brief field testing for neurotoxicity. *Neurobehav Toxicol Teratol* 7(4):387–393.

Gamberale, F (1985) The use of behavioral performance tests in the assessment of solvent toxicity. *Scand J Work Environ Health [Suppl]* 27:206–212.

Gessell, A and Amatruda, CS (1947) *Developmental Diagnosis* (2nd ed). New York: Hoeber-Harper.

Ghent, L (1956) Perception of overlapping and imbedded figures by children of different ages. *Am J Psychol* 69:576–587.

Gordon, EW and Terrell, MD (1981) The changed social context of testing. *Am Psychol* 36(10):1167–1171.

Gould, SJ (1981) *The Mismeasure of Man.* New York: WW Norton.

Green, BF (1981) A primer of testing. *Am Psychol* 36(10):1001–1011.

Green, BF (1983) Computer testing (Letters). *Science* 222:1181.

Halstead, WC (1947) *Brain and Intelligence.* Chicago: University of Chicago Press.

Hänninen, H and Lindström, K (1976) *A Battery for Toxipsychological Evaluation.* Helsinki: Institute of Occupational Health.

Hänninen, H, Hernberg, S, Mantere, P, et al. (1978) Psychological performance of subjects with low exposure to lead. *J Occup Med* 20:683–689.

Hathaway, SR and McKinley, JC (1942) A multiphasic personality schedule (Minnesota) III. The measurement of symptomatic depression. *J Psychol* 14:73–84.

Johnson, BL (ed) (1987) *Prevention of Neurotoxic Illness in Working Populations.* New York: John Wiley & Sons.

Lachar, D (1983) *The MMPI: Clinical Assessment and Automatic Interpretation.* Los Angeles: Western Psychological Services.

Lacks, P (1984) *Bender Gestalt Screening for Brain Dysfunction.* New York: John Wiley & Sons.

Lezak, MD (1976) *Neuropsychological Assessment.* New York: Oxford University Press.

Luria, AR (1966) *Higher Cortical Functions in Man.* New York: Basic Books.

Luria AR (1973) *The Working Brain.* New York: Basic Books.

Luria, AR and Majowski, LV (1977) Basic approaches used in American and Soviet clinical neuropsychology. *Am Psychol* 32:959–968.

Matarazzo, JD (1972) *Wechsler's Measurement and Appraisal of Adult Intelligence* (5th ed). Baltimore: Williams & Wilkins.

Matarazzo, JD (1981) Obituary: David Wechsler (1896–1981). *Am Psychol* 36:1542–1543.

Matarazzo, JD (1983) Computerized psychological testing (Editorial). *Science* 221:323.

Messik, S (1980) Test validity and ethics of assessment. *Am Psychol* 35:1012–1027.

New York Times (1984) Obituary: Dr. Starke R. Hathaway, 80: Invented a Psychological Test. Thursday, July 5.

Olmedo, E (1981) Testing linguistic minorities. *Am Psychol* 36:1078–1085.

Osmon, DC (1983) The use of test batteries in clinical neuropsychology. In *Foundations of Clinical Neuropsychology,* CJ Golden and RJ Vincente (eds). New York: Plenum Press, pp. 113–141.

Reitan, RM and Davidson, LA (eds) (1974) *Clinical Neuropsychology: Current Status and Applications.* New York: Halsted.

Reitan, RM and Davison, LA (1974) *Clinical Neuropsychology: Clinical Status and Applications.* New York: Winston/Wiley.

Valciukas, JA (1984) A decade of behavioral toxicology: Impressions of a NIOSH–WHO workshop in Cincinnati, Ohio, May 1983. *Am J Ind Med* 5:405–406.

Valciukas, JA and Lilis, R (1980) Psychometric techniques in environmental research. *Environ Res* 21:275–297.

Valciukas, JA and Singer, RM (1982) An embedded figure test in environmental and occupational neurotoxicology. *Environ Res* 28:183–198.

Williams, E (Principal investigator) (1979) *Behavioral Test Battery for Health Hazard Evaluation. Report to the National Institute for Occupational Safety and Health.* Washington, DC: NIOSH.

World Health Organization (1986) *Principles and Methods for the Assessment of Neurotoxicity Associated with Exposure to Chemicals.* Geneva, WHO.

SUGGESTED READINGS

Acker, W (1980) In support of microcomputer based automated testing: A description of the Maudsley Automated Psychological Screening test (MAPS). *Br J Alcoholism* 15:144–147.

Adler, T (1989) Revision brings test 'to the 21st century' [MMPI-2]. *Psychol Monit* 20(11), November.

American Psychological Association (1974) *Standards for Educational and Psychological Tests.* Washington, DC: APA.

American Psychological Association (1986) *Guidelines for Computer-Based Tests and Interpretations.* Washington, DC: APA.

Anger, WK (1985) Overview of NIOSH neurobehavioral testing/research. *Neurobehav Toxicol Teratol* 7(4):289–290.

Baumring, D (1985) Research using intentional deception. *Am J Psychol* Vol. 2 Feb, 165–174.

Bender, L (1938) *A Visual Motor Gestalt Test and Its Clinical Use.* New York: American Orthopsychiatric Association.

Bender, MB (1952) *Disorders in Perception.* Springfield, IL: Charles C. Thomas.

Benton, AL (1974) *Revised Visual Retention Test Manual.* New York: Psychological Corporation.

Benton, AL, Des Hamsher, K, Varney, NR, et al. (1983) *Contributions to Neuropsychological Assessment.* New York: Oxford University Press.

Bittner, AC, Smith, MG, Kennedy, RS, et al. (1985) Automated portable test (APT) system: Overview and prospects. *Behav Res Methods Inst Comput* 17(2):217–221.

Bittner, AC, Carter, RC, Kennedy, RS, et al. (1986) Performance evaluation tests for environmental research (PETER): Evaluation of 114 measures. *Percept Motor Skills* 63:683–708.

Bowler, RM, Thaler, CD, and Becker, CE (1986) California Neuropsychological Screening Battery (CNS/BI & II). *J Clin Psychol* 42(6):946–955.

Branconier, RJ (1985) Dementia in human populations exposed to neurotoxic agents: A portable microcomputerized dementia screening battery. *Neurobehav Toxicol Teratol* 7(4):379–386.

Bridgman, PW (1927) *The Logics of Modern Physics.* New York: Crowell-Collier-Macmillan.

Buros, OK (ed) (1970) *Personality Tests and Reviews I.* Lincoln: University of Nebraska, Buros Institute of Mental Measurement.

Chapman, PD (1988) *Schools as Sorters: Lewis M Terman, Applied Psychology and the Intelligence Testing Movement, 1890–1930.* New York: New York University Press.

Cherry, N, Waldron, HA, Wells, GG, et al. (1980) An investigation of the acute behavioral effects of styrene on factory workers. *Br J Ind Med* 37:234–240.

Ciminero, AR, Calhoun, KS, and Adams, HE (eds) (1986) *Handbook of Behavioral Assessment* (2nd ed). New York: John Wiley & Sons.

Delaney, RC (1982) Screening for organicity: The problem of subtle neuropsychological deficit and diagnosis. *J Clin Psychol* 38:843–846.

Derner, GF, Aborn, M, and Canter, AH (1950) The reliability of the Wechsler Bellevue subtests and scales. *Consult Psychol* 14:172–179.

Dick, RB (1988) Short duration exposures to organic solvents: The relationship between neurobehavioral test results and other indicators. *Neurotoxicol Teratol* 10(1):39–50.

Eckerman, ED (Principal investigator) (1982) *Progress Report for the Appletox Project.* Chapel Hill: Department of Psychology, The University of North Carolina.

Erickson, RC and Scott, ML (1977) Clinical memory testing: A review. *Psychol Bull* 84:1130.

Eskelinen, L, Luisto, M, Tenkanen, L, et al. (1986) Neuropsychological methods in the differentiation of organic solvent intoxication from certain neurological conditions. *J Clin Exp Neuropsychol* 8(3):239–256.

Fleishman, EA and Quaintance, MK (1984) *Taxonomies of Human Performance: The Description of Human Tasks.* New York: Academic Press.

Frankenburg, WK, Camp, BW, and Van Natta, PA (1971) Validity of the Denver Developmental Screening Test. *Child Dev* 42:475–485.

Gamberale, F and Hultengren, M (1973) Methylchloroform exposure: II. Psychophysiological functions. *Work Environ Health* 10:82–92.

Gamberale, F, Annwall, G, and Olson, BA (1976) Exposure to trichloroethylene: III. Psychological functions. *Scand J Work Environ Health* 4:220–224.

Gamberale, F, Annwall, G, and Hultengren, M (1978) Exposure to xylene and ethylbenzene: III. Effects on central nervous functions. *Scand J Work Environ Health* 4:204–211.

Golden, CJ, Hammeke, TA, and Purisch, A (1980) *The Luria–Nebraska Neuropsychological Battery: A Manual for Clinical and Experimental Uses.* Lincoln: University of Nebraska Press.

Golden, CJ, Osmon, DC, Moses, JA, et al. (1981) *Interpretation of the Halstead–Reitan Neuropsychological Test Battery: A casebook approach.* New York: Grune & Stratton.

Hall, JA (1978) Gender effects in decoding nonverbal cues. *Psychol Bull* 85:845–857.

Haney, W (1981) Validity, vaudeville, and values: A

short history of social concerns over standardized testing. *Am Psychol* 36:1021–1034.

Hänninen, H (1985) Twenty-five years of behaviorial toxicology within occupation medicine: A personal account. *Am J Ind Med* 7:19–30.

Hänninen, H (1988) The psychological performance profile in occupational intoxication. *Neurotoxicol Teratol* 10(5):485–488.

Hänninen, H, Eskelinen, L, Husman, K, et al. (1976) Behavioral effects of long-term exposure to a mixture of organic solvents. *Scand J Work Environ Health* 4:240–255.

Harbeson, MM, Bittner, AC, Kennedy, RS, et al. (1983) Performance evaluation tests for environmental research (PETER). *Bibl Percept Motor Skills* 57:283–293.

Harbeson, MM, Krause, M, Kennedy, RS, et al. (1982) The Stroop as a performance evaluation test for environmental research. *J Psychol* 111:223–233.

Hinton, HL (1988) *Lewis M Terman: Pioneer in Psychological Testing.* New York: New York University Press.

Jensen, AR (1980) *Bias in Mental Testing.* New York: The Free Press.

Jensen, AR and Rohwer, WD (1966) The Stroop color–word test: A review. *Acta Psychol* 25:36–93.

Johnson, JH and Johnson, KN (1981) Psychological considerations related to the development of testing stations. *Behav Res Methods Instr* 13:421.

Jones, MB, Kennedy, RS, and Bittner, AC (1981) A video game for performance testing. *Am J Psychol* 94:143–152.

Kamin, LJ (1974) *The Science and Politics of IQ.* Potomac, MD: Lawrence Erlbaum.

Kaplan, RM and Sacuzzo, DP (1988) *Psychological Testing* (2nd ed). Pacific Grove, CA: Brooks/Cole.

Kennedy, RS, Bittner, AC, Harbeson, MM, et al. (1982) Television-computer games: A "new look" in performance testing. *Aviation Space Environ Med* 53:49–53.

Kennedy, RS, Wilkes, RL, Dunlap, WP, et al. (1987) Development of an automated performance test system for environmental and behavioral toxicology. *Percept Motor Skills* 65(3):947–962.

Koppitz, E (1975) *The Bender–Gestalt Test for Young Children,* Vol. II. New York: Grune & Stratton.

LaBarba, RC (1981) *Foundations of Developmental Psychology.* New York: Academic Press.

Letz, R and Baker, EL (1986) Computer-administered neurobehavioral testing in occupational health. *Semin Occup Med* 1(3):197–203.

Lindström, K (1973) Psychological performance of workers exposed to various solvents. *Work Environ Health* 10:151–155.

Lord, MR and Novick, M (1968) *The Statistical Theory of Mental Tests Scores.* Reading, MA: Addison-Wesley.

Malgady, RG and Rogler, LH (1987) Ethocultural and linguistic bias in mental health evaluation of Hispanics. *Am Psychol* 42:228–234.

Mantere, P, Hänninen, H, and Hernberg, S (1982) Subclinical neurotoxic lead effects: Two-year follow-up studies with psychological test methods. *Neurobehav Toxicol Teratol* 4(6):725–727.

Matarazzo, JD (1986) Computerized clinical psychological test interpretations: Unvalidated plus all mean and no sigma. *Am Psychol* 41:14–24.

McReynolds, P and Chelune, GJ (eds) (1984) *Advances in Psychological Assessment.* San Francisco, CA: Jossey-Bass.

Minton, HL (1988) *Lewis M Terman: Pioneer in Psychological Testing.* New York: New York University Press.

Mira y Lopez, E (1965) *Myokinetische Psychodiagnostik.* Berne: Hans Huber.

Piaget, J (1947) *The Psychology of Intelligence.* London: Routledge and Kegan Paul.

Pikivi, L and Hänninen, H (1989) Subjective symptoms and psychological performance of chlorine-alkali workers. *Scand J Work Environ Health* 15(1):69–74.

Purdue Research Foundation (1948) *Examiner Manual for the Purdue Pegboard.* Chicago: Science Research Associates.

Ray, A (1964) *L'Examen Clinique in Psychologie.* Paris: Presses Universitaires de France.

Reitan, RM (1958) The validity of the trail making test as an indicator of organic brain damage. *Percept Motor Skills* 8:271.

Research and Education Association (1981) *Handbook of Psychiatric Rating Scales.* New York: REA.

Ryan, CM, Morrow, L, Bromet, EL, et al. (1987) Assessment of neuropsychological dysfunction in the workplace: Normative data from the Pittsburgh Occupational Exposure Test Battery. *J Clin Exp Psychol* 9(6):665–679.

Snyderman, M and Rothman, S (1988) *The IQ Controversy, the Media and Public Policy.* New Brunswick, NJ: Transaction Books.

Sokal, MM (ed) (1984) *Psychological Testing and American Society.* New Brunswick, NJ: Rutgers University Press.

Teuber, H-L (1960) Perception. In *Handbook of Physiology,* Sect 1, Vol III, *Neurophysiology,* J Field, HW Magoun, and VE Hall (eds) pp. 1595–1668. Washington, DC: American Physiological Society.

Teuber, H-L, Battersby, WS, and Bender, MB (1949) Changes in visual searching performance following cerebral lesions. *Am J Physiol* 159:592.

Teuber, H-L, Battersby, WS, and Bender, MB (1951) Performance of complex visual tasks after cerebral lesions. *J Nerv Ment Dis* 114:413–420.

Tiffin, J (1968) *Manual for Purdue Pegboard.* Chicago, IL: Science Research Associates.

Valciukas, JA (1984) Occupational neurotoxicology: A recent monograph reviewing the state of the art and emerging trends. *Am J Ind Med* 6:395–396.

Valciukas, JA (1987) *Principles and Methods for the Assessment of Neurotoxicity Associated with Exposure to Chemicals* (book review). Environ Res 43:441–443.

Vorhees, CV (1987) Reliability, sensitivity and validity of behavioral indices of neurotoxicity. *Neurotoxicol Teratol* 9(6):445–464.

Wechsler, D (1958) *The Measurement and Appraisal of Adult Intelligence* (4th ed). Baltimore: Williams & Wilkins.

Wechsler, D (1974) *Manual: Wechsler Intelligence Scale for Children—Revised.* New York: The Psychological Corporation.

World Health Organization (1985) *Neurobehavioral Methods in Occupational and Environmental Health.* Copenhagen: World Health Organization, Regional Office for Europe.

Yerkes, RM (ed) (1925) *Psychological Examining in the United States Army: Memoirs of the National Academy of Sciences,* Vol. 15. Washington, DC: Government Printing Office.

5

Electrophysiological Procedures

The history of using electrophysiological procedures for the understanding of how neurotoxic agents affect nervous system function is intertwined with that of the neurobiology of neurotoxic disease. Thus, electrophysiological procedures have also evolved along three distinctive levels discussed previously: gross morphological, cellular, and molecular. This chapter is a review of the essential features of several electrophysiological procedures that have either already been used or been proposed as having potential for the objective evaluation of neurotoxic illness. These include electroencephalography, evoked potentials, event-related potentials, electromyography, nerve conduction velocities, oculography, and other techniques. The chapter ends with an evaluation of the significance of electrophysiological procedures for epidemiological studies of toxin-induced neurological illness.

The second edition of the book *Electrodiagnosis in Clinical Neurology* (Aminoff 1986a) is an excellent comprehensive review of these techniques.

We are fortunate that the history of neurophysiology has been preserved in a variety of sources (Boring 1950; Brazier 1984, 1986). Galvani's *hanging frogs' legs from a fence during a storm to observe his specimen's twitches is probably a vivid picture in the minds of many. But Galvani's studies on animal electricity—as well as many other discoveries of the electrical properties of neural tissue in the 19th century and the beginning of the 20th—had little bearing on neurotoxicological research.*

As early as 1809, Magendie performed studies on the action of "arrow poisons" (curare) and the mechanisms of strychnine action on the nervous system. In the 1850s, Claude Bernard continued these studies as well as the study of the effects of carbon monoxide on nervous system function. However, it is unlikely that Magendie or Bernard held a strong interest in occupational and environmental neurotoxicology as we know it today (Doull and Bruce 1986). As will be seen in Chapter 38, England and Germany were forced to deal with matters of occupational hygiene in the middle of the 19th century as a result of episodes of severe chemical poisoning, notably carbon monoxide and carbon disulfide—the unwanted price these nations had to pay for the birth of industry.

The major event that left a mark on many neurotoxicological investigations to come was Hans Berger's discovery of the electrical rhythms of the brain in 1929. This discovery led to the development of electroencephalography and later to the application of this technique to the study of how neurotoxic agents in the workplace might affect brain functions.

Hans Berger (1873–1941) discovered in 1929 that the human brain exhibited synchronous rhythmic activity (similar experiments were conducted in animals 50 years earlier). By the middle of the 1950s, electrophysiological techniques came into use around the world. Searching for the first scientist who used electroencephalographic techniques for the investigation of the effects of environmental and occupational agents is probably a fruitless effort, however. National histories of the field exist from both Western and Eastern European countries, and the United States and Japan have traced their own accounts (WHO 1986).

For each electrophysiological procedure discussed below, this chapter provides brief technical information on how it is performed or the record is obtained, its physiological basis, the information it provides, representative studies, and an evaluation of the state of the art.

ELECTROENCEPHALOGRAPHY

An *electroencephalogram* (EEG for short) is a permanent record of the spontaneous electrical activity of the brain; in the clinic, an *electroencephalograph* is the equipment used to obtain such a record. (The term "EEG" is often used interchangeably to designate the technique and the record derived from this technique.) A *polygraph* is an apparatus used under laboratory conditions in which many other physiological measures are simultaneously recorded in addition to the EEG—eg, heartbeat, blood pressure, skin electrical conductance, breathing rate, eye movements, and stimulus conditions present during the recording session.

Electroencephalography, which is the technique for the recording, analysis, and interpretation of human EEGs, was a well-developed clinical and research tool by the middle of the 1950s, and the principles of recording and interpretation have remained fairly unchanged since.

In the international 10–20 system of electrode placement, active electrodes are glued to the scalp, and a neutral electrode placed in an area removed from the recording site. With adequate amplification and filtering of unwanted signals (eg, those of muscle activity, which may result from clenching of the teeth), a characteristic pattern of electrical waves ranging from 0.5 to 50 Hz (cycles per second) is obtained (Fig. 5.1). Typical voltages range from 20 to 100 microvolts (μV). The appearance of an EEG results from the positioning of the recording electrodes on different areas on the right and left hemispheres of the brain. In certain types of human clinical experimentation, up to two dozen or more electrodes can be employed.

Among the two most widely used maneuvers employed to unveil abnormal EEG patterns are hyperventilation and photic stimulation. In the former, the subject is asked to breath forcefully with the mouth open for 3 minutes. In the latter, subjects see a high-intensity flicker stimulation at close range. Both methods are known to elicit abnormal EEG patterns, such as those characteristic of several forms of epilepsy, in subjects who would not exhibit them during passive recording.

There are many sources dealing with the technical aspects of EEG recordings (Niedermeyer and Lopez da Silva 1982). Aminoff (1986b) and Tharp (1986) are the most recent comprehensive reviews of this technique.

The Electroencephalogram's Physiological Basis

The EEG is the expression of the sum of the activity of individual cortical cells. At one time, it was thought that the EEG was related to the action potential of cortical cells. Now, it is generally accepted that the EEG is a record of the extracellular current flow originating from a particular variety of neurons called pyramidal cells. Pyramidal cells are arranged at right angles to the surface of the skull, their dendrites being close to the surface. The potential that gives rise to the EEG

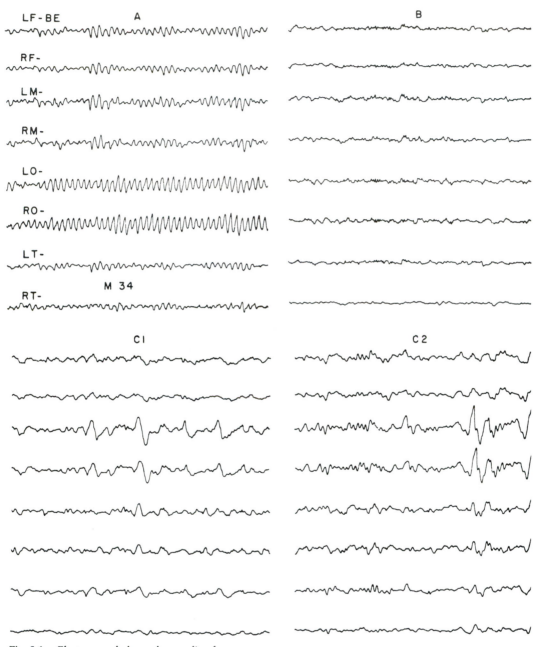

Fig. 5.1. Electroencephalograph recording from a normal subject. (Kooi et al. 1978.)

is the summed synaptic potential originating in the dendrites of these cells.

Many other neural structures contribute to the EEG, particularly the ascending reticular formation, a nucleus that extends from the brainstem to the thalamus (see Chapter 1), and most sensory systems (eg, auditory, visual, somatosensory). Stimulation of the latter will produce a pattern of electrical activity (the sensory evoked potential, to be reviewed below) in primary and secondary sensory processing areas of the brain.

Information Provided by the Electroencephalogram

The EEG ranges in frequencies from 0.5 to 30 Hz. However, the prevailing EEG rhythm ranges from 8 to 13 Hz, the *alpha rhythm*. The alpha rhythm is associated with a behavioral state of relaxed wakefulness. Faster and slower rhythms are observed in other behavioral states. For example, beta waves (13 to 30 Hz) are often observed in the frontal lobe or in many regions of the brain as a result of attentive concentration. Delta (0.5 to 4 Hz) and theta (4 to 7 Hz) are associated with stages of sleep and have the largest voltages.

Unfortunately, correlations between behavioral states and EEG events are poor. In the early years of electroencephalography, many scientific and popular accounts described EEG findings as if such correlations existed. Indeed, experienced electroencephalographists develop a "sense" of what a human subject—or any experimental animal—might be doing at a particular moment by looking at the record only. But when this "sense" is subjected to strict scientific scrutiny, the facts do not support the claims. (This point is developed further at the end of this section.)

In the middle 1950s, electronic devices that helped to display the spectral composition of EEG waves became available (Fig. 5.2). Microcomputers attached to EEG-recording equipment now are used for the same purposes. Thus, it has been possible for many years to ascertain whether a given neurotoxic agent—such as a pesticide—changes the spectral distribution of EEG waves in exposed individuals. Surprisingly, these well-known technical developments are still described as "new" in the most recent neurotoxicological literature.

The value of traditional EEG recordings using scalp electrodes to localize regions of the brain that might be affected by a neurotoxic agent is limited when compared with new imaging techniques (Chapter 6). As a rule, neurotoxic agents cause symmetrical

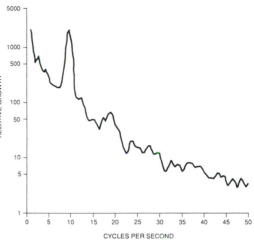

Fig. 5.2. A spectral analysis of an EEG. (Adapted from Kooi et al. 1978.)

damage to the nervous system. Disruption of the symmetrical pattern of EEG activity is of paramount importance in the analysis and interpretation of the recordings.

The EEG is a noninvasive electrophysiological procedure and a well-established diagnostic tool for well-defined purposes. Coupled with eye movement recordings (described below), EEG can be used to monitor the level of medical anesthesia during surgery and for the diagnosis of epilepsy in both children and adults. The EEG has also received wide public attention in connection with the definition of clinical death. The total absence of the electrical activity of the brain defines such a state (Chatrian 1986).

A wealth of information is available regarding EEG correlates of normal and abnormal behavior. An EEG represents the integrated activity of all neurons and neural circuits of the brain. Thus, it is the best example of a holistic view of research, namely, the study of the activity of the brain as a whole.

Although the introduction of EEG for the evaluation of subclinical effects of neurotoxic agents marked a new era in neurotoxicology, its original potential as a clinical screening procedure has yet to materialize. Both the expert visual inspection of the EEG and the analysis of its spectral composition are too insensitive to detect subclinical or preclinical manifestations of neurotoxic illness. As in the case of other techniques for the assessment of toxin-induced brain changes, EEG changes are not specific for any known chemical compound.

Representative Studies

Ørbæck et al. (1985) performed one of the most comprehensive studies among painters with long-term exposure to solvents. In addition to clinical neurological evaluation, clinical chemistry, psychometric, peripheral nerve conduction velocity, and regional cerebral blood flow measurements, a detailed EEG study of exposed subjects and controls was made. One of the salient aspects of this study is that the quantitative EEG frequency analysis used in the study did not involve subjective evaluation of the records except for excluding periods of failing vigilance or artifacts during the examination. Figure 5.3 is the result of fast Fourier analysis of the EEG recordings as processed on line via a computer. Fourier analysis is a mathematical

technique allowing the analysis of a complex wave into its sinusoidal components. Twenty spectra (left row) were averaged, each of which was constructed from 30 seconds of EEG recording. Monitoring of individual spectra makes it possible to check for fluctuations in vigilance and artifacts.

A good source of additional EEG studies on the toxicity of industrial agents in humans is the monograph published by the World Health Organization in 1986.

The Electroencephalogram and Its Interpreter

As a measure of brain activity, EEG techniques have been plagued by numerous data collection problems particularly obvious in early reports (1955–1975). Some of the issues have been adequately addressed only recently (Gevins 1986).

Some problems associated with the use and interpretation of EEG data are inherent in all attempts at sampling-over-time procedures. For example, what is a "typical" sample of EEG in a given human? The brain's spon-

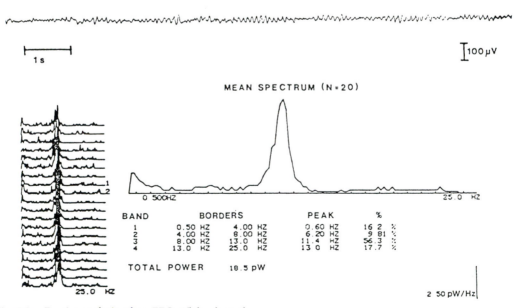

Fig. 5.3. Fourier analysis of an EEG. (Ørbæck et al. 1985.)

Table 5.1. Agreement of Two Raters on Category Using a Method of Concise Clinical EEG Classification ($N = 307$)

Rater 1	Rater 2						
	Normal	Borderline	Abnormal Slow	Abnormal Fast	Abnormal Paroxysmal	Subtotals	
Normal	95	7	15	2	4	123	40.1%
Borderline	1	2	5			8	2.6%
Abnormal slow	9	5	126		1	141	46.0%
Abnormal fast				3			0.9%
Abnormal paroxysmal			8		24	32	10.4%
Subtotals	105	14	154	5	29		
	34.2%	4.6%	50.2%	1.6%	9.4%		

From Gevins (1986).

taneous electrical activity changes over time, and, for research purposes, the selection of the segment of an EEG record representative of the experimental conditions under which the record was obtained is essentially subjective. During a particularly long session lasting several hours, and while recording the EEG of a healthy individual, it is possible to observe large fluctuations, some of which might be abnormal. The decision on whether an EEG recording is "normal" or "abnormal" is difficult and in this case is based on the same statistical principles of sampling theory: "normal" features are expected to be observed more frequently than "abnormal."

The EEG record needs to be interpreted. (In fact, this is also true of the outcome of all techniques described in this work.) The interpreter judges whether the patterns of waveforms are "normal" or "abnormal." Experts with a "trained eye" using "clinical judgment" can recognize the EEG patterns associated with various normal stages of sleep, brain tumors, and sometimes various types of epilepsy. In spite of the shortcomings, the agreement between independent raters is very good (Table 5.1). Recently, decision trees have been proposed which use EEG in clinical diagnosis.

Assessment of the State of the Art

There is an important distinction between a *data-gathering device,* which provides information on the functional status of the brain and behavior, and *data-analytical strategies,* by means of which the information furnished by data-gathering devices is transformed into variables adequate for statistical analysis. The conclusion that a specific chemical compound is neurotoxic is **never** arrived at on the basis of information furnished by a specific data-gathering device; a human being makes such a conclusion—an alert observer, a trained professional. This is so because an EEG is not designed for such a task, and if it were, it would certainly not be specific, a fate that EEG techniques share with all equipment designed to record nervous system function and behavior. Toxic causation is based on data-analytical procedures (a topic that is discussed in Chapters 15 to 19).

As a data-gathering device and a tool used by an expert clinician, the EEG has achieved a great deal of sophistication in the arsenal of current techniques used in the clinic for evaluation of numerous neurological conditions of diverse etiology. This has not been so in human neurotoxicological research. Thus far, the data-analytical strategies used in analysis of possible dose–response relationships between EEG and human toxic exposures have remained considerably behind the standards reached by other techniques of nervous system assessment, notably psychometric techniques.

Let us first examine the assessment of human exposure and dose (the independent variable). In almost all studies in which EEG has been used, "occupational group" is used as a proxy for "toxic exposure," which, as seen in Chapters 10 and 14, represents the lowest level of quantification of human dose. Adequate measures of human toxic dose (for example, based on industrial hygiene procedures) and the assessment of absorption of dose are virtually absent in studies in which EEG changes have been used as a measure of outcome.

When EEG is the outcome (or dependent) variable, the vast majority of neurotoxicological studies define outcome as "normal" EEG and "abnormal" EEG. From the data-analytical point of view, "normal EEG," versus "abnormal EEG" represents a dichotomy. However, one wonders whether EEG information that generates continua—such as the magnitude of the peaks in the power spectrum analysis—are not more suitable for the evaluation of EEG as an outcome variable in the context of toxic dose–EEG response evaluations. It is as if only a fraction of the wealth of information that EEG techniques currently furnish is being used in the search for possible toxic causation. Evoked potentials, described in the next section, eliminated in part the dilemma of deciding which are the more appropriate measures of outcome.

The search for possible links between toxic exposure and EEG changes has been guided by strategies that are appropriate for treatment of the EEG changes as a dichotomous variable. For example, causation is generally and primarily established on the basis of testing a null hypothesis, the hypothesis of no EEG differences or abnormalities between the exposed and the control group. However, in

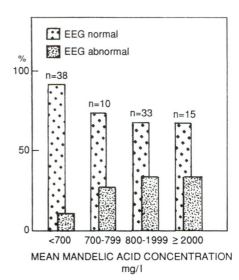

Fig. 5.4. Relative frequencies of normal and abnormal EEGs of styrene-exposed subjects according to the subjects' urinary mandelic acid concentrations. (From Harkonen et al. 1978.)

the 1970s dose–response relationships between objective measures of exposure and EEG changes began to be reported (Fig. 5.4).

EVOKED POTENTIALS

Since the discovery of the electroencephalogram by Berger in 1929, many investigators have used sensory stimulation to study the resulting changes in the EEG recordings. These electrical changes became known as *evoked potentials* (EP).

The term "evoked potential" has several meanings. In humans, it is the electrical response arising in the cerebral cortex as a result of a specific stimulation of a specific sensory system. Thus, visual, auditory, or somatosensory stimulation will induce a visual evoked potential (VEP), an auditory evoked potential (AEP), or a somatosensory evoked potential (SEP), respectively. In animals studied under laboratory conditions, evoked potentials can be produced by electrical stimulation of sensory systems, sometimes via implanted electrodes, and the evoked potential can be recorded as it passes through several neural relay stations. These evoked potentials can be recorded anywhere along the sensory neural pathway.

Evoked potentials can result from specific cognitive acts, in which case they are called event-related potentials (ERP), the next topic in this chapter. Evoked potentials can also be recorded before a motor act is initiated (the readiness potential described by Kornhuber and Deecke in 1965).

There are several good sources dealing with the background and technical and interpretive aspects of EP. A good comprehensive source is Aminoff (1986a), containing articles by Sokol (1986), Stockard et al. (1986), Picton et al. (1986), and by Eisen and Aminoff (1986). More advanced sources reviewing experimental studies in human and animals are Barber (1980) and Bodis-Wollner (1982).

The Neurophysiological Basis of Evoked Potentials

A sensory system consists of receptors, neural pathways, relay nuclei, and centers of neural integration. A sensory system is biologically designed to obtain information from the external and internal world and to make appropriate adjustments in the organism's physiology and behavior. Sensory systems are the basis of perception. However, "sensation" is no longer contrasted with "perception." As seen in the classical psychological literature prevailing until approximately 1950, "sensation" was conceived of as information provided by "primary sensory pathways" and "perception" as that which resulted from a process of cortical integration.

Electrophysiologists study the electrical signals as they travel from the receptors to their final destination in the cerebral cortex. If cochlear receptors are activated by their specific stimulus (ie, sound) or by a mild electric shock, receptors give rise to the generator potential. As stated in Chapter 2, the generator potential is a graded potential that, after achieving a certain level (the firing threshold) is capable of initiating the action potential.

Several individual action potentials derived from single receptors and their associated single fibers form the compound sensory potential. The action potential travels via afferent nerves to sensory ganglia located outside the spinal cord. Then the sensory message penetrates the spinal cord in well-defined regions that correspond to the body's stimulation site. Inside the spinal cord the electrical signal takes an upward direction. At the level of the medulla oblongata at the upper level of the spinal cord, which corresponds approximately to the lower section of the neck, the compound action potential finds its first relay station. The message, now carried by a second neuron, continues toward the brain, reaching the third neuron in the thalamus. From specific thalamic nuclei, the electrical signal then reaches the cortex, where an electrode placed on the scalp picks up the message. The electronic superposition of 10 to 1000 such signals—commonly called "averaging"—is necessary to "see" an evoked potential in the midst of EEG background waves.

Information Provided by the Evoked Potential

Evoked potential assessment is a firmly established ancillary technique in clinical neurology and animal experimental research. As Chiappa (1983) has stated,

The clinical utility of EPs is based on their ability (1) to demonstrate abnormal sensory system function when the history and/or neurological examination are equivocal, (2) to reveal the presence of clinically unsuspected malfunctioning of a sensory system when demyelinating disease is suspected because of symptoms and/or signs in another area of the central nervous system . . . (3) to help define the anatomic distribution of a disease process, and (4) to monitor objective changes in a patient's status.

In animal research, sensory evoked potentials are essential for the ascertainment of neuropathological mechanisms of neurotoxic diseases.

In pediatrics, evoked potentials are used to assess possible blindness or deafness when no behavioral techniques can be used for these two purposes because of the infant's age (Picton et al. 1986).

Representative Research

Araki and collaborators (1980, 1986, 1987; Araki and Honma 1976) have used electrophysiological sensory evoked potentials in the context of clinical neurology to ascertain the extent of the alterations caused by lead within the neural pathways mediating somatosensory functions in humans. They studied subclinical central and peripheral nervous system dysfunction among lead-exposed workers by measuring short-latency somatosensory evoked potentials (SSEP) and maximal motor and sensory nerve conduction velocities (MCV and SCV) following stimulation of the median nerve at the wrist. The examinations were conducted in 20 gun-metal foundry workers exposed to lead, zinc, copper, and tin. Blood lead levels ranged from 16 to 64 μg/dL with a mean of 42 μg/dL.

These investigators found that among the metal-exposed workers, the interpeak latency of SSEP in the cervicospinobulbar region was significantly prolonged and the MCV and SCV in the forearm significantly slowed. Multiple regression analysis revealed that the yield of urinary lead following challenge with calcium disodium ethylenediamine tetraacetate (CaEDTA) and packed red blood cell volume were the major factors associated with the lengthening of the SSEP latency in the cervicospinobulbar region. In addition, the interpeak latency in the upper central nervous system was inversely related to the zinc concentration in erythrocytes. Finally, the MCV

and SCV in the palm were positively related to erythrocyte zinc concentrations and blood plasma copper concentrations, respectively.

According to the authors, these findings suggest that the subclinical neurophysiological effects of lead occur not only in the peripheral nerves but also in the central nervous system. It appears that zinc antagonizes the central and peripheral neurological dysfunction caused by lead; similarly, copper antagonized the peripheral sensory nerve dysfunction.

Arezzo and Schaumburg have published numerous animal studies on the effects of neurotoxic agents on sensory pathways by means of evoked potentials (Arezzo et al. 1985; Schaumburg et al. 1974). This group, based at Albert Einstein College of Medicine in New York City, has performed numerous other anatomic, neuropathological, and psychophysical investigations on the status of the nervous system resulting from neurotoxic insults.

Evoked Potentials in Neurotoxicological Research: An Evaluation

Although numerous comprehensive reviews on evoked potentials are available, few address their value for neurotoxicological research. Critical reviews are almost totally absent. To quote Arezzo et al. (1985):

> Although powerful, EPs do not appear at this time to be a reasonable "first-line" method for screening large at-risk populations. They are relatively expensive and time-consuming; they require sophisticated equipment and technical recording for analyzing data. The proper niche for EPs in the field of neurotoxicology is still evolving and will be shaped by future morphological and electrophysiological research.

Truly neurotoxicological EP studies with adequate strategies for data analysis have already appeared in the literature. For example, in the studies by Araki (reviewed above), the yield of urinary lead following challenge with calcium disodium ethylenediamine tetraacetate (CaEDTA) and packed red blood cell volume are the objective independent variables, and the lengthening of the SSEP latency in the cervicospinobulbar region is the objective dependent variable. Then, the main effects of the independent variables on the dependent variables are studied by multiregression analysis accounting for possible confounders. This degree of sophistication in defining exposures and determining toxic causation by means of EP techniques is rare in the human neurotoxicological literature.

EVENT-RELATED POTENTIALS

Evoked sensory potentials are electrical responses produced by external stimulation (visual, auditory, touch, vibration, olfactory, etc). In contrast, *event-related potentials* (ERP) are electrical events associated with internal events or mental processes in the brain. Two types of event-related potentials are recognized: exogenous ERP are electrical processes evoked by external stimuli, whereas endogenous ERP are electrical processes initiated by the subject being examined. Event-related potentials were independently discovered by Gray Walter and his colleagues (1964) and Kornhuber and Deecke (1965).

The three most prominent features of ERPs are the contingent negative variation (CNV) (a negative wave that occurs before the initiation of a motor act, eg, the intention to move the hand), the readiness potential (RP) (also a negative wave occurring about 1 second before the initiation of a stereotyped movement; temporally the readiness potential occurs after the contingent negative variation), and the P300 wave (a rather large positive wave so named because it starts 300 msec after the initiation of the sensory stimulus and has a peak between 300 and 600 msec).

Goodin (1986) provides a good introduction to the subject. The book edited by Otto

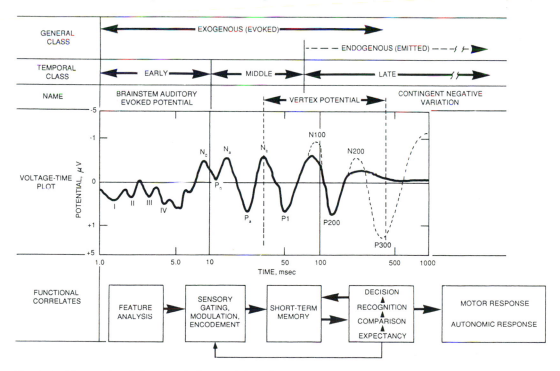

Fig. 5.5. Temporal and functional characteristics of event-related brain potentials. (Adapted from Hillyard and Woods 1979 and Otto 1983.)

(1978) contains numerous descriptions of techniques for the study of ERP in laboratory animals and humans, and a section of that publication (Chapter VII) is devoted to the significance of ERP in environmental neurotoxicology.

Evoked event-related potentials are obtained by averaging a large number of evoked potentials accompanying electrophysiological stimulation or planned behavioral acts. Recording of slow potentials of the brain was not possible until the late 1950s and early 1960s. At that time, both technical improvements in the recording devices—in particular, amplifiers specially designed to amplify such waveforms—and techniques to store electrical responses resulting from large numbers of successive trials became available. Figure 5.5 is an illustration of the temporal relationship of ERP to other potentials in the brain. The ERPs are usually termed "slow" potentials because they occur much later—measured in milliseconds—after the sensory evoked potentials occur. The typical latency of endogenous ERPs are 100 msec or more after the onset of the stimulus.

Information Provided by Event-Related Potentials

Rebert (1980) speculates that the functional significance of an ERP occurs at two levels: neuronal activity and gross behavioral acts. During the late 1970s there was a strong suspicion that there was a neurochemical basis for the origin of ERPs. But the excitement about the possibility that these slowly occurring potentials might explain a variety of psychological functions has largely disappeared. At the time of their discovery, it was thought that ERPs provided the physiological basis for volitional acts, information processing, memory, moods, and anxiety.

Representative Research

Otto and collaborators (1978) from the US Department of Environmental Protection and the University of North Carolina at Chapel Hill have studied how ERPs are affected by neurotoxic agents and have reviewed the literature on the subject. This group has per-

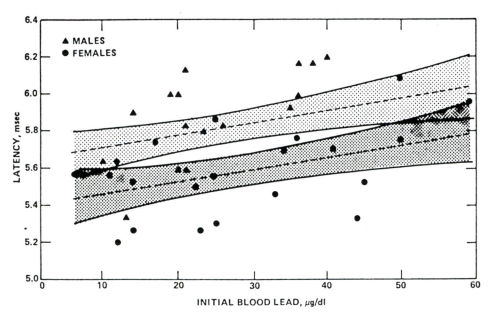

Fig. 5.6. Relationship between ESRPs and Pb-B. (From Otto 1985.)

formed studies on the effects of lead on ERP in children. A relationship has been found between these slow-wave voltages and blood lead levels during sensory conditioning. This work is significant in that the authors claim that changes in ERP are observed to occur at 30 µg/dL of lead in blood, a level that, at the time of their publication, was below the maximum recommended exposure to lead for children (50 µg/dL of blood). The results could be indicative of neural damage or impaired sensory conditioning. Figure 5.6 shows a dose–response relationship between blood lead levels and ERSPs (event-related sensory potentials) among children.

As Otto (1983) stated, "... very little is known about the anatomical, physiological, or chemical substrate of these intriguing waveforms. Even the psychological and behavioral significance of ERSPs remains a subject of lively debate."

State of the Art

Otto has evaluated the potential usefulness of recording ERP for occupational and environmental neurotoxicology. He cites as shortcomings lack of uniformity in the testing situations in different laboratories, lack of group norms, and numerous data collection problems—ie, eye and body movement artifacts and the need for eye fixation, which in children is difficult, particularly in those whose cognition and behavior have been altered by neurotoxic agents. The promises of ERPs in human neurotoxicological research have yet to be fulfilled.

ELECTROMYOGRAPHY

Electromyography is a term applied to a collection of techniques for the recording of the electrical activity of muscles. More appropriately, electromyography (EMG) techniques, as they are generally known, are electrophysiological techniques to determine the degree of intactness of the motor unit and its four major components: its cell body, located in the ventral horn of the spinal cord; its axon; the neuromuscular junction; and the muscle fibers innervated by that neuron (Fig. 5.7). The EMG techniques cannot easily be separated from *electroneuronography* (ENG), the measurement of nerve conduction velocities, the next topic in this chapter. *Electroneuromyography* (ENMG) is a term that has been developed to accommodate the electro-

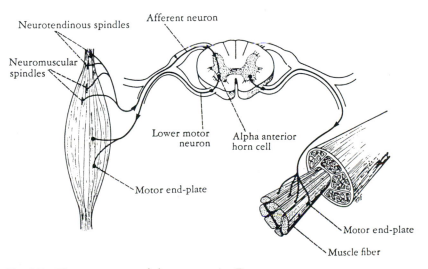

Fig. 5.7. The components of the motor unit. (From Snell 1987.)

diagnosis of the motor unit, which involves both muscle and nerve activity. But the term EMG continues to be widely used in the neurotoxicological literature. (The term "EMG" is often used interchangeably to designate the technique and the record derived from this technique.)

The electrical activity of the muscle is studied by inserting a recording electrode directly into the muscle. The electrode is a concentric needle electrode consisting of a pointed steel cannula within which runs a fine silver, steel, or platinum wire that is insulated except for the tip. The voltage originates from the potential difference between the outer cannula and the inner wire. The bioelectrical potentials are then amplified and displayed on an oscilloscope for their visual analysis; amplified potentials are very often sent to a loudspeaker for acoustical monitoring. The firing rate of normal or abnormal muscle activity is thus characterized acoustically.

The needle electrode is inserted into the muscle on the basis of the patient's neurological signs and symptoms. The electrophysiologist then systematically explores the muscle activity, observing the insertion activity—the activity of the relaxed muscle at the moment the needle is inserted—and firing rates.

Information Provided by an Electromyography Examination

An EMG is an invasive and painful procedure confined to the clinic. With the aid of an EMG examination, a trained neurologist can ascertain whether a disease is likely to be affecting a motor neuron located in the spinal cord or peripheral nerves outside the vertebral column. Neurologists can also determine whether the disease is typical of the lower motor unit (characteristic in flaccid paralysis) or typical of disease of the upper motor unit (where upper regions of the brain no longer exert their inhibitory action on lower regions of the spinal cord, creating a permanent contraction of the muscle).

Representative Research

Many neurotoxic agents—most notably organic solvents such as n-hexane and certain metals such as lead and mercury—have a particular affinity for the peripheral nervous system. Therefore, a thorough EMG study is often essential for the clinical evaluation of the effects of neurotoxic agents.

Allen and collaborators (1975) described an industrial outbreak of toxic neuropathy caused by methyl n-butyl ketone (MBK). This report is a model describing details of strategies, the manner in which uniformity of the research protocol was obtained, how screening of workers was performed, how differential diagnosis was established, the description of the occupational environment, and the relationship of clinical findings to animal experimentation. Their work is cited here as a representative example because EMG techniques were used as a screening procedure in conjunction with a physical and neurological examination.

The medical and EMG examinations were performed on 1157 employees in a plant producing vinyl-coated fabrics. Printshop workers were exposed to methyl ethyl ketone (MEK) and methyl n-butyl ketone (MBK). On the basis of these examinations, 194 workers were suspected of having toxic neuropathy. These workers were referred for further neurological evaluation. On the basis of symptoms, findings in the neurological evaluation, and EMG studies, 86 workers were diagnosed as having MBK-related distal polyneuropathy. Among these 86 workers and on the basis of EMG findings, 11 were classified as moderate to severe, 38 mild, and 37 minimal. The rating scale for electrodiagnostic studies was as follows:

- Score 1 was given to any abnormalities of the EMG in one or more normally vulnerable muscles, positive waves in one or more muscles, and fasciculation.
- Score 2 was given to one of more fibrillations and multiple muscle involvement.

- Score 3 was given to abnormal motor unit potentials or a decreased number of potentials and borderline distal latency of nerve conduction velocities.
- Score 4 corresponded to increased distal latency.
- Score 5 referred to a decrease in nerve conduction velocity.

The causative agent (MBK) was ascertained after a detailed examination of work practices and the reproduction of neurological findings in experimental animals.

State of the Art

In the clinic, EMG is a technique of choice for making the differential diagnosis of neurological illness, that is, ruling out the presence of neurological conditions that might explain the patient's findings. This technique has never been recommended for screening. Because they are painful, scientific studies (that is, studies carried out primarily to gain knowledge) need to be performed with adherence to ethical standards for human studies.

NERVE CONDUCTION VELOCITY STUDIES

The historical background of the development of attempts to ascertain how fast nerves conduct electricity is interesting and sometimes amusing. Picture Albrecht von Haller in 1762 trying to determine the velocity of nerve conduction by reading the Aeneid aloud. He counted how many letters he could pronounce within 1 minute. Among the 1500 letters per minute, 'R' was assumed to require 10 successive contractions of the styloglossus muscle, indicating that a muscle can contract and relax 15,000 times per minute. From this he assumed that each contraction lasted 2 msec to travel the 10 cm from the brain to the muscle. Thereby, he concluded that the velocity was about 50 m/sec, very close to the real value as measured by contemporary electroneurono-

graphic studies, which is between 40 to 60 m/sec depending on the nerves, age, and temperature (this study is cited in Buchthal and Rosenfalck 1966).

In 1796, the astronomer Maskelyne dismissed his assistant because the latter observed the times of stellar transit almost a second later than Maskelyne. This seemingly trivial event was the background for the study of the "personal equation" and, later on, "reaction time" (Boring 1950).

However, the first convincing measure of the nerve conduction velocity of sensory nerves was obtained in the 1950s when signal-averaging techniques began to be developed, allowing the measurement of the latency of the nerve's evoked potential.

Nerve conduction velocities (NCVs) are determined with the aid of the electromyograph. Figure 5.8 shows the placement of stimulating and recording electrodes for the determination of the motor conduction velocity of the median nerve. Three key features of the electrical response are recorded: the latency of the response, its amplitude, and the distance from the stimulating and recording electrode (Fig. 5.9). The NCV is a measure obtained by dividing the latency by the distance between the two electrodes.

In epidemiological studies in which large numbers of individuals are studied, sometimes under slightly different conditions, the recording of skin temperature is essential. The

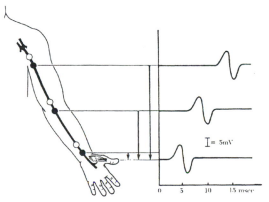

Fig. 5.8. Placement of electrodes for the recording of the conduction velocity of the median nerve. (From Oh 1984.)

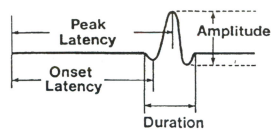

Fig. 5.9. Components of the nerve evoked potential. (From Oh 1984.)

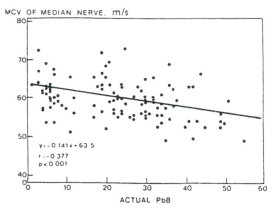

Fig. 5.10. Dose–response relationships between blood lead levels and nerve conduction velocity. (From Sepäläinen and Hernberg 1980.)

lower the skin temperature, the slower the nerve conduction velocity. (Statistical procedures involving the use of regression equations are used to rule out the presence of this confounder.)

Age is another important confounder: the older the individual, the slower the NCVs. The reason why this is so is still unclear; morphological, general, and biochemical explanations have been advanced.

Information Provided by Nerve Conduction Velocity Studies

Nerve conduction velocities are used as a clinical and research tool. Clinical neurologists use NCVs as part of their EMG study; it is essential for the diagnosis of the nature and locus of neurological diseases, particularly those affecting the peripheral nervous system. As a result of extensive normative data, in recent years a quantitative approach for the evaluation of NCV abnormalities has appeared (Oh 1984). Nerve conduction velocities have been successfully used for the assessment of the dose–response relationship between toxic agents and the status of the peripheral nervous system (Fig. 5.10).

Buchthal, Behse, and Rosenfalck from the Institute of Neurophysiology, University of Copenhagen in Denmark and the Rigshopital in Copenhagen have performed the most exhaustive NCV studies in large unexposed groups to date. These investigators have provided data on NCV of numerous nerves under various sets of stimulation and recording

conditions among neurotoxically unexposed people (Buchthal 1982a,b; Buchthal and Behse 1979; Buchthal and Rosenfalck 1966; Buchthal et al. 1975).

An important piece of information derived from this monumental effort is how NCVs change with age, as determined cross-sectionally, that is, with individuals of different ages studied at one point in time. The numerical values of the constants of the linear regression equations are valuable for calculating discrepancies between expected and actual values for a given individual.

Age adjustments and temperature adjustments are now possible because of the availability of this information. It is important to note that most of the measurements of NCV and the study of the effects of neurotoxic agents on NCV have not adopted this rigorous treatment of the data.

Variability of Nerve Conduction Velocities in Normal Persons

Honet and collaborators (1968) studied 27 healthy persons to measure variations in nerve conduction velocities of three motor nerves—median, ulnar, and peroneal—and two sensory nerves—median and ulnar. Physiological variability and observer variability were studied under three conditions: (1) reading the latencies from stimulation to response from photographic pictures, (2) studying the differences between keeping the electrodes stationary and moving and placing the electrodes in position, and (3) increasing the interval of time between measurements.

The standard deviation of readers' blind measurement of the same picture ranged between 2 and 3 m/sec. The availability of computer-generated cursors that "navigate" on the waveform until locked by the observer at a desired position has probably reduced this source of error to even lower figures.

A comparatively more serious source of error in the measurement of NCVs is the one generated in measuring the length of two points along the limb. Variations of a few millimeters can cause large variations in the calculated nerve conduction velocity. (This source of error is often overlooked in the literature on NCVs.) The variability caused by removal and replacement of electrodes after a 5-minute period is greater if electrodes are left in place. However, the numerical value of the variability achieves statistical significance only in one nerve (the ulnar). Measures over time intervals of more than a week increase the variability of the measures. The maximum standard deviation observed during repeated measures was 5.8 m/sec.

Ruling out the Presence of Confounders in the Analysis of Group Data

Critical readers of the neurotoxicological literature pay attention to how investigators deal with known confounders such as age and temperature in judging the quality of the scientific reports. For example, in countries where the use of air conditioning is not as prevalent as in the United States, summer measurements of controls and winter measurements of study groups might explain group differences. Either the limb needs to be warmed up to a known and constant temperature (eg, 30°C) or the temperature effects need to be controlled for a posteriori by means of statistical procedures. As a confounder, the influence of age is also quite marked, as observed in cross-sectional studies. In case–control studies, most investigators deal with age as a confounder by examining whether the mean differences in age are statistically significant. It has long been recognized, however, that the mean is not the best descriptor for a statistical frequency distribution. Moreover, in a clinically oriented study involving 20 to 25 patients, the distributions are very unlikely to be normal, ie, to have the mean and the median overlap. This is the reason why either the median of the two groups must be calculated or more information on the distributions (ie, skewness, kurtosis) should be available.

Contrast between Psychophysical and Electrophysiological Procedures for the Assessment of Peripheral Nervous System Function

Sensory nerve conduction velocity determinations are more closely related to psychophysical determinations of vibratory and thermal thresholds than to the inherently insensitive clinical examination of touch and temperature sensations. Arezzo and his coworkers, who have conducted considerable research on this subject, conclude that when electrophysiological procedures are contrasted to psychophysical procedures, the latter compete very favorably with the former.

The actual procedure for obtaining a sensory nerve conduction velocity is often described as being noninvasive. For some, however, it is uncomfortable if not painful, particularly when sensory nerves need to be stimulated. Sensory nerves carry the sensations of pain. A psychophysical determination of threshold is truly noninvasive and, we might add, is even interesting for the subject. Both electrophysiological and psychophysical procedures have been used for the assessment of subclinical and preclinical manifestations of neurotoxic illness and for monitoring purposes. Because of the noninvasive nature of the latter, its advantages, particularly in prospective studies, are clear.

Human Nerve Conduction Velocity Studies under Clinical Conditions

Dr. Anna Maria Seppäläinen, formerly at the Institute of Occupational Health in Helsinki, Finland, and now at the Department of Neurology of the University of Helsinki, is one of the world leaders in the use of electrophysiological procedures for the assessment of clinical and subclinical manifestations of neurotoxic illness of occupational origin. The pioneering work performed by her and her collaborators in Finland is extensive and could well be used to illustrate exemplary research in many sections of this chapter. Her publications on subclinical electrophysiological indicators of neurotoxin-induced neuropathies (Seppäläinen and Hernberg 1972; Seppäläinen et al. 1975, 1979) are classics in the field.

Although reports indicating a reduction in NCVs in lead-exposed workers were already published by the middle 1960s, Seppäläinen and her co-workers studied the problem not only from a neurological point of view but also from the viewpoint of prevention. From their work, it was possible to ascertain how safe the recommended "safe" maximal blood lead levels were among workers occupationally exposed to lead. (At the time of her writings it was 70 μg/dL in Finland. The present United States standard is 40 μg/dL. There is some evidence that lead exposure actually has no threshold limit for its neurophysiological effects.)

Seppäläinen and co-workers measured the motor conduction velocity (MCV) of the median, ulnar, peroneal, and posterior tibial nerves, the conduction velocities of the slower motor fibers (CVSF) of the ulnar and peroneal nerves, as well as the sensory conduction velocity (SCV) of the median, ulnar, and sural nerves. The MCVs and SCVs were increasingly slower with increasing levels of lead in blood. This dose–response relationship was particularly noticeable in the arm nerves. Then they focused their attention on individuals with blood lead levels below 70 μg/dL of blood. They found that at this "safe level," MCVs and CVSF's were slower than those of healthy controls.

In addition, they performed an analysis that, later on, was to be adopted by other investigators in their studies of subclinical effects of occupational neurotoxic agents. A correlational analysis between blood lead levels and NCVs showed that a dose response was still present even at values below those then considered "safe" (70 μg/dL). This work was extensively reviewed and discussed when a new standard for lead was adopted in the United States.

Nerve Conduction Velocity Studies under Field Conditions

Because of the issues associated with medical field surveys (discussed in chapters dealing with basic epidemiological concepts), representative studies of NCVs under field conditions need to be reviewed under a special heading. The fact that this type of research can be carried out at all is in part because of recent technical advances in equipment design and manufacture. The stimulation/recording equipment is now small and rugged. Microprocessors allow the immediate printout of the status of switches at the moment of testing and the NCV values then obtained. Two environmental/occupational agents have been selected for discussion in the following: the herbicides 2,4,5-trichlorophenoxyacetic acid (2,4,5-T) and 2,4-dichlorophenoxyacetic acid (2,4-D).

The potential adverse health effects of 2,4,5-T and 2,4-D are still a highly emotionally charged issue. Agent Orange, used in the United States' military involvement in Vietnam from 1965 to 1970, contained a combination of 2,4,5-T and 2,4-D. The historical background for this research is found in a report by Singer and collaborators (1982). In their study, NCVs of the median motor, median sensory, and sural nerves were measured in 56 workers employed in the manufacture of 2,4,5-T and 2,4-D. The control group consisted of 25 subjects without exposure to neurotoxic agents. All NCV values were adjusted for age and temperature and standardized (transformed to Z values). The exposed group showed a statistically significant slowing of the sural and median motor nerves. Duration of employment was significantly correlated with slowing of the NCV of the sural nerve. As a group, the chemical workers had one or more slowed NCVs as compared with controls (46% versus 5%). In spite of these findings, it is as difficult to conclude that 2,4,5-T and 2,4-D are the causative agents of a slowing of NCV as to say that they are not. An important source of information—the biological indicators of exposure—was impossible to obtain. The best evidence was based on group differences.

Boeri and his collaborators in Italy (Boeri et al. 1978) performed the first epidemiological studies in which NCV determinations were part of the neurological evaluation. This study was carried out in response to the environmental tragedy in the Seveso region where, on July 10, 1976, as a result of an explosion in a chemical factory, TCDD (2,3,7,8-tetrachlorodibenzo-p-dioxin) was released into the environment.

Singer, Valciukas, and Lilis (1983) studied the effects of lead on the differential time course of sensory and motor nerve effects among 40 automobile production workers. The NCV of the median motor, median sensory, peroneal motor, and sural nerves were measured along with indicators of lead exposure—blood lead—and zinc protoporphyrin levels. A group of 31 workers not exposed to lead served as controls. All NCV values were adjusted for age and temperature. Lead-exposed workers had slower median sensory and slower sural NCV than the controls. The lead-exposed group was then divided into two subsamples based on duration of employment: equal or less than 10 years and longer than 10 years. The correlation between blood lead and zinc protoporphyrin levels and sural NCV was stronger in the subsample with the longer duration of employment. Within the known constraints inherent in cross-sectional studies, it was concluded that slowing of sensory NCVs was likely to occur earlier than slowing of motor NCVs.

The Determination of Nerve Conduction Velocities in Prospective Studies

Bornschein and Rabinowitz (1985), in an issue of the journal *Environmental Research* devoted entirely to prospective studies of lead, stated that "... by the late 1970s it became apparent that it was necessary to move beyond cross-sectional studies in order to better characterize the level of timing of exposure and to monitor the development process during and after the exposure period(s)." Although the journal issue is devoted only to prospective studies of lead, this statement can be generalized to encompass other neurotoxic agents.

Seppäläinen and Hernberg (1982) carried out the first prospective study of NCVs among lead workers. Until then, the time course of onset of NCV findings was inferred from cross-sectional studies. The initial cohort consisted of all 89 new employees entering a storage battery plant for the first time. None of them had been previously exposed to lead. The turnover rate was high: of the 89 workers, 23 were available for examination the following year. It was found that the distal motor NCV of the medial nerve and distal sensory NCV of the median nerve were slower among lead workers during the first year of exposure. Impairment in NCVs was observed among workers whose blood lead levels had risen from 30 μg/dL to a maximal blood lead level of 48 μg/dL. Those workers whose blood lead levels remained below 30 µg/dL had NCVs similar to the controls.

Electrophysiological Studies of Local Neurotoxicity

Local neurotoxicity is a neurotoxic effect observed or felt in a circumscribed area of the body—eg, loss of sensitivity after injection of anesthesia to treat a tooth; temporary (or permanent) loss of sensitivity after a nerve is accidentally cut. In occupational neurotoxicology, local neurotoxicity is often observed in the limbs. In humans, it is characterized by paresthesia (subjective feeling of abnormal sensation), numbness, and, sometimes, dermatitis in fingers.

Seppäläinen and Rajaniemi (1984) studied the local neurotoxicity of methyl methacrylate exposure among dental technicians, who suffered these conditions as a result of absorption of methyl methacrylate through the skin. Dental technicians often handle this substance with their bare hands before polymerization reactions take place. The NCVs were determined in 20 technicians having neurological complaints and 18 healthy controls. Dental technicians were found to have significantly slower distal sensory NCVs than controls. These findings may represent mild axonal degeneration in areas with the closest and most frequent contact with methyl methacrylate.

OCULOGRAPHY

Oculography is a generic term used for a large variety of techniques for the stimulation of the oculomotor system and recording of eye movements. Technically, oculography belongs to the family of electrophysiological procedures—the topic of this chapter—when eye movements are recorded by taking advantage of the electrical events associated with such movements. In the clinical literature dealing with disorders of eye movements caused by pathological conditions, including neurotoxic agents, oculography is also known as electrooculography (EOG) or electronystagmography (ENG).

Eye movements are executed by very small muscles, the extraoculomotor muscles. The neural pathways leading to these muscles are extremely complex with neural centers in the brainstem (the vestibular nuclei), the cerebellum, and the cortex. Eye movements are initiated by a variety of sensory inputs, including visual and vestibular, the otolithic organs and the semicircular canals. The *oculogram* is the record of the eyes as they follow visual stimuli in the horizontal plane.

In the past, ingenious devices have been designed to study eye movements based on mechanical, optical, and infrared principles. Infrared devices, included those described below, have the advantage of producing almost artifact-free recordings in complete darkness. Eye movements need to be recorded under dark conditions for the subject to avoid "locking" his vision onto room objects. Some eye movement abnormalities are not observed in a normally lit room.

We still do not have an oculographic technique suitable for large-scale studies of humans, required in epidemiological studies of neurotoxic agents. One study has been reported by the group at Mount Sinai Medical School where eye movements were studied under field conditions using an infrared technique (Glickman et al. 1984).

Eliciting and Recording Eye Movements

There is no unified method for eliciting eye movements; each laboratory, and sometimes each group within the same laboratory, has developed its own procedures. The following is the one developed at the Mount Sinai Medical School in New York City to elicit saccadic eye movements. A programmable visual display consisting of six light sources located in the horizontal plane is mounted in such a way that one of the light sources is at the center of the visual field and the others at visual angles of 7.5°, 15°, and 30° to the

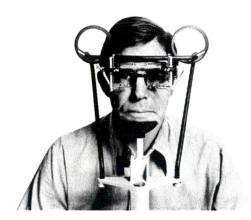

Fig. 5.11. An infrared technique for recording eye movements. (By permission Narco Bio-Systems.)

right and to the left of the visual center target. The lights are switched on and off by means of a silent programmable switch. The order of presentation of visual stimuli, the duration of the light-on periods, and the interstimulus interval vary randomly.

Horizontal saccadic eye movements for a total of 66 stimuli are recorded for each subject. Head position is fixed using a chin and head rest with an adjustable head holder. An infrared reflection system is used to record saccadic eye movements (Fig. 5.11). Eye movements are recorded monoocularly from the right eye on a polygraph. Features of the saccadic eye movement quantified are saccadic accuracy, which results from counting the number of eye movements executed to reach the 66 targets, overshoots, that is, eye movements that are 2° greater than the target amplitude followed by a corrective movement back to the target, and saccadic maximum velocity, which is the amplitude of recorded eye movements when plotted as a function of maximum velocity for each subject.

Representative Research

Glickman and collaborators (1984) conducted a field study to determine whether automobile assembly plant workers exposed to lead exhibited eye movement abnormalities. The investigation was prompted by the well-established fact that lead has an affinity for cerebellar structures. It was argued that since eye movements are dependent on the intactness of cerebellar structure, eye movement abnormalities among individuals with high levels of lead absorption should be demonstrable.

A group of workers exposed to lead in an auto body shop was the study group. Workers were exposed to lead while filling gaps between panels with lead and grinding the excessive lead for smoothness before painting. Controls were people of similar demographic characteristics and age but not occupationally exposed to lead or other neurotoxic agents.

The results indicated that workers exposed to inorganic lead did indeed show a decrease in saccade accuracy and an increase in overshoots compared with controls, but the differences were just short of statistical significance. Correlations between measures of saccadic eye movements and indicators of lead absorption—blood lead and zinc protoporphyrin levels—were analyzed in the lead-exposed workers. Saccade accuracy was negatively correlated with both blood lead and zinc protoporphyrin levels. Saccadic maximum velocity was not correlated with blood lead levels. However, there was a significant correlation with zinc protoporphyrin levels. In addition, saccadic eye movements in younger workers below 30 years of age were more affected by exposure to inorganic lead than were saccadic eye movements in workers 50 years and older.

This pattern of lead exposure reflected job assignments based on age: the younger workers were assigned to the dirtiest jobs. These findings are consistent with the selective neuropathological abnormalities found to be caused by lead in humans and in experimental animals. Cerebellar abnormalities have been found to occur at gross morphological, cellular, and neuropharmacological levels.

In 1953 an episode of methylmercury poisoning occurred around Minamata Bay in southwest Kyushu, Japan. Inhabitants of the

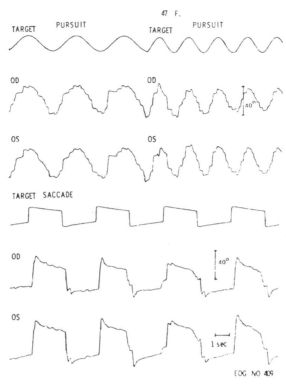

Fig. 5.12.   Alterations of eye movements in Minamata disease. (From Tsutsui 1980.)

area ate fish and shellfish contaminated with methylmercury discharges from a chemical plant in Minamata city. In acute, serious cases, the clinical picture included sensory disturbances, ataxia (disorder of normal coordinated movement), constrictions of the visual fields, confusion, and coma. Tsutsui (1980) conducted a neuroopthalmological examination that included visual acuity, critical flicker frequency (CFF), visual field determinations, pupil reaction, and electrooculography. The electrooculographic examination included pursuit eye movements, saccades, and the examination of the vestibuloocular reflex (Fig. 5.12). (The vestibuloocular reflex is elicited by rotating the subject with an oscillatory movement in the dark.) In patients in whom the diagnosis of Minamata disease was made, 73% of 276 cases exhibited abnormal pursuit eye movements. The prevalence of eye movement abnormalities was 92% among the most severe cases. Abnormal sac-

cadic eye movements were found in 50% in cases where signs of cerebellar involvement could be detected and in 30% in those without cerebellar signs. The vestibuloocular reflex was abnormal in 12% of the adult cases but severely impaired in the "fetal cases," where methylmercury occurred in utero. These findings concurred with neuropathological observations. In the adult brain, single-cell necrosis is localized, particularly in the calcarine, the precentral cortices, and in the granular layer of the cerebellum. In fetal cases, lesions are more diffuse, extending over the cerebellar cortex and the cerebellum.

Ödkvist and collaborators from Lindkoping, Sweden, published a review in 1980 of several studies on the effects of industrial solvents on the vestibulooculomotor system in the rabbit, cat, and humans. Spontaneous nystagmus (a constantly present repetitive movement of the eye), positional nystagmus in lateral positions, nystagmus induced by rotatory acceleration, and optokinetic nystagmus were assessed by means of electronystagmographic (ENG) techniques. In animals, ENG is recorded by inserting needle electrodes subcutaneously at the eyes' outer canthi. Positional nystagmus was elicited in rabbits after intravenous injection of the solvents xylene, styrene, methylchloroform, and trichloroethylene. The fast phase of position nystagmus was left-beating in the right lateral position and right-beating in the left lateral position. These findings, as well as many others published in their 1980 review, are consistent with a possible influence of hydrocarbon solvents on the vestibulooculomotor system.

OTHER TECHNIQUES

Electroretinography

The *electroretinogram* (ERG) represents the retina's electrical response to photic stimulation (Fig. 5.13). In humans, it is obtained by means of two electrodes, one attached to a contact lens applied on the cornea and one a reference attached to any part of the head

(eg, ears). Many different technical procedures are utilized to obtain ERG from laboratory animals (there is an abundance of information on the ERG of invertebrates).

Originally it was thought that the ERG was the electrical response of the retina's photoreceptors—rods and cones—but later investigations disproved this. Now, ERG is thought to be the expression of the retinal neural network's electrical activity. As is the case in many other electrophysiological techniques described in this chapter, the ERG is used both in the clinical—particularly in the diagnosis of neuroophthalmological disorders—and as a research tool for the understanding of the retina's basic neurophysiological processes. But contrary to the expectations of many, ERG has not been systematically used for the study of the effects of neurotoxic agents.

Agents such as solvents (particularly anesthetics) have been used by Granit (1955) to study the fundamental components of this electrical response. More recently, Grant (1980), an authority on the subject of the neurotoxicology of the eye, recommended ERG as an ancillary procedure. The ERG may not be suitable for screening procedures, but

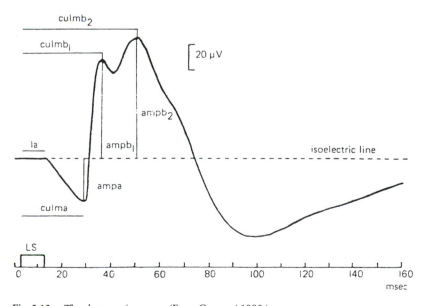

Fig. 5.13.   The electroretinogram. (From Gramoni 1980.)

it is suitable for the assessment of subclinical or preclinical manifestations of neurotoxic illness (eg, those resulting from solvent exposure). Little literature is available that has a direct bearing on occupational and environmental neurotoxicology.

Electrocardiography

The *electrocardiogram* (ECG) is a record of the activity of the heart. The heart is innervated by the autonomic branch of the nervous system; heartbeat changes resulting from acute or chronic exposure to neurotoxic agents acting on the autonomic nervous system can be monitored in experimental animals. Electrocardiogram techniques have been extensively used in pharmacology for understanding the mechanisms of action of many toxic substances and drugs on the heart muscles and the vascular system (Goodman Gilman et al., 1980, chapters on cardiovascular drugs).

There is very little information on the cardiotoxic effects of environmental and occupational neurotoxic agents in humans. Clinically, workers exposed to solvents often complain of pounding heartbeat (tachycardia), but a careful differential diagnosis must be made, since tachycardia is often observed among chronic alcoholics and heavy smokers.

CONCLUSIONS

Electrophysiological techniques are increasingly being used in health surveys of possible adverse effects associated with chemical exposure. This is the result of the following changes:

1. The need to use objective techniques to study neurotoxic effects sometimes associated with subjective complaints such as headaches, dizziness, lack of concentration, memory problems, personality changes, nausea, etc.

2. The expansion of the notion of targets. First, the brain alone was conceived as the primary target, and objective techniques were limited to electroencephalography and psychometric procedures. Now, assessment of peripheral neuropathies—requiring the measurement of nerve conduction velocities of peripheral nerves under field conditions—are commonplace.

3. Technical developments, particularly miniaturization, allow the transport to the field of equipment that until recently was restricted to a permanent setting such as the clinic. With the aid of a single apparatus that can be carried by one person, it is now possible to obtain EEGs, EPs, ERPs, EMGs, NCVs, and EOGs in the field.

Within the constraints of limited budgets, experts are often called on to decide what specific electrophysiological techniques are appropriate for the evaluation of specific health problems or exposures to specific toxic chemicals. Neurophysiological techniques are often deemed to be the quintessence of the objective techniques. But are they?

A physiological technique is never completely objective because data are collected by a device; it is objective because a scientist or group of scientists have demonstrated that it is sensitive, reliable, valid, and, rarely, specific for the assessment of the neurotoxic effects of a given chemical compound. However, no technique is totally free from human judgment. Human minds create techniques, plan experiments, select animal models, interpret data, and persuade audiences.

Electrophysiological techniques are not error-free and sometimes require considerable experience to know when and how an involuntary error has occurred.

*   A polygraph that was calibrated at the time the study group was tested may no longer be calibrated at the time the control group is tested. Thus, study and con-

trol differences may reflect equipment artifacts.

- A claim that nerve conduction velocities are correlated with duration of toxic exposure may in fact be the result of incorrect adjustment for age effects.
- Biased record selection should never be excluded. There are no guidelines for selection of a given record to show an electrophysiological abnormality.
- An applied neurotoxicologist needs to know the difference between an experimental technique that shows promise and a state-of-the-art technique. Sometimes this decision is difficult.
- Changes of the electrical conductance of the skin associated with emotional states have been known for many decades. It is conceivable that an investigator may want to study changes in skin galvanic responses (SGR) in people exposed to neurotoxic agents and in ones not exposed. The SGR is here an experimental, "objective" technique but hardly state of the art.
- Some EEG changes are measurable because of the wide availability of equipment to make such records. Thus, EEG is a state-of-the-art technique for the evaluation of diffuse brain pathology. But EEG is hardly appropriate as a component of a screening battery for the study of subclinical changes associated with acute or chronic neurotoxic exposures. It lacks sensitivity.
- The ERP is sensitive but is still experimental.

An experimental technique sometimes becomes the state of the art. The determination of nerve conduction velocities—first an experimental, then a clinical technique to assess peripheral neuropathies—is now the state of the art in environmental and occupational neurotoxicology.

Sometimes the process is the opposite. The EEG, once the state of the art for the assessment of neurotoxicity, is being largely replaced by more sensitive techniques such as the measurement of visual or auditory evoked potentials and the measurement of slow potentials such as ERPs. However, judging from recent sources (World Health Organization 1986), the EEG is still the state of the art in the Soviet Union and in many Eastern European countries.

In medical field surveys performed to assess possible neurotoxic effects of toxic exposure, electrophysiological techniques do not replace either the observational skills required for clinical judgments or the assessment of changes in performance documented by psychometric techniques: they complement them. A medical field survey conducted only with the aid of electrophysiological procedures may be biased and incomplete.

REFERENCES

Allen, N, Mendell, JR, Billimaier, DJ, et al. (1975) Toxic polyneuropathy due to *n*-butyl ketone: An industrial outbreak. *Arch Neurol* 32:209.

Aminoff, MJ (ed) (1986a) *Electrodiagnosis in Clinical Neurology.* New York: Churchill Livingstone.

Aminoff, MJ (1986b) Electroencephalography: General principles and clinical applications. In *Electrodiagnosis in Clinical Neurology* (2nd ed), MJ Aminoff (ed) pp. 21–75. New York: Churchill Livingstone.

Araki, S and Honma, T (1976) Relationship between lead absorption and peripheral nerve conduction velocities in lead workers. *Scand J Work Environ Health* 4:225–231.

Araki, S, Honma, T, Yanagihara, S, et al. (1980) Recovery of slowed nerve conduction velocity in lead-exposed workers. *Int Arch Occup Environ Health* 46:151–157.

Araki, S, Murata, K, and Aono, H (1986) Subclinical servico-spino-bulbar effects of lead: A study of short-latency somatosensory evoked potentials in workers exposed to lead, zinc, and copper. *Am J Ind Med* 10:163–175.

Araki, S, Murata, K, and Aono, H (1987) Central and peripheral nervous system dysfunction in workers exposed to lead, zinc and copper: A follow-up study of visual and somatosensory evoked potential. *Int Arch Occup Environ Health* 59:177–187.

Arezzo, JC, Simpson, R, and Brennan, NE (1985) Evoked potentials in the assessment of neurotoxicity in humans. *Neurobehav Toxicol Teratol* 7(4):299–304.

Barber, C (ed) (1980) *Evoked Potentials: Proceedings*

of an International Evoked Potential Symposium Held in Nottingham, England. Baltimore: University Park Press.

Bodis-Wollner, I (ed) (1982) *Evoked Potentials, Annals of the New York Academy of Sciences,* Vol. 388. New York: New York Academy of Sciences.

Boeri, E, Bordo, B, Crenna, P, et al. (1978) Preliminary results of a neurological investigation of the population exposed to TCDD in the Seveso region. *Riv Pat Ner Ment* 99:111–128.

Boring, EG (1950) *A History of Experimental Psychology.* New York: Appleton-Century-Crofts.

Bornschein, RL and Rabinowitz, MB (1985) Foreword. *Environ Res* 38:1–2.

Brazier, MAB (1984) *A History of Neurophysiology in the 17th and 18th Centuries: From Concept to Experiment.* New York: Raven Press.

Brazier, MAB (1986) The emergence of electrophysiology as an aid to neurology. In *Electrodiagnosis in Clinical Neurology* (2nd ed), MJ Aminoff (ed). pp. 1–19. New York: Churchill Livingstone.

Buchthal, F (1982a) Human nerve potentials evoked by tactile stimuli: I. Maximum conduction and properties of compound potentials. *Acta Physiol Scand [Suppl]* 502:5–18.

Buchthal, F (1982b) Human nerve potentials evoked by tactile stimuli: II. Stimulus parameters and recruitment of components. *Acta Physiol Scand [Suppl]:* 502:19–32.

Buchthal, F and Behse, F (1979) Electrophysiology and nerve biopsy in men exposed to lead. *Br J Ind Med* 36:135–147.

Buchthal, F and Rosenfalck, A (1966) Evoked action potential and conduction velocity in human sensory nerves. *Brain Res* 3:1–122.

Buchthal, F, Rosenfalck, A, and Behse, F (1975) Sensory potentials of normal and diseased nerves. In *Peripheral Neuropathy,* PJ Dycke, PK Thomas, and EH Lambert (eds) pp. 442–464. Philadelphia: WB Saunders.

Burchfiel, JL, Duffey, FH, Bartels, PH et al. (1980) The combined discriminating power of quantitative electroencephalography and neuropsychological measures in evaluating central nervous system effects of lead at low levels. In *Low Level Lead Exposure,* HL Needleman (ed) pp. 91–119. New York: Raven Press.

Chatrian, G-E (1986) Electrophysiology: Evaluation of brain death. In *Electrodiagnosis in Clinical Neurology* (2nd ed), MJ Aminoff (ed) pp. 669–736. New York: Churchill Livingstone.

Chiappa, KH (1983) *Evoked Potentials in Clinical Medicine.* New York: Raven Press.

Doull, J and Bruce, MC (1986) Origin and scope of toxicology. In *Casarett and Doull's Toxicology: The Basic Science of Poisons* (3rd ed), CD Klaasen, MO Amdur, and J Doull, (eds) pp. 3–10. New York: Macmillan.

Eisen, A and Aminoff, MJ (1986) Somatosensory evoked potentials. In *Electrodiagnosis in Clinical Neurology* (2nd ed), MJ Aminoff (ed) pp. 535–595. New York: Churchill Livingstone.

Gevins, AS (1986) Quantitative aspects of EEG and evoked potentials. In *Electrodiagnosis in Clinical Neurology* (2nd ed), MJ Aminoff (ed) pp. 149–203. New York: Churchill Livingstone.

Glickman, L, Valciukas, JA, Lilis, R, et al. (1984) Occupational lead exposure: Effects on saccadic eye movements. *Int Arch Occup Environ Health* 54:115–125.

Goodin, DS (1986) Event-related (endogenous) potentials. In *Electrodiagnosis in Clinical Neurology,* MJ Aminoff (ed) pp. 575–595. New York: Churchill Livingstone.

Goodman Gilman, A, Goodman, LS, and Gilman, A (1980) *Goodman-Gilman's The Pharmacological Basis of Therapeutics* (6th ed). New York: Macmillan.

Gramoni, R (1980) Retinal function of rats exposed to organomercurials. In *Neurotoxicity of the Visual System,* WH Merigan and B Weiss (eds) pp. 101–111. New York: Raven Press.

Granit, R (1955) *Receptors and Sensory Perception.* New Haven: Yale University Press.

Grant, WM (1980) The peripheral visual system as a target. In *Experimental and Clinical Neurotoxicology,* P Spencer and HH Schaumberg (eds) pp. 77–91.

He, F, Zhang, S, Wang, H et al. (1989) Neurological and electroneuromyographic assessment of the adverse effects of acrylamide on occupational exposed workers. *Scand J Work Environ Health* 15(2):125–129.

Hillyard, SA and Woods, DL (1979) Electrophysiological analysis of human brain function. In *Handbook of Behavioral Neurobiology,* Vol 2, *Neuropsychology,* MS Gazzaniga (ed) pp. 345–378. New York: Plenum Press.

Honet, JC, Jebsen, RH, and Perrin, EB (1968) Variability of nerve conduction determinations in normal persons. *Arch Physiol Med Rehab* 650–654.

Kooi, KA, Tucker, RP, and Marshall, RE (1978) *Fundamentals of Electroencephalography* (2nd ed). New York: Harper & Row.

Kimura, J (1989) *Electrodiagnosis in Diseases of Nerve and Muscle: Principles and Practice.* Philadelphia, PA: FA Davis.

Kornhuber, HH and Deecke, L (1965) Hirnpotentialanderungen bei wilkurbewegungen und passiven Bewegungen des Menschen, Bereitschaftpotential und reafferente Potential. *Pflugers Arch* 284:1–17.

Langauer-Lewowicka, H and Kazibutowska, Z (1989) Multimodal evoked potentials in occupational exposure to metallic mercury. *Polish J Occup Med* 2(2):192–199.

Ma, DM and Liverson, JA (1983) *Nerve Conduction Handbook*. Philadelphia, PA: FA Davis.

Niedermeyer, E and Lopez da Silva, F (1982) *Electroencephalography: Basic principles, clinical applications and related fields*. Baltimore: Urban & Schawartzenberg.

Ödkvist, LM, Larsby, B, Fredrickson, JMF, et al. (1980) Vestibular and oculomotor disturbances caused by industrial solvents. *J Otolaryngol* 9(1):53–59.

Oh, SJ (1984) *Clinical Electromyography: Nerve Conduction Studies*. Baltimore: University Park Press.

Ørbæck, H, Risberg, J, Rosén, I et al. (1985) Effect of long-term exposure to solvents in the paint industry. *Scand J Work Environ Health* 11(Suppl 2):16.

Otto, D (ed) (1978) *Multidisciplinary Perspectives in Event-Related Potential Research, Proceedings of the Fourth International Congress on Event-Related Slow Potentials of the Brain (EPICIV), Hendersonville, North Carolina, April 4–10, 1976*. Washington, DC: United States Environmental Protection Agency, Office of Research and Development, Environmental Research Information Center, Cincinnati, Ohio, Publication No EPA-600 9-77-043.

Otto, DA (1983) The application of event-related slow brain potentials in occupational medicine. In *Neurobehavioral Methods in Occupational Health*, R Giglidi, MG Cassito, and V Foà (eds) pp. 71–78. New York: Pergamon Press.

Otto, DA, Robinson, G, Bauman, S, et al. (1985) 5-Year follow-up study of children with low-to-moderate lead absorption: Electrophysiological evaluation. *Environ Res* 38:168–186.

Picton, TW, Taylor, MJ, Durieux-Smith, A, et al. (1986) Brainstem auditory evoked potentials in pediatrics. In *Electrodiagnosis in Clinical Neurology* (2nd ed), MJ Aminoff (ed) pp. 505–534. New York: Churchill Livingstone.

Piikivi, L and Tolonen, U (1989) EEG findings in chlor-alkali workers subjected to long-term exposure to mercury vapors. *Brit J Ind Med* 46(6):370–375.

Rebert, CS (1980) The brain stem auditory evoked response as a tool in neurobehavioral toxicology and medicine. In *Motivation, Motor and Sensory Processes of the Brain: Progress in Brain Research*, Vol. 54, HH Kornhuber and L Deeke (eds) pp. 458–461. Amsterdam: Elsevier.

Schaumburg HH, Wisniewski, H, and Spencer, PS (1974) Ultrastructural studies of the dying-back process: I. Peripheral nerve terminal and axon degeneration in systemic acrylamide intoxication. *J Neuropathol Exp Neurol* 33:260–284.

Seppäläinen, AM and Hernberg, S (1972) Sensitive techniques for detecting subclinical lead neuropathy. *Br J Ind Med* 29:443–449.

Seppäläinen, AM and Hernberg, S (1980) Subclinical lead neuropathy. *Am J Ind Med* 1:413–420.

Seppäläinen, A and Hernberg, S (1982) A follow-up study of nerve conduction velocity in lead exposed workers. *Neurobehavioral Toxicol Teratol* 4:721–722.

Seppäläinen, AM and Rajaniemi, R (1984) Local neurotoxicity of methyl methacrylate among dental technicians. *Am J Ind Med* 5(6):471–477.

Seppäläinen, AM, Tola, S, Hernberg, S et al. (1975) Subclinical neuropathy at "safe" levels of lead exposure. *Arch Environ Health* 30:180–183.

Seppäläinen, AM, Hernberg, S, and Kock, B (1979) Relationship between blood lead levels and nerve conduction velocities. *Neurotoxicol* 1:313–332.

Singer, R, Moses, H, Valciukas, JA et al. (1982) Nerve conduction velocity studies of workers employed in the manufacture of phenoxy herbicides. *Environ Res* 29:297–311.

Singer, R, Valciukas, JA, and Lilis, R (1983) Lead exposure and nerve conduction velocity: The differential time course of sensory and motor nerve effects. *Neurotoxicology* 4(2):193–202.

Snell, RS (1987) *Clinical Neuroanatomy for Medical Students*. Boston: Little, Brown & Co.

Sokol, S (1986) Visual evoked potentials. In *Electrodiagnosis in Clinical Neurobiology* (2nd ed), MJ Aminoff (ed) pp. 441–466. New York: Churchill Livingstone.

Stockard, JJ, Stockard, JE, and Sharbrough, FW (1986) Brainstem auditory potentials in neurology: Methodology, interpretation, and clinical application. In *Electrodiagnosis in Clinical Neurology* (2nd ed), MJ Aminoff (ed) pp. 467–503. New York: Churchill Livingstone.

Tharp, BR (1986) Neonatal and pediatric electroencephalography. In *Electrodiagnosis in Clinical Neurology* (2nd ed), MJ Aminoff (ed) pp. 77–124. New York: Churchill Livingstone.

Tsutsui, J (1980) Clinical and pathological studies of eye movement disorders in Minamata disease. In *Neurotoxicity of the Visual System*, WH Merigan and B Weiss (eds) pp. 187–202. New York: Raven Press.

Walter, WG, Cooper, R, Aldridge, VJ, et al. (1964) Contingent negative variation: An electric sign of sensori-motor association and expectancy in the human brain. *Nature* 203:380–384.

World Health Organization (1986) *Principles and Methods for the Assessment of Neurotoxicity Associated with Exposure to Chemicals*. Geneva: World Health Organization.

SUGGESTED READINGS

Ajmone-Marsan, C (1986) Depth electrography and electrocorticography. In *Electrodiagnosis in Clinical Neurology* (2nd ed), MJ Aminoff (ed) pp. 205–230. New York: Churchill Livingstone.

Anderson, P and Kaada, BR (1953) The electroencephalogram in poisoning by lacquer thinner (butyl acetate and toluene). *Acta Pharmacol Toxicol* 9:125–130.

Arezzo, JC, Schaumburg, HH, and Spencer, PS (1982) Structure and function of the somatosensory system: A neurotoxicological perspective. *Environ Health Perspect* 44:23–30.

Arezzo, JC, Schaumburg, HH, Vaughan, et al. (1982) Hind limb somatosensory evoked potentials in the monkey: The effects of distal axonopathy. *Ann Neurol* 12:24–32.

Armington, JC (1974) *The Electroretinogram.* New York: Academic Press.

Babel, J, Stangos, N, Korol, S, et al. (1977) *Ocular Electrophysiology: A Clinical and Experimental Study of Electroretinogram, Electro-Oculogram, Visual Evoked Response.* Stuttgart: Georg Thieme.

Barret, L, Arsac, P, Vincent, M, et al. (1982) Evoked trigeminal nerve potential in chronic trichloethylene intoxication. *J Toxicol* 19(4):419–423.

Barret, L, Garrel, S, Daniel, V, et al. (1987) Chronic trichloroethylene intoxication: A new approach by trigeminal-evoked potentials? *Arch Environ Health* 42(5):297–302.

Basmajian, JV (1972) Electromyography comes of age. *Science* 176:603–609.

Beck, EC, Dustman, RE, and Lewis, EG (1975) The use of the averaged evoked potentials in the evaluation of central nervous system disorders. *Int J Neurol* 9:211–232.

Behse, F and Buchthal, F (1978) Sensory action potentials and biopsy of the sural nerve in neuropathy. *Brain* 101:473–493.

Beningnus, VA (1984) EEG as a cross species indicator of neurotoxicity. *Neurobehav Toxicol Teratol* 6(6):473–483.

Bennet, MH and Janetta, PJ (1980) Trigeminal evoked potentials in humans. *Electroencephalogr Clin Neurophysiol* 48:517–526.

Bolton, CF, Carter, K, and Koval, JJ (1982) Temperature effects on conduction studies of normal and abnormal nerve. *Muscle Nerve* 5:S145–S147.

Boyes, W, and Dyer, R (1983) Pattern reversal and flash evoked potentials following acute triethylin exposure. *Neurobehav Toxicol Teratol* 5:571–577.

Boyes, WK, Jenkins, DE, and Dyer, RS (1985) Chlordiform produces contrast-dependent changes in visual-evoked potentials in hooded rats. *Exp Neurol* 89:391–407.

Brazier, MAB (1987) *A History of Neurophysiology in the 19th Century.* New York: Raven Press.

Brown, HW (1971) Electroencephalographic changes and disturbance of brain function following human organophosphate exposure. *Northwest Med* 70:845–846.

Brown, WS, Marsh, JT and LaRue, A (1983) Exponential electrophysiological aging: P3 latency. *Electroencephalogr Clin Neurophysiol* 55:277–285.

Burchfiel, JL and Duffy, FH (1982) Organophosphate neurotoxicity: Chronic effects of sarin on the electroencephalogram of monkey and man. *Neurobehav Toxicol Teratol* 4(6):767–778.

Callaway, E, Tueting, P, and Celesia, GG (eds) (1978) *Event-Related Brain Potentials in Man.* New York: Academic Press.

Campbell, WW, Ward, LC, and Swift, TR (1981) Nerve conduction velocity varies inversely with height. *Muscle Nerve* 4:520–323.

Cerra, D and Johnson, EW (1962) Motor nerve conduction velocity in premature infants. *Arch Physiol Med Rehab* 43:160–164.

Chalupa, B, Synková, S, and Sevcík, M (1960) The assessment of electroencephalographic changes and memory disturbances in acute intoxications with industrial poisons. *Br J Ind Med* 17:238–241.

Chen, RC, Sung, SM, Chen, CF, et al. (1978) Normal motor nerve conduction velocity amongst Chinese in Taiwan. *J Formos Med Assoc* 77:394–401.

Courjon, J, Mauguiere, F, and Revol, M (1982) *Advances in Neurology,* Vol. 32: *Clinical Applications of Evoked Potentials in Neurology.* New York: Raven Press.

Cruz Martinez, AS, Barrio, M, Perez Conde, MC et al. (1978) Electrophysiological aspects of sensory conduction velocity in healthy adults. II. Ratio between the amplitude of sensory evoked potentials at the wrist on stimulating different fingers in both hands. *J Neurol Neurosurg Psychiatry* 41:1097–1101.

Daube, J (1980) Nerve conduction studies. In *Electrodiagnosis in Clinical Neurology,* J Aminoff (ed) pp. 229–264. New York: Churchill Livingstone.

Dawson, GD (1951) A summation technique for detecting small signals in a large irregular background. *J Physiol (Lond)* 115:2P–3P.

Deecke, L, Becker, W, Grozinger, B, et al. (1973) Human brain potentials preceding voluntary limb movement. *Electroencephalogr Clin Neurophysiol [Suppl]* 33:87–94.

Deecke, L, Grozinger, B, and Kornhuber, HH (1976) Voluntary finger movements in man: Cerebral potentials and theory. *Biol Cybernet* 23:99–119.

Deecke, L, Scheid, P, and Kornhuber, HH (1969) Distribution of readiness potential, pre-motion positivity, and motor potential of the human cerebral cortex. *Exp Brain Res* 7:158–168.

DeJesus, PV, Hausmanowa-Petrusewicz, I, and Barchi, RL (1973) The effect of temperature on nerve conduction of human slow and fast nerve fibers. *Neurology (Minneap)* 23:1182–1189.

DeJesus, CPV, and Pleasure, DE (1973) Hexachlorophene neuropathy. *Arch Neurol* 29:180.

Dorfman, IJ and Bosely, TM (1979) Age related changes in peripheral and central nerve conduction in man. *Neurology (Minneap)* 29:38–44.

Drenth, HJ, Ensberg, IFG, Roberts, DV, et al. (1972)

Neuromuscular function in agriculture workers using pesticides. *Arch Environ Health* 25:395–398.

Duffy, FH, Burchfiel, JL, Bartels, PM, et al. (1979) Long-term effects of an organophosphate upon the human electroencephalogram. *Toxicol Appl Pharmacol* 47:161–176.

Duncan-Johnson, CC and Donchin, E (1982) The P300 component of the event-related potential as an index of information processing. *Biol Psychol* 14:1–52.

Dyer, RS (1980) Effects of prenatal and postnatal exposure to carbon monoxide on visually-evoked responses in rats. In *Neurotoxicity of the Visual System*, B Weiss and W Merigan (eds) pp. 17–33. New York: Raven Press.

Dyer, RS (1985a) The use of sensory-evoked potentials in toxicology. *Fund Appl Toxicol* 5:24–40.

Eccles, CU (1988) EEG correlates of neurotoxicity. *Neurotoxicol Teratol* 10(5):423–428.

Evarts, EV, Shinoka, Y, and Wise, SP (1984) *Neurophysiological Approaches to Higher Brain Function*. New York: John Wiley & Sons.

Ewert, T, Beginn, U, Winneke, G, et al. (1986) Sensory nerve conduction and visual and somatosensory evoked potentials in children exposed to lead. *Nervenartz* 57(8):465–471.

Feldman, RG (1986) Nerve conduction measures in occupational medicine. *Semin Occup Med* 1(3):163–173.

Feldman, RG, Hayes, MK, Younes, R, et al. (1977) Lead neuropathy in adults and children. *Arch Neurol* 34:481–488.

Feldman, RG, Niles, CA, Kelley-Hayes, M, et al. (1979) Peripheral neuropathy in arsenic smelter workers. *Neurology (Minneap)* 29:930–944.

Ford, JM, Roth, WT, Mohs, RC, et al. (1979) Event-related potentials recorded from young and old adults during a memory retrieval task. *Electroencephalogr Clin Neurophysiol* 47:450–459.

Fox, DA, Lowndes, HE, and Bierpkamper, GG (1982) Electrophysiological techniques in neurotoxicology. In *Nervous System Toxicology,* CL Mitchell (ed) pp. 299–335. New York: Raven Press.

Gevins, AS Morgan, NH, Bressler, SL, et al. (1987) Human neuroelectric patterns predict performance accuracy. *Science* 235:580–585.

Gilliatt, RW (1982) Electrophysiology of peripheral neuropathies: An overview. *Muscle Nerve* 5:S108–116.

Goodgold, J and Eberstein, A (1983) *Electrodiagnosis of Neuromuscular Diseases*. Baltimore: Williams & Wilkins.

Halliday, AM (1982) *Evoked Potentials in Clinical Testing*. Bath: Churchill Livingstone.

Harbin, TJ (1985) The late positive component of the evoked cortical potential: Application to neurotoxicity testing. *Neurobehav Toxicol Teratol* 7:339–344.

Harbin TJ, Beningnus, VA, Muller, KE, et al. (1988)

The effects of low-level carbon monoxide exposure upon evoked cortical potentials in young and elderly men. *Neurotoxicol Teratol* 10(2):93–100.

Hari, R and Lounasmaa, OV (1989) Recording and interpretation of cerebral magnetic fields. *Science* 244:432–436.

Heffly, E, Foote, B, Mui, T, et al. (1985) PEARL II: Portable laboratory computer system for psychophysiological assessment using event related brain potentials. *Neurobehav Toxicol Teratol* 7:399–407.

Horvath, M and Frantik, E (1979) Industrial chemicals and drugs lowering central nervous system activation level: Quantitative assessment of hazards in man and animals. *Acta Nerv Super (Praha)* 21:269–272.

Horvath, M and Michalova, C (1956) Changes of EEG in experimental exposure to carbon disulfide in the light of Vedensky's theory of parabiosis. *Arch Gewerbepathol* 15:131–136.

Hosko, M (1970) The effect of carbon monoxide on the visual evoked potential and the spontaneous electroencephalogram. *Arch Environ Health* 21:174–180.

Hughes, JR (1982) *EEG in Clinical Practice*. Boston: Butterworths.

Iida, M, Yamamura, Y, and Sobue, I (1969) Electromyography findings and conduction velocity on *n*-hexane polyneuropathy. *Electromyography* 9:247.

Jabre, JF and Hacken, ER (1983) *EMG Manual*. Springfield, IL: Charles C Thomas.

John, ER, Prichep, LS, Fridman, J, et al. (1988) Neurometrics: Computer-assisted differential diagnosis of brain dysfunctions. *Science* 239:162–169.

Johnson, BL (1980) Electrophysiological methods in neurotoxicity testing. In *Experimental and Clinical Neurotoxicology,* PS Spencer and HH Schaumburg (eds) pp. 726–742. Baltimore: Williams & Wilkins.

Johnson, EW (1980) *Practical Electromyography*. Baltimore: Williams & Wilkins.

Kellaway, P and Petersin, I (1974) *Automation of Clinical Electroencephalography*. New York: Raven Press.

Kimura, J (1976) Collison techniques: Physiological block of nerve impulses in studies of motor nerve conduction velocity. *Neurology (Minneap)* 26:680–682.

Kimura, J (1984) Principles and pitfalls of nerve conduction studies. *Ann Neurol* 16:415–429.

Kimura, J (1989) *Electrodiagnosis in Diseases of Nerve and Muscle: Principles and Practice*. Philadelphia, PA: FA Davis.

Knott, JR and Irwin, DA (1973) Anxiety, stress and the contingent negative variation. *Arch Gen Psychiatry* 29:538–541.

Krarup, C and Buchthal, F (1980) Conduction studies in peripheral nerve. *Neurobehav Toxicol Teratol* 7:319–323.

Kutas, M, McCarthy, G, and Donchin, E (1977) Augmenting mental chronometry: The P300 as a measure of stimulus evaluation time. *Science* 197:792–795.

LeQuesne, PM (1978) Neurophysiological investigation of subclinical and minimal toxic neuropathies. *Muscle Nerve* 1:392.

LeQuesne, PM (1978) Clinical expression of neurotoxic injury and diagnostic use of electromyography. *Environ Health Persp* 26:89–95.

Liveson, JA and Spielholz, NI (1979) *Peripheral Neurology.* Philadelphia: FA Davis.

Loeb, GE and Parker, C (1986) *Electromyography for Experimentalists.* Chicago: University of Chicago Press.

Lopez da Silva, FH and Storm Van Leeuwen, W (eds) (1986) *Handbook of Electroencephalography and Clinical Neurophysiology.* Amsterdam: Elsevier.

Low, MD, Borda, RP, and Kellaway, P (1966) Contingent negative variation in rhesus monkeys: An EEG sign of a specific mental process. *Percept Mot Skills* 22:443–446.

Lowndes, HE (ed) (1987) *Electrophysiology in Neurotoxicology.* Boca Raton: FL: CRC Press.

Lukas, E (1983) Electroneurography: A review with regard to personal experience with antidromic sensory conduction velocity of N ulnaris and N medianus and H-reflex velocity of N tibialis. *Adv Biosc* 46:17–25.

Ma, DM and Liverson, JA (1983) *Nerve Conduction Handbook.* Philadelphia, PA: FA Davis.

Manu, P, Lilis, R, Landranjan, I, et al. (1970) The value of electromyographic changes in the early diagnosis of carbon disulphide neuropathy. *Med Lavoro* 61(2):102–108.

Mattson, JL and Albee, RR (1988) Sensory evoked potentials in neurotoxicology. *Neurotoxicol Teratol* 10(5):435–443.

McCarthy, G, and Donchin, E (1981) A metric for thought: A comparison of P300 latency and reaction time. *Science* 211:77–80.

Mendell, JR, Saida, K, Ganansia, MF, et al. (1974) Toxic polyneuropathy produced by methyl-*n*-butyl ketone. *Science* 185:787–789.

Metcalf, DR and Holmes, JH (1969) EEG, psychological and neurological alterations in humans with organophosphorus exposure. *Ann NY Acad Sci* 160:375–385.

Montanini, R and Torrigiani, G (1962) Valeur et limites de l'électroencéphalografie dans les intoxications professionalles. *Scapel* 115:51.

Moody, L, Arezzo, J, and Otto, D (1986) Evaluation of workers for easy peripheral neuropathy: The role of existing diagnostic tools. *Semin Occup Med* 1(3):153–162.

Muiser, H, Hoogendijk, EMG, Hooisma, J (1987) Lead exposure during demolition of a steel structure coated with lead-based paints: II. Reversible changes in the conduction velocity of the motor nerves in tran-

siently exposed workers. *Scand J Work Environ Health* 13:56–61.

Nielsen, VK (1973) Sensory and motor nerve conduction in the median nerve in normal subjects. *Acta Med Scand* 194:435–443.

Norris, AH, Schock, NW, and Wagman, IH (1953) Age changes in the maximum conduction velocity of motor fibers of human ulnar nerves. *J Appl Physiol* 5:589–593.

Nuciante Cesaro, A and Salvini, M (1953) Osservazioni elettroencefalografici nei sulfo carbonismo professionale. *Folia Med (Napoli)* 36:409.

Nunez, PL (1981) *Electric Fields in the Brain: The Neurophysics of EEG.* New York: Raven Press.

Ochoa, J (1980) Criteria for the assessment of polyneuropathy. In *Experimental and Clinical Neurotoxicology,* PS Spencer and HH Schaumburg (eds) pp. 681–707. Baltimore: Williams & Wilkins.

Otto, DA (1986) The use of evoked potentials in neurotoxicity testing of workers. *Semin Occup Med* 1(3):175–183.

Otto, DA, Beningnus, VA, Muller, KE, et al. (1981) Effects of age and body lead on CNS function in young children: I. Slow cortical potentials. *Electrophysiol Clin Neurophysiol* 52:229–471.

Otto, D, Baumann, S, and Robinson, G (1985) Application of portable microprocessor-based system for electrophysiological field testing of neurotoxicity. *Neurobehav Toxicol Teratol* 7:409–414.

Pazderova-Vejlupkova, J, Nemcova, M, Pickova, J, et al. (1981) The development and prognosis of chronic intoxication by tetrachlordibenzo-*p*-dioxin in men. *Arch Environ Health* 36:5–11.

Rebert, CS (1983) Multisensory evoked potentials in experimental and applied neurotoxicology. *Neurobehav Toxicol Teratol* 5:659–672.

Rebert, CS, McAdam, DW, Knott, JR, et al. (1967) Slow potential change in human brain related with level of motivation. *J Comp Physiol Psychol* 63:20–23.

Redmond, A (ed) (1977) *EEG Informatics: A Didactic Review and Applications of EEG Data Processing.* Amsterdam: Elsevier.

Roberts, DV (1977) A longitudinal electromyographic study of six men occupationally exposed to organophosphorus compounds. *Int Arch Occup Environ Health* 38:221–229.

Rose, DF, Smith, PD, and Sato, S (1987) Magnetoencephalography and epilepsy research. *Science* 238:329–335.

Rosenman, KD, Valciukas, JA, Glickman, L, et al. (1986) Sensitive indicators of inorganic mercury toxicity. *Arch Environ Res* 41(4):208–215.

Roth, B, and Klimkova-Deutschova, E (1963) The effect of the chronic action of industrial poisons on the electroencephalogram of man. *Rev Czech Med* 9:217–227.

Rowland, LP (1985) Diseases of the motor unit: The

motor neuron, peripheral nerve and muscle. In *Principles of Neural Science* (2nd ed), ER Kandel and JH Schwartz (eds) pp. 196–208. New York: Elsevier.

Ruchtin, DA and Glaser, EM (1976) *Principles of Neurobiological Signal Analysis.* New York: Academic Press.

Schaumburg, HH, Spencer, PS, and Thomas, PK (1983) *Disorder of Peripheral Nerves.* Philadelphia: FA Davis.

Schuchmann, JA (1977) Sural nerve conduction: A standardized technique. *Arch Phys Med Rehab* 58:166–168.

Seppäläinen, AM (1973) Neurotoxic effects of industrial solvents. *Electroencephalogr Clin Neurophysiology* 34:702–703.

Seppäläinen, AM (1975) Applications of neurophysiological methods in occupational medicine: A review. *Scand J Work Environ Health* 1:1–14.

Seppäläinen AM (1984) Electrophysiological evaluation of central and peripheral neural effects of lead exposure. *Neurotoxicology* 5(3):43–52.

Serra, C and Ambrosio, L (1961) L'Elettroencefalogramma in Medicina de Lavoro. Naples: Acta Neurologica.

Shapiro, IM, Summer, AJ, Spitz, LR, et al. (1982) Neurophysiological and neuropsychological function in mercury exposed dentists. *Lancet* 1:1147–1150.

Stohr, M, and Petruch, F (1979) Somatosensory evoked potentials following stimulation of the trigeminal nerve in man. *J Neurol* 220:95–98.

Stylová, V (1977) Electroencephalography in the diagnosis of early cerebral changes due to carbon disulfide [in German]. *Int Arch Occup Environ Health* 48:263–282.

Tecce, JJ (1972) Contigent negative variation (CNV) and psychological processes in man. *Psychol Bull* 77:73–108.

Waldrop, MM (1989) Biomagnetism attracts diverse crowd. *Science* 245:1041–1046.

Walter, WG (1967) Slow potentials changes in the human brain associated with expectancy, decision and intention. *Electroencephalogr Clin Neurophysiol [Suppl]* 26:123–130.

Xintaras, C, Johnson, BL, Ulrich, CE, et al. (1966) Application of the evoked resonse technique in air polution toxicology. *Toxicol Appl Pharmacol* 8:77–87.

Zilm, DH, Huskar, L, Carlen, PL, et al. (1980) EEG correlates of the alcohol-induced organic brain syndrome in man. *Clin Toxicol* 16(3):345–358.

6

Imaging of the Nervous System

An *imaging technique* is one that allows the visualization of structural features of the nervous system or pharmacological processes resulting from the use of specially treated chemical substances. Until recently, the location and extent of neural lesions was primarily a judgment based on the neurological examination, the interpretation of signs and symptoms, and the use of imaging techniques of poor resolution such as X-ray.

The urge to know what happens inside the brain when one thinks has captured the interest of many since the brain was first conceived as the site of thinking. There are well-documented Greek and Roman sources about these speculations. But anthropological evidence suggests that this yearning has an even earlier origin—ie, Egyptian, Chinese, and American Indian cultures. The fascinating story of the search for a visual image of the nervous system has rarely been told to nonspecialists; the little gem of a book by Oldendorf (1980) is a rare exception. However interesting their historical backgrounds, not all imaging techniques have been used in neurotoxicological research. Most importantly, not all have shown promise in the past or at the present time for this purpose.

Major breakthroughs and technical developments resulting in improved imaging techniques have occurred in no particular pattern and have sometimes coexisted without influencing each other very much. The term "imaging" is one of recent coinage. Only when this diverse collection of techniques is lumped within the framework of "imaging" can both their common features and their fundamental differences be appreciated.

X-RAY-BASED TECHNIQUES

The discovery of the X-ray by Roentgen in 1895 was translated into practical use the very next year. In 1896 the first radiography of the skull was obtained. However, much to the disappointment of those who had hoped this technique would reveal new features of brain structure, no such visualization resulted.

Angiography

Injecting opaque substances into the vascular system of cadavers (1896 to 1926) and the visualization of blood vessels by X-ray gave rise to *angiography*. However, it was not until 1926 that Egas-Moniz, a Portugese neurosurgeon, performed an angiogram in a live patient for the first time.

Early X-ray imaging techniques were hazardous. Technical personnel, scientists, and physicians died from radiation exposure; radiation was not recognized as a health hazard until people began to die from it. X-ray angiography can also result in hemorrhage and blood clotting, and the opaque material can produce allergies or deprive the brain cells of oxygen (anoxia), leading to brain damage.

Pneumoencephalography

Pneumoencephalography (PEG) involves the injection of air into the cavities of the nervous system for imaging purposes ("pneumo" means "air" in Greek). Pneumoencephalography began with the accidental introduction of air into the brain ventricles—cavities in the central nervous system filled with liquid—of a man who suffered head trauma. Since air is about 800 times less dense to X-rays than water, an air bubble is clearly visible in the patient's brain X-ray image. Air bubbles in the brain had been observed toward the end of the 19th century, but the year 1912 marked the beginning of its use in imaging. The first injection of air into the head of a patient to visualize cerebral ventricles was performed by Dandy in 1918. Because of its risks and the advent of new imaging procedures, PEG is no longer in use.

ECHOENCEPHALOGRAPHY

The tragic sinking of the Titanic in 1912 motivated the search for better methods of locating icebergs. Echolocation of objects was proposed about that time, but the effective use of sound echoes by sonar was not accomplished until around the time of World War II.

Echoencephalography was short-lived as a brain-imaging technique. It was first used in 1956 to detect shifts in the brain's midline structures. Morphologically, the brain is a fairly symmetrical structure. If the skull were transparent, the left hemisphere of the brain would be the mirror image of the right. The midline of the brain is the site where the left and right hemispheres are joined. Should a mass exert pressure on the right side, the acoustic picture of the midline will be seen as shifted to the left. Until the 1970s echolocalization was used fairly effectively for that purpose. However, it faded away when improved imaging techniques, such as computer-assisted tomography (CAT), were shown to have superior image resolution capabilities.

Ultrasound has long been successfully used in the imaging of unborn fetuses. This is an important research tool in teratology, where gross effects of neurotoxic agents in the unborn can sometimes be assessed. However, neurotoxicological studies in which the ultrasound image of the fetus is used are limited to case reports. Thus far, no large-scale epidemiological or neurotoxicological studies have been reported.

Radiography, pneumoencephalography, angiography, and ultrasound imaging are not common tools for everyday use in neurotoxicological research, either in humans or in animals. An exception to this is the clinical assessment of the overt picture of poisoning, where fairly symmetrical swelling of neural structures can often occur.

Modern imaging techniques are important clinical and research tools, but they are rather expensive, and many countries around the world do not have access to them. Traditional X-ray-based procedures are still effective aids for judging neurotoxicity (ie, whether or not a neurotoxic effect is occurring) and in the differential diagnosis of neurological diseases (ie, whether the patient is suffering from a chronic disease of occupational origin or the signs and symptoms are consistent with, for example, a degenerative disease).

ISOTOPE SCANNING

A fundamental correspondence between the brain's functional activity and its metabolism was postulated about a century ago (Roy and Sherrington 1890). The development of radioisotopes succeeded in establishing this connection, so long postulated on theoretical grounds only. Two historical events are worth noting: the discovery of the blood–brain barrier and the early use of gamma-emitting isotopes.

Paul Ehrlich first noted in the 1880s that when a mouse was injected with an aniline dye, the whole animal was quickly stained except the brain and the spinal cord. This extraordinary observation was interpreted as proof that the central nervous system had a selected protection against foreign substances. Brain capillaries—small blood vessels—were identified as providing a successful barrier.

Many myths have been shattered since this early discovery. Some of the tragedies resulting from the lack of understanding on how the blood–brain barrier operates, such as the thalidomide episode, are discussed in Chapter 9. It is now widely accepted that the blood–brain barrier is not impenetrable but rather **selectively** permeable. Moreover, it is now known that pathological conditions may affect this selective permeability. Tracers (radiolabeled substances) used to study the brain's blood flow and the brain's metabolic activity were found to bypass the blood–brain barrier.

The second historical event of importance was the intravenous injection of fluorescein for the detection of tumors during surgery, used first in 1947 (Oldendorf 1980). After injection of the fluorescein dye a brain tumor removed for biopsy fluoresced when illuminated by ultraviolet light, while the healthy neural tissue surrounding the tumor did not. Soon, fluorescein was replaced by radioactive isotopes for visualizing tumors.

An *isotope* is any one of the many forms of an element. Isotopes have the same or very similar properties as the common form of an element but with different atomic weights from the usual form. When radioisotopes decay, they give off gamma rays to gain their original state of equilibrium. The decay process

is defined in half-life units. *Half-life* is the time when half of the atoms have decayed to the original state. Isotope scanning methods have already been used to understand the effects of occupational and environmental agents in vitro (ie, in cells observed in laboratory dishes) or in vivo (ie, in laboratory animals while they are still alive).

Representative Research

Risberg and Hagtadius (1983) investigated whether measurements of regional cerebral blood flow (rCBF) could provide useful information in the description of changes of brain functions related to solvent exposure. The study group included 50 male workers from a paint factory ranging in age from 26 to 62 years who had been exposed to organic solvents—ketones, aromatic hydrocarbons, ethers, alcohols, etc.—for at least 10 years. The controls were 50 workers from a sugar refinery not exposed to such solvents. On the basis of current and past exposure data, subjects in the study group were divided into three "dose" groups: low, medium, and high. The regional cerebral blood flow was determined by a xenon-133 inhalation technique. Subjects inhaled the tracer mixed with air for 1 minute followed by 10 minutes of normal air breathing.

Each subject was measured first under conditions of rest and then during a mental task. The task consisted of learning visually presented word pairs on six slides with 10 word pairs each. Subjects were asked to recall one member of the pair immediately after rCBF measurements.

The mean rCBF of the total exposed group was significantly reduced when compared to controls. The workers in the high-dose group showed the greatest reduction, the low-dose group the least, and the medium group an intermediate value. The rCBF also declined with age. Although not statistically significant, mean test scores on the word-pair associates were lower in the exposed than in the control group.

The investigators reported that the highest-exposure group showed a significant increase in parietal, parietooccipital, and premotor activities in both brain hemispheres and that the regions showing signs of increased activity agreed well with earlier findings in normal subjects performing similar types of mental tasks. In addition, they concluded that these observations might be interpreted as reflecting a somewhat accelerated aging process in the brains of exposed workers.

Isotope scanning is still very much in use. From an historical point of view, the early attempts at isotope scanning of brain tissues in vitro and in vivo provided the necessary background for the development of instrumentation of modern imaging techniques such as positron emission tomography (PET; reviewed below).

COMPUTER-ASSISTED TOMOGRAPHY

It has often been said that isotope scanning and PET provide a chemical picture of the brain in vivo. The fact is that they are used primarily to detect morphological, not chemical, abnormalities. *Computer-assisted tomography* (CAT or CAT scanning; the original term was "computer-axial tomography," but the acronym CAT remained the same) was specifically developed for the study of the structure of the whole body, not primarily for the brain. But neurotoxic agents can cause morphological changes in the brain under special and often extreme circumstances—for example, brain malformations may be produced by organic mercury in children exposed to this neurotoxic agent in utero (Minamata disease). However, CAT scanning is hardly the technique of choice for the study of subclinical neurological changes associated with long-term low-level occupational or environmental exposure to neurotoxic agents. For one thing, CAT scanners cannot detect the important and essential difference between the brain's gray matter (neural cells) and white matter (fibers). Nevertheless, as discussed below, CAT scanning provided the

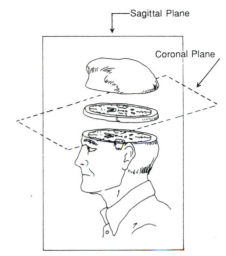

Fig. 6.1. Illustration of the image of the brain obtained by tomography and spatial planes. (From Gregory 1987.)

first striking evidence that occupational exposure to organic solvents can produce brain atrophy.

CAT scans are also known as X-ray computer tomographs (XCT) to differentiate them from other imaging techniques based on different principles. Tomography derives from the Greek "tomos" (a slice or a piece cut off) and "graphos" (to write, to represent). It is an imaging technique by which a single cross-sectional plane of an organ (in this case, the brain) is outlined, eliminating the planes of other adjacent structures (Fig. 6.1). Visually, a tomogram of the brain is a slice of someone's brain obtained in vivo!

The principles of CAT scanning can be broken down into five basic steps (Oldendorf 1980):

1. Collimation of the X-ray beam (ie, "focusing" of the X-ray into a beam).
2. X-ray interaction with brain tissue.
3. Detection of X-rays.
4. Reconstruction of the image via a computer.
5. Two-dimensional display of the final picture.

Picture in your mind an X-ray source placed in front of your head and an X-ray detector in the back, both on a straight line. Let the source–detector axis rotate around your head in a full horizontal plane, beaming X-rays and detecting them at a succession of points in the circle. The chair where you are sitting is elevated a few millimeters, and the procedure is repeated. This is the procedure underlying all tomographs.

Neural structures exist as different levels of opacity to X-rays. As a result, the energy of the X-ray beam reaches the detector at varying levels of intensity. The CAT scanner evolved from the original single beam detector. Now, fan-like arrays of hundreds of source–detector pairs are utilized, with the X-rays originating from a single source. The electrical signals generated from the array of X-ray-sensing devices are fed into a computer, which keeps track of the position and direction of movement of each detector. The computer reconstructs the signals by two basic procedures: (1) the information on the relative opacity to X-rays of various brain structures is stored in a computer, and (2) the tomogram—the "brain slice"—is calculated and visualized on the computer screen by means of "reconstruction algorithms," techniques based on integral calculus. In one circular passage around the brain's coronal ("crown-like") plane, the CAT scanner and the computer, fed with density data and reconstruction algorithms, reproduce a slice of the brain of a living person.

Computer-assisted tomographic scanners are invaluable sources of information for observing structural features of the brain such as tumors, brain anomalies produced by strokes, atrophy caused by degenerative diseases, and traumatic changes. In neurotoxicological research, they have also proved useful for the demonstration of atrophic changes in the brain produced by chronic alcoholism and chronic occupational exposure to industrial solvents. These morphological changes are, however, likely to be observed only in advanced stages of the neurotoxin-induced disease.

CAT scanners may be hazardous. High emissions of ionizing radiation have resulted in several recalls since 1977 (Portugal 1984). Concerns about whole-body X-ray radiations, on the other hand, have been minimized as a result of technical improvements in instrumentation (specifically, shielding and scanning speed).

POSITRON EMISSION TOMOGRAPHY

Pharmacological techniques taking advantage of a few isotopes that decay while emitting positrons have been available since the middle 1950s. But it is only since the middle 1980s that these techniques have been grouped under the common name of *positron emission tomography,* also known by its acronym PET. The tracers most frequently used are carbon 11, nitrogen 13, oxygen 15, and fluorine 18.

Positron emission tomography scanning involves four distinctive processes (Ter-Pogossian 1985):

1. Labeling a selected compound—oxygen, glucose, fatty and amino acids, drugs, body fluids, gases, etc.
2. Administering the compound by injection into the bloodstream.
3. Imaging the regional distribution of positron activity in the brain as a function of decay time by means of special instrumentation.
4. Reconstructing the tomogram by means of a procedure such as the one described for CAT—storage of computer density values and reconstruction algorithms.

In CAT scanning, the image is that of the attenuation of the radiation in tissues—ie, how tissues filter energy passing through. In PET scanning the image is that of the distribution of positron-emitting radionuclides. In PET scanning, as in many other scanning techniques, tissue "filtering" is also a factor to be considered. (Biological tissues "filter" the radiating energy by absorbing part of it; different tissues absorb different wavelengths.) In clinical studies, PET images for measuring oxygen and glucose consumption and protein synthesis are the most extensively used.

PET scanning has already been successfully used in the exploration of etiological factors of many brain disorders including psychiatric diseases (eg, schizophrenia) and neurological disorders (eg, epilepsy and Alzheimer's disease) and to study cognitive function in healthy and mentally or emotionally disturbed individuals.

How local cerebral glucose uptake is related to regional changes in brain function was demonstrated by the fundamental work of Sokoloff et al. (1977). First measured in laboratory animals, local cerebral glucose consumption was soon observed in humans (Reivich et al. 1979).

PET scanning shows great promise as a new technology for providing information on the brain's organization and function. PET scanning, for example, may have definite advantages over lesion studies. In lesion studies, the function of a region of the brain is inferred after the region is removed. In experimental lesion studies, a piece of brain tissue from a laboratory animal is surgically aspirated, burned, or rendered chemically nonfunctional, and the resulting behavior of the animal is observed (Lashley 1929). Clinical studies based on the observation of the effect of traumatic or surgical lesions on human behavior have similar limitations. Conclusions of lesion studies are based on observations of a brain functioning abnormally and are therefore perhaps not wholly appropriate for an understanding of the operation of the intact brain. PET scanning is appropriate, on the other hand, because it allows the observation of the brain of the intact, sometimes actively functioning, individual.

PET scanning allows the study of direct effects of stimuli on fundamental metabolic processes of the intact brain. It also makes possible the study of changes in brain metabolism during self-generated cognitive stimuli—ie, the process of recall of previously presented visual stimuli or the visual representation of mental images in one's memory.

Greenberg et al. (1981) studied subjects who were listening to and recalling a taped factual story delivered through a single earphone placed over one ear. To motivate them, subjects were told that they would get paid in proportion to the detail they could remember. PET results showed that the glucose metabolic rate of the auditory cortex contralateral to the side with the earphone was higher than that of the auditory cortex of the same side. This is in agreement with our current knowledge of the anatomy and physiology of the auditory pathways. Similar findings were obtained using visual and somatosensory stimulation and cognitive tasks (Gur and Reivich 1980). A good review of "normal" studies on cerebral metabolic effects resulting from differential glucose consumption in the brain is found in Reivich and Gur (1985).

PET is an invasive technique, and subjects suffer considerable anxiety as a consequence of the necessary arterial and venous catherization, the injection of the isotope, and the actual process of scanning. Radiological studies of the brain, echolocalization, and CAT scanning on the other hand can, for all practical purposes, be considered noninvasive. However, they are of limited value for neurotoxicological research.

MAGNETIC RESONANCE IMAGING

Magnetic resonance imaging (MRI) scanners have often been described as dream machines. Unlike CAT scanners and other X-ray-based techniques, MRI scanners can "see" through the thickest of bones (Fig. 6.2). No contrasting material is required. Moreover, MRI scanners can differentiate between gray and white matter, a distinction that CAT scanners cannot make.

The imaging principle of MRI scanning is based on the magnetic properties of element nuclei containing an odd number of protons. These nuclei behave like tiny spinning magnets. The heart of the MRI imager is a large superconducting magnet weighing about 6 tons. The magnet itself costs hundreds of

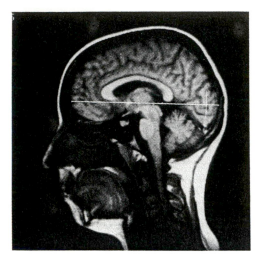

Fig. 6.2. An MRI tomograph (sagittal plane). (From Gregory 1987.)

thousands of dollars, representing 30% of the system's cost. When these "spinning magnets" are placed inside the very strong magnetic field generated by the magnet, the vast majority of the nuclei line up in the direction of that field. The nuclei also wobble around the axis very much like spinning tops. Different nuclei wobble at different frequencies.

A second magnetic field of alternating radiofrequency in the order of megahertz is then applied at right angles to the first. As a result of this alternating magnetic field added to the steady one, some nuclei move into a new alignment. If the frequency of the alternating magnetic field matches that of the natural wobbling frequency, the nuclei are "in resonance." This phenomenon is similar to making a tuning fork "hum" by hitting it with a sound having the fork's natural resonance frequency.

When the rapidly oscillating magnetic field is turned off, the resonating nuclei return to their original aligned position relative to the steady magnetic field. In the process of returning to their original aligned position, they release energy, with decay characteristics for each element. The signal is detected by coils and processed by a computer. The computer performs a mathematical process called Fourier transform aimed at analyzing the sig-

nal's distribution of frequencies and their relative strengths. A color code is then used to create a density map of the brain.

MRI scanners generate a density map of hydrogen, which, contained in water, makes up 75% of the composition of the human body. But MRI scanners also promise the imaging of sodium and phosophorus, not available with other imaging techniques (Duel et al. 1985). Phosphorus is involved in the energy-yielding mechanisms of all living processes and most living cells generate chemical processes involving this element. Thus, techniques to image this key element hold great promise.

The phenomenon of nuclear magnetic resonance, or NMR for short, was first described in 1946. Felix Block and Edward Purcell won the Nobel Prize in physics in 1952 for showing how MRI techniques could be used to study atomic nuclei. Further development of NMR imagers occurred in the early 1970s. Just who conceived the imaging principles first is a matter of controversy. In 1972 R. Damadian obtained a US patent for this invention; in 1973 F. Lauterbur described a similar principle.

Assessment of Magnetic Resonance Imaging Technology

Developers of MRI still face some problems. Exposure to magnetic fields is harmless except under conditions described below. However, it is dangerous for those wearing cardiac pacemakers or surgical metal clips. Also, the long-term consequences of exposure to high magnetic fields are unknown. Thus, the Food and Drug Administration (FDA) has limited the strength of the magnetic fields to 2 teslas. (A tesla equals 10,000 gauss, a unit of magnetic force.)

MRI scanners pose other, more dramatically dangerous conditions. "Otherwise innocuous objects, like hairpins, keys, and mechanical pencils fly toward the magnet as though shot from a rifle—with the same deadly effect on whoever happens to be in the way" (Portugal 1984).

MRI scanners are very expensive, their present costs being over a million dollars. When and if their price becomes reduced, we will see their true potential in competing with other imaging devices, particularly those based on ultrasound. The anatomic detail of images obtained in aborted fetuses by MRI scanning is better than that obtained by ultrasound. As stated earlier, safe, noninvasive techniques are badly needed in the study of the possible effects of exposure to neurotoxic effects in the unborn.

In a Consensus Development Conference that met in Bethesda, Maryland October 26 through 28, 1987, MRI was given high marks as a clinical and research tool. It was concluded that ". . . for diagnosing some diseases, especially those involving the brain and spinal cord . . . MRI is now superior to older techniques such as computer-assisted tomography (CT)" (Marks 1987). In addition, the panel concluded that ". . . [MRI] is roughly equivalent to CT for detecting most brain tumors, and superior to CT for diagnosing tumors located at the rear and base of the skull." CAT scanning still has an edge in detecting brain hemorrhages, an advantage that still makes it the method of choice for examining patients with possible strokes. A promising area of investigation, the panel concluded, is magnetic resonance spectography, which can be used to obtain information about metabolic states of tissues rather than their anatomy.

BRAIN ELECTRICAL ACTIVITY

Brain electrical activity mapping (BEAM) and its display on a color computer monitor are now possible. This mapping technique was developed when it became obvious that long-latency evoked potentials (event-related potentials, ERP, described in Chapter 5) were sensitive to background variations of brain activity. Duffy (1982) used 20 recording sites in the head with a standard electroencephalographic electrode positioner. Voltage frequencies detected at each electrode site are split on an equal-interval scale.

Two codes are employed: a "gray-scale" code in which the values of each frequency range are assigned to different gradations of gray between white and black (or different intensities of a single color) and a "pseudo-color" scheme in which each range of frequency values is assigned to a separate color.

BEAM scanning belongs both to the imaging techniques already discussed in this chapter and to that reviewed in the previous chapter dealing with electrophysiological procedures. BEAM scanning does not compete with CAT, PET, or NMR scanning. It is essentially a much-welcomed data-reduction technique in electroencephalographic and evoked potentials research. Because it is noninvasive, BEAM scanning has a distinct potential for neurotoxicological research both in field situations and in clinical studies.

INFRARED IMAGING

Infrared (IR) imaging, developed over the past 25 years as a result of military and industrial needs, has already been used in human neurotoxicological research for the assessment of eye movements in lead-exposed workers in the dark (Glickman et al. 1984).

Four wavelength regions of the infrared spectrum are used. These include the near-infrared wavelengths at about 1 μm and other "windows" at 2 to 2.5, 3.5 to 4.2, and 8 to 14 μm. In sensing equipment that has appeared in the market only a few years ago, windows are selected electronically. The thermal image of the whole body or restricted areas such as one eye can be observed in motion, "frozen," and stored. Infrared imaging offers great potential for assessing the effect of neurotoxic agents on the autonomic nervous system—for example, in perceiving alterations in the time course of recovery from cold stimulation which is indicative of alterations in autonomic innervation of blood vessels. Ravich (1986) has written a good technical review on the subject.

OTHER IMAGING TECHNIQUES

The concept of "imaging" can be stretched to include classical photography and motion and television pictures. Television cameras, for example, have been successfully used for the study of impaired eye movements as a result of methylmercury posioning (Tsutsui et al. 1972). *Acoustic imaging* has been used for the study of the development of the blinking reflex in the child. The blinking reflex is an unconditioned response—a reflex one is born with—of closing the eyes as a result of a sudden and loud noise. The suspicion that young babies do not hear is prompted by the absence of this blinking reflex. The blinking reflex can be elicited in the fetus at as early as 24 weeks of gestation by the use of acoustic imaging.

Image processing (IP) is the recording, digitation, storage, display, modification, and computer analysis of visual information obtained from optical scanners. Few reports are available on the use of these powerful techniques in the study of the toxic effects of chemical agents.

Imaging techniques used in *thermography* have potential for the study of the effects of neurotoxic agents on the autonomic system. Sweat glands are innervated by autonomic fibers, and forced sweating—by subjecting the patient to sauna-like conditions—can be used to assess the autonomic system function. In addition, a mixture of starch and iodine can be used to cover the patient's body to observe regional perspiration. The mixture turns to a blue-black color when the skin becomes moist.

CONCLUSIONS

In neurobiology, an imaging technique is one that allows the visualization of structural features of the nervous system or pharmacological processes resulting from the use of specially treated chemical substances. New imaging techniques available in the late 1980s are noninvasive and relatively safe, although extremely expensive. They are now being increasingly used to understand how neurotoxic agents affect the structure and pharmacological action of neural cells.

REFERENCES

Duel, RK, Yue, GM, Sherman, WR, et al. (1985) Monitoring the time course of cerebral deoxyglucose metabolism by 31-P nuclear magnetic resonance spectroscopy. *Science* 228:1329–1331.

Duffy, FH (1982) Topographic display of evoked potentials: Clinical applications of brain electrical activity mapping (BEAM). In *Evoked Potentials,* I Bodis-Wollner (ed) pp. 183–196. New York: The New York Academy of Sciences.

Glickman, L, Valciukas, JA, Lilis, R, et al. (1984) Occupational lead exposure: Effects on saccadic eye movements. *Int Arch Occup Environ Health* 54:115–125.

Greenberg, J, Reivich, M, Alavi, A, et al. (1981) Metabolic mapping of functional activity in human subjects with the (^{18}F)-fluorodeoxyglucose technique. *Science* 212:678–680.

Gregory R (1987) *Oxford Companion to the Mind.* Oxford: Oxford University Press.

Gur, RC and Reivich, M (1980) Cognitive task effects on hemispheric blood flow in humans: Evidence for individual differences in hemispheric activation. *Brain Lang* 9:78–92.

Lashley, KS (1929) *Brain Mechanisms and Intelligence.* Chicago: University of Chicago Press.

Marks, JL (1987) Imaging techniques passes muster. *Science* 238:888–889.

Oldendorf, WH (1980) *The Quest for an Image of the Brain: Computerized Tomography in the Perspective of Past and Future.* New York: Raven Press.

Portugal, FH (1984) NMR: Promises to keep. *High Tech* August, pp. 66–73.

Ravich, LE (1986) Thermal imaging: A review. *Laser Focus/Electro-Optics,* February, 98–110.

Reivich, M and Gur, R (1985) Cerebral metabolic effects of sensory and cognitive stimuli in normal subjects. In *Positron Emission Tomography,* M Reibich and A Alavi (eds) pp. 329–344. New York: Alan R Liss.

Reivich, M, Kuhl, D, Wolf, A, et al. (1979) The ^{18}F-fluorodeoxyglucose method for the measurement of local cerebral utilization in man. *Circ Res* 33:127–137.

Risberg, J and Hagstadius S (1983) Effects on regional cerebral flow of long-term exposure to organic solvents. *Acta Psychiatr Scand (Suppl)* 303:92–99.

Roy, CS and Sherrington, MB (1890) On the regulation of the blood supply in the brain. *J Physiol* (Lond) 1:85–108.

Sokoloff, L, Rivich, M, Kennedy, C, et al. (1977) The (^{14}C)deoxyglucose method for the assessment of local glucose utilization: Theory, procedures and normal values in the conscious and anesthetized albino rat. *J Neurochem* 28:897–916.

Ter-Pogossian, M (1985) Positron emission tomography instrumentation. In *Positron Emission Tomography,* M Reivich and A Alavi (eds) pp. 329–344. New York: Alan R Liss.

Tsutsui, J, Teruya, M, Murata, T, et al. (1972) Pupillary reflex in Minamata disease recorded with video-pupillography (in Japanese). *J Kumatoma Med Soc* 46:551–665.

SUGGESTED READINGS

Aichmer, F, Gerstenbrand, F, and Grevic, N (1989) *Neuroimaging II.* New York: VCH Publishers.

Andreasen, N (1988) Brain imaging: Applications in psychiatry. *Science* 239:1381–1388.

Andrew, ER (1984) A historical review of NMR and its clinical applications. *Br Med Bull* 40:115–119.

Berland, LL (1987) *Practical CT: Technology and Techniques.* New York: Raven Press.

Bergman, K (1983) Application and results of whole body autoradiography in distribution studies of organic solvents. *CRC Crit Rev Toxicol* 12:59–118.

Bigler, ED, Yeo, RA, and Turkheimer, E (eds)(1989) *Neuropsychological Function and Brain Imaging.* New York: Plenum Press.

Birnholtz, JC and Benacerraf, BR (1983) The development of the human fetal hearing. *Science* 222:516–518.

Budinger, TF (1985) Quantitative single-photon emission tomograph for cerebral flow and receptor distribution imaging. In *Positron Emission Tomography,* M Reivich and A Alavi (eds) pp. 227–240. New York: Alan R Liss.

Chugani, HT and Phelps, ME (1986) Maturational changes in cerebral function in infants determined by ^{18}FDG positron emission tomography. *Science* 231:840–843.

Drummond, PD and Lance, JW (1984) Thermographic changes in cluster headache. *Neurology* 34:1292–1298.

Gadian, DG (1982) *Nuclear Magnetic Resonance and Its Applications to Living Systems.* Oxford: Clarendon Press.

Gibbons, A (1990) New maps of the human brain. *Science* 249:122–123.

Gur, D, Good, WF, Wolfson, SK et al. (1982) In vivo mapping of local cerebral blood flow by xenon-enhanced computer tomography. *Science* 213:1267–1268.

Hagstadius, S, Ørbæck, P, Risberg, J et al. (1989) Regional cerebral blood flow at the time of diagnosis of chronic encephalopathy induced by organic-solvent exposure and after cessation of exposure. *Scand J Work Environ Health* 15(2):130–135.

Harms, ST and Kramer, DM (1985) Fundamentals of magnetic resonance imaging. In *Critical Reviews in Diagnostic Imaging,* Y Wang, J Edeiken, and MK Loken (eds) pp. 79–111. Boca Raton, FL: CRC Press.

Heiss, W-D and Phelps, ME (eds)(1983) *Positron Emission Tomography of the Brain.* New York: Springer-Verlag.

Hibbard, LS, Mc Glone, JS, Davis, DW, et al. (1987) Three dimensional representation and analysis of brain energy metabolism. *Science* 236:1641–1646.

Ikeda, T, Kondo, T, Mogami, H, et al (1978) Computerized tomography in cases of acute carbon monoxide poisoning. *Med J Osaka Univ* 29:253–262.

Juntunen, J, Hernberg, S, Eistola, P, et al. (1980) Exposure to industrial solvents and brain atrophy. *Eur Neurol* 19:366.

Kessler, LW (1988) *Acoustical Imaging.* New York: Plenum Press.

Moore, WS (1984) Basic physics and relaxation mechanisms. *Br Med Bull* 40:120–124.

Phelphs, ME and Mazziotta, JC (1985) Positron emission tomography: Human brain function and biochemistry. *Science* 228:799–809.

Phelps, ME, Mizziotta, JC, and Schelbert, HR (1986) *Positron Emission Tomography and Autoradiography: Principles and Applications for the Brain and the Heart.* New York: Raven Press.

Pritchard, JW and Schulman RG (1986) NMR spectroscopy of brain metabolism in vivo. *Annu Rev Neurosci* 9:61–85.

Radda, GK (1986) The use of NMR spectroscopy for ther understanding of disease. *Science* 233:640–645.

Ramsey, RG (1987) *Neuroradiology* (2nd ed). Philadelphia: WB Saunders.

Rechle, ME (1983) Positron emission tomography. *Annu Rev Neurosci* 6:249–267.

Rechle, ME (1986) Neuroimaging. *Trends Neurosci* 9:525–529.

Reivich, M And Alavi, A (eds)(1985) *Positron Emission Tomography.* New York: Alan R Liss.

Robb, RA (1985) *Three-Dimensional Biomedical Imaging.* Boca Raton, FL: CRC Press.

Trimble, MR (ed)(1986) *New Brain Imaging Techniques in Psychopharmacology.* New York: Oxford University Press.

Valk, J (1987) *MRI of the Brain, Head, Neck and Spine.* Boston: Martinus Nijhoff.

Wagner, HN, Burns, DH, Dannals, RF, et al. (1983) Imaging dopamine receptors in the human brain by positron tomography. *Science* 221:1264–1266.

Part II

Neurotoxic Chemical Compounds and Drugs

7

The Neurotoxic Environment

A chemical substance is called neurotoxic when it can cause a harmful change in an individual's nervous system. In this book, the *neurotoxic environment* is the sum of all the chemical compounds present in the human habitat that have a potential of creating a neurotoxic health hazard to humans. This chapter deals with helpful definitions of terms used throughout the book and the difficulties of naming—or even classifying—all neurotoxic agents present in the human habitat. First, some definitions are necessary.

DEFINITIONS

Poison is any agent that is capable of producing a deleterious response in a biological system or capable of destroying life or seriously injuring function (Klaassen et al. 1986). Cyanide is an example of poison.

Toxic is a synonym of "poisonous," the latter now rarely in use. A substance that is toxic has the property of producing a harmful or lethal effect. Asbestos is a toxic substance, but asbestos is not known to be neurotoxic.

A *neurotoxic substance* is capable of producing a deleterious effect on the nervous system at the structural (macroscopic or molecular) or functional (behavioral or psycho-logical) level. Methylmercury, for example, is a powerful neurotoxic agent.

The *neurotoxicity* of a given chemical compound relates, among other factors to be examined in Chapter 9, to its amount and concentration. Zinc, for example, is often listed appropriately as a neurotoxic metal. Yet zinc is also a vital nutrient that is required in only very small quantities.

The level of organization at which neurotoxicity can be demonstrated is important. Neurotoxic effects can occur at the gross morphological, cellular, or molecular level of organization. These levels of organization are described in Chapter 2, dealing with the neurobiology of toxic illnesses. Often, compendia of toxic chemicals list "neurotoxic agents" irrespective of the level of organization at which their toxicity has been demonstrated. For example, a powerful neurotoxic agent capable of producing human death instantly may be described alongside another that has been found to produce pharmacological alterations only in the glia of the spinal cord of chicken embryos in vitro.

The neurotoxic properties of many compounds may be overlooked in lists where the primary target of toxicity is cited. For example, some drugs whose primary target is the cardiovascular system are also neurotoxic. Digitalis, for example, increases the force of contraction of the myocardium, but at toxic levels it can also cause blurred vision, loss of visual acuity, and disturbances in color perception. Most toxic agents have multiple targets of toxicity.

The intrinsic association between a group of chemical compounds and neurotoxic properties should never be suggested or implied without clinical, experimental, or epidemiological evidence. For example, many industrial solvents are neurotoxic. But one should not infer that all solvents are neurotoxic. Thus, though water is generally regarded as the "universal solvent," only under exceptional circumstances is water toxic. Water is toxic when—as a result of ingestion of large amounts, often by mentally disturbed individuals—an imbalance in electrolytes vital for neural transmission occurs.

A *neurotoxin* is any toxic substance that occurs naturally in the environment, or is produced by living organisms, which is capable of producing a biological effect on the nervous system. In many cases, neurotoxins are part of a plant or animal's defensive or offensive mechanism. Nicotine and caffeine, for example, occur naturally in plants, protecting them against predators. Neurotoxins can also kill. The sting of some spiders, such as the black widow, can produce human death. Some neurotoxic agents such as anthrax and botulism, although naturally occurring, are also part of the arsenal in human chemical warfare. Though a neurotoxin is generally an organic, naturally occurring compound (eg, the venom contained in the sting of the marine animal Portuguese man-of-war), toxins can also be produced synthetically or by means of genetic engineering in the laboratory.

The term neurotoxin should not be taken as implying that the nervous system is the only target. For example, snake venoms are often classified separately as neurotoxins, cardiotoxins, hemotoxins, cytotoxins, myotoxins, and the like. Yet, snake venoms appear to affect many membranes and perhaps most tissues of the body. A *neurotoxicant* is

a term designating any neurotoxin, neurotoxic agent, or neurotoxic drug. Although the term is useful for its broad connotations, it is not widely used in the environmental and occupational toxicology literature.

A *neurotoxic drug* is:

- A naturally occurring substance or, more frequently, a manufactured chemical compound developed for therapeutic purposes to alleviate medical conditions [such as the use of acetylsalicylic acid (aspirin) to relieve pain].
- A chemical compound used to arrest the progress of a neurological disease: L-dopa, for example, which is used to halt the devastating degenerative effects of Parkinson's disease.
- A chemical substance that can control behavioral changes, such as the use of lithium to alleviate severe swings in mood.

A *xenobiotic agent* is any chemical compound developed by humans; the Greek word "xenos" means "foreign," indicating that the compound is not part of our natural habitat. But not all xenobiotic agents are harmful. In fact, the vast majority of chemical compounds and drugs created by humans have beneficial effects on humans or have directly or indirectly improved the quality of our lives.

Neurotoxic agents are chemical compounds capable of producing a temporary or permanent change in nervous system function. The term refers to a large family of chemical compounds that is used or has been developed for useful purposes in industry, agriculture, or the household but are inadvertently harmful to humans. There may be several interrelated factors explaining why they may be harmful: (1) their dangerous neurotoxic properties may be unknown—for example, until their accidental release in the environment, polybrominated biphenyls (PBBs) were not known to be toxic; (2) their presence in the human habitat may be unsuspected—for example, children have died after consuming insecticide with the thought that it was sugar; (3) they may be inadequately handled—for example, mercury used as a fungicide to protect wheat seed intended for planting caused devastating health effects in Iraq when, during a period of famine, these seeds were used to make bread (Bakir et al. 1973).

NEUROTOXIC AGENTS IN THE HUMAN HABITAT

The compilation of comprehensive databases on all toxic agents, their uses in work environments, and their presence in the living environment of humans is a formidable task. In the United States, one of the most comprehensive databanks is the chemical information system of the National Institutes of Health/Environmental Protection Agency, which at its installation in 1982 contained 200,000 entries. It is generally estimated that more than one fourth of all the toxic agents listed are neurotoxic (Anger and Johnson 1985).

Many such databases guide the user to locate additional information. But one needs to read the information critically. The following are some guiding questions.

1. **Which neurotoxic agents have in fact been proven to be so?** There may not be a clear answer to this question. At the time of this writing, the most comprehensive list of neurotoxic agents is that of Anger and Johnson published in 1985, containing approximately 850 entries. However, since no firm neurotoxicity testing protocol has yet been agreed on, information on the neurotoxic properties of a given chemical compound may not be available simply because no such testing has ever been performed. For example, very little is known about the effects of toxic agents on olfaction because studies of neurotoxin-induced olfactory changes in humans are rarely performed.

2. **What are the most likely uses?** "Typical" uses of great numbers of neurotoxic agents are now available. These compilations are essential for the development of health preservation programs. But knowledge of "atypical" uses of a given toxic agent is equally important. An accident, for instance, may constitute an "atypical" use of the toxic compound. For example, in 1973 many chemists knew the use of polybrominated biphenyls (PBBs) as a flame retardant, but for health scientists in Michigan it took a great deal of creative research to identify their accidental presence in farm animals' feed (Anderson et al. 1979).

Selikoff (1984) has warned of the important distinction between product manufacture, product use, and environmental exposure when evaluating people at risk. Until recently, the primary exposure that occurred as a result of product manufacture was the principal—if not the only—object of concern. A case in point is the "lead worker," a category of risk which is gradually disappearing. Instead, far larger groups of product users are at risk. The vast majority of neurotoxic exposures now occur as a result of product use or environmental exposure. The environmental persistence of such neurotoxic agents as lead, DDT, PBBs, dioxins, etc. is of greatest concern.

3. **Under what conditions might people be exposed to the neurotoxic agent in the environment?** Neurotoxic agents may be present in air, soil, or water. They might be inhaled, ingested, or absorbed through the skin. The design of relational databases allowing the generation of exposure information without the need of compiling all possible permutations is now possible. A relational database is a computer-based filing procedure in which several columns containing information can be linked by following certain rules.

Experts operate on the concept of *principles*. In an empirical science such as environmental and occupational neurotoxicology, a principle is an educated judgment resulting from familiarity with one's field. In an environmental accident where no causative agent is originally known, such as in the massive killing of fish, experts may entertain several hypotheses until a causative agent(s) of death is found. The body of universally accepted scientific laws in environmental health sciences is yet to be compiled.

4. In which occupations are they likely to be found? This is a variation of Ramazzini's question: "What trade are you of?" In contemporary society "occupations" have lost their old connotation of a fixed activity performed through life. In a typical lifetime, people either engage in multiple occupations or switch jobs several times or both. In addition, in the very highest and the very lowest socioeconomic strata, people often do not have "jobs" as we understand them. Thus, matching jobs and neurotoxic agents is often an unrewarding task. The US Department of Health, Education, and Welfare published a valuable guide: *Occupational Diseases: A Guide to their Recognition,* last updated in 1977.

This is why fixed, a priori preconceptions about which neurotoxic agents are expected to be found in which occupations should be avoided. Databases generated as a result of this effort may produce an oversimplified picture of the prevalence of toxic agents in work environments. Further, fixed databases may inhibit the investigation of novel combinations or patterns of use of neurotoxic agents. Two examples are the cases of trichloroethylene and DDT. Trichloroethylene is frequently listed (correctly) as an industrial solvent; in fact it can be found almost anywhere, including drycleaning establishments and offices in "white-out" agents (to cover typographical mistakes while writing). DDT was banned long ago, but it is estimated that in at least 10,000 homes, DDT persists (Lipske 1986); from time to time the use of DDT is authorized in the United States and abroad to combat pests resistant to other agents.

The neurotoxic environment of the child and the deadly neurotoxic agents released during chemical warfare are two aspects of the human habitat that have not been adequately covered in environmental and occupational neurotoxicology. These are reviewed below.

The Neurotoxic World of the Child

Neurotoxic poisoning of children has been the object of intense study around the world since the late 19th century. Although the vast literature on this subject deals particularly with the pernicious effects of lead, many other naturally occurring toxins and industrial neurotoxic agents are present in a child's habitat.

- Snake bites, for instance, occur primarily in children.
- Accidents in which adults have ingested neurotoxic agents by food consumption—eg, Minamata disease produced by methylmercury-contaminated fish—are likely to affect children as well, sometimes even more severely, because doses are larger relative to smaller body weights.
- Children sometimes are targets of neurotoxic epidemics. In 1984, in Argentina, for example, babies were exposed to organic mercury when their diapers were washed by a commercial company that used the chemical compound as a fungicide.

There are several reasons why the neurotoxic environment of the child has to be considered in a category of its own:

1. The mother's womb is the child's first living environment; the task of identification of neurotoxic agents in that early environment is far from understood.
2. As we discuss in Chapter 20, on the effects of neurotoxic agents on the developing brain, children are more susceptible than adults to the effects of neurotoxic agents. Thus, recommended standards that have been developed for

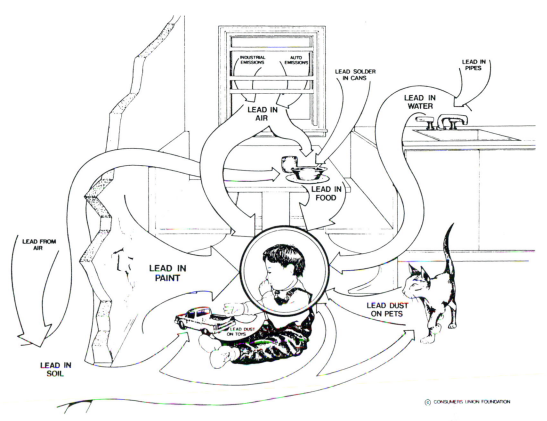

Fig. 7.1. Child in a leaded environment. (Copyrighted material of Consumers Union of US, Inc, Mount Ver-non, NY 10553. Reprinted by permission from Consumers Union Foundation.)

regulation and control of maximal exposures to neurotoxic agents at the workplace, intended for adults, may not be applicable to the child.

3. While engaging in such normal practices as teething, the child greatly increases his or her vulnerability to neurotoxic exposure in an otherwise innocuous environment.

4. Normal child play (eg, building toy houses in waste dumps with elements collected in the area) and curiosity and exploration (eg, descending into sewage systems) put children at risk. The general fact that a child walks close to the floor and can reach places where adults cannot reach or are not interested in reaching are factors to be considered in the description

of the special hazardous environments of the child (see Fig. 7.1).

5. Children in the household may be inadvertently exposed to neurotoxic agents brought in by parents on their shoes or clothing. This is called *bystander exposure*. Children have been known to be exposed to lead and pesticides in this manner.

6. Lastly, in many countries of the world there are children who work. As a result of the rapid increase in world population and poverty, the trend of child labor has recently been said to be on the increase. The system of apprenticeship—still existing in underdeveloped countries—forces the child to be in contact with toxic agents early in life.

Neurotoxic Agents Used in Chemical Warfare

Many neurotoxic agents are specifically designed to kill humans: neurotoxic agents are commonly part of a country's chemical ammunition arsenal. (Chapter 35 contains a more detailed discussion of this topic.)

There are two main types of neurotoxic agents used as ammunition: *neutralizing agents*—a euphemism for an agent aimed to kill—and *incapacitating agents*—agents designed to destroy the combat effectiveness of enemy troops without inflicting permanent injury or death. Organophosphorus compounds—organic chemicals containing phosphorus—were among the first man-made insecticides. Nerve gas, a neutralizing agent, belongs to this group of compounds. Nerve "gas" is a misnomer because not all neurotoxic agents used in chemical warfare are gases. Some of them are still known by their code names used in World War I, such as the "G" agents, including Tabun (GA), Sarin (GB), and Soman (GD). These agents are anticholinesterase agents: they kill by inhibiting neurotransmission by affecting essential enzymatic processes.

There is documented evidence that in many countries, including the United States, research on incapacitating agents took place using prisoners of war or experimental subjects who did not know they were participating in such experiments. One such substance was lysergic acid diethylamide (LSD). These experiments were made public in connection with a lawsuit by a private citizen against the US Army. The lawsuit culminated in a 1987 Supreme Court ruling that the Army could not be sued for its responsibility in these experiments.

CLASSIFICATION OF NEUROTOXIC AGENTS

A *classification* is a system of arranging objects into groups according to factors common to each. No classification of all known neurotoxic agents by chemical structure is yet possible. This is because it has been only in the past 30 years or so that chemical structures and pharmacological actions of many neurotoxic agents and drugs have been actively investigated. Thus, when industrial and commercially available neurotoxic drugs are listed alongside naturally occurring neurotoxins and neurotoxic drugs, there is no rational basis for such grouping based on chemical structure. The next chapter reviews current attempts to find a rational basis for these groupings by considering neural targets. For a review of the problems of determining correlation between structure and activity as a predictive tool in toxicology—particularly in cancer-causing chemical agents—see Goldberg (1983). The book by Solomon H. Snyder, *Drugs and the Brain,* published in 1986 contains an enlightening historical account of the development of a large family of neurotoxic drugs.

Abbreviated List of Neurotoxicants

There have been numerous different listings of neurotoxicants. As stated above, the most comprehensive enumeration to date is that of Anger and Johnson (1985), where names—including trade names—of close to 850 industrial and commercial neurotoxic substances, their mode of action, and bibliographic sources are given. In its original source, the list encompasses 71 pages. The following is a summary adapted from that source.

Alloys, see also Electronics, Glass making, Metallurgy, Optics, Paints (bismuth, cadmium, cobalt, indium, manganese tetraoxide, nickel carbonyl)

Anesthetics (halothane, nitrous oxide)

Antifreeze, coolants, also found as a wine additive to increase sweetness (ethylene glycol, propylene glycol, trichlorofluoromethane)

Beverages, see also Antifreeze [caffeine, ethyl alcohol (ethanol)]

Combustion products (carbon monoxide)

Degreasers, see Solvents

Detergents (alkyl ethoxylates)

Diving as a profession or sport (nitrogen, oxygen)

Dyes (acid violet S, aminobenzene, benzathrone, dimethyl sulfate, dinitrobenzene 2,4-dinitrophenol, 6-ethoxybenz-1-3-thiazo-2-thionium chloride, nitrophenol, p-phenylenediamine, quinoline, rhodanine)

Electronics industry (barium, cadmium, polychlorinated biphenyls, rubidium)

Electroplating, see also Optics (cadmium, chromium)

Explosives (cyclonite, nitroglycerine, ethylene glycol dinitrite, hydrazoin acid, dynamite)

Fertilizers (ammonia, ammonia salts, calcium cyanamide, ethyl formate)

Fire extinguishers (chlorobromoethane)

Fire retardants (cresyldiphenyl phosphate, polybrominated biphenyls)

Food and beverages, including substances used in food and beverage preparation, preservatives, flavoring, additives, decoration, etc. (ammonium glycyrrhizate, ammonium sulfide, butyl acetates, butyl alcohol, butylated hydroxyanisole, butyric acid, cuprizone, jequinity beam, malic acid, menthol, oil of peppermint, Teflon™, potassium sulfide, valeric acid)

Fuels (benzene, decarborane, 1,1-dimethylhydrazine, ethyl benzene, hexane-1, propylene dinitrate, propylnitrate, tetranitromethane)

Gasoline additives [bromide, ethylene dibromide, manganese, tetraethyl lead (TEL), tetramethyl lead (TML)]

Glass making, see also Optics, Electronics industry (barium, bismuth, palladium, polymethylmethacrylate, selenium, tellurium derivatives, thallium)

High-quality metals, production of (iron carbonyl, manganese carbonyl)

Insect attractants (cyclohexane carboxylates, cyclohexane acetate)

Insect repellents (w-chloroacetaphenone, di-(2-hexoxyethyl) succinate, oil of citronella)

Insecticides, see Plaguicides below

Jewelry (gold, poisonous seeds used as collars, bracelets, dress accessories, children playing with and chewing such ornaments)

Mining and metallurgy, see also Alloys, Metals (aluminum, cyanide, molybdenum, iron, inorganic lead, manganese, metallic mercury, nickel, nickel carbonyl, tellurium, organic tin, tin salts, vanadium)

Moth balls (naphthalene)

Munitions (methyl nitrate)

Natural sources (nitrogen, oxygen, ozone)

Paints, see also Solvents (aluminum, barium, lead, cobalt, mercury, polymethylmethacrylate)

Paint removers, see Solvents

Petrochemicals, petrochemical fuels (benzene, butane, butylene glycols, crude oil, ethylene, n-heptane, isopentene, isopropene, kerosene, methane, isobutane, naphthalene, n-octane, propylethylene, unrefined petroleum, propadiene, propane, propylene)

Photography (p-aminophenol, hydroquinone)

Plastics manufacture industry, plasticizers (alkyl oxyalkyl, phthalates, camphor, cresyldiphenyl phosphate, dimethylphthalate, methyl acrylonitrile, methyl methocrolate, styrene, tributyl phosphate, vinyl bromide, vinyl chloride, vinyl toluene)

Refrigerants (Freon-12™)

Rubber, chemicals used in the rubber industry (barium, butadiene, carbon disulfide, furfuramide, perchlorobutadiene)

Seed disinfectants (alkyl mercuric chlorides)

Smelting, Metals, Metallurgy

Soaps (acetyl ethyl tetramethyl tetralin)

Solvents (reviewed below)

Textiles, chemicals used in the textile industry (alkylbenzene sulfonates, carbon disulfide, quinone)

Veterinary medicine (arecoline, bismuth, n-butyl chloride)

Waterproofing (acrylamide)

Welding (manganese)

GROUPINGS

Neurotoxic agents can be grouped as agents of natural origin, neurotoxic metals, metal salts and metalloids, plaguicides, household products, and neurotoxic drugs.

Neurotoxic Agents of Natural Origin

Natural neurotoxins are broadly subdivided into phytotoxins, of plant origin—including fungi, although fungi are not plants—and neurotoxins, of animal origin. Toxins of plant origin do not follow any particular botanical taxonomic pattern. Among the most common are akee, castor and fava beans, hemlock, certain varieties of mushrooms, poison ivy, etc. The seeds of many edible fruits such as the apple, cherry, peach, apricot, and plum contain glycosides that release cyanide on digestion.

Neurotoxins of animal origin include powerful venoms formed by marine animals, arachnids, insects, and reptiles. Marine animals include shellfish—ie, mussels, clams, and oysters—that may become poisonous during the warm season and fish (eg, stingray, scorpion fish). Among the arachnids, the poisonous properties of a powerful neurotoxin secreted by the black widow spider is well known. In desert areas scorpions are found whose lethal sting has been known since antiquity. Reptiles that secrete venoms include snakes of the crotaid (eg, rattlesnake), viperid (European vipers), and elapid (eg, cobra) families. The gila monster, also a reptile, is the only known poisonous lizard. A large number of poisonous insects secret neurotoxins. Some of them act as individuals and are capable of producing serious neurological disorders. Others need to act in swarms to affect an adult's health (eg, bees, wasps). Because the toxicity depends on the nature of the neurotoxin, the dose, the body weight of the victim, and the victim's physiological state, the size of the swarm necessary to produce a harmful effect varies from case to case.

A good pocket-sized source of information on prevention, diagnosis, and treatment of naturally occurring poisonous plants and animals—as well as a rather comprehensive list of poison centers in the country and around the world—is Dreisbach's *Handbook of Poisoning* (10th edition, 1980).

Neurotoxic poisons have long been used as research tools in clinical neuropharmacology. This important point of view is well represented in the book edited by Simpson and Curtis (1971), *Neuropoisons: Their Pathophysiological Actions*. Volume 1 deals with poisons of animal origin, and Volume 2 with poisons of plant origin.

Neurotoxic Metals, Metalloids, and Metals That Have Neurotoxic Salts

Published information is available on the following: aluminum, arsenic, barium, bismuth, cadmium, gold, iron, lead, lithium, manganese, mercury, molybdenum, nickel, palladium, selenium, tellurium, thallium, tin, tungsten, uranium, vanadium, and zinc. In the literature, it is sometimes stated or implied that "heavy" metals are neurotoxic. The use of this term should be discouraged, because not all neurotoxic metals are "heavy." Metals such as tin are not neurotoxic, but their salts are.

For further information, Anger and Johnson (1985) is recommended.

Solvents

Solvents are a large number of chemical compounds having the common ability to dissolve and readily disperse fats, oils, waxes, paints, pigments, varnishes, rubber and many other materials (Lilis 1986). The following are examples of solvents that have demonstrated neurotoxicity:

Acetone
Benzyl alcohol
Bromobenzene
1-Butanol

2-Butanol
t-Butyl alcohol
Butylene glycol mono-*n*-butyl ether
Butylene glycol monoethyl ether
t-Butyltoluene
Carbon tetrachloride
Chlorobenzene
Cyclohexane
Diacetone alcohol
o-Dichlorobenzene
1,2-Dichloroethane
Diethyl ether
Diethylene glycol
Diethylene oxide
Dimethylformamide
Dioxane
Dipropylene glycol
Dipropylene glycol monomethyl ether
2-Ethoxyethanol
Ethyl *n*-butyl ketone
Ethylene glycol diethyl ether
Ethylene glycol dimethyl ether
Ethylene glycol monobutyl ether
Ethylene glycol monoethyl ether acetate
Ethylene glycol monoisobutyl ether
Ethylene glycol monoethyl ether
Furfural
Hexanol
Isopropyl chloride
Isopropyl ether
2-Methoxyethanol
Methyl *n*-amyl ketone (MAK)
Methyl *n*-butyl ketone (MBK)
Methylchloroform
Methylcyclohexane
Methylcyclohexanol
o-Methylcyclohexanone
Methylene bromide
Methyl ethyl ketone (MEK)
Methyl isobutyl ketone (MIBK)
Methyl *n*-propyl ketone
Nitromethane
2-Nitropropane
Nonyl alcohol
2-Octanol
2-Octanone
Pentachloroethane
Petroleum ethane
Petroleum ether

Pine oil
Pluronic polyols
n-Propyl alcohol
Propylbenzene
Propylene dichloride
Propylene glycol allyl ether
Propylene glycol monoacrylate
Propylene glycol mono-*n*-butyl ether
Propylene glycol monoethyl ether
Propylene glycol monoisopropyl ether
Propylene glycol monomethyl ether
Propylene glycol *n*-monopropyl ether
Propylene glycol monoesterate
Propylene glycol phenyl ether
Styrene
1,1,2,2-Tetrachloroethane
Tetrachlorethylene
Tetraethylene glycol monophenyl ether
Tetrahydrofuran
Toluene
1,1,2-Trichloroethane
Trichloroethylene
2,2,4-Trimethyl-1,3-pentanediol diisobutirate
Tripropylene glycol monomethyl ether
Turpentine
Xylene

For additional information, see *Kirk-Othmer Encyclopedia of Chemical Technology* (1984) and Lilis (1986).

Chemical Plaguicides

"Plagues" are groups of plants or animals that are a human health hazard or may cause economic loss. A *plaguicide* is any chemical compound designed to kill such plant or animal species. Rachel Carson (1962), in her book *Silent Spring*, first called attention to the relative meaning of the term "plague," ie, the danger of killing species without consideration of the global ecology. Among the chemical plaguicides are acaricides, or miticides (to control mites and ticks), baits (to attract or trap pests in order to destroy them by other means), defoliants, desiccants, foaming agents, foggers, fungicides, growth regulators, herbicides, insecticides, rodenticides, soil fumigants, and sprays.

One tends to associate agricultural neurotoxic agents with pesticides/plaguicides. However, pesticides are used in various other circumstances, most commonly in the household. Wood treaters, people who work in the construction industry handling pesticide-treated woods, sportspeople, particularly golf players who walk over a recently pesticide-spread lawn, fishermen who eat newly caught fish coming from heavily contaminated waters, and compulsive housewives who use exaggerated amounts of insect killers are among those exposed to plaguicides. Lipske (1986), for example, refers to the case of the Seattle woman who used five insecticide bombs to attack fleas. The gas was so concentrated that windows and the roof blew out, ignited by the pilot light of her stove.

A partial list of plaguicides includes the following:

Aldicarb
Aldrin
Alkyl tin
Allethrin
Azinphos-methyl
Barium carbonate
Benzimidazole fungicides
Carbaryl
Carbophenothion
Chlordane
Chlordecone
2-Chloroethanol
Chlorophenols
Chlorovinyl phosphate
Chlorthion™
Coumaphos
Cresol
Cyanide
Dihydroacetic acid
Diallate
Dibrom™
1,2-Dibromo-3-chloropropane (DBCP)
p-Dichlorobenzene
Dichlorodiphenyltrichloroethane (DDT)
2,4-Dichlorophenyl benzenesulfonate

2,4-Dichlorophenoxyacetic acid (2,4-D)
O-(2,4-Dichlorophenyl)-O-diethyl phosphorothionates (VC-13, Nematocide)
O-(2,4-Dichlorophenyl)-O-methyl isopropylphosphoamidothiate (DMPA)
4,4′-Dichloro-alpha-trichloromethyl benzhydrol
Dichlorvos
Dicrotophos
Dieldrin
Diisopropylfluorophosphate (DFP)
DMPA (Zytron™)
Dimefox
Dimetan
Dimethoate
Dimetilan
Diphenyl (biphenyl)
Diquat
Diquat dibromide
Dursban™
Disulfoton
Dodecylguanidine acetate (Cyprex)
Endosulfan
Endrin
Ethion
Ethyl mercuric phosphate
O-Ethyl O-p-nitrophenyl phenylphosphonothiate (EPN)
Fenamiphos
Fensulfothion
Fenthion
Ferbam
Fonofos
Heptachlor
Herban
Hexachloroethane
Imidan
Isobenzan
Isolan™
Leptophos
Lindane
Malathion
Metaldehyde
Methyl demeton
Methomyl
Methyl parathion
Mipafox
Mirex

Monocrotophos
Nicotine
Octyl ammonium metharsonate
Organophosphates
Paraquat
Parathion
Pentachlorophenol
Phorate
Propachlor
Pyrolan
Ronnel
Ryania
Sabadilla
Schradan
Sodium xanthate
Squill
Sulprofos
Tetraethyl dithionopyrophosphate (TEDP)
Tetraethylpyrophosphate (TEPP)
Thionacin
Thioquinox
Thiram
Thynol
Toxophene
Triacetin
S,S,S-Tributyl phosphorotrithioate (DEF)
Trichlorobenzene
2,3,6-Trichlorobenzoic acid
2,4,5-Trichlorophenoxy acetic acid (2,4,5-D)
Trichlorophon

Recommended sources include Anger and Johnson (1985) and the *Pesticide Applicator Training Manual* (Cornell University 1990).

Household Neurotoxic Products

Among the most common toxic products in the household are pest-control chemicals (insecticides, flea and roach powder, weed killer, etc), solvents (paint thinners, turpentine, nail polish remover, furniture stripper), and drugs (prescription medications that can be accidentally ingested by persons other than the one the medication is prescribed for).

Recommended sources include Golden Empire Health Planning Center (1990), *Household Hazard Waste: Solving the Disposal Dilemma;* and the information kit gathered by the League of Women Voters of Massachusetts (1990).

Neurotoxic Drugs

A *drug* is any substance used as a medicine for the alleviation or treatment of diseases and conditions. A neurotoxic drug is a chemical compound that has the nervous system as a primary target of its effect.

Medical uses of these drugs include the following:

- Analgesics such as aminopyrine, antipyrine, oxyphenbutazone, and phylbutazone, which in large doses can stimulate the nervous system.
- Local anesthetics such as cocaine, procaine, and others.
- General anesthetics, including such volatile and gaseous agents as ether, chloroform, divinyl ether, ethyl chloride, halothane, methoxyflorane, trifluoroethylvinyl ether, ethylene, cyclopropane, and nitrous oxide.
- Depressants, including sedatives, hypnotics, and anticonvulsants.
- Narcotic analgesics such as codeine, heroin, methadone, morphine, and opium.
- Drugs affecting the autonomic nervous system, such as atropine, belladonna, scopolamine, and synthetic substitutes—sympathomimetic agents such as epinephrine, amphetamine, and related drugs such as ergot and derivatives.
- Cardiovascular drugs such as digitalis, and beta blockers to control hypertension.
- Stimulants, depressants, and psychotomimetic agents—anxiolytics and antipsychotic drugs.

There are numerous drugs that are used in research to gain knowledge of the fundamental chemical and physiological processes of the nervous system. They are named for the neurotransmitter with which they interact—cholinergic, adrenergic, and serotonergic drugs. A recent area of intensive research is newly discovered neurotransmitters, notably amino acids and peptides.

Recommended sources for further information include Goodman Gilman et al. (1980) and Feldman and Quenzer (1984).

CONCLUSIONS

There is no universally accepted rationale for classifying, grouping, or even listing all neurotoxic substances present in the environment and the workplace that are potentially harmful to humans. Further, because sometimes environmental disasters and occupational accidents may call attention to previously unknown neurotoxic properties of chemical compounds, a rigid view of the possible links between neurotoxic agents and occupations is unwarranted.

REFERENCES

Anderson, HA, Wolff, MS, Lilis, R, et al. (1979) Symptoms and clinical abnormalities following ingestion of polybrominated-biphenyl-contaminated food products. *Ann NY Acad Sci* 320:684–702.

Anger, WK and Johnson, BJ (1985) Chemicals affecting behavior. In *Neurotoxicity of Industrial and Commercial Chemicals,* Vol II, JK O'Donoghue (ed) pp. 51–148. Boca Raton, FL: CRC Press.

Bakir, F, Damluji, SF, Amin-Zaki, L, et al. (1973) Methylmercury poisoning in Iraq: An inter-university report. *Science* 18:230–241.

Carson, R (1962) *Silent Spring.* Greenwich, CT: Fawcett Publications.

Cornell University, Chemical Pesticides Program (1990) *Pesticide Applicator Training Manual.* Ithaca, NY: Cornell University Press.

Dreisbach (1980) *Handbook of Poisoning: Prevention, Diagnosis and Treatment* (10th ed). Los Altos, CA: Lange Medical Publications.

Feldman, RS and Quenzer, LF (1984) *Fundamentals of Neuropsychopharmacology.* Sunderland, MA: Sinauer Associates.

Goldberg, L (ed) (1983) *Structure–Activity Correlation as a Predictive Tool in Toxicology: Fundamentals,* *Methods and Applications.* Washington, DC: Hemisphere.

Golden Empire Health Planner (1990) *Household Hazard Waste: Solving the Disposal Dilemma.* Sacramento, CA: Golden Empire.

Goodman Gilman, A, Goodman, LS, and Gilman, A (eds) (1980) *Goodman and Gilman's The Pharmacological Basis of Therapeutics.* New York: Macmillan.

Kirk-Othmer Encyclopedia of Chemical Technology (1984) HF Mark, M Grayson, and D Ecroth (eds) New York: John Wiley & Sons.

Klaassen, CD, Amdur, MO, and Doull, J (1986) *Casarett and Doull's Toxicology: The Basic Science of Poisons* (3rd ed). New York: Macmillan.

League of Women Voters of Massachusetts (1990) Information kit on toxic household products. Boston: League of Women Voters.

Lilis, R (1986) Organic compounds. In *Maxcy and Rosenau Public Health and Preventive Medicine,* John M Last (ed) pp. 617–656. Norwalk, CT: Appleton-Century-Crofts.

Lipske, M (1986) Danger: Are you throwing poisons into the trash? *Nat Wildlife* Aug–Sept, pp. 20–23.

Selikoff, IJ (1984) Twenty lessons from asbestos. *EPA* 10(4):21–24.

Simpson, LL and Curtis, DR (1971) *Neuropoisons: Their Pathophysiological Action,* Vol 1, *Poisons of Animal Origin;* Vol 2, *Poisons of Plant Origin.* New York: Plenum Press.

Snyder, SH (1986) *Drugs and the Brain.* New York: Scientific American Books.

US Department of Health, Education, and Welfare, Public Health Service (1977) *Occupational Diseases: A Guide to their Recognition.* Washington, DC: US Government Printing Office.

SUGGESTED READINGS

Biery, TL (1978) *Venomous Arthropods Handbook.* Washington, DC: US Government Printing Office.

Borbely, F (1947) *Erkennung und Behandlung der organischen Lösungsmittelvergiftungen.* Bern: Medizinischer Verlag Hans Huber.

Boudou, A and Ribeyre, F (1989) *Aquatic Ecotoxicology: Fundamental Concepts and Methodologies.* Boca Raton, FL: CRC Press.

Bové, FJ (1970) *The Story of Ergot.* Basel: S Karger.

Bowen, HJM (1979) *Environmental Chemistry of the Elements.* New York: Academic Press.

Bower, DJ, Hart, RJ, Matthews, PA, et al. (1981) Nonprotein neurotoxins. *Clin Toxicol* 18(7):813–863.

Broockneel, W and Blau, GE (1985) *Environmental Exposure to Chemicals.* Boca Raton, FL: CRC Press.

Browning, F (1985) *Toxicity and Metabolism of Industrial Solvents.* Amsterdam: Elsevier.

Carson, PA and Mumford, CJ (1988) *The Safe Handling of Chemicals in Industry*. New York: John Wiley & Sons.

Cheeke, PR (1989) *Toxicants of Plant Origin*. Boca Raton, FL: CRC Press.

Clarke, L (1989) *Acceptable Risk? Making Decisions in a Toxic Environment*. Berkeley, CA: University of California Press.

Clements, JF and Pietrusko, RG (1979) Pit viper snakebite envenomation in the United States. *Clin Toxicol* 14(5):515–538.

Cohen, EN (1980) *Anesthetic Exposure in the Workplace*. Littleton, MA: PSG Publishing Co.

Committee for the Working Conference on Principles and Protocols for Evaluating Chemicals in the Environment (1975) *Principles for Evaluating Chemicals in the Environment*. Washington, DC: National Academy of Sciences.

Committee on Methods for the In Vivo Toxicity Testing of Complex Mixtures, Board on Environmental Studies and Toxicology, Commission on Life Sciences, National Research Council (1988) *Complex Mixtures: Methods for In Vivo Toxicity Testing*. Washington, DC: National Academy Press.

Committee to Survey Opportunities in Chemical Sciences (1985) *Opportunities in Chemistry*. Washington, DC: National Academy Press.

Cralley, LJ, and Cralley, LV (eds) (1985) *Patty's Industrial Hygiene and Toxicology, Vol III, Theory and Rationale of Industrial Hygiene Practice* (2nd ed), 3A, *The Work Environment*. New York: John Wiley & Sons.

Duke (1985) *Handbook of Medicinal Herbs*. Boca Raton, FL: CRC Press.

Farm Chemicals (1990) *Farm Chemical Handbook*. Willoughby, OH: Farm Chemicals.

Finkel, AJ (ed) (1983) *Hamilton and Hardy's Industrial Toxicology* (4th ed). Boston: John Wright.

Fergusson, JE (1990) *The Heavy Elements: Chemistry, Environmental Impact and Health Effects*. New York: Pergamon Press.

Froines, JR, Baron, S, Wegman, DH, et al. (1990) Characterization of the airborne concentrations of lead in US industry. *Am J Ind Med* 18:1–17.

Grover, R (1990) *Environmental Chemistry of Herbicides*. Boca Raton, FL: CRC Press.

Hardy, DL (1986) Fatal rattlesnake envenomation in Arizona: 1969–1984. *J Toxicol* 24(1):1–10.

Hayes, AW (1980) Mycotoxins: A review of biological effects and their role in human diseases. *Clin Toxicol* 17(1):45–83.

Howard, PH (1989) *Handbook of Environmental Fate and Exposure Data for Organic Chemcials, Vol 1, Large Production and Priority Pollutants*. Chelsea, MI: Lewis.

IARC Working Group (1990) Phenoxy herbicides and contaminants: Description of the IARC international register of workers. *Am J Ind Med* 18:39–45.

Inoue, T, Takeuchi, Y, Hisanaga, N, et al. (1983) A nationwide survey on organic solvent compounds in various solvent products, Part I. Homogeneous products such as thinners, degreasers and reagents. *Ind Health* 21:175–183.

Inoue, T, Takeuchi, Y, Hisanaga, N, et al. (1983) A nationwide survey on organic solvent compounds in various solvent products, Part II. Heterogeneous products such as paints, inks and adhesives. *Ind Health* 21:185–197.

Jensen, AA, Breum, NO, and Wynder, EL (1990) Occupational exposures to styrene in Denmark 1955–1988. *Am J Ind Med* 17:593–606.

Kamrin, MA and Rodgers, PW (1985) *Dioxins in the Environment*. New York: Hemisphere.

Keeler, RF and Tu, AT (1983) *Handbook of Natural Toxins, Vol 1: Plant and Fungal Toxins*. New York: Marcel Dekker.

Kizer, KW (1983) Marine envenomations. *J Toxicol* 21:527–555.

Klaasen, CU and Doull, J (1980) Evaluation of safety: Toxicological evaluation. In *Casarett and Doull's Toxicology, The Basic Sciences of Poisons* (2nd ed), J. Doull, CD Klaassen, and MO Amdur (eds) pp. 11–27. New York: Macmillan.

Kunkel, DB, Curry, SC, Vance, MV, et al. (1983) Reptile envenomations. *J Toxicol* 21:503–526.

Lampe, KF (1979) Toxic fungi. *Annu Rev Pharmacol Toxicol* 19:85–104.

Lauwerys, RR (1983) *Industrial Chemical Exposure: Guidelines for Biological Monitoring*. Davis, CA: Biomedical Publications.

Lenihan, J and Fletcher, WW (1981) *The Chemical Environment*. New York: Academic Press.

Lu, FC (1985) *Basic Toxicology: Fundamentals, Target Organs, and Risk Assessment*. New York: Hemisphere.

Mackison, FW and Stricoff, LJ (1978) *NIOSH/OSHA Pocket Guide to Chemical Hazards*. Washington, DC: US Department of Health, Education and Welfare, Public Health Service, Center for Disease Control, National Institute for Occupational Safety and Health/US Department of Labor, Occupational and Safety Administration.

Maltoni, C and Selikoff, IJ (eds) (1988) *Living in a Chemical World: Occupational and Environmental Significance of Industrial Carcinogens*. New York: Annals of the New York Academy of Sciences, Vol. 434.

Manahan, SE (1989) *Toxicological Chemistry*. Chelsea, MI: Lewis Publishers.

Marks, G and Beatty, WK (1971) *The Medical Garden*. New York: Charles Scribner's Sons.

McIntyre, AR (1947) *Curare: Its History, Nature and Clinical Use*. Chicago: University of Chicago Press.

Merck (1983) *The Merck Index* (10th ed). Rahway, NJ: Merck & Co.

Milne, GWA, Fisk, CL, Heller, SR, et al. (1982) Environmental uses of the NIH–EPA chemical information system. *Sciences* 215:371–375.

Minton, SA (1970) Identification of poisonous snakes. *Clin Toxicol* 3(3):347–362.

Neely, WB and Blau, GE (1985) *Environmental Exposure from Chemicals*. Boca Raton, FL: CRC Press.

O'Donoghue, JL (ed)(1985) *Neurotoxicity of Industrial and Commercial Chemicals*. Boca Raton, FL: CRC Press.

Rand, GM and Petrocelli, SR (1984) *Fundamentals of Aquatic Toxicology: Methods and Applications*. New York: Hemisphere.

Rauber, A (1983) Black widow bites. *J Toxicol* 21:473–485.

Rowe, WD (1983) *Evaluation Methods for Environmental Standards*. Boca Raton, FL: CRC Press.

Royal Society of Chemistry for the Commission of European Communities (1988) *Solvents in Common Use: Health Risks to Workers*. Boca Raton, FL: CRC Press.

Russell, FE (1965) *Marine Toxins and Venomous and Poisonous Marine Animals*. New York: Academic Press.

Sax, NI (ed) (1984) *Dangerous Properties of Industrial Materials* (6th ed). New York: Van Nostrand.

Schuck, PH (1986) *Agent Orange on Trial: Mass Toxic Disasters in the Courts*. Cambridge: Beknap/Harvard University Press.

Schurr, GG (1981) Paint. In *Kirk-Othmer Encyclopedia of Chemical Technology*, Vol 16, pp. 742–768. New York: John Wiley & Sons.

Schwarts, BS and Golstein, MD (1990) Lyme disease in outdoor workers: risk factors, preventive measures, and tick removal methods. *Am J Epidemiol* 131(5):877–885.

Slimak, M and Delos, C (1983) Environmental pathways of exposure to 129 priority pollutants. *J Toxicol* 21:39–63.

Smith, PF, Benach, JL, White, DJ, et al. (1988) Occupational risk of Lyme disease in endemic areas of New York State. *Ann NY Acad Sci* 539:289–301.

Southcott, RV (1970) Human injuries from invertebrate animals in the Australian seas. *Clin Toxicol* 3(4):617–636.

Spoerke, DG and Smolinske, SC (1990) *Toxicity of Houseplants*. Boca Raton, FL: CRC Press.

Steering Committee on Identification of Toxic and Potentially Toxic Chemicals, Board on Toxicology and Environmental Health Hazards, Commission on Life Sciences, and National Research Council (1984) *Toxicity Testing: Strategies to Determine Needs and Priorities*. Washington, DC: National Academy Press.

Streifler, M and Cohn, DF (1981) Chronic central nervous system toxicity of the chicken pea *Lathyrus sativus*. *Clin Toxicol* 18(12):1513–1517.

Terrill, JB, Montgomery, RR, and Reinhardt, CF (1978) Toxic gases from fires. *Science* 200:1343–1347.

Travis, CC and Hattemer-Frey, HA (eds) (1990) *Health Effects of Municipal Waste Incineration*. Boca Raton, FL: CRC Press.

Tu, AT (ed) (1988) *Handbook of Natural Toxins:* Vol 1, *Plant and Fungal Toxins;* Vol 2, *Insect Poisons, Allergens and Other Invertebrate Venoms;* Vol 3, *Marine Toxins and Venoms*. New York: Marcel Dekker.

US Department of Health, Education and Welfare, Public Health Service, Center for Disease Control, National Institute for Occupational Safety and Health (1973) *The Industrial Environment: Its Evaluation and Control*. Washington, DC: US Government Printing Office.

US Environmental Protection Agency (1988) *Superfund Chemical Profiles: Extremely Hazardous Chemicals*. Park Ridge, NJ: Noyes.

US Navy, Bureau of Medicine and Surgery (1968) *Poisonous Snakes of the World* (rev ed). Washington, DC: US Government Printing Office.

Wexler, P (1987) *Information Resources in Toxicology* (2nd ed). New York: Elsevier Science Publishing.

8

Classification of Neurotoxic Substances

Four taxonomies (classification schemes) of neurotoxic substances can be recognized:

- by occupation of victim
- by neuropathological changes to the gross morphology of nervous tissue
- by neuropathological alterations at the cellular level
- by neuropharmacological action at the molecular level

From the outset, it needs to be emphasized that some of these taxonomic systems are not, strictly speaking, classifications. In science, a *taxonomy* is the arrangement of all the data or facts according to a system. In the biological sciences, for example, all living organisms are grouped by phylum, class, order, family, genus, species, and variety according to their structure and natural relationship. In past and current taxonomies for neurotoxic substances, either the proposed classification is not comprehensive or the system on which the classification is based has not been clearly specified.

CLASSIFICATION BY VICTIM'S OCCUPATION

Until the Industrial Revolution there was a rigid conception about people's occupations,

and people had little job mobility. People who performed manual labor were commonly seen at the bottom of a hierarchy. The Greeks, for example, thought that "In the activity of thinking, man attains his highest felicity or blessedness; the happiness which man can attain through practical virtue is secondary and is associated with the life he is compelled to lead in dealing with the world's external things" (Bataglia 1973).

In Florence, the state system of the Italian Renaissance (circa AD 1500) recognized three principal social groups: the nobility, the commoners, and the masses. A system of guilds and municipal ordinance defined a socially invisible class of workers. When at that time the great humanists—such as Machiavelli—revealed their sympathy for common people, the sympathy did not include laborers.

Bernardino Ramazzini (1633–1714) recognized that the health of workers was a genuine domain of medicine. Ramazzini, the founder of occupational medicine, firmly established a tradition of taking people's occupations as proxies of exposure. In his book *Diseases of Workers* (Ramazzini 1713), one finds a long list of occupations and exposures including those of miners of metals, gilders, chemists, potters, tinsmiths, glass workers and mirror makers, painters, sulfur workers, blacksmiths, workers with gypsum and lime, apothecaries, cleaners of cesspits, fullers, oil pressers, tanners, cheese makers and other workers, tobacco workers, corpse bearers, midwives, wet nurses, vintners and brewers, bakers and millers, starch makers, sifters and measurers of grain, and many others.

Historically, such characterizations have been favored when the causes of diseases were not known. But sometimes when the causes and mechanisms of diseases are understood, occupations are still considered proxies for toxic exposure. For example, occupational physicians deal with "farmer's lung," "miner's nystagmus," "writer's cramps," etc. Some neurological signs have been linked to occupations as well—eg, "hatter shakes" (caused by mercury exposure). A polyneuropathy—ie, a neuropathological condition in which several components of the nervous system are affected at the same time—has been linked to chronic exposure to solvents, namely, "the chronic painter syndrome" (Arlien-Søborg et al. 1979).

CLASSIFICATION BY NEUROPATHOLOGICAL CHANGES TO GROSS MORPHOLOGY

Classical pathological syndromes evolved from the clinical study of very sick people and from postmortem examinations. Under those circumstances, the large components of the nervous system—eg, peripheral, central, autonomic—served as the basis of this classification scheme (Virchow, 1893) (Fig. 8.1). Historically, many of these signs and syndromes were named after those who described them (eg, Korsakoff's psychosis, Babinski's sign, Moro's reflex). Now, it is common to label syndromes after the most prominent feature of a toxic disease. Lead, for example, is often described as producing peripheral neuropathy, a prominent but not the only feature of lead neurotoxicity. Chronic occupational exposure to organic solvents is said to produce a toxic encephalopathy—a brain dysfunction—a term that does not fully capture the involvement of the peripheral nervous system.

Neuropathology has also contributed its view of systems and organs as targets of neurotoxicity: "toxicology of the eye," "ototoxicity" (toxicology of the ear), etc. The cerebellum is said to be a target in chronic alcohol intoxication. In neurotoxicology, the neuropathological classification of diseases by target systems and organs is now seen as too general if not misleading. For example, the term "toxicology of the eye" does not make clear the role of eye movements in visual perception. The classification of certain naturally occurring toxins as "cardiotoxic" may wrongfully imply that its neurotoxic effects are of secondary importance.

CLASSIFICATION BY NEUROPATHOLOGICAL ALTERATIONS AT THE CELLULAR LEVEL

Experimental neuropathologists are among the few who have explicitly used the term "taxonomy" in their proposed classification of neuropathological mechanisms. The core of this classification is the target cellular site where neurotoxic agents have an effect and "process disease," ie, whether these changes occur at proximal or distal portions of the neuron (Spencer and Schaumburg 1980).

As the neuropathological effects of neurotoxic agents begin to be understood, it is now possible to describe where changes occur in the neural cell. Figure 8.2 illustrates a simplified version of the classification scheme proposed by Spencer and Schaumburg in the late 1970s. Neurotoxin-induced morphological changes are seen as producing a breakdown of the neuron's cell body (neuronopathy), its axon (axonopathy), or its nerve sheath (myelinopathy). Certain solvents, such as n-hexane, produce distal axonopathies: the end of the axon dies first in a process called "dying back." Vascular changes and changes in the permeability of the blood–brain barrier are placed in a category by themselves.

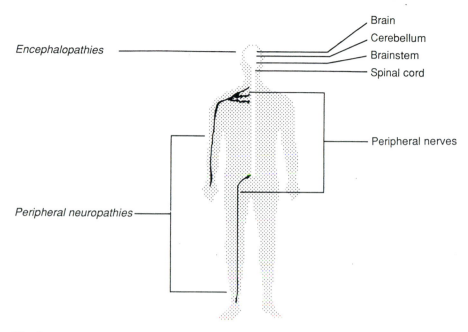

Fig. 8.1. Classification scheme of neuropathology at the gross morphological level.

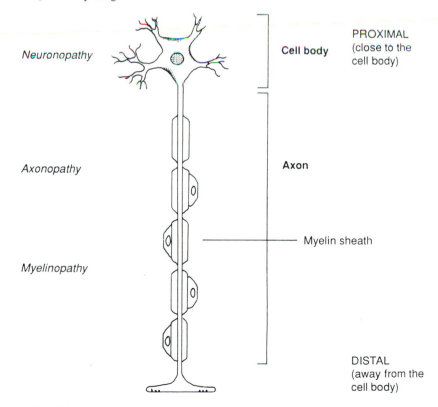

Fig. 8.2. Spencer and Schaumburg classification of neurotoxic agents by their effects at the cellular (neuronal) level.

NEUROPHARMACOLOGICAL CLASSIFICATION

Considerable advances have been made in the precise identification of the locus of many neurotoxins and drugs. The venom of the black widow spider, for example, is known to cause massive release of neurotransmitters by promoting fusion of synaptic vesicles at sites outside the normally active zones. But in the vast majority of cases, the pharmacological action of many environmental and occupational neurotoxic agents whose clinical manifestations have been known for generations is still poorly understood.

Chapter 2 contains a discussion of the different mechanisms of action of neurotoxic agents on neurotransmission—namely, that a toxic agent could act as a receptor blocker, a blocker of the synthesis of neurotransmitters, an accelerator of the release of the neurotransmitter into the synaptic cleft, etc. These mechanisms provide the basis for a pharmacological classification of neurotoxic agents and drugs. A schematic drawing of sites of action of several biological toxins in the neuroeffector junction as described by Price and Griffin (1980) is shown in Figure 8.3.

It is unfortunate that the term "neuropharmacological" is frequently associated with "acute," "transient," "functional," and "reversible," whereas "morphological" is linked with "chronic" and "irreversible." While proposing their own morphological taxonomy of neurotoxic sub-

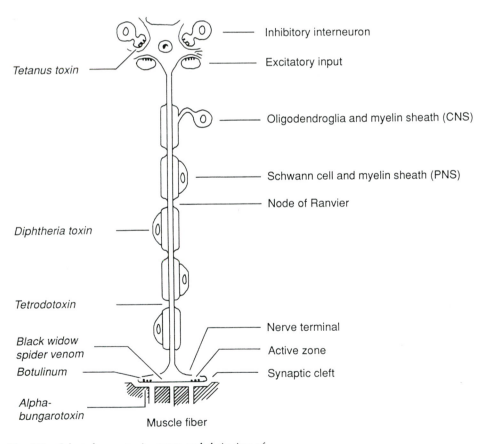

Fig. 8.3. Selected neurotoxic agents and their sites of action. CSN, central nervous system; PNS, peripheral nervous system.

stances, Spencer and Schaumburg (1980) wrote: "[Our classification] deals exclusively with those toxins which produce structural changes in the nervous system and ignores the acute, rapidly reversible effects of drugs, or high concentration of solvents, which, at the present time, are best categorized by the pharmacologist and behavioral toxicologist" (pp. 94–95).

REFERENCES

Arlien-Søborg, P, Bruhn, P, Gyldensted, C, et al. (1979) Chronic painter's syndrome: Chronic toxic encephalopathy in house painters. *Acta Neurol Scand* 60:149–156.

Bataglia, F (1973) Work. In *Dictionary of the History of Ideas: Studies of Selected Pivotal Ideas,* PP Wie-

ner (ed) pp. 530–535. New York: Charles Scribner's Sons.

Price, DL and Griffin, JW (1980) Neurons and ensheathing cells as targets of disease processes. In *Experimental and Clinical Neurotoxicology,* PS Spencer and HH Schaumberg (eds) pp. 2–23. Baltimore: Williams & Wilkins.

Ramazzini, B (1713) *De Morbis Artificum Diatriba* [translated as *Diseases of Workers*]. New York: New York Academy of Medicine.

Spencer, PS and Schaumburg, HH (1980) Classification of neurotoxic disease: A morphological approach. In *Experimental and Clinical Neurotoxicology,* PS Spencer and HH Schaumberg (eds) pp. 92–99. Baltimore: Williams & Wilkins.

Virchow, R (1893) The position of pathology among biological studies, lecture delivered in the theater of the London University, March 16. In *Post Mortem Examinations.* Metuchen, NJ: Scarecrow Reprint Corporation.

Part III

Pharmacology, Toxicology, and Occupational Health

9

Absorption, Distribution, and Excretion of Neurotoxic Agents

The mere presence of a neurotoxicant in the environment is not necessarily a cause of neurotoxic illness: the chemical compound must enter the body and reach a target somewhere in the nervous system. In the previous chapters chemical compounds that are neurotoxic were discussed; in this chapter we will understand *why* they are neurotoxic by considering their absorption, distribution, metabolism, and excretion. In environmental and occupational health sciences, this information is essential for designing effective strategies for biological monitoring and for accurate reconstruction of the workers' occupational history (the topic of Chapter 11).

ABSORPTION

Neurotoxic agents can enter the body through various routes. Some of these routes may not be suspected, and thus it is important to identify them so that inadvertent exposure does not occur. For example, a weekend gardener working in his shorts may absorb a significant amount of pesticides via testicular absorption, which is as effective in causing illness as oral absorption for certain pesticides. Cigarette smoking at a lead smelting facility, for another example, is a practice that may result in increased levels of lead absorption. Lead particles may be inhaled along with the cigarette smoke. Lead deposited on the cigarette paper as a result of handling the cigarette with contaminated hands may be both inhaled and ingested.

The locus of action needs to be recognized. A *local effect* is the direct effect of a toxic agent at the site of the contact between the toxicant and the biological tissue. A chemical compound may thus be caustic to the stomach; some others are lung irritants. The nerves of the peripheral nervous system can be affected locally as a result of percutaneous absorption. A *systemic effect* is one requiring absorption and distribution of the toxicant from its entry point to a distant site at which deleterious effects might occur. For example, the alcohol ingested by a partygoer or solvents inhaled by a professional painter produce their neurotoxic effects when the toxicants reach the brain. Figure 9.1 is a simplified view of the absorption, transport, and fate of neurotoxicants.

Inhalation

Many environmental and occupational neurotoxic agents are absorbed through the lungs.

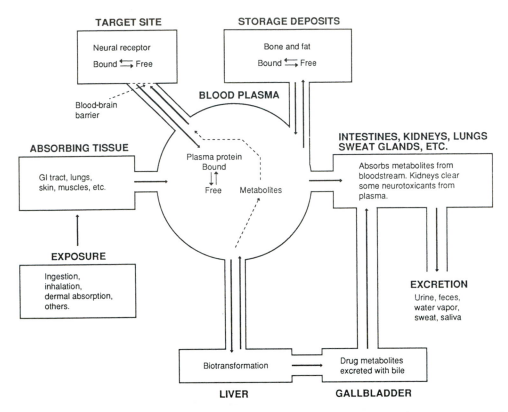

Fig. 9.1. Absorption, transport, and fate of neurotoxicants. (Modified from Feldman and Quenzer (1984), reproduced by permission of Sinauer Associates Inc., Sunderland, MA.

Volatile and gaseous toxic agents, such as industrial and commercial solvents, may be inhaled via the nose and mouth and enter the circulatory system through the mucous membranes of the respiratory tract. In the lungs, the area of absorption is very large, and access to blood circulation is rapid.

Physically, the agents may be present as either dusts or droplets in air (aerosols). Auto body shop workers who remove excessive lead applied to gaps by sanding, painters exposed to organic solvents in paints, and chemical workers who manufacture psychoactive drugs (mind modifiers) may be occupationally exposed through this mechanism. The snorting of cocaine, occurring at the olfactory epithelium, is an example of local absorption of soluble dusts.

Ingestion

Oral absorption is an important route of neurotoxic absorption in children. Lead intoxication, for example, can occur as a result of mouthing contaminated soil. It is also a possible route of entry for workers exposed to neurotoxic dusts, such as miners and smelter workers, in whom ingestion may take place without the individual realizing it as, for example, when workers eat in a contaminated workplace.

There are numerous factors that regulate gastrointestinal absorption:

- The **physicochemical properties** of the neurotoxic agents or drugs, especially lipid solubility. The greater the ability of an agent or drug to be dissolved in fat, the greater are its chances of being absorbed.

- The **physiological factors** involved at the particular site of the gastrointestinal tract. For example, many drugs and environmental and occupational toxicants are absorbed more readily in the small intestine than in the stomach because of favorable pH, enzymatic activity, and intestinal motility.
- The amount of **surface area** exposed to the neurotoxic agent; the greater the surface area, the greater is the absorption. Factors that affect surface area are the intestinal flora present and whether the individual has eaten food that could inhibit absorption.
- The **concentration** of the neurotoxic agent or drug at the site of absorption; this is fundamental.
- The **maturational state of the individual;** children have a much greater rate of gastrointestinal absorption than adults.

Dermal Absorption

Some neurotoxic agents readily penetrate the skin; these include a large number of solvents and pesticides. Workers who continually use degreasers for personal cleansing, eg, acetone, may absorb these agents dermally and later show neurotoxic illness. Improper design of protective gloves and shoes may actually maximize dermal absorption by trapping toxic substances between the inner surface of the glove or the shoe and the skin. In hot environments, rolling up the sleeves or pants legs of clothing designed to protect the skin can also increase dermal absorption.

The skin is not a homogeneous organ; several areas of the body have a different potential for dermal absorption. Factors such as skin thickness and local blood circulation play important roles; the thicker the skin, the less the absorption. The skin of the back, for instance, is thick, whereas that of the lips is very thin. The skin on the genital organs of men and women is an example of thin, highly vascularized tissue, favoring dermal absorption.

Sublingual Absorption

This route of entry is encountered in drug administration for therapeutic purposes. Though the surface area on the tongue is relatively small, the tongue cannot be overlooked as a possible route for occupational exposures. For example, nitroglycerin is taken sublingually to treat heart conditions. Despite the tongue's small surface area, this drug is effective because it is potent and has a high lipid solubility; ie, few molecules are needed to produce the desired therapeutic effect.

Local Absorption

This is also called "area" or "topical" (from the Greek, topos, meaning place) absorption. Some occupational exposures occur as the result of the direct contact of neurotoxic agents on peripheral nerves. Dental assistants, for example, may expose peripheral nerves in their hands to methyl methacrylate when manually preparing amalgam, an alloy used for filling cavities. Topical application on mucous membranes of the nose is another example of local absorption. This route of entry is common in illegal drug administration, such as in cocaine snorting, or in solvent addiction, such as toluene.

Other Routes of Entry

In medicine as well as in drug addiction, other routes of entry include injection either subcutaneously, intramuscularly, or intravenously. Intraperitoneal administration, meaning injecting the drug or neurotoxic agent directly into the outer limits of the abdominal cavity, is often used in laboratory animals. Rectal administration is used for therapeutic doses of drugs when oral administration is impossible because of vomiting or when the patient is unconscious. This route is also preferred when the drug is destroyed by digestive enzymes. To circumvent the blood–brain barrier (discussed below), some drugs are administered directly into the cerebrospinal fluid, as in the case of spinal anesthesia during difficult childbirths. In experimental studies of drug action in laboratory animals, sometimes drugs or toxic agents are injected into the brain with the aid of positioning equipment and microsyringes.

Factors Affecting Susceptibility

Age. Neurotoxic agents and drugs have a differential effect on children, adults, and the elderly. This is primarily because of differences in the rate of absorption in the gastrointestinal tract and the liver's capacity to metabolize chemical substances. For a large number of neurotoxic agents and psychoactive drugs, children and the elderly are more susceptible to the toxic effects than mature adults. Experimental work with laboratory animals such as the rat have shown that, in the case of lead, the neonate's gastrointestinal tract surface is more permeable than the adult's. The likelihood and danger that some neurotoxic agents, such as polybrominated biphenyls, can be released from the mother through breast feeding and absorbed by the neonate is an issue that has been raised.

Gender. In epidemiological studies of neurotoxic illness, biological factors associated with ingestion, distribution, and metabolism and psychological and cultural factors such as eating habits are sometimes difficult to disentangle. Neurotoxic agents can accumulate in fat and bones. Fat deposition, for example, is genetically different in males and females. During pregnancy, massive toxic doses of lead may be released from fat and bone deposits into the bloodstream. But eating habits are primarily determined by culture. Male North American Indians, for example, eat muskrats, which may be contaminated with methylmercury; females rarely eat them. The source of methylmercury is the fish that muskrats eat.

Race. Scientists have, in the past, attributed apparent racial variations in toxic absorption to genetic predisposition. A classic example involved the occupational absorption of asbestos among insulators. Until a generation ago, asbestosis was thought to be a disease of whites. It was argued that blacks were genetically "less susceptible" than whites to the toxic effects of asbestos, when in fact it was eventually realized that because of long-standing discriminating job practices, blacks were less likely to be engaged as insulators. Thus, the lower prevalence of asbestosis in blacks had no genetic basis.

In other epidemiological studies, racial/genetic factors have also been targeted. Particularly, black workers have been found to have higher blood levels of many neurotoxicants than white communities, and so it has been concluded that blacks are "more susceptible" than whites to absorption of these toxins. But a closer look may reveal that blacks are merely more often assigned jobs that give greater exposure to neurotoxic contaminants.

It has been well established, however, that certain racial groups do exhibit greater absorption of particular toxins. For instance, people of Chinese ancestry lack the enzyme aldehyde hydrogenase necessary for ethanol metabolism. Minimal ingestion of alcoholic beverages may result in illness and sudden rash developing in these people.

Body Size. Some quantitative aspects of the absorption and distribution of toxic chemicals depend on physical properties of the body considered as a single compartment. The *volume of distribution* within such a compartment is assumed to be relatively uniform or not of practical consequence if not uniform. A given amount of chemical compound will be in a relatively higher concentration in someone with a small body than in someone with a larger body. This is why "toxic dose" is specified as a unite of volume per weight.

In addition to body weight, in epidemiological studies it is necessary to know *body mass*. For certain toxic agents, such as DDT, the greater the body mass, the greater is the statistical likelihood of increased accumulation of toxin in fat. There are several anthropometric measures of body mass, one of which is the *Quetelet index* (or body mass index), relating height and weight. The Quetelet index is defined as weight ÷ (height^2). This measure correlates highly with skinfold thickness or body density. The presence of fat can be ascertained by means of anthropometric techniques, as, for example, the use of calipers to measure natural skin foldings.

Effects of Physiological Conditions

The physiological activity of an individual at the moment of examination is important in the estimation of the pharmacological properties of neurotoxic agents. Feeding, physical exercise, and emotional state are examples of physiological conditions that have been extensively investigated.

Feeding is a factor: people who drink milk before alcoholic beverages, for example, retard the process of ethanol ingestion by reducing the available surface for gastrointestinal absorption.

In general, **physical exercise** increases the rate of absorption of neurotoxic agents. Numerous animal and human studies support the role of physical exercise in neurotoxic absorption.

Emotional states are factors that affect drug and toxicant absorption; emotions are difficult to measure and interpret. Emotional states seem to have an effect on a neurotoxic agent's rate of absorption in three ways. First, an emotional state may be associated with agitation and increased respiratory rate, leading to more effective inhalation of gaseous agents. Second, an emotional state such as depression may lead to apathy and failure to take precautions about possible sources of con-

tamination. Third, emotional states are complex neurobehavioral phenomena controlled by the hypothalamic–autonomic system; the possibility that emotional states physiologically modulate absorption has long been envisioned but not yet adequately studied.

DISTRIBUTION

Neurotoxic agents are absorbed, metabolized, and excreted through mechanisms that can be described at the cellular, pharmacological, and molecular level. The following is a brief review of principles of pharmacology and toxicology that are essential for the understanding of why toxic agents produce their effects on the nervous system.

Transport of Neurotoxic Agents across Membranes

Although a direct effect of neurotoxic agents on the nervous system is possible (as, for example, in the case of local anesthesics or methyl methacrylate) the vast majority of drugs and neurotoxic agents reach their target via the bloodstream. Once in the blood, the process of transport into the cells is accomplished via cell membranes. Membranes are responsible for maintaining the integrity of the cells by regulating the migration of materials into and out of their interior. Four basic chemical principles underlie the transport of neurotoxic agents: active transport (to be discussed below), passive diffusion, lipid solubility, and ionization.

Passive diffusion. Dissolved substances move from regions of higher concentrations to those of lower concentration following the passive process called diffusion. No energy is required in this process. Once a state of equilibrium is achieved, diffusion ceases. The effects of many drugs and neurotoxic agents can be predicted on the basis of their concentration gradient and the richness of area blood flow. Chemical substances are absorbed as long as a gradient exists between a higher concentration in the gastrointestinal tract and the circulating blood.

Lipid solubility. Chemical compounds that have the characteristic of fats (lipids) are more readily metabolized than the ones dissolved in water. The ability of a substance to dissolve in oils or fats is a basic chemical property. The partition coefficient of a chemical substance is the ratio of the drug concentration in oil over its concentration in water. The chemical compound's relative affinity for water or for oil will determine how readily it will reach the brain and other areas of the nervous system. Neurotoxic agents that have a high affinity for oil or fats are called *lipophilic*.

Some neurotoxic agents—notably, degreasers—have been industrially developed to dissolve oils or fats. They have the capacity to dissolve fatty membranes and other neural structures rich in fat, such as the myelin sheaths covering the axons of nerve cells, or to destroy olfactory receptor cells.

Ionization. Water solubility and ionization are related concepts. The molecules of water-soluble chemical substances are formed by ionic bonding of atoms. Ions can be positively charged (cations) or negatively charged (anions). Table salt—sodium chloride—is formed by an ion of positively charged sodium and an ion of negatively charged chlorine. Ionization is a fundamental pharmacological mechanism because it determines the percentage of positively charged hydrogen ions in a substance, expressed as *pH*. The pH is the negative logarithm of the concentration of hydrogen ions (H^+) in a water solution.

Different parts of the gastrointestinal tract and different regions of the body differ in their pH. For example, gastric juice of the stomach is very acidic and has a pH of 1.0, whereas the small intestine has a pH varying from 5.0 to 6.0. The capacity of a chemical compound to diffuse through membranes and the ultimate fate of a neurotoxic agent depend both on the ionization state of the agent and the medium through which it travels. There are important interactions between the

lipid solubility and the state of ionization of chemical compounds.

The transport of chemical compounds and drugs may sometimes be inhibited by the presence of natural defense mechanisms. The blood–brain barrier is an example of one such mechanism.

The Blood–Brain Barrier

The concept of a barrier between the blood and the brain was proposed by Paul Ehrlich in 1882. He noted that when trypan blue—a common stain used in histology—was injected into the bloodstream of experimental animals, it infiltrated most tissues, leaving nervous tissue relatively unstained. He argued that this barrier must be the brain's natural defense mechanism against the migration of unwanted substances. It was later shown that trypan blue does not reach the brain because it binds to albumin, a large molecule that cannot pass the blood–brain barrier. But these findings do not alter the validity of his observations. Ehrlich's concept remained virtually unchallenged until the episode of thalidomide proved to be the tragic exception.

A good grasp of how the brain barrier operates is essential for the understanding of how drugs accomplish their therapeutic effects and how environmental or occupational chemical agents become neurotoxic (to be reviewed below in this chapter) and why the unborn and the young are so vulnerable to brain damage during the early stages of central nervous system development (to be discussed in Chapter 20, dealing with the effect of chemical compounds on the developing brain).

The brain–blood barrier can be manipulated by drugs to allow the entrance of therapeutic drugs and imaging substances, that is, substances that allow the visualization of brain structure.

Figure 9.2 shows the structural features of the brain capillaries (small blood vessels) and

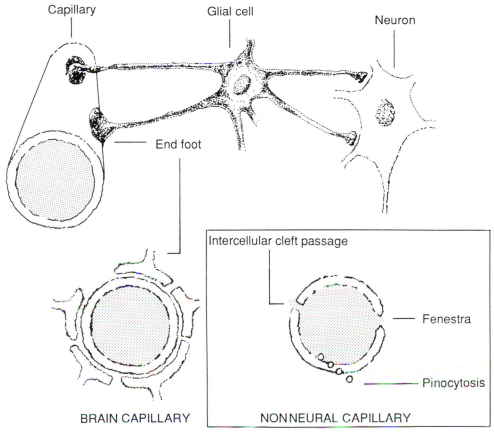

Capillary   Glial cell   Neuron

End foot

Intercellular cleft passage

Fenestra

Pinocytosis

BRAIN CAPILLARY   NONNEURAL CAPILLARY

Fig. 9.2. Relationships among capillaries, glial cells, and neurons.

nerve cells of the blood–brain barrier and the spatial relationships existing among capillaries, glia, and neurons. There are two types of capillaries—the nonneural and neural capillaries—and they are structurally different. In nonneural capillaries, present in any structure except the brain, small molecules can pass to surrounding tissues through passive diffusion, intercellular cleft passages, fenestrae (openings), and pinocytosis. (*Pinocytosis* is the active uptake of molecules by means of vesicles that envelop and transport large molecules through the walls of capillaries.) In neural capillaries intercellular clefts and fenestrae are absent, and pinocytosis is rare.

Large molecules leave and enter neurons through their membranes without disrupting their struc-

tural characteristics. Two major processes are involved: exocytosis, by which molecules leave the neuron, and endocytosis, by which molecules enter the neuron. Exocytosis involves several steps, which are illustrated in Figure 9.3. In step 1, a vacuole within the neuron containing its own membrane approaches the neuron's membrane. In step 2, the vacuole touches the neuron membrane without fusing with it. In step 3, the membrane of the vacuole and that of the neuron fuse, forming a single one. Finally, the fused membrane breaks, delivering the vacuole's contents into the cell exterior.

Endocytosis is the reverse of exocytosis. A vacuole from another cell outside the neuron approaches it and the vacuole membrane fuses with the neuron membrane. The vacuole produces an invagination in the neuron, and eventually a membrane will cover the site where the vacuole entered. One form of endocytosis is phagocytosis, *in which*

Exterior

Neuron
Interior

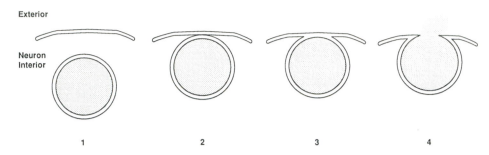

1   2   3   4

Fig. 9.3.   Expulsion of molecules through neuron membrane by exocytosis (see text).

the cell acts as a scavenger eating bacteria, dead tissue, etc.

The processes of exocytosis and endocytosis play a fundamental role in the absorption, distribution, and excretion of neurotoxicants, the transport of substances through the blood–brain barrier, and the release of neurotransmitter at the axon terminal.

Once it was thought that the molecular weight of a chemical compound was the property that dictated its migration into the nervous tissue: the larger the molecular weight, the less the likelihood of its entry. However, it is now understood that several combinations of factors may be involved in the migration of chemical compounds. Relatively large lipophilic neurotoxic agents, for example, may enter the brain readily, whereas relatively small water-soluble molecules may not.

There are places in the capillary–brain interface where small molecules are naturally allowed to pass into the brain. These include the *area postrema,* the *median eminence,* the *choroid plexus,* and the *pineal gland.* Some of these centers are strategically located near reflex centers responsible for important defensive and hormonal regulatory balance. For example, the area postrema is located in the vicinity of the chemical trigger zone in the medulla oblongata, a zone that induces the neural reflex of vomiting when chemically activated by certain poisonous chemicals. Vomiting is a beneficial reaction for the body allowing the rejection of harmful substances; it is often but, very importantly, not always a sign of intoxication.

The choroid plexus secretes the cerebral spinal fluid (CSF). As stated earlier, sometimes a drug is administered directly into the CSF, thus circumventing the blood–brain barrier. The choroid plexus also performs what is called a "sink function," being one of the several routes by which chemical substances are stored once they are allowed to penetrate the nerve tissue.

RECEPTORS

A *receptor* is a place where any biologically active agent is capable of producing a molecular, structural, or physiological change. The exact configurations of most pharmacological receptors are not known or are still in dispute. D.K. de Jongh (1964) wrote: "To most modern pharmacologists the receptor is like a beautiful remote lady. He has written to her many a letter, and quite often she has answered . . . From (which he) . . . has built himself an image."

The reader has to be alerted that the term "receptor" is used in many disciplines with slight variations in meaning. In this chapter, the term "receptor" is used with its pharmacological connotation only; in Part V (The Targets of Neurotoxicity), sensory receptors—such as rods and cones of the retina, hair cells in the vestibular and auditory apparatus—will be discussed with their neurophysiological connotation.

In pharmacology, there are two fundamental principles regarding the functioning of receptors: (1) receptor physiology follows *the law of mass action*; and (2) there is a *dose–response relationship* between dose and receptor effect. These fundamental processes are several steps removed from behavioral changes or psychological manifestations of neurotoxic diseases.

The two principles—the law of mass action and dose–response relationship—are intimately related. In the simplest of cases, it is believed that once a neurotoxic agent reaches its receptor, the effects it causes are proportional to the fraction of receptors entering into the reaction. Further, it is assumed that the binding of the agent with its receptor is reversible, the molecules binding and breaking away. In symbols:

Agent (A) + Receptor (R) $\rightleftharpoons$ AR $\rightarrow$ Pharmacological effect

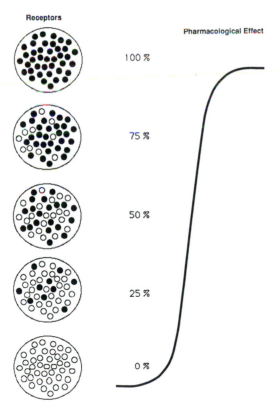

Fig. 9.4. Receptor recruitment and dose–response relationships. Open circles represent unaffected receptors (a function of low dosage); filled circles represent affected receptors, the number of which increases with increasing dosage.

The *dose–response curve* describes the changes in pharmacological action in proportion to the concentration of the agent present at the receptor (Fig. 9.4). At low doses, few receptors are involved, and the pharmacological effects are minimal. As the dose is increased, more and more receptors become involved. The pharmacological effects eventually reach a saturation point where a further increase in the dose no longer leads to an increased pharmacological effect (seen at the top, as the flat portion of the curve).

Plasma protein, muscle, and fat—and, in general, various organs well supplied with blood—are targets of neurotoxic agents. They are also potential regions for storage. But because no pharmacological effects are readily observed, they are called *silent receptors*. DDT, which accumulates in fat tissues, may go unnoticed for many years, until the individual loses weight as a result of a medical condition or through a crash diet, releasing the agent.

EXCRETION AND BIOTRANSFORMATION

Drugs and neurotoxic agents are secreted from the body either unchanged or as *metabolites*. In environmental and occupational neurotoxicology, knowledge of whether a neurotoxic agent is excreted unchanged or is biotransformed (metabolized) is important. This physiological fact supports the concept of biological monitoring (BM), to be reviewed in the following chapter dealing with the toxicological basis of environmental and occupational health sciences. Biological monitoring is essential for the control of toxic agents in the environment and the workplace. Most of the excretion of a toxic substance from the body is by the kidney or by biotransformation by the liver.

Renal Excretion

The kidneys excrete the end products of body metabolism (urea) as well as any excess of vital substance, such as sodium, potassium, and chloride. They also maintain a balance of water and sodium, an essential process under the control of hormones generated by the hypothalamus. The kidneys perform these functions in three major ways: glomerular filtration, reabsorption, and tubular excretion.

The functional unit of the kidney is the *nephron,* a long, unbranched tubule extending from a capsule-like structure, the *Bowman's capsule,* encircling a network of capillaries, the *glomerulus.* There are one to three million nephrons per kidney, totaling about 35 miles of tubules. The internal/external fluid exchange is facilitated by the close contact between blood vessels and the tubules. The glomerulus has pores 70 to 80 angstroms (Å) in diameter, and under normal positive hydrostatic conditions in the glomerulus, all molecules smaller than molecular weight 20,000 are filtered. Thus, large proteins or protein-bound drugs and neurotoxic agents remain in the plasma.

The glomerular filtrate contains many essential body constituents such as water and glucose. These—along with lipid-soluble drugs or neurotoxic agents—are reabsorbed back into the blood plasma. There are many factors influencing this process, the pH of the filtrate being one of them.

Elimination of liquid waste as urine occurs via the collecting ducts, which converge into the ureters. Tubular excretion of foreign compounds may be accomplished by active secretion into the renal tubules by anion and cation carrier processes. Urine analysis is important for the detection of the presence of drugs and neurotoxic agents or their metabolites.

Liver Metabolism

Although biotransformation can occur in the kidney, spleen, intestine, blood, lung, brain, and skin, the greatest amount is accomplished by the liver. The end product of liver activity is the production of single inactive and active metabolites. Active metabolites are important since drugs or neurotoxic agents may not, by themselves, produce a neurotoxic effect, but their metabolites may. An illustration of how active metabolites are generated in the blood-forming mechanisms as a consequence of lead absorption is given below.

Drugs and neurotoxic agents are biotransformed by *enzymes.* The ability of an enzyme to alter a drug or neurotoxic agent is dependent on the liver's ability to form an enzyme–agent interaction. The principles underlying these chemical and pharmacokinetic processes are very similar to those governing the formation of receptor–agent bonds, discussed above.

The molecules of drugs or neurotoxic agents can be modified by two processes: synthetic and nonsynthetic reactions. A *synthetic reaction* is the chemical bonding of a drug or neurotoxic agent, or its metabolite(s), with naturally occurring molecules provided by the body. The result of this process is the formation of a pharmacologically inert, generally water-soluble product that is readily excreted from the kidney. In pharmacology, this process is also known as *conjugation.*

Four major chemical groups make synthetic reactions possible; these include carbonyl (COOH), hydroxyl (OH), amino (NH_2), and sulfhydryl (SH) groups. For conjugation to occur, one of these chemical groups must be present. A drug or neurotoxic agent may undergo a nonsynthetic reaction before conjugation if there is not a site for the pharmacological bond to occur, that is, if none of these four chemical compounds is present.

Nonsynthetic reactions involve oxidation, reduction, or hydrolysis. Oxidation is a chemical reaction by which a carbon atom increases its covalent bonds to either oxygen or nitrogen. In a reduction, a carbon atom reduces the number of its bonds to oxygen or nitrogen. In hydrolysis, water molecules take an active part in the biotransformation of the drug or neurotoxic agent. The end result of a nonsynthetic reaction may be the formation of an active metabolite more potent (more toxic) than the original drug or neurotoxic agent.

Drugs and neurotoxic agents are metabolized by liver enzymes located in the smooth endoplasmic reticulum. The enzymes perform primarily nonsynthetic reactions of oxidation, reduction, and hydrolysis. Among their functions is conjugation with glucuronic acid. A detailed review of the numerous liver enzymes, the chemical processes in which they are involved, and the effects of drugs and agents on enzymatic activity of the liver is beyond the scope of this chapter. The chapter by Neal (1980) is a good introduction to the subject.

Repeated exposure to certain drugs, such as mood modifiers, changes the enzymatic activity of the liver. Tolerance to drugs (see below) is explained by this mechanism.

Other Routes of Excretion

Neurotoxic agents may be found in feces, expired air, sweat, saliva, vomitus, tears, milk, nails, and hair. Health investigators who need to monitor the quality of people's health often study the fate of chemicals or their metabolites by analyzing these products.

The chemical analysis of expired air is important in metabolic studies of the effects of industrial solvents in humans. These studies are usually performed under laboratory conditions, where a known amount of a solvent is inhaled, and then the exhaled air is collected in plastic bags for further analysis.

Droz and Guillemin (1986) have reviewed the value of breath analysis for monitoring exposure to solvents at the workplace. Breath analysis has an advantage over other biological monitoring procedures in that the method is noninvasive and can be applied to a large range of compounds. Breath analysis is the only means of biological monitoring for several inert compounds. The presence of solvents, for example, can be detected by means of chromatographic procedures. Chromatography is an analytical chemical technique that allows the separation of closely related compounds by allowing a solution or mixture to seep through an absorbent material such as clay or paper. Each compound becomes absorbed in a separate, often distinctly colored layer. The appropriate layer can be "developed" with a reagent that produces a colored product, which can then be chemically analyzed.

Milk excretion is important in neuroteratological studies. Drugs and neurotoxic agents may be secreted via this route, causing health problems in infants whose livers lack fully developed metabolizing enzymes to biotransform them.

Analysis of hair samples has received considerable attention, for example, in archeological research and forensic toxicology. Hair samples of ancient mummies have been studied for their lead content. The levels of arsenic and other metals can be examined in people who have died hundreds of years ago. Secretion and storage of neurotoxic agents can also occur in animal fur. Knowledge of this route of excretion is essential in veterinary toxicology.

For many years it was thought that effective lead monitoring could be achieved by hair sampling. However, the results have proved to be disappointing because in the actual sample it is not possible to separate endogenous or stored lead from airborne lead deposited in hair.

BLOOD LEAD LEVELS AS A PREDICTOR OF NEUROTOXICITY

Lead is known to have toxic effects on blood and blood-forming organs. It is because of these alterations that lead becomes neurotoxic. The neurotoxicity of lead is not paradigmatic for the study of other neurotoxic agents and other metabolic processes. But because the neurotoxic properties of lead have been studied for so long, and so much is now known about how lead becomes neurotoxic, a special section is devoted to this topic.

Porphyrins are a group of compounds found in all living matter which are the basis of respiratory pigments in both animals and plants. One porphyrin—heme—is an important constituent of hemoglobin (a respiratory pigment occurring in the red blood cells of vertebrates).

Although the existence of naturally occurring porphyrins has been known since the early 1940s thanks to the pioneering work of Heinrich Klüver (1897–1979), it is only recently that porphyrins have been linked to the toxic effects of lead. Silbergeld and Lamon, in an admirable article written in 1980, traced the possible metabolic pathways that lead can follow to produce its neurotoxic effects. Klüver observed that in numerous animals the fluorescence spectrum of the white matter of the central nervous system revealed a well-defined emission band at 630 to 620 nm.

In the middle 1970s Lamola—then a young man—and collaborators produced a fundamental work leading to the measuring of this spectral band in blood (Lamola and Yamane 1974; Lamola et al. 1975). William Blumberg and Joseph Eisinger at the Bell Laboratories in Murray Hill, New Jersey, developed the hematofluorometer, more familiarly known as the ZPP meter (Blumberg et al. 1977). The hematofluorometer measures the levels of zinc protoporphyrin (ZPP) by exposing a blood sample obtained by a pin prick to a blue light. Since the intensity of the resulting fluorescence is proportional to the presence of ZPP, after adequate calibration procedures, it was possible to calculate the concentration of ZPP in minute amounts of blood. Blumberg and Eisinger obtained a patent for their invention.

Fischbein, Lilis, and this author did preliminary work on the application of the hematofluorometer for the screening of groups occupationally exposed to lead (Fischbein et al., 1976; Lilis et al. 1977, 1978; Valciukas et al. 1978). It was found that ZPP was more closely related to lead-induced central nervous dysfunctions than blood lead levels. Similar findings were obtained early with free erythrocyte porphyrin (FEP). But the technical procedures to analyze FEP are costly. The hematofluorometer has the advantage that once the equipment is obtained, the ZPP meter can be used by almost anyone at essentially no additional cost.

Why Lead Is Neurotoxic

Several metabolic consequences of lead's ability to inhibit heme (the oxygen-carrying constituent of hemoglobin) synthesis are used as indications of lead absorption. These include increased levels of the porphyrin precursor δ-aminolevulinic acid (ALA), increased concentrations of the heme precursor protoporphyrin in red cells, and decreased activity of the enzyme ALA dehydrase in red cells.

Silbergeld and Lamon (1980) speculated that the toxic effects of lead may be mediated by (1) certain intermediates of heme biosynthesis that accumulate in excess as a result of the lead-induced inhibition of ALA dehydrase and ferrochelatase and (2) decreased availability of heme because of these blocks in the pathway adversely affecting the function of other biochemical systems dependent on heme. By citing evidence derived from their own work and research reports in the scientific literature, they concluded that ALA itself may be neurotoxic. They state, "When lead is added in vitro to cultures of sympathetic ganglion and caudate tissue, the production of fluorescent compounds is increased, suggesting that acute lead exposures can increase production and accumulation of porphyrins. Thus, ALA levels in brain may rise in lead poisoning by action of lead in situ on brain heme synthesis." The authors conclude that "The possibility that altered heme metabolism may be responsible for the neurotoxic manifestations of lead poisoning may provide an explanation of the well-described neurological similarities between lead poisoning and the acute attack forms of porphyria."

TOLERANCE

Tolerance is the reduction of potency of a drug or the toxicity of an agent following repeated administration of that drug or repeated exposure to the agent. Tolerance is a function of the organism, not the chemical compound. As a result, increasing levels of the drug or toxic agent are needed to produce the same effect. Sometimes, there can be a dissociation in the development of different tolerance effects. With repeated oral ingestion of chlordiazepoxide (Librium), for example, tolerance develops to its sedative properties while its antianxiety properties remain unchanged. Repeated ingestion of barbiturates may reduce their sedative properties or even produce insomnia, but the property of dangerously inhibiting the respiratory centers does not show tolerance. Although strongly suspected, there are little clinical data on tolerance to environmental and occupational neurotoxic agents.

Several forms of tolerance are recognized (Feldman and Quenzer 1987). *Cross tolerance* is the development of tolerance to a drug or neurotoxic agent by repeated exposure to a second drug or neurotoxic agent. Cross tolerance to alcohol has been extensively studied, for example. Phenobarbital, an anticonvulsant drug, is more potent in patients who have developed tolerance to alcohol than in patients who have not. Cross tolerance exists among many hallucinogenic drugs, such as LSD, psilocybin, and mescaline.

Drug disposition tolerance is the induction of tolerance to a drug or neurotoxic agent through the increased presence of metabolizing enzymes in the liver. This is also called *metabolic tolerance*. It is presumed that the drug creates a reduction of effect at its receptor by decreasing the effective concentration of the agonists or by reducing the reactivity of the receptor.

Cellular tolerance is an adaptation to the effects of a drug or environmental or occupational toxic agent even when the plasma levels of the drug are high. It is also called *pharmacodynamic tolerance*. It is thought that the tolerance is produced through diminished numbers of receptors or lower affinity of the receptors for the chemical compound. The most common form of pharmacological tolerance, for example, is that to opiates such as morphine and heroin.

Behavioral tolerance is a behavioral adaptation to a drug's effects following repeated administration. A person who suffers from severe alcoholism, for example, learns to compensate for the acute effects of alcohol; while intoxicated he or she can get the car keys and perform the complex coordination action involved in driving home.

CONCLUSIONS

Neurotoxic agents in the environment and the workplace enter the body through various routes. This results in pharmacological effects on neural targets, effects that may depend on easily recognizable factors such as age, gender, and body size.

Neurotoxic agents and drugs are excreted from the body either unchanged or transformed and then excreted as metabolites. The kidney and the liver are the principal organs involved in this process of biotransformation. Repeated administration of a drug and repeated exposure to a neurotoxic agent can lead to tolerance, wherein the body responds less and less to a given dose. The mechanisms of several instances of tolerance are now understood.

REFERENCES

Blumberg, WE, Eisinger, J, Lamola, AA, et al. (1977) The hematofluorometer. *Clin Chem* 23:270–274.

De Jongh, DK (1964) Introduction. In *Molecular Pharmacology*, Vol I, EJ Ariens (ed) pp. 13–16. New York: Academic Press.

Droz, PO and Guillemin, MP (1986) Occupational exposure monitoring using breath analysis. *J Occup Med* 28(8):593–602.

Feldman, RS and Quenzer, LF (1984) *Fundamentals of Neuropsychopharmacology*. Sunderland, MA: Sinauer Associates.

Fischbein, A, Eisinger, J, and Blumberg, WE (1976) Zinc protoporphyrin determination: A rapid screening test for the detection of lead poisoning. *Mount Sinai J Med* 43(3): 294–299.

Klüver, H (1944) On naturally occurring porphyrins in the central nervous system. *Science* 99:482–484.

Lamola, AA, Joselow, M, and Yamane, T (1975) Zinc protoporphyrin (ZPP): A simple, sensitive fluorometric screening test for lead poisoning. *Clin Chem* 21:93–97.

Lamola, AA and Yamane, T (1974) Zinc protoporphyrin in the erythrocytes of patients with lead intoxication and iron deficiency anemia. *Science* 186:936–938.

Lilis, R, Eisinger, J, Blumberg, W, et al. (1978) Hemoglobin, serum ion, and zinc protoporphyrin in lead-exposed workers. *Environ Health Perspect* 25:97–102.

Lilis, R, Fischbein, A, Eisinger, J, et al. (1977) Prevalence of lead disease among secondary smelter workers with biological indicators of lead exposure. *Environ Res* 14:255–285.

Neal, RA (1980) Metabolism of toxic substances. In *Casarett and Doulls' Toxicology: The Basic Science of Poisons*, J Doull, CD Klaassen, and MO Amdur (eds) pp. 56–69. New York: Macmillan.

Silbergeld, EK and Lamon, JM (1980) Role of altered heme synthesis in lead neurotoxicity. *J Occup Med* 22(10):680–684.

Valciukas, JA, Lilis, R, Eisinger, J, et al. (1978) Behavioral indicators of lead neurotoxicity: Results of a clinical field study. *Int Arch Occup Environ Health* 41:217–235.

SUGGESTED READINGS

Ahlgren, L, Heager-Aronson, B, Mattsson, S, et al. (1980) In vivo determination of lead in the skeleton following occupational exposure. *Br J Ind Med* 37:109–113.

Aito, A, Pekari, K, and Järvisalo, J (1984) Skin absorption as a source of error in biological monitoring. *Scan J Work Environ Health* 10:317–320.

Aldridge, WN (1986) The biological basis and measurement of thresholds. *Annu Rev Pharmacol Toxicol* 26:39–58.

Barnes, JM (1968) Percutaneous toxicity. In *Modern Trends in Toxicology*, E Boyland and R Goulding (eds), pp. 18–38. London: Butterworths.

Baselt, RC (ed) (1989) *Biological Monitoring Methods for Industrial Chemicals*. Boca Raton, FL: CRC Press.

Bénard, P, Burgat, V, and Rico, AG (1985) Application of whole-body autoradiography in toxicology. *Crit Rev Toxicol* 15(2):181–215.

Bergman, K (1983) Application and results of the whole-body autoradiography in distribution studies of organic solvents. *Crit Rev Toxicol* 12(1):59–118.

Betz, AL, Firth, JA, and Goldstein, GW (1980) Polarity of the blood-barrier: Distribution of enzymes between the luminal and antiluminal membranes of brain capillary endothelial cells. *Brain Res* 192:17–28.

Bouldin, TW, Mushak, P, O'Tuama, LA, et al. (1975) Blood–brain barrier dysfunction in acute lead en-

cephalopathy: A reappraisal. *Environ Health Perspect* 12:81–88.

Bradbury, M (1979) *The Concept of a Blood–Brain Barrier*. New York: John Wiley & Sons.

Bronaugh, RL and Maibach, HI (1985) In vitro models for human percutaneous absorption. In *Models in Dermatology*, Vol 2, HI Maibach and NJ Lowe (eds) pp. 178–188. Basel: Karger.

Brown, HS and Hattis, D (1989) The role of skin absorption as a route of exposure to volatile organic compounds in household tap water: A simulated kinetic approach. *J Am Coll Toxicol* 8(5):839–851.

Brunekreef, B (1984) The relationship between air lead and blood lead in children: A critical review. *Sci Total Environ* 38:79–123.

Christoffersson, JO, Ahlgren, L, Schütz, A, et al. (1986) Decrease of skeletal lead levels in man after end of occupational exposure. *Arch Environ Health* 41(5):312–318.

Cohen, GM (ed) (1986) *Target Organ Toxicity*, Vols 1 and 2. Boca Raton: FL: CRC Press.

Cooper JR, Bloom, FE, and Roth, RH (1986) *The Biological Basis of Neuropharmacology* (5th ed). New York: Oxford University Press.

Cullen, MR (ed) (1987) Workers with multiple chemical sensitivities. Philadelphia, PA: Hanley and Belfuls.

DeBruin, A (1976) *Biochemical Toxicology of Environmental Agents*. Amsterdam: Elsevier.

Doss, M (1978) *Diagnosis and Therapy of Porphyrias and Lead Intoxication*. New York: Springer-Verlag.

Durkiewicz, T and Tyras, H (1968) Skin absorption of toluene, styrene and xylene by man. *Br J Ind Med* 25:243.

Ecobichon, D (1982) *Pesticides and Neurological Diseases*. Boca Raton, FL: CRC Press.

Engström, K, Husman, K, and Riihimaki, V (1977) Percutaneous absorption of *m*-xylene in man. *Int Arch Occup Environ Health* 39:181–189.

Fiserova-Bergerova, V, Pierce, JT, and Droz, PO (1990) Dermal absorption potential of industrial chemicals: Criteria for skin notation. *Am J Ind Med* 17:617–635.

Forbes, GB and Reina, JC (1972) Effect of age on gastrointestinal absorption (Fe, Sr, Pb) in the rat. *J Nutr* 102:647–652.

Franklin, CA, Somers, DA, and Chu, I (1989) Use of percutaneous absorption data in risk assessment. *J Am Coll Toxicol* 8(5):815–827.

Froines, JR, Liu, W-CV, Hinds, WC, et al. (1986) Effect of aerosol size on the blood lead distribution of industrial workers. *Am J Ind Med* 9:227–237.

Gad, SC and Chengelis, CP (1988) *Acute Toxicology Testing: Perspectives and Horizons*. Caldwell, NJ: Telford.

Goldberg, L (1983) *Structure Activity Correlation as a Predictive Tool in Toxicology: Fundamentals, Methods, and Applications*. New York: Hemisphere.

Goldstein, GW and Betz, AL (1986) The blood–brain barrier. *Sci Am* 255:74–83.

Goodman Gilman, A, Goodman, LS, and Gilman, A (ed) (1980) *Goodman and Gilman's The Pharmacological Basis of Therapeutics.* New York: Macmillan.

Gralla, EJ (1981) *Scientific Considerations in Monitoring and Evaluating Toxicological Research.* New York: Hemisphere.

Grandjean, P (1979) Occupational lead exposure in Denmark: Screening with the haemotofluorometer. *Br J Med* 36:52–58.

Grandjean, P, Berlin, A, Gilbert, M, et al. (1988) Preventing percutaneous absorption of industrial chemicals: The "skin" denotation. *Am J Ind Med* 14:97–107.

Gross, PM and Weindl, A (1987) Peering through the windows of the brain. *J Cereb Blood Flow Metab* 7:663–672.

Guillemin, M, Murset, JC, Lob, M, et al. (1974) Simple method to determine the efficiency of a cream used for skin protection against solvents. *Br J Ind Med* 31:310–316.

Hattis, D (1978) *Analysis of Available Evidence on Blood Lead–Air Lead Relationships Relevant to the Selection of Permissible Exposure Limit for Lead in Air.* Cambridge, MA: Massachusetts Institute of Technology, Center for Policy Alternatives.

Haxton, J, Linddsay, DG, Hislop, J, et al. (1979) Duplicate diet study of fishery communities in the United Kingdom: Mercury exposure in a critical group. *Environ Res* 10:351–358.

Hayes, AW (1984) *Principles and Methods of Toxicology, Student Edition.* New York: Raven Press.

Hayes, WJ (1982) *Pesticides Studied in Man.* Baltimore: Williams & Wilkins.

Hedden, KF (1983) Multimedia fate and transport models: An overview. *J Toxicol* 21:65–95.

Ho, JK (1987) *Toxicology of CNS Depressants.* Boca Raton, FL: CRC Press.

Hogstedt, C and Stahl, R (1980) Skin absorption and protective gloves in dynamic work. *Am Ind Hyg Assoc J* 41:367–372.

Hunter, DJ, Morris, JS, Chute, CG, et al. (1990) Predictors of selenium concentration in human toenail. *Am J Epidemiol* 132(1):114–122.

Hursh, JB, Clarckson, TW, Miles, EF, et al. (1989) Percutaneous absorption of mercury vapor by man. *Arch Environ Health* 44(2):120–127.

Inoue, O, Seiji, K, Kawai, T, et al. (1989) Relationship between vapor exposure and urinary metabolite excretion among workers exposed to trichloroethylene. *Am. J Ind Med* 15:103–110.

Johanson, CE (1989) Ontogeny of the blood–brain barrier. In *Implications of the Blood–Brain Barrier and its Manipulation,* Vol 1, *Basic Science Aspects,* EA Neuwelt (ed) pp. 101–129. New York: Plenum Press.

Kalow, W, Goedde, HW, and Agarwal, DP (eds) (1986) *Ethnic Differences in Reactions to Drugs and Xenobiotics.* New York: Alan R. Liss.

Kaplan, J (1980) Neurotoxicity of selected biological toxins. In *Experimental and Clinical Neurotoxicology,* PS Spencer and HH Schaumburg (eds) pp. 631–648. Baltimore: Williams & Wilkins.

Klaassen, CD (1975) Biliary excretion of xenobiotics. *Crit Rev Toxicol* 4(1):1–29.

Klaassen, CD, Amdur, MO, and Doull, J (eds) (1986) *Casarett and Doull's Toxicology: The Basic Science of Poisons,* 3rd ed. New York: Macmillan.

Kononen, DW, Kinter, HJ, and Bivol, KR (1989) Air lead exposures and blood lead levels within a large automobile manufacturing workforce, 1980–1985. *Arch Environ Health* 44(4):244–251.

Li, AP (ed) (1985) *Toxicity Testing: New Approaches and Applications in Human Risk Assessment.* New York: Raven Press.

Lloyd, WE (1986) *Safety Evaluation of Drugs and Chemicals.* New York: Hemisphere.

Maibach, HI and Wester, RC (1989) Percutaneous absorption: In vivo methods in humans and animals. *J Am Coll Toxicol* 8(5):803–813.

Manahan, SE (1989) *Toxicological Chemistry: A Guide to Toxic Substances in Chemistry.* Chelsee, Michigan: Lewis.

Mann, T and Lutwak-Mann, C (1982) Passage of chemicals into human and animal semen: Mechanisms and significance. *Crit Rev Toxicol* 11(1):1–32.

Marino, PH, Franzblau, A, Lilis, R, and Landrigan, PJ (1989) Acute lead poisoning in construction workers: The failure of current protective standards. *Arch Environ Health* 44(2):140–145.

Masuda, Y, Kagawa, R, Kuroki, H, et al. (1978) Transfer of polychlorinated biphenyls from mothers to foetuses and infants. *Bull Environ Contam Toxicol* 16:543–546.

Mayer, SE, Melmon, KL, and Gilman, AG (1980) Introduction: The Dynamics of Drug Absorption, Distribution, and Elimination. In *Goodman and Gilman's The Pharmacological Basis of Therapeutics,* A Goodman Gilman, LS Goodman, and A Gilman (eds) pp. 1–27. New York: Macmillan.

Meuling, WJA, Bragt, PC and Braun, CLJ (1990) Biological monitoring of carbon disulfide. *Am J Ind Med* 17:247–254.

Milby, TH (1971) Prevention and management of organophosphate poisoning. *JAMA* 216:2131–2133.

Miller, RW (1977) Pollutants in breast milk. *J Pediatr* 90:510–512.

Moore, TJ, Lione, AP, Sugda, MC, et al. (1976) Beta-hydroxybutyrate transport in rat brain: Developmental and dietary modulations. *Am J Physiol* 230:619–636.

Namba, T, Nolte, CT, Jackrel, J, et al. (1971) Poisoning due to organophosphate insecticide: Acute and chronic manifestation. *Am J Med* 50:475–492.

Nomiyama, K and Nomiyama, H (1974) Respiratory

retention uptake and excretion of organic solvents in man. *Int Arch Arbeitsmed* 32:75–83.

Nomiyama, K and Nomiyama, H (1974) Respiratory elimination of organic solvents in man. *Int Arch Arbeitsmed* 32:86–91.

Nordberg, GF (ed) (1976) *Effects and Dose–Response Relationships of Toxic Metals, Proceeding from an International Meeting organized by the Subcommittee on the Toxicology of Metals of the Permanent Commission and International Associations on Occupational Health, Tokyo, November 18–23, 1974.*

Oehmem FW (1980) Absorption, biotransformation and excretion of environmental chemicals. *Clin Toxicol* 17(1):147–158.

Olendorf, WH (1975) Permeability of the blood–brain barrier. In *The Nervous System,* Vol 1, *The Basic Neurosciences,* DB Tower (ed) pp. 279–289. New York: Raven Press.

Ong, CN, Chia, KS, Koh, D, et al. (1989) Neurochemical effect of lead exposure: A study of cathecholamine metabolism. *Am J Ind Med* 16:667–673.

Pardridge, WM, Connor, JD, and Crawford, IL (1975) Permeability changes in the blood–brain barrier: Causes and consequences. *Crit Rev Toxicol* 3(1):159–199.

Quarterman, J and Morrison, E (1978) The effect of age on the absorption and excretion of lead. *Environ Res* 17:78–83.

Rabinowitz, MB, Wetherill, GW, and Kopple, JD (1977) Magnitude of lead intake from respiration by normal man. *J Lab Clin Med* 90:238–248.

Rapoport, SI (1976) *Blood–Brain Barrier in Physiology and Medicine.* New York: Raven Press.

Roels, HA, Balis-Jacques, MN, Buchet, JP, et al. (1979) The influence of sex and of chelation therapy on erythrocyte protoporphyrin and urinary delta-aminolevulinic acid in lead-exposed workers. *J Occup Med* 21:527–539.

Sato, A and Nakajima, T (1987) Pharmacokinetics of organic solvent vapors in relation to their toxicity. *Scand J Work Environ Health* 13:81–93.

Scheuplin, T (1978) The skin as a barrier. In *The Physiology and Pathology of the Skin,* Vol 5, A Jarret (ed) pp. 1669–1692. London: Academic Press.

Scheuplin, T and Blanke, IH (1971) Permeability of the skin. *Physiol Rev* 51:702–747.

Seppäläinen, AM and Rajaniemi, R (1984) Local neurotoxicity of methyl methacrylate among dental technicians. *Am J Ind Med* 5:471–477.

Silbergeld, EK and Fowler, BA (eds) (1987) Mechanisms of chemical-induced porphyrinopathies. *Ann NY Acad Sci* 514:1–35.

Spector, R and Johanson, CE (1989) The mammalian choroid plexus, *Sci Am* 261(5):68–74.

Sterman, AB and Schaumburg, HH (1980) Neurotoxicity of selected drugs. In *Experimental and Clinical Neurotoxicology,* PS Spencer and HH Schaumberg (eds) pp. 593–612. Baltimore: Williams & Wilkins.

Suckling, AJ, Rumsky, MG, and Bradbury, MWB (eds) (1986) *The Blood–Brain Barrier in Health and Disease.* New York: VCH Publishers.

Suskind, RR (1977) Environment and the skin. *Environ Health Perspect* 20:27–37.

Tola, S (1977) The effect of blood lead concentration, age, sex, and time of exposure upon erythrocyte delta-aminolevulinic acide dehydratase activity. *Work Environ Health* 10:26–35.

Toriumi, H and Kawai, M (1981) Free erythrocyte protoporphyrin (FEP) in a general population, workers exposed to low-level lead, and organic-solvent workers. *Environ Res* 25:310–316.

Vinson, LJ, Singer, EJ, Koehler, WR, et al. (1965) The nature of the epidermal barrier and some factors influencing skin permeability. *Toxicol Appl Pharmacol* Supp 2, 7–19.

Vitale, LF, Joselow, MM, and Wedeen, RP (1975) Blood lead—an inadequate measure of occupational exposure. *J Occup Med* 17:155–156.

Waldron, HA (1974) The blood lead threshold. *Arch Environ Health* 29:271–273.

Wallace, LA, Pellizzari, ED, Hartwell, TD, et al. (1989) The influence of personal activities on exposure to volatile organic compounds. *Environ Res* 50:37–55.

Wallen, M, Holm, S, and Byfält Nordqvist, M (1985) Coexposure to toluene and *p*-xylene in man: Uptake and elimination. *Br J Ind Med* 42:111–116.

Webster, RC and Maibach, HI (1989) Human skin binding and absorption of contaminants from ground and surface water during swimming and bathing. *J Am Coll Toxicol* 8(5):853–859.

Weiss, B and Simon, W (1974) Quantitative perspectives on the long-term toxicity of methylmercury and similar poisons. In *Behavioral Toxicology,* B. Weiss and VG Laties (eds) pp. 429–437. New York: Plenum Press.

Wielopolski, L, Ellis, KJ, Vaswani, AN, et al. (1986) In vivo bone lead measurements: A rapid monitoring method for cumulative lead exposure. *Am J Ind Med* 9:221–226.

Wildt, K, Berlin, M, and Isberg, PE (1987) Monitoring of zinc protoporphyrin levels in blood following occupational lead exposure. *Am J Ind Med* 12:385–398.

Williams, PL and Burson, JL (1985) *Industrial Toxicology: Safety and Health Applications in the Workplace.* New York: Van Nostrand Reinhold.

Wright, JLC, Boyd, RK, de Freitas, ASW, et al. (1989) Identification of domoic acid, a neuroexcitatory amino acid, in toxic mussels from eastern Prince Edward Island. *Can J Chem* 67:481–490.

Zielhuis, RL (1984) Biological monitoring. In *Assessment of Toxic Agents at the Workplace: Role of Ambient and Biological Monitoring,* A Berlin, EE Eodaiken, and BA Henman (eds) pp. 84–94. The Hague: Martinus Nijhoff.

10

Toxicology and the Environmental and Occupational Health Sciences

The disciplines of human toxicology and the environmental and occupational (E & O) health sciences are rapidly converging. It is generally perceived that for the E & O health sciences to be on a firm footing, toxicological principles must be adopted. This chapter is devoted to a review of the common language that has already developed between these two disciplines.

THE LANGUAGE OF TOXICOLOGY

Every chemical substance can be classified as to its potency or toxicity. Traditionally, six basic classes of potency are recognized: extremely toxic, highly toxic, moderately toxic, slightly toxic, relatively nontoxic, and relatively harmless. Poison is a chemical term referring to extremely or highly toxic.

What makes an agent neurotoxic is its ability to reach, react with, and pharmacologically affect some branch of the nervous system. As has been seen in the previous chapter dealing with the absorption, distribution, metabolism, and excretion of chemical compounds (processes linked under the name *pharmacokinesis*), a neurotoxic agent can affect the nervous system locally—as when an esthetics are injected by dentists into the gums without affecting other portions of the mouth—and systemically—as when the toxic agent needs to travel some distance to produce its toxic effects.

Some of the effects can be direct, and some others indirect. Halothane, an anesthetic, has a direct effect on the nervous system producing narcosis. *Narcosis* is profound loss of consciousness provoked by a drug. Some others produce indirect effects on the nervous system through their primary action on the kidney, liver, blood-forming mechanisms, or pulmonary action. Sometimes a toxic agent causes physical changes and traumatic alterations in the nervous system.

The effects of a neurotoxic agent can also be acute or chronic. *Acute* is a term used to indicate both a short period of time—minutes, hours, days, and even weeks; the term is often used to indicate that the toxic effect is reversible.

The period of time for the production of an acute effect cannot always be precisely defined. Thus, the acute effects of certain neurotoxic agents are measured either in milliseconds—such as in certain neurophysiological preparations involving experimental laboratory animals—or in minutes, hours, days, and even weeks, such as the time a human takes to recuperate from poisoning by certain snakes.

A *chronic effect* is one where there is permanent damage to the nervous system, and the term is used to label a phenomenon that lasts a long period of time—months or years—and is largely irreversible. The effect of exposure to methylmercury in utero, for example, causes chronic damage to the child's nervous system (Minamata disease) associated with profound mental retardation.

Most investigators agree that long-term, low-level exposure to a neurotoxic agent needs a distinct term. The term subchronic has been proposed to describe such a pattern of toxic exposure. But the reader needs to ascertain how a particular author uses this term in the literature. The expression "long-term low-level exposure" is used throughout this volume in order not to contribute to this confusion.

In Chapter 3, dealing with the clinical manifestations of neurotoxic diseases, two terms used in neurology were introduced: subclinical and preclinical. *Subclinical* indicates a pharmacological, neurophysiological—or even a behavioral or psychological—change that is not detected during the course of the clinical examination of the subject at a given point in time. Certain electrophysiological and psychometric procedures are useful to detect changes that are not observed by examining physicians and, sometimes, by the subjects themselves.

Preclinical signs, symptoms, or syndromes are those that occur before the appearance of the overt manifestation of neurotoxic illness. Thus, in the term preclinical, "pre" indicates time. "Preclinical" is a useful term in preventive medicine to indicate cases where if conditions are left by themselves and without control, a clinical manifestation of neurotoxic disease is likely to appear.

Neurotoxic effects may be observed immediately after the inhalation, ingestion, injection, or topical application of the agent, or, on the other hand, after several days. The latter is called *delayed neurotoxicity*. Certain pesticides, such as triorthocresyl phosphate

(TOCP), leptofos, and mipafox are capable of producing *delayed toxic neuropathies*—that is, delayed effects on the peripheral nervous system producing paralysis and sensory alterations first in lower limbs and then in upper limbs.

There are numerous terms describing the manner in which chemicals interact with each other. The following is a partial list; some others may be found in Klaassen (1986). The environmental or occupational toxic agent, or the drug, can be administered to an experimental animal under laboratory conditions, or humans may be exposed to it as the result of its presence in the environment or the workplace.

An *additive effect* is one in which the combined effect of two chemicals is approximately the sum of the effect of each individual agent. The simultaneous presence of several organophosphorus pesticides appears to be additive and is explained in terms of the additive effects of the rate of inhibition of cholinesterase (an enzyme) by each pesticide.

A *synergistic effect* is one in which the effect of two chemical compounds is much greater than the simple sum of their single effects. Ethanol (alcohol) produces a synergistic effect when present along with many drugs and industrial solvents.

Potentiation describes an effect in which a chemical compound itself may not be able to produce a toxic effect but, when added to another, makes the latter much more toxic.

Antagonism describes the inhibitory effects that two chemicals have when they are simultaneously present. *Antidote,* with its original meaning of being capable of arresting or negating the effects of a poison, is now rarely used in the scientific literature.

Mortality Toxicology

Human toxicologists and epidemiologists perform essentially two types of studies: mortality (dealing with death) and morbidity (dealing with illness). In mortality studies, one of the basic measurements is the ascertainment of the lethal dose. The concept of *lethal dose* is well rooted in statistical thinking. When a single dose—that is, the concentration per unit weight of a given toxic agent—is administered to a group of cells, bacteria, or experimental animals, the percentage of individuals who will die increases with the dose. At a lower concentration, for example, 30% of the individuals may die; at a higher dose, 75%. Thus, lethal dose is a relative term.

During the initial stages of an experimental investigation, several different percentages of lethal dose are plotted. Theoretically, and depending on financial and human resources, one could ascertain the percentage of dead individuals for increasing doses of the chemical agent in very fine steps. But this is both impractical and unnecessary. A few well-chosen steps—usually in logarithmic incremental units—can give a good idea of the overall statistical trends for the group. The LD_{50}, that is, the dose capable of killing 50% of the individuals, is a common reference point and is ascertained by mathematical extrapolation of empirical data.

The concept of lethal dose is basic in classical toxicology and epidemiology studies dealing with mortality—for example, in toxicological studies of cancer. In neurotoxicology, however, the terms used in "morbidity toxicology" are important. As a result, we will have little use for the concept of lethal dose except for how lethal dose is related to effective dose (ED) and toxic dose (TD), to be examined later in this chapter. What follows is a brief introduction to the terminology of "morbidity toxicology."

Morbidity Toxicology

A *threshold* is the minimal amount of energy, either physical or chemical, just sufficient to produce an observable effect. Physicochemists, pharmacologists, and neurophysiologists determine at what concentration (or dose) a given chemical substance appears to produce a physical, chemical, physiological, or behavioral change. Both the stimulus and the effects are intertwined. For example, slowing of the electrical conduction velocity of a nerve (the *effect*) is related to the stimulus—the oral administration of methyl mercury (the *cause*). The effect is defined in terms of the levels of the stimulus (the cause), that is, at which level of ingested levels of methyl mercury a statistically significant reduction of the nerve conduction velocity is observed.

"Threshold" as a scientific concept has existed since the middle of the 19th century. Weber (1795–1878), a physiologist, performed the classic experiment to determine the magnitude of the physical stimulus just sufficient to produce specific sensations (eg, pain). Fechner (1801–1887) concluded that the magnitude of the sensation and the physical stimuli required to produce the effect were related by a logarithmic law, called the Weber–Fechner law. The branch of experimental psychology dealing with the study of stimulus–response relationships in the sensory systems is called psychophysics (Boring 1950).

When and why psychophysicists and toxicologists parted and went their own ways is difficult to ascertain. Psychophysics and toxicology had a common ancestor and a common language in the German science of the last century. Physics was taught alongside chemistry and the physiological sciences, and psychology, then a new discipline, was well rooted in physiology. In addition, most scientists of the period had a particular inclination for philosophy; some of them, such as Fechner, considered themselves "experimental philosophers" and performed their experiments to test or prove philosophical ideas.

There is a great deal of overlap between psychophysics and theoretical toxicology, the branch of toxicology that deals with the scientific foundations of this discipline. Psychophysics is a discipline that studies the relationships between psychological events—particularly sensation—and the physical world. Toxicology deals with the scientific study of the relations between the "chemical world" and its pharmacological, physiological, behavioral, or psychological effects on humans.

Threshold limit value is almost a tautology, as is the expression "the hazardous effects of dangerous substances." Threshold *is* a limit. However, "limit" has the connotation of "ceiling," the maximum allowable levels of a substance recommended in the environment or the workplace. Threshold limit values (TLVs) for a large number of substances have been calculated. The best source for current information is *TLV's™*, *Threshold Limit Values and Biological Exposure Indices for 1985–1986* published by the American Conferences of Governmental and Industrial Hygienists. The significance of threshold limit values for regulation and control of environmental and occupational neurotoxic agents is clear. But, sometimes thresholds ascertained under laboratory conditions in nonhuman species are used to extrapolate to the human environment or the workplace.

How and under what conditions these extrapolations from animals to humans should be made is the subject of chemical risk analysis, a discipline still in its infancy. A separate branch of risk analysis dealing with neurotoxic effects was envisioned by Weiss and Simon in 1974. But the basic premise of that theory—that intellectual function is related to neural cell density—is not supported by the neurosciences.

Threshold limit values are necessary but inadequate. The most serious problem with TLVs is that certain toxic agents—most notably asbestos and neurotoxic substances such as lead—do not seem to have a threshold. That is, there is no "safe" limit of exposure. Moreover, TLVs need to be complemented by other concepts. The concept of a *no-effect level* (NEL) is obviously inadequate because, by "effect," one may mean changes in the physical appearance of nerve cells in vitro, changes in the selective permeability of membranes, slowing of conduction of peripheral nerves, or reduction in reaction time. The possibility of delayed neurotoxicity (described above) may need to be taken into account as well. Finally, the concept of a no-effect level is subjective and depends very much on who does the observing. Thus, the concept

of no-effect levels has been upgraded to include the use of techniques that could be available for public scrutiny, giving rise to the concept of *nonobservable-effect level* (NOEL). But, how important would knowledge of the physiological properties of a toxic substance be if no adverse health effects for humans or animals could be demonstrated? The concept of *nonobservable-adverse-effect levels* (NOAEL) originated in response to this criticism.

Dose–Response Relationships

The concept of dose–response relationship is fundamental in experimental pharmacology, human toxicology, and E & O health sciences. Toxicologists view the dose and response as causally related, whereas epidemiologists tend to be more cautious, speaking of statistical associations between exposure levels and neurological signs and symptoms or the results of electrophysiological and psychometric tests. This distinction has enormous legal consequences that are the object of current debates.

THE LANGUAGE OF ENVIRONMENTAL AND OCCUPATIONAL HEALTH

The fields of environmental health and occupational health are rapidly expanding. One of the major objectives of these disciplines is the prevention of environmentally or occupationally induced toxic illnesses. As stated earlier, there have been many individual attempts to link many of the principles of environmental and occupational health to firmly rooted pharmacological and toxicological principles. However, a literal translation is practically impossible and does not always satisfy the large number of professionals with different backgrounds.

Some of the most basic concepts are "drug" and "toxic agent." Drugs and toxic agents follow the same pharmacokinetic and pharmacodynamic laws, but the conditions of "administration" are radically different: Drugs are **administered** under clinical conditions for their therapeutic value, and the individual who takes the drug (or his or her relatives) agrees to the drug administration; people are **involuntarily exposed** to toxic agents in the environment or the workplace—in many cases, people who are affected by environmental or occupational toxic exposure do not even know about the existence of such exposures. There is current discussion about a common terminology that applies to both fields.

Following are three essential concepts that have originated in the environmental and occupational health sciences. Zielhuis, in an editorial published in 1985, urged the proper use of these terms. Quotations are taken from that source and from Berlin et al. (1984).

1. *Environmental monitoring* (EM) is the "measurement and assessment of agents at the workplace and evaluates ambient exposure and health risk compared to an appropriate reference."
2. *Biological monitoring* (BM) is the "measurement and assessment of workplace agents or their metabolites either in tissues, secreta, excreta, expired air, or any combinations of these to evaluate exposures and health risk compared to an appropriate measure."
3. *Health surveillance* (health effects monitoring, HEM) is the "periodic medicophysiological examination of exposed workers with the objective of protecting health and preventing occupationally related disease."

Both the external and the internal (within the body) environments are monitored. Industrial hygienists, while measuring ambient levels of a chemical compound in the workplace, make an evaluation of the external environment. Biological monitoring measures humans' internal indications of absorption (blood lead levels) or internal indicators of effects (eg, ZPP, ALA-D, ALA-U). These are

sometimes called biological markers of absorption (or effects). Some of these indicators are agent-specific: zinc protoporphyrin for lead and cholinesterase for exposure to cholinesterase-inhibiting chemical compounds. Some others at are non-agent-specific, since many chemical compounds may produce the same biological response, for example, anemia.

The American Conference of Government Industrial Hygienists (ACGIH) published in 1986 a list of biological exposure indices (BEI) with meanings similar to biological monitors. A committee of the Deutsche Forschungs Gemeinschaft proposed the concept of biologically acceptable limits of occupational exposure.

REFERENCES

American Conference of Governmental and Industrial Hygienists (1986) *TLVs®: Threshold Limit Values and Biological Indices for 1985–86*. Cincinnati, OH: ACGIH.

Berlin, A, Yodaiken, RE, and Henman, BA (eds) (1984) *Assessment of Toxic Agents at the Workplace: Role of Ambient and Biological Monitoring*. The Hague: Martinus Nijhoff.

Boring, EG (1950) *A History of Experimental Psychology*. New York: Appleton-Century-Crofts.

Klaassen, CD (1986) Principles of toxicology. In *Casarett and Doull's Toxicology: The Basic Science of Poisons,* 3rd ed. CD Klaassen, MO Amdur, and J Doull (eds) pp. 11–32. New York: Macmillan.

Weiss, B and Simon, W (1974) Quantitative perspectives on the long-term toxicity of methylmercury and similar poisons. In *Behavioral Toxicology,* B Weiss and VG Laties (eds) pp. 429–437. New York: Plenum Press.

Zielhuis, RL (1985) Editorial: Biological monitoring: Confusion in terminology. *Am J Ind Med* 8:515–516.

SUGGESTED READINGS

Aitio, A, Riihimaki, V, and Vainio, H (1984) *Biological Monitoring and Surveillance of Workers Exposed to Chemicals.* New York: Hemisphere.

Aldridge, WN (1986) The biological basis and measurement of thresholds. *Annu Rev Pharmacol Toxicol* 26:39–58.

Berlin A, Wolff, AH, and Hasegawa Y (eds) (1979) *The Use of Biological Specimens for the Assessment of*

Human Exposure to Environmental Pollutants. The Hague: Martinus Nijhoff.

Castleman, BI and Ziem, GE (1988) Corporate influence on threshold limit values. *Am J Ind Med* 13:531–559.

DeBruin, A (1976) *Biochemical Toxicology of Environmental Agents.* Amsterdam: Elsevier.

Gralla, EJ (1981) *Scientific Considerations in Monitoring and Evaluating Toxicological Research.* New York: Hemisphere.

Hayes, AW (1984) *Principles and Methods of Toxicology, Student Edition.* New York: Raven Press.

Klaassen, CD, Amdur, MO, and Doull, J (eds) (1986) *Casarett and Doull's Toxicology: The Basic Science of Poisons,* 3rd ed. New York: Macmillan.

Lave, LB and Upton, AC (eds) (1987) *Toxic Chemicals, Health and the Environment.* Baltimore: The Johns Hopkins University Press.

Lauwerys, RR (1983) *Industrial Chemical Exposure: Guidelines for Biological Monitoring.* Davis, CA: Biomedical Publications.

Matsumara, F, Boush, GM, and Misato, T (1972) *Environmental Toxicology of Pesticides.* New York: Academic Press.

Nordberg, GF (ed) (1976) *Effects and Dose–Response Relationships of Toxic Metals, Proceedings from an International Meeting organized by the Subcommittee on the Toxicology of Metals of the Perma*nent Commission and International Associations on Occupational Health, Tokyo, November 18–23, 1974.

Schulte, PA (1987) Methodologic issues in the use of biological markers in epidemiologic research. *Am J Epidemiol* 126(6):1006–1016.

Smyth, HS (1962) A toxicologist's view of threshold limits. *Am Ind Hyg Assoc J* 23:37–44.

Williams, PL and Burson, JL (1985) *Industrial Toxicology: Safety and Health Applications in the Workplace.* New York: Van Nostrand Reinhold.

Zielhuis, RL (1971) Interrelation of biochemical responses to the absorption of inorganic lead. *Arch Environ Health* 23:299–311.

Zielhuis, RL (1975) Dose–response relationship for inorganic lead. *Int Arch Occup Health* 35:1–18.

Zielhuis, RL (1984) Biological monitoring. In *Assessment of Toxic Agents at the Workplace: Role of Ambient and Biological Monitoring,* A Berlin, EE Yodaiken, and BA Henman (eds) pp. 84–94. The Hague: Martinus Nijhoff.

Zielhuis, RL and Henderson, PT (1986) Definitions of monitoring activities and their relevance for the practice of occupational health. *Int Arch Occup Environ Health* 57:249–257.

Zielhuis, RL and Wibowo, AE (1989) Standard setting in occupational health: "Philosophical" issues. *Am J Ind Med* 16:569–598.

11

Occupational History

Occupational history is a chronological account of all the jobs a person has had since he or she entered the work force. It includes exposures, use of protective equipment, and hygiene practices. The occupational history is taken by many: professionals during clinical examinations; health scientists during epidemiological surveys; scientists who perform experimental studies with human subjects under laboratory conditions; and forensic professionals who evaluate objective findings, signs, and symptoms in court cases involving claims of occupation-induced neurotoxic illness.

In environmental and occupational neurotoxicology, assessment of human dose is made by essentially two types of data: measurements of environmental levels of chemical compounds and exposure estimates abstracted from the occupational history. (A discussion of techniques of sampling and continuous monitoring of environmental chemicals in air, water, and soil, techniques for continuous personal monitoring, and chemical analytical techniques for analysis of these samples is beyond the scope of this book.) Measurement of environmental levels of toxic substances is not always possible; eg, management does not allow these measurements

to be made on the premises; the product that is suspected to cause a health problem is no longer in use; there is no accepted technology for such assessments. Therefore, sometimes the occupational history is the only source of information of the possible causes of health problems. In Chapter 15 a more detailed analysis of how this information is further quantified is found.

An occupational history that is taken by an experienced interviewer and abstracted by a professional well trained in both job practices and data-reduction procedures can produce the following information:

- The classification of an entire work force by job categories and further by process division or task duties—eg, custodians, pipe fitters, painters, mechanics, office workers.
- A ranking of jobs by exposure—eg, lead smelters (heaviest exposure to lead), packers and workers in the unloading deck carrying batteries to the smelter (intermediate exposure), and workers in the shipping department (minimal exposure).
- Quantitative estimates of length of service in the industry—ie, duration of toxic exposure. This information can lead to es-

timates of turnover rates (how quickly workers quit their jobs and why) and whether these turnover rates are related to changes in environmental conditions.

- When the information derived from the occupational history is related to measures of biological markers of exposures, quantitative dose estimates are sometimes possible—eg, levels of lead in blood and levels of metabolites known to be associated with toxic agents such as mandelic acid as a result of exposure to styrene.

INFORMATION CONTAINED IN THE OCCUPATIONAL HISTORY

The importance of the occupational history in the evaluation of human neurotoxic effects cannot be overestimated. As seen in the Introduction to this book, dealing with the historical roots of occupational and environmental neurotoxicology, it was Ramazzini who first recommended that his students add to the "anamnesis" (the medical history) the important question "In which trade are you in?" or "What is your occupation?" (See Fig. 11.1 for an example of a contemporary occupational history questionnaire.)

Today workers change occupations many times in their lifetimes. As a result, the relationship between job and health is complicated, and these suspected links need to be established by careful probes into the past work history as well as the present occupation. The actual probing is an art. All the professional and personal skills of an interviewer—ie, ability to establish a professional but frank communication with the worker, patient, victim of an environmental disaster, the plaintiff or defendant in court, etc—are required for this task. In the clinic, the physician or the neuropsychologist takes this information during the initial visit. Current guidelines for occupational history taking (Johnson 1987) include both past occupational history (dates, occupations, places of employment, job tasks, exposures, use of personal protective equipment, and personal hygiene practices) and present occupation (place of employment, month and year when current job began, job tasks, exposures, use of personal protective equipment, and personal hygiene practices).

The spouse's occupation is often overlooked, but the interviewee may suffer *bystander toxic exposure*—eg, bystander exposure to pesticides, lead, etc, leading to illness or even death.

Sometimes the occupation of the interviewee's parents is important—eg, as in the possibility of bystander exposure at home with lead brought in on a parent's clothing. The child sometimes helps his or her parents in farming, hobbies, or small shops, and these activities may be overlooked during the course of a pediatric examination.

One needs to be familiar with work practices and have a knowledge of the toxicity of numerous chemical compounds to be able to obtain additional information on exposures. For example, if the person being interviewed says that he/she engaged in cabinet making as a hobby, questions about the use of glues, varnishes, and solvents are necessary. However, intelligent decisions must to be made when probing the depth of a particular activity. A bulky occupational history of several pages collected by an inexperienced interviewer is not necessarily more useful than a terse one obtained by an experienced industrial hygienist.

There are numerous scientific reports dealing with such important matters as the validity and reliability of the occupational history and intraobserver and interobserver variability. *Recall bias* is an important factor as well. There have been numerous attempts to minimize these factors by suggesting the use of fixed protocols in which all the interviewers ask the same questions. However, attempting to use fixed occupational history protocols when one needs to perform a medical survey under emergency conditions in unknown regions of the country or the world is a futile exercise.

Computer-based procedures may also be misleading. These procedures are developed for highly structured working conditions existing notably in the United States. It is easy to overlook a pattern of exposure among foreign-born workers or job practices engaged in by artisans and craftmen.

Written notes with examples are preferred. The actual questionnaire to document the work history and present employment can be very simple. The probe usually begins with the question "What is the first job you have ever had?" or "What were your parents' occupations at the time of your birth?" Notes need to be taken as the information is gathered. Occupational histories do not look alike even from people in small towns living and working under similar conditions and performing the same activity.

A "job" cannot be conceived of as a rigid entity. Besides, people have different perceptions about how dangerous their environment is. As a result, unusually anxious people may volunteer the names of an extraordinary array of chemicals they have been exposed to; others, having a more stoic attitude toward work, may perceive actual dangerous working conditions as innocuous.

The publication *Occupational Outlook Handbook,* published every year by the US Department of Labor, Bureau of Labor Statistics, contains a Dictionary of Occupational Titles and a Statistical Occupational Classification (US Department of Labor 1986).

Occupational analysis is performed during the following operations:

1. Job training—eg, when a particular job such as "use of cranes" is broken down into basic units; the individual is then tested in the skills required for the mastery of these skills.
2. Employee's selection—eg, whether the skills and knowledge of the prospective candidate for a job match the job profile.
3. Ergonomic studies—eg, motion and time studies performed to ascertain physical attributes of the environment, its architectural features, workers' postures, and the overall estimate of the cost/efficiency of the operations.

There are courses and manuals in which workers are taught the proper handling of neurotoxic agents. Pesticide applicators are trained in the identification and proper use of pesticides, environmental conditions needed to be taken into account, and use of protective equipment. *The Pesticide Applicator Training Manual* published by Cornell University is a good example. Some labor organizations have developed safety and training programs that rival similar courses offered at technical schools and specialized 2-year colleges. An example is the course in welding safety and health offered by the American Welding Society.

OCCUPATIONAL ANALYSIS

The aims and methods used for the documentation of an occupational history and present employment should not be confused with available methods of occupational analysis and vocational training. The latter is performed in a quite different context, and, in the vast majority of cases, occupational analysis does not include exposure data. Because of this possible confusion, occupational analysis needs to be characterized briefly.

CONCLUSIONS

In E & O neurotoxicology, assessment of human dose is made by essentially two types of data: measurements of environmental levels of chemical compounds and exposure estimates abstracted from the occupational history. Because measurements of environmental levels of toxic substances are not always possible, data derived from analysis of the occupational history of individuals or groups of people often become the only information

ENVIRONMENTAL SCIENCES LABORATORY
MOUNT SINAI SCHOOL OF MEDICINE OF THE CITY UNIVERSITY OF NEW YORK

0 A

1   2   3   4   5   6

OCCUPATIONAL HISTORY

INTERVIEWER
IDENTIFICATION

□ □
7   8

CURRENT EMPLOYMENT

INSTRUCTIONS: Provide a brief sketch of current employment. Include: type of industry; description of various jobs; materials handled. Use codes in left column. If you have questions, ask section chief or consult separate instruction/example sheet.

EMPLOYMENT CATEGORY
1. secretarial/clerical
2. service/sales
3. management
4. professional
5. labor
6. self-employed
7. other

SELECTED OCCUPATIONS
01. unemployed/laid off
02. disabled illness
03. homemaker
04. no previous employ
05. farming/general
06. farming/dairy
07. farming/livestock
08. farming/orchard, fruit
09. fishing/processing
10. grain handling
11. animal feed prep.
12. manufacturing/general
13. manufacturing/vehicles
14. manufacturing furniture
15. manufacturing/electronics
16. manufacturing/chemicals
17. plastics industry
18. refinery
19. pharmaceuticals
20. dry cleaning
21. metal smelting
22. foundry, iron/steel
23. shipyards
24. construction
25. painting trades
26. mining/milling ores
27. pulp/paper industry
28. printing industry
29. textile industry
99. other

SELECTED EXPOSURES
01. none of below
02. don't know
03. unk. smoke/fume/vapor
04. unk. dust
05. unk. eye/nose irritants
06. acids/alkali
07. asbestos
08. talc
09. insulation work
10. brake repair
11. dry wall taping
12. maintenance work
13. silica
14. sand blasting
15. rock crushing/drilling
16. coal
17. powerhouse work
18. lead
19. mercury
20. beryllium
21. cadmium
22. grinding/drilling metal
23. arsenic
24. pesticides/herbicides
25. chemical handling
26. solvents/degreasers
27. benzene
28. CCL_4, TCE, PCE, Chloroform
29. ionizing radiation
30. noise/protection required
31. vibrating equipment
32. welding

Current employment status:

1 = employed/full   6 = disabled
2 = multiple jobs   7 = laid off
3 = employed part.   8 = retired
4 = homemaker   9 = student
5 = unemployed

If 1-3, write 99.
If 4-9, list year status began.

If 4-9, go to PREVIOUS EMPLOYMENT section on page 2.

Current employment _____

_____

_____

On your current job, what materials do you work with, or are you exposed to? List below. Code only those on selected exposures list to left.

_____

_____

_____

On your current job, is safety equipment provided? 1 = yes
                              2 = no
                              3 = not applicable

IF YES: What type of equipment? Do you use it?

equipment code   use code
1 = mask respirator   1 = never
2 = air supply resp.   2 = sometimes
3 = gloves/any kind   3 = always
4 = coveralls/company
5 = safety glasses
6 = hearing protect
7 = other

□
9

□ □
10   11

□   employment
12   category

□ □   occupation
13 14 code

□ □   year began
15 16 employment

selected   selected
exposure   exposure

□ □   □ □
17 18 19 20

□ □   □ □
21 22 23 24

□ □
25 26

□
27

□ equip □
28 ment 29 use

□ equip □
30 ment 31 use

□   □
32   33 use

□ equip □
34 ment 35 use

□ equip □
36 ment 37 use

Fig. 11.1. An occupational history questionnaire (by permission of Dr. Irving J. Selikoff).

INSTRUCTIONS: Provide a brief sketch of each employment period. Include: type of industry; description of various jobs; materials handled. Use codes in left-hand column. If you have questions, ask section chief or consult instruction example sheet.

PREVIOUS EMPLOYMENT*

1st employment _____

_____

2nd employment_____

_____

3rd employment _____

_____

4th employment _____

_____

5th employment _____

_____

6th employment _____

_____

7th employment _____

_____

8th employment _____

_____

***Interviewer, please copy patient's
I.D. number in these boxes**

9th employment _____

_____

10th employment _____

_____

*Please check if patient's I.D. is copied correctly before going on.

EMPLOYMENT CATEGORY
1. secretarial/clerical
2. service/sales
3. management
4. professional
5. labor
6. self-employed
7. other

SELECTED OCCUPATIONS
01. unemployed/laid off
02. disabled illness
03. homemaker
04. no previous employ
05. farming/general
06. farming/dairy
07. farming/livestock
08. farming/orchard, fruit
09. fishing/processing
10. grain handling
11. animal feed prep.
12. manufacturing/general
13. manufacturing/vehicles
14. manufacturing/furniture
15. manufacturing/electronics
16. manufacturing/chemicals
17. plastics industry
18. refinery
19. pharmaceuticals
20. dry cleaning
21. metal smelting
22. foundry, iron/steel
23. shipyards
24. construction
25. painting trades
26. mining/milling ores
27. pulp/paper industry
28. printing industry
29. textile industry
99. other

SELECTED EXPOSURES
01. none of below
02. don't know
03. unk. smoke/fume vapor
04. unk. dust
05. unk. eye/nose irritants
06. acids/alkali
07. asbestos
08. talc
09. insulation work
10. brake repair
11. dry wall taping
12. maintenance work
13. silica
14. sand blasting
15. rock crushing/drilling
16. coal
17. powerhouse work
18. lead
19. mercury
20. beryllium
21. cadmium
22. grinding/drilling metal
23. arsenic
24. pesticides/herbicides
25. chemical handling
26. solvents/degreasers
27. benzene
28. CCL₄, TCE, PCE, Chloroform
29. ionizing radiation
30. noise/protection required
31. vibrating equipment
32. welding

KEY

employment category   occupation code

38   39 40

year began employment
41 42

43   44 45

46 47

48   49 50

51 52

53   54 55

56 57

58   59 60

61 62

63   64 65

66 67

68   69 70

71 72

73   74 75

76 77

OB
1 2 3 4 5 6

7   8 9

10 11

12   13 14

15 16

for qualitative and quantitative estimates of toxic exposures.

REFERENCES

Cornell University Chemical Pesticides Program (1990) *Pesticide Applicator Training Manual.* Ithaca, NY: Cornell University Press.

Johnson, BL (ed) (1987) *Prevention of Neurotoxic Illness in Working Populations.* New York: John Wiley & Sons.

US Department of Labor (1986) *Dictionary of Occupational Titles.* Washington, DC: Department of Labor.

US Department of Labor, Bureau of Labor Statistics (annual) *Occupational Outlook Handbook.* Washington, DC: Department of Labor.

SUGGESTED READINGS

Baumgarten, M, Siemiatycki, J, and Gibbs, GW (1983) Validity of work histories obtained by interview for epidemiologic purposes. *Am J Epidemiol* 118(4):583–591.

Brune, DK and Edling, C (1989) *Occupational Hazards in the Health Professions.* Boca Raton, FL: CRC Press.

Committee for the Working Conference on Principles and Protocols for Evaluating Chemicals in the Environment (1975) *Principles for Evaluating Chemicals in the Environment.* Washington, DC: National Academy of Sciences.

Cralley, LJ and Cralley, LV (ed) (1985) *Patty's Industrial Hygiene and Toxicology,* Vol III, *Theory and Rationale of Industrial Hygiene Practice,* 2nd ed, 3A, *The Work Environment.* New York: John Wiley & Sons.

Felton, JS (1980) The occupational history: A neglected area in the clinical history. *J Fam Pract* 11(1):33–39.

Fryklund, VC (1970) *Occupational Analysis: Techniques and Procedures.* New York: Bruce.

Goldman, RH and Peters, JM (1981) The occupational and environmental health history. *JAMA* 246(24):2831–2836.

Gottfreson, GD and Holland, JL (1989) *Dictionary of Holland Occupational Codes,* 2nd ed. Odessa, FL: Psychological Assessment Resources.

Held, BJ and Kotowski, MJ (1985) Personal protective equipment. In *Patty's Industrial Hygiene and Toxicology,* Vol III, *Theory and Rational for Industrial Hygiene Practice,* 2nd ed, 3A, *The Work Environment,* LJ Cralley and LV Cralley (eds) pp. 655–715. New York: John Wiley & Sons.

Holden, M and Sletten, I (1970) The patient as an information source. *Clin Toxicol* 3(2):195–203.

Hunt, VR (1979) *Work and the Health of Women.* Boca Raton, FL: CRC Press.

International Labor Office (1968) *International Classification of Occupations.* Washington, DC: ILO.

Kurlychek, RT (1987) Neuropsychological evaluation of workers exposed to industrial neurotoxins. *Am J Forens Psychol* 5(4):55–66.

Kusnetz, S and Huchison, M (1979) *A Guide to Work-Relatedness of Disease* (rev ed). Rockville, MD: US Dept Health, Educ & Welfare, PHS, Center for Disease Control, NIOSH 79-116.

Luckens, MM (1967) The occupational hygiene survey: Principles, practice, significance. *Am Ind Hyg Assoc J* 28:179–183.

Lynch, JR (1985) Measurement of worker exposure. In *Patty's Industrial Hygiene and Toxicology,* Vol III, *Theory and Rational for Industrial Hygiene Practice,* 2nd ed, 3A, *The Work Environment,* LJ Cralley and LV Cralley (eds) pp. 569–615. New York: John Wiley & Sons.

Polakoff, PL (1984) The occupational history: How to close the information gap. *Occup Health Safety* November 53(9):34–35.

Proctor, NH, Hughes, JP, and Fischman, ML (1989) *Chemical Hazards of the Workplace,* 2nd ed. Philadelphia: JB Lippincott (distributed by Van Nostrand Reinhold).

Rosenstock, L, Logerfo, J, Heyer, NJ, et al. (1984) Development and validation of a self-administered occupational health history questionnaire. *J Occup Med* 26(1):50–54.

Stewart, WF, Tonascia, JA, and Matanoski, GM (1987) The validity of questionnaire-reported work history in live respondents. *J Occup Med* 29:795–800.

Ulfvarson, U (1983) Limitations to the use of employee exposure data on air contaminants in epidemiologic studies. *Int Arch Occup Environ Health* 52:285–300.

US Department of Health, Education and Welfare, Public Health Service, Center for Disease Control, National Institute for Occupational Safety and Health (1973) *The Industrial Environment: Its Evaluation and Control.* Washington, DC: US Government Printing Office.

Walker, AM and Blettner, M (1985) Comparing imperfect measures of exposure. *Am J Epidemiol* 121(6):783–790.

Part IV

Methods of Data Analysis

12

The Epidemiological Study of Neurotoxic Diseases

The large majority of human studies in which a neurotoxic dose has been linked to levels of neuropsychological functioning has been performed in the context of epidemiological surveys and with the aid of statistical thinking. That is the reason for the emphasis on these methods in this section. Experimental human studies on the effects of neurotoxic agents on behavior and psychological function are possible, but this approach has practically been abandoned, at least in the United States, because of the important ethical questions they pose.

EPIDEMIOLOGY DEFINED

There exist no flawless methods for the study of people in their daily lives. What substitutes for decisive, aristocratic perfection in research design is a more-or-less crude rule of the majority. The data accumulate; from report to report the numbers are never quite the same; there's almost always something that doesn't quite fit. But the trend emerges. It's as though you had a dozen compasses, no two of which pointed in quite the same direction. You would still be willing to hazard a guess which way was north.
William Ira Bennett, *The New York Times,* January 10, 1988.

According to Last (1983), *epidemiology* is "the study of the distribution and determinants of health-related states and events in populations, and the application of this study to control the health problems." This chapter is devoted to the review of the application of epidemiological methods to the study of neurotoxic illness in a large number of people.

THE WIDENING PERSPECTIVES OF ENVIRONMENTAL AND OCCUPATIONAL EPIDEMIOLOGY

Epidemiology is experiencing a growth spurt. Traditionally focused in the study of infectious agents, the scope and the areas of study of this discipline have now expanded to cover a large variety of environmental and occupational health problems. Interestingly, this growth is possible thanks to the methods borrowed from many other disciplines including statistics, computer sciences, toxicology, psychology, neurology, and pediatrics, to name a few.

The following is an example of the use of epidemiological methods for the study of toxic agents in the environment and the workplace.

The Accidental PBB Contamination in Michigan

Sadly, the toxic properties of chemical compounds are sometimes studied *after* their accidental release into the environment, producing their catastrophic effects. A good example is the release of polybrominated biphenyls (PBBs) in Michigan in 1973.

Polybrominated biphenyls are chemical mixtures, usually four to eight bromines per molecule, which are used as fire retardants in thermoplastic resins. One such mixture, Firemaster FF-1™, mainly hexobromobiphenyl, caused widespread contamination of livestock including dairy and beef cattle, poultry, and eggs after an accidental introduction into the animals' feed in Michigan during 1973 (Jackson and Halbert 1974; Kay 1977).

At the time the accident was detected, the toxic properties of PBBs were recorded in logs in private laboratories, and no guidelines existed for allowable limits of PBBs in food for human consumption. Under intervention of federal and state agencies, more than 500 farms were found to have cattle and/or milk over a quickly established "action limit." Over 23,000 dairy cattle and 1.6 million chickens died or were destroyed. Before the cause and dimensions of the tragedy were fully appreciated, contamination of milk, beef, pork, eggs, and poultry had already occurred, and ingestion of these foodstuffs resulted in PBB absorption by those who ate the products. Farm families used to eating their own produce were the first and most heavily exposed. In the interval of more than 9 months between the accident and the identification of its cause, the beginning of statewide testing, and the establishment of quarantines, contaminated commercial products had entered the food chain.

By April 1976, the Michigan Department of Agriculture had characterized the extent of PBB contamination in 1039 farms. Considerable information was available, including farm owners' names and addresses, dates and types of sampling, serial test results, size of herd, data and length of quarantines, and the number of contaminated animals dead or destroyed. Utilizing these lists, a medical field study was carried out by the Environmental Sciences Laboratory of Mount Sinai Medical School under the direction of Dr. Irving J. Selikoff.

On the basis of this information, four subgroups were identified: group 1, families randomly chosen from the Michigan Department of Agriculture's list of tested farms; group 2, consumers of products purchased directly from participating farms; group 3, self-selected Michigan families; and group 4, Wisconsin dairy farmers not exposed to PBBs. More detailed information of these groups is found in Anderson et al. (1979).

A total of 1221 adults and children from Michigan and 228 from Wisconsin—the control group—participated in the medical field survey. The major findings were that: 96% of the Michigan population had detectable levels of PBB in their blood serum; significant differences in subjective symptoms and objective medical findings were observed between the PBB-exposed population and the Wisconsin control group; there was no observable dose–response relationship between PBB levels and subjective and objective medical findings; and symptoms were correlated with biochemical abnormalities.

The Mount Sinai Medical School team (Anderson et al. 1979) also conducted the first neurobehavioral study of a subset of the PBB-intoxicated group from Michigan and of the controls from Wisconsin. The prevalence and incidence of neurological symptoms were analyzed in 626 adults from Michigan and 153 from Wisconsin. The subsample, examined by means of performance tests, consisted of 95 males and 67 females from Michigan and 50 males and 43 females from Wisconsin.

Neurological symptoms, particularly depression, were the earliest and most prominent symptoms in Michigan residents exposed to PBB. The possible role of stress in the determination of depression was never underestimated, but stress could not have been the sole causative agent. For example, consumer groups—who had undergone no economic loss and were not involved in legal actions, and who were not aware of the extent of their exposure at the time of examination—exhibited similar patterns to that of exposed farmers.

Among Michigan residents, particularly males, those with the most marked symptoms tended to show diminished performance as assessed by means of neurobehavioral tests. There were no dose–response relationships between neurological signs and symptoms and results of performance testing and PBB levels. Low indices of performance were also significantly correlated with intake of home produce foodstuffs, particularly during the years 1972 to 1974, and store-bought products during the years 1975 to 1976. Further details of this study are found in Valciukas et al. (1979).

Epidemiological Studies of Neurotoxic Agents in the Workplace

The toxic properties of many chemical compounds are sometimes first observed as workers become ill as the result of occupational exposure. Landrigan (1985) recognized an orderly progression between the detection of a sudden occupational health problem and its ultimate link to a neurotoxic agent. The neurotoxic properties of three agents—DMAPN, chlordecone, and BHMH—have been painstakingly documented in this manner.

Briefly, DMAPN (dimethylaminopropionitrile) is used as a catalyst in the production of polyurethane. Its absorption is associated with bladder neuropathy (Kreiss et al. 1980). Chlordecone is a pesticide; occupational exposure during its manufacture causes tremors, ataxia, memory disturbances, and weight loss (Cannon et al. 1978). BHMH (2-t-butylazo-2-hydroxy-5-methylhexane) is a foaming agent

that causes sensorimotor peripheral neuropathy, slowed nerve conduction velocities, visual disturbances including blurring vision and diminished night and color vision, diminished peripheral vision, ataxia, bladder and bowel dysfunction, and loss of recent memory and learning ability.

The first step in conducting an epidemiological study is usually the clinical description of the manifestations of a syndrome, leading to the development of plausible causal hypotheses about their etiology. These hypotheses are often developed after a careful analysis of the workers' occupational histories. Often, before workers look for help, they already know the causal link between exposures and symptoms. These isolated albeit significant cases that alert us to the presence of a wider health problem have been termed "sentinel health events," a single event indicative of a larger problem.

The second step is the epidemiological assessment of the syndrome through the description of the pattern of occurrence of cases. A common time of onset, a similar time course of evolution of signs and symptoms, or a peculiar geographic distribution in a plant may indicate a link between a recently introduced neurotoxic exposure in one part of the plant and a recently observed neurological or neuropsychological syndrome.

The third step is the confirmatory proof, that is, the toxicological corroboration that the chemical agent(s) in question can produce a neuropsychological syndrome in experimental animals similar to that observed in humans. One proof of causality is the demonstration of an anatomic or biochemical mechanism that explains the illnesses.

The Epidemiology of Accidents

Epidemiological studies sometimes cannot be planned—for example, in epidemiological studies of environmental disasters or occupational accidents. Epidemiologists learn as much from environmental disasters and occupational accidents as from studies whose planning and execution may take several years. It takes an educated mind to understand an accident: epidemiologists strive for organized thought even in the midst of chaos.

Human neurotoxicology has achieved the prominence that it has on the basis of the study of human accidents. Accidents do not occur in an orderly manner. Accidents put a large number of individuals at risk in almost any conceivable circumstance. For example, we would not think of studying farmers for exposure to fire retardants. However, in the accident that occurred in the state of Michigan in 1973 (reviewed above), farmers were accidentally exposed to PBBs—a fire retardant—in the food chain. A serious student of the epidemiology of neurotoxic agents is conversant with all the details of planned and organized research as well as the almost unteachable skills required to deal with the realities of unpredictable accidents.

Schoenberg coined the term neuroepidemiology *to describe a discipline that estimates the burden of neurological diseases in the population, the accurate pictures of their natural history, the evaluation of the effectiveness of health programs aimed at their prevention and treatment, and ways of planning for the needs of the individuals affected. The two most important considerations for the neuroepidemiologist are representativeness of the population studied and accuracy of the diagnosis.*

The field of neuroepidemiology has been proposed to compensate for the fact that epidemiological investigations of neurological diseases have lagged behind epidemiological studies of other disorders such as heart disease or cancer. However, as described by Schoenberg (1978), the program of neuroepidemiology is really a subdivision of general epidemiology. In addition, it is not certain that the already excessive fragmentation and superspecialization of knowledge will, in the end, have beneficial effects on the health sciences and society.

Pharmacoepidemiology *is the epidemiological study of drugs. According to Ray and Griffin (1989), "current methods used in pharmacoepidemiology include spontaneous reporting systems,* correlational studies of associations between secular trends of morbid events and medication use, special-purpose prospective follow-up studies of newly marketed drugs, prescription event monitoring, systematic and ad hoc case-control studies of events that are possibly drug related, prospective cohort studies of specific drugs such as oral contraceptives, and systems of automatic medical records for defined populations, including health maintenance organizations, and Medicaid programs."*

RESEARCH PLANS AND STUDY DESIGNS

All research, regardless of whether observational or experimental, requires a plan. In a research plan, sometimes called *research protocol*, the objective of the research is stated, the subjects to be studied are identified, and the techniques to be employed are described. In addition, the research protocol includes a description of how techniques are to be used, how data will be collected, how the analysis of data will be performed, and what conclusions are expected to be drawn. Sometimes the significance of the proposed research for science and society is expected to be stated. Increasingly, ethical aspects of record keeping and informed consent are part of the research plan.

The fundamental difference between epidemiological studies in humans and toxicological experiments in animals is the degree of control of the independent variable. For example, epidemiologists observe whether pesticides found in the water of a local river—the independent variable—affect the health of the inhabitants who consume fish from the contaminated water. Toxicologists administer pesticides to laboratory animals in food to study changes in motor behavior.

Because of ethical considerations, human research is very limited and is confined to clinical trials and the study of acute effects of neurotoxic agents under laboratory conditions. Epidemiological investigations are thus, in most cases, observational, and the independent variables are almost never under the control of the investigator. It is best to refer to the plan of epidemiological studies as "study design." The term "experimental design" refers to a situation in which the independent variables are under experimental control, such as those found in toxicological experiments.

Epidemiological studies, including medical field surveys, are more apt to be called quasi-experiments. The "treatment effects" are studied as they exist, that is, as a result of environmental and/or occupational exposure to toxic agents. Subjects cannot be randomly assigned to different treatment groups: the selection of "high," "intermediate," and "low" exposures is made a posteriori. The effects of confounding variables (such as age, ethnic background, education, socioeconomic status, language, etc.) are adequately controlled for or treated with appropriate statistical procedures.

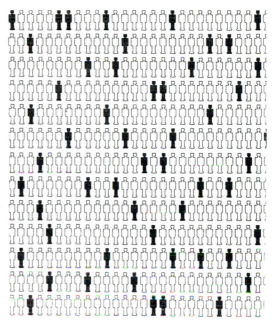

Fig. 12.1. Pictorial representation of the prevalence of a condition in the general population. The shaded figures represent affected individuals; the nonshaded figures represent unaffected individuals.

THE THREE TYPES OF STUDY DESIGN

The most common types of study design encountered in published reports in E & O neurotoxicology are cross-sectional, case–control, and, most recently, cohort studies.

Cross-Sectional Studies

A *cross-sectional study* is the examination of a group of people at one point in time in order to ascertain the relationship between disease—the "dependent" variable—and the neurotoxic exposure—eg, solvent use. A cross-sectional study is also called a morbidity survey, disease frequency survey, or prevalence study. The relationship between dependent and independent variables is investigated in terms of the prevalence of neurological signs or symptoms, presence of neuropsychological dysfunctions as determined by means of psychometric or electrophysiological procedures, biochemical abnormalities, etc at dif-

ferent levels of the independent variable. A cross-sectional study is sometimes the "case" study of a case–control design. Finally, a cross-sectional study can be the base-line study (year 1) of a prospective study lasting several years. Figure 12.1 is a visual representation of the notion of prevalence of a condition in the general population.

According to Last (1983), a field survey is "the planned collection of data in 'the field'— ie, usually among noninstitutionalized persons in the general population." It is also "a method of establishing a relationship between two or more variables in a population in numerical terms by eliciting and collating information from existing sources." Medical health surveys occupy a unique niche in the science and art of study design. They are called quasi-experiments because the treatment effects, such as the amount of solvent absorption by a worker, are not under the control of the experimenter.

Medical field surveys are often carried out to meet urgent needs such as in the case of an epidemic or occupational accident of catastrophic consequences. As a result, they fulfill an important need in occupational health as long as their biases in subject selection are recognized. "Bias" is intimately related to "fallacy," an error in judgment resulting from illogical reasoning or incomplete understanding of factors that need to be considered during the course of a scientific investigation.

Case–Control Studies

According to Last (1983), a *case–control study* is one that "starts with the identification of persons with the disease (or other outcome variable) of interest, and a suitable control population (comparison, reference) group of persons without the disease. The relationship of an attribute to the disease is examined by comparing the diseased and nondiseased with regard to how frequently the attribute is present or the levels of the attribute in each of the groups" (Fig. 12.2). This study design is also known under other names, such as case–comparison or case–referent.

The assessment of neurological and behavioral changes as a result of exposure to neurotoxic agents can be made by contrasting the symptoms or results of psychological and neurophysiological tests of either one individual and a reference group, or one group known to be exposed to a neurotoxic agent and another group not so exposed. Comparing the performance of an individual with the performance of controls is the essence of individual neuropsychological or neurophysiological evaluation. For example, one can measure the performance or neurophysiological function of an individual exposed to lead, and then this can be compared to the mean values found in a non-lead-exposed but otherwise similar group. We can ask, for example, whether the performance test results of a 23-year-old caucasian woman with 2 years of college education exposed to solvents as a laboratory technician and living in a small town are different from those of a reference group. That reference group will be

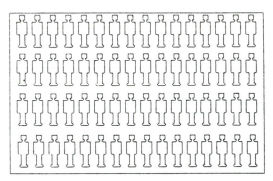

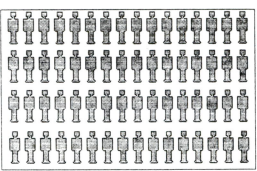

Fig. 12.2. The case–control design, in which a group of affected individuals (the cases) are compared with a group of unaffected individuals (the controls).

a group of women of approximately the same age, perhaps within a maximum of a 3-year range above or below the actual age, with similar education, with a similar socioeconomic status, and living in a small town.

However, this method is not restricted to clinical settings. Discriminant analysis (explained in Chapter 19) is a statistical technique that can be used to assess the probability that a single individual belongs to a control group. Thus, discriminant analysis can be used as a "diagnostic" tool as well.

In epidemiological research, the most common case is the second example: the comparison between a group exposed to neurotoxic agents and another group not so exposed. This type of research model is relatively easy to grasp but in practice is very difficult to carry out successfully. It is difficult to compare study groups to reference groups because of the problem of matching for confounding variables. The most important confounding variables are gender, ethnic background, age, education, income, and socioeconomic status, an abstract variable arrived at by multiplying years of schooling and income.

In general, each one of these demographic variables has an effect on performance. They contribute a positive or negative load to the total measurable characteristics of performance and sometimes neurological signs and symptoms and even results of neurophysiological tests. For example, skin temperature is a confounding variable in determinations of nerve conduction velocity but of little consequence (except in extreme values of body temperature range) for assessment of behavior. The level of education and native language are definite factors in the evaluation of language-dependent intellectual functions but irrelevant for the evaluation of visually evoked potentials. It is not possible to summarize here the wealth of knowledge that has accumulated as a result of experimental work regarding the effects of these variables.

The definition of a reference group is one that shares levels of confounding (demographic) variables with the study group but is different in that the control or reference group is not exposed to neurotoxic agents. In all other possible variables such as age, gender, ethnic background, etc, an effort to "match" the control with the study group is made. It is extremely difficult, however, to identify a reference group with absolutely no exposure to any neurotoxic agent. Considerable effort has to be directed toward extracting information about possible neurotoxic effects by holding other confounding effects constant.

Experts in the field of neurotoxicology have yet to agree on what the "ideal" control group is. Are a group of poeple absolutely not exposed to any neurotoxic agent a "real" group? Among a blue-collar population, are we to dismiss anyone who drinks alcoholic beverages? If we set an upper limit on ingestion or intake as a rejection criterion, are we not eliminating subjects who might have become alcoholics as a result of the realization of intellectual decline—a consequence, perhaps,

of chronic exposure to neurotoxic agents? If we find such an ideal group, are we not bound to find the greatest number of abnormalities in nervous system function? Is it not the case that the "ideal" group is a sociological curiosity rather than a pragmatic anchor point to establish research work on a firm footing?

Prospective Studies

In the *prospective study,* also called a *cohort study,* or a follow-up study, a group of people—a cohort—is studied over long periods of time at fixed intervals (Fig. 12.3). The cohort is its own control; ie, each specific subject is his or her own control.

Prospective studies are analyzed by making statistical assumptions different from those made for cross-sectional studies. With everything else held constant—something that is difficult if not impossible in epidemiological research—the variation in observed behavior, the number and kinds of neurological symptoms, the results of psychological and/or neurophysiological tests between two individuals is called the "between-subjects variation." This variation should be contrasted with that observed in the same individual examined on two separate occasions, "the within-subject variation."

Prospective studies are invaluable in reconstructing the time course of development of a disease. Such reconstructions can be made from cross-sectional studies, but in this case an intuitive process is used, and serious biases are present. Aging effects, for example, stud-

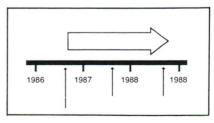

Fig. 12.3. The prospective (or cohort) study design. In this example, the first cross-sectional study (thin arrow) is conducted in the summer of 1987; the cohort is then studied again at the end of each summer following (broad arrow).

ied prospectively often lead to different conclusions when studied cross-sectionally. Aging effects determined prospectively are less pronounced than those ascertained by cross-sectional studies.

Prospective studies are valuable because they yield data in which the "within-subject variation" is low. As a result, the likelihood of detecting a neurotoxic effect when one is present is maximized. Identical twins are subjects for whom the "between-subject variation" almost approaches the "within-subject variation." Identical twins reared apart have been extensively studied in an attempt to extract the genetic from the environmental components of behavior. A less-than-ideal (but more practical) procedure is to reduce the "between-subject variation" by one-to-one matching.

Prospective Studies on the Effects of Lead on Child Development. Epidemiological methods have been utilized to investigate the effects of lead on the growth and psychological development of children. As of 1985, several prospective studies have been completed in various cities: Boston (Bellinger et al. 1985), Cincinnati (Bornschein et al. 1985), Cleveland (Ernhart et al. 1985), Glasgow, Scotland (Moore et al. 1985), Nordenham, Germany (Winneke et al. 1985), Chapel Hill, North Carolina (Otto et al. 1985), and Port Pirie, Australia (Vimpani et al. 1985). All these studies are reviewed in detail in Chapter 20, dealing with the effects of toxic agents on the developing brain.

All of these studies share the common characteristics of being follow-up studies. It is now well recognized that cross-sectional studies are of limited value for the study of effects of neurotoxic agents on child development. In cross-sectional studies, physical growth and psychological development are inferred from the one-time examination of children of different ages. Follow-up studies are designed to study the effects of neurotoxic agents by examining the same child over long periods of time.

The Second International Conference on Prospective Studies of Lead (which last met in Cincinnati in April, 1984) was a forum where methodological issues, study protocols, confounding factors, assessment techniques, and the results of several world surveys were discussed (Bornschein and Rabinowitz 1985).

MIXED STUDY DESIGNS

Retrospective Studies as an Example of Mixed Study Design

Health investigators sometimes use two or more research strategies. The following illustrate how a retrospective study can be conducted during the course of a cross-sectional study or a case–control study.

According to Last (1983), a *retrospective study* is "a research design which is used to test etiological hypotheses in which inferences about exposure to the putative causal factor(s) are derived from data relating to characteristics of the persons under study or to events or experiences in their past." Retrospective studies are based on a simple premise: among those who at the present time are suffering from a similar condition such as peripheral neuropathy, common factors in the past associated with the present condition can sometimes be ascertained. For example, among those who suffer from brain tumors in a certain trade, is it possible to link these tumors to specific exposures at the workplace at a time prior to the appearance of the tumor?

The information derived from retrospective studies is unique and can rarely be gathered by the use of any other experimental design. In most experimental designs, we have access to the independent, dependent, and confounding variables. In retrospective studies, the dependent variable (or the outcome variable) is under experimental control: the effects of independent and confounding variables back in time have to be inferred. A

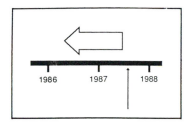

Fig. 12.4. Relationship between a cross-sectional and a retrospective epidemiological study. In this example, a cross-sectional study (thin arrow) examines the summer of 1987 exclusively, whereas a retrospective study (broad arrow) examines events that happened over the course of the entire year between the summmer of 1986 and the summer of 1987.

widely recognized weakness of retrospective studies is that they must rely on historical information, ill-documented facts, and often unreliable memories of past events.

A retrospective study can be conducted as a result of a cross-sectional study. (Figure 12.4 is a diagram that illustrates the relationship between a cross-sectional and a retrospective study.) In a retrospective study, "the essential feature is that some of the persons under study have the disease or other outcome conditions of interest, and their characteristics and past experiences are compared with those of other, unaffected persons" (Last 1983). Thus, retrospective studies can also be conducted as a result of a case–control study.

Convergence of Study Designs in Testing Hypotheses of Environmental Causation

In 1987, a report in *Science* by Peter S. Spencer and collaborators presented evidence for the notion that certain neurological diseases—such as Parkinson's, Alzheimer's, and motoneuron diseases—may be caused by environmental toxins. This study is reviewed here in order to provide an important convergence between epidemiological and neuropathological methods in testing hypotheses about causation of neurotoxic illness. They write:

Amyotrophic lateral sclerosis (ALS) is a progressive, fatal disorder of adults stemming from degeneration of the anterior horns of the spinal cord, certain motor nuclei of the brain stem, and neurons in the motor cortex. Elucidation of the etiology of ALS has been sought for over 35 years through intensive longitudinal studies of indigenous (Chamorro) populations of the Marianas islands of Guam and Rota, where there is a high prevalence of this disease, as well as a parkinsonism–dementia (PD) clinical variant thereof. In the 1950s, ALS prevalence ratios and death rates of Chamorro residents of Guam or Rota were 50 to 100 times the estimates for the continental United States and other developed countries. The decline of ALS after 1955 on Guam and the absence of demonstrable inherited or viral factors in this disease led to the search for environmental agents that might have been decreasing as the Chamorro population has become more Americanized.

An early suggestion incriminated the highly toxic seed of the false sago palm (*Cycas circinalis* L.), which was used in food and traditional medicine until the acculturation of these people after World War II to the contemporary practices of the continental United States, resulting in the decline of cycad use. Descriptions of a degenerative locomotor disease in animals grazing on cycad species fueled interest in the possible etiological role of this plant in Guam ALS–PD.

Laboratory investigation of the *C. circinalis* revealed the presence of various glycosides, including cycasin, and an "unusual" nonprotein amino acid, α-amino-β-methyl-aminoproprionic acid (synonym, β-*N*-methylamino-L-alanine or L-BMAA), an agent that possessed certain neurotoxic properties but failed to induce an experimental disorder akin to ALS–PD. Cycad research in relation to Guam ALS–PD was then abandoned as animal models failed to show the main components of the syndrome.

In 1987, Spencer and his collaborators reported a study in which repeated doses of the amino acid BMAA led to the development in monkeys of corticomotoneural dysfunction, parkinsonian features, and behavioral anomalies with degenerative changes of motor neurons in the cerebral cortex and spinal cord. Thus, the monkeys displayed many of the symptoms characteristic of the neurological syndrome of the Chamorro people of Guam.

This investigation not only lent support to the hypothesis that cycad exposure plays an important role in the etiology of Guam disease but was of broader significance in that it suggested that certain motor diseases, such as Huntington's chorea, Parkinson's disease, and olivopontocerebellar atrophy and Alzheimer's disease might also be related to exposure to environmental neurotoxic agents.

SOURCES OF BIAS IN MEDICAL FIELD SURVEYS

Bias is a systematic error. This error can result from the study design, the sampling method, the characteristics of the instruments that are used to gather the data, the manner in which these instruments are used, the individual who uses them, and the subject under observation. Like many other types of surveys, medical surveys are also subject to bias.

Bias can occur during selection (sampling) of the subjects. A *sampling bias* can occur when certain characteristics of one group are either an overestimate or an underestimate of the true value of that characteristic in the general population. For example, the fraction of people over 65 years of age may be underestimated because of the difficulty of getting in touch with this age group, particularly if individuals live alone.

Sampling bias can be compounded by the impossibility of estimating the proportion of people of a certain demographic profile in a given geographical area. For example, the proportion of Hispanics in New York City is difficult to estimate; investigators also disagree how a "Hispanic" is defined.

Sampling bias occurs during the design of an epidemiological study. The proportion of Hispanics selected to be contacted for a survey questionnaire, for example, is expected to match the proportion of Hispanic people estimated for a given geographical area. Before the execution of the study, the investigator(s) need to test whether this is true by means of appropriate statistical procedures. (In Chapter 18, a reference is made to these procedures.)

Participation bias may occur during the execution of the study. The investigator(s) may have sampled the estimated proportion of Hispanic people in the target geographical area, but the actual proportion of Hispanics that come to the testing site or return a mail questionnaire, for example, is less than the expected proportion.

Certain questionnaires have an inherent *response bias,* which is a reflection of the subjects' consistent mode of behavior (his or her personality). For example, in a questionnaire in which attitudes toward the environment are rated, some individuals may rate all items with minimal scores, whereas other individuals may rate all items with maximal scores. There are statistical procedures to correct for response bias before the data are analyzed.

Some of people's biases are well known. The interviewer may impose his/her own bias in the observation of human behavior (*interviewer* or *observer bias*). Among 10 interviewers participating in a medical field survey, for example, interviewer 5 may be bossy and push people around. When data are subsequently analyzed by interviewer code, the psychometric test scores may be found to be lower than the means of all other interviewers combined. (This interviewer's examinees left the testing site as quickly as they could, not really trying to perform well in the test.) The investigator in charge of the entire medical survey or important segments of it may have his/her own bias in postulating hypotheses, analyzing and interpreting the data obtained during the medical field surveys, reporting the findings to the public, or in hoping to prove a personal, political, theoretical, or philosophical point. Conflicting findings may not be examined in detail or may not be reported.

In medical field surveys some of the biases are insidious. For example, a person whose health is affected may be afraid to participate because of fear of losing his or her job. Often, the investigator cannot influence the decision process as to whether or not a particular individual will agree to participate in a medical field survey. The selected individual—particularly if affected by a neurotoxic agent altering cognition—may be too sick to read or understand the meaning of the letter of invitation. The investigator may then be studying the potentially least important subjects. (This bias is called "survivorship bias.") Finally, a person who is chronically ill may use a medical field survey for a free medical examination.

A discussion of whether bias has been recognized and controlled often arises when the results of surveys are discussed in a legal context. The detailed discussion of these biases is beyond the scope of this chapter. (Parenthetically, some claim that the noun "bias" has no plural; however, "biases" is widely used in the epidemiological literature.) Many textbooks of epidemiology, such as those listed under Suggested Readings, contain both an intuitive description and, sometimes, a mathematical treatment on how these biases can influence the interpretation of findings.

SAMPLING

Epidemiological surveys were originally unreliable because of a lack of understanding of the statistical properties of sampling and the biases introduced by the diverse methods of data collection. In the past 40 years, theoretical research performed on the statistical properties of samples has resulted in a marked improvement in the accuracy of predictions made on the basis of sampling. Current state-of-the-art polling techniques claim to accurately reflect the attributes of the U.S. population, within a 3% to 5% margin of error.

Sampling is related to the logic of scientific investigation. Theorists of science recognize that there are two fundamental modes of seeking new knowledge: by means of inductive and deductive inference. Sampling is part of the inductive process that proceeds from the specific to the general. Toxicology is essentially an empirical and inductive science; our truths derive from the observation of facts, from which we establish universal truths. But science can also be deductive—as in mathematics—proceeding from the general to the specific: an explanatory theory is provided first and is followed by predictions on the basis of that theory. Scientists deduce as part of their daily thinking, not from a general theory but from pockets of well-organized knowledge. (Little theoretical work has been performed in toxicology, which mainly uses an inductive approach.)

Toxicology is a discipline that aims at both universal and individual truths. An example of a universal truth is that lead—in a certain chemical form, in certain amounts, and when incorporated into the human body—is a powerful neurotoxic agent. The individual truth is that different people anywhere in the world exposed to lead, such as lead miners, secondary lead smelters, auto body shop workers, cable splicers, cable manufacturers, police who shoot arms indoors, or babies who eat lead-containing paint chips, are all at risk of a serious toxic illness.

In environmental and occupational health sciences, the *universe* is all people who have a common trait—eg, all lead workers—or meet a criterion—eg, all babies born from mothers who were exposed to mercury. ("Universe" is applied to nonhuman entities as well, such as the "universe of all chemical compounds.") The universe cannot be studied directly because it is so large; thus, the universe is only a mental construct. The sample can be studied properly, as it is only a portion of the universe—eg, all lead miners in Middletown. A representative sample is one that has been obtained in such a manner that what is true for the sample is probably true for the universe. There are several types of samples.

A *grab sample* is the way "people-on-the-streets" surveys are carried out. They are also called samples of convenience. Most of the laboratory studies carried out with volunteers—college students or laboratory personnel—are grab samples. Findings obtained through the use of grab samples cannot be generalized to the universe because of the bias imposed in the selection of the individuals. Modifications of grab samples are sometimes useful. In real estate, for example, one of the criteria taken to value a property is the demographic profile of the people who pass in front of that property or enter or exit the facilities.

In a *cluster sample,* the selected unit is a group of individuals—eg, all members of a given local union of a given city or all persons in a given city block. Most community-based toxicological studies are based on cluster samples.

A *probability sample* is a sample in which all the individuals have the same known chance of being included in the sample. For example, if the universe consists of 10,000 individuals, a probability sample of 1000 can be obtained by listing all the names by last name and then picking up every 10th name.

If a list of 10,000 union members contains few blacks, and in the sample of 1000, 35 blacks are found, any generalization about blacks would be subject to a large error. More sampling needs to be performed among blacks. *Stratified sampling* involves dividing the universe into distinct subgroups—in this example, by race—and selecting a random sample for each group.

Sampling Errors

A survey contains several elements acting as internal quality control checking. One of them is an estimate of the magnitude of possible bias. An important phase in survey design is the estimation of sampling errors. The error in sampling is the difference between the "true" value of a measure in the universe (eg, the reaction time in milliseconds of all shipyard painters in the United States) and the empirical value obtained in a sample of shipyard painters.

For the sake of argument, let's assume that the universe of painters is 5000 and that a list of 170 names is a representative sample of that universe. When those individuals are approached, 135 individuals agree to have their reaction times measured, while 35 are nonrespondents. The proportion of respondents is 0.79 (135 over 170); the proportion of nonrespondents is 0.21 (35 over 170). The *sampling error* is proportional to the number of nonrespondents and to the difference between the empirical value and the true value in the universe.

The difference between the true value and the empirical value is always an estimate. Since nonrespondents create a bias that may affect inferences about the generality of findings, it is important to report both the levels of nonresponse and, whenever possible, the demographic profile of the nonresponse group. Different profiles among respondents and nonrespondents may create a bias.

There are important practical considerations in the sampling occurring in medical field surveys. The number of people who can be examined in a medical field survey is dictated by the medical and technical personnel, equipment, time, and space available. The maximum number of people that can be examined in such surveys usually ranges between 50 and 100 participants a day depending on the combination of these four primary factors. In some medical field surveys involving a larger number of medical/technical personnel, fewer forms, and a limited scope of medical examinations, hundreds or even thousands of individuals can be examined each day.

Sampling and Bias

Import fallacies arise because of failure to interpret the concept of sampling.

The *occupational link fallacy* occurs when the rate of illness that is characteristic of the population in general or the community in particular is interpreted as related to the jobs workers have. Figure 12.5 is an illustration

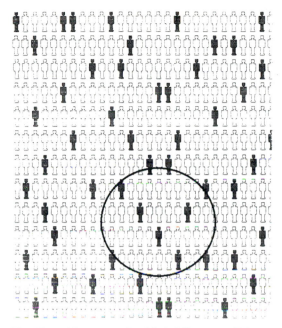

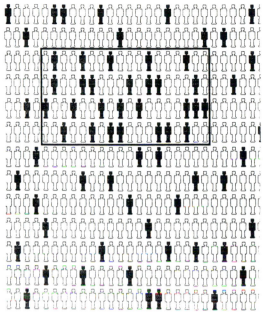

Fig. 12.5. The occupational link fallacy, in which an illness is erroneously associated with a particular occupation (individuals within circle) when in fact the illness exists throughout the population.

Fig. 12.6. Self-selection bias. When a particular profession experiences a high rate of occurrence of an illness, the condition may be related not to the profession per se, but rather to a circumstance that is common in—but not exclusive to—the profession. [Note that the prevalence of affected individuals is much higher within the given profession (boxed area), but the condition is not restricted to the profession.]

of this still common fallacy. The increasing availability of data on rates of neurological signs and symptoms and, more recently, psychometric testing performance of large segments of the population has greatly reduced the possibility of incurring this serious error in judgment.

Self-selection bias arises because there are jobs that are filled by people having common characteristics (Fig. 12.6). Two examples follow.

Should we need to design a neuropsychological study on the effects of anesthetic gases among physician anesthetists, we would have to be prepared to find that most anesthetists are very intelligent, the result of a long selection that occurred first at college, then at medical school, and then when they finally obtained the positions they hold now. Should we find that anesthetists perform better than a group of controls, we would not conclude that anesthetic gases cause an increase in intelligence.

However, neurotoxic causation and self-selection in jobs that may be filled with people of lower intelligence are sometimes more difficult to disentangle. Should we need to study cognitive effects of pesticides among lettuce pickers in the state of California, and should we find that performance is worse than in a control group, the conclusion that pesticides cause a reduction in cognitive function is not necessarily warranted.

These two examples also illustrate the serious limitations of case–control studies in the search for possible toxic causation and why dose–response relationships are necessary to establish that causation, a topic discussed in Chapter 19.

The *healthy worker effect* is seen in mortality studies, particularly at the beginning of prospective studies. Workers usually exhibit lower overall death rates than the general population because severely ill or disabled

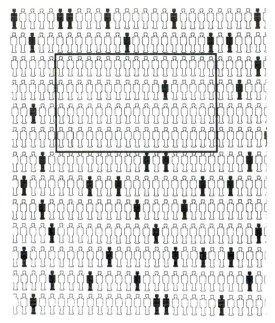

Fig. 12.7. The healthy worker effect. Workers within a given profession (boxed area) will probably be less likely than the general population to succumb to an illness, as the more vulnerable members of a community, such as the severely ill or disabled, tend not to be in the workforce.

people cannot hold certain jobs (Fig. 12.7). The healthy worker effect is also observed in morbidity studies on the effects of chemical agents on neural function. For example, should we need to study the motor performance of athletics instructors, we would probably find them healthier as a group than teachers engaged in other activities.

CONCLUSIONS

The traditional view of conducting epidemiological research was that the epidemiologist participates in the study plan and the collection of data, whereas the statistician contributes to the analytical phase of the study. This stereotype is rapidly disappearing. Epidemiology and statistics are experiencing a larger and larger degree of overlap, and both are contributing methods for human studies of E & O toxic agents.

REFERENCES

Anderson, HA, Wolff, MS, Lilis, R, et al. (1979) Symptoms and clinical abnormalities following ingestion of polybrominated-biphenyl-contaminated food products. In *The Scientific Basis for the Public Control of Environmental Health Hazards,* WJ Nicholson and JA Moore (eds) pp. 684–702. New York: The New York Academy of Sciences.

Bellinger, D, Leviton, A, Waternaux, C, et al. (1985) Methodological issues in modelling the relationship between low-level lead exposure and infant development: Examples from the Boston Lead Study. *Environ Res* 38:119–129.

Bennett, WI (1988) Letter. *The New York Times,* January 10.

Bornschein, RL, Hammond, PB, Dietrich, KN, et al. (1985) The Cincinnati prospective study of low-level exposure and its effects on child development: Protocol and status report. *Environ Res* 38:4–18.

Bornschein, RL and Rabinowitz, MB (eds) (1985) The Second International Conference on Prospective Studies of Lead. *Environ Res* 38(1):1–210.

Cannon, SB, Veazey, JM, Jackson, RS, et al. (1978) Epidemic Kepone poisoning in chemical workers. *Am J Epidemiol* 107:529.

Ernhart, CB, Wolf, AW, Sokol, RJ, et al. (1985) Fetal lead exposure: Antenatal factors. *Environ Res* 38:54–66.

Jackson, TF and Halbert, FL (1974) A toxic syndrome associated with the feeding of polybrominated biphenyls-contaminated concentrate to dairy cattle. *J Am Vet Med Assoc* 165:437–439.

Kay, K (1977) Polybrominated biphenyls (PBB), environmental contamination in Michigan 1973–1976. *Environ Res* 13:64–93.

Kreiss, K, Wegman, DH, Niles, CA, et al. (1980) Neurological dysfunction of the bladder in workers exposed to dimethylaminopropinonitrile. *JAMA* 243:741.

Landrigan, PJ (1985) The uses of epidemiology in the study of neurotoxic pollutants: Lessons from the workplace. *Int J Men Health* 14(3):44–63.

Last, JM (1983) *A Dictionary of Epidemiology.* New York: Oxford University Press.

Moore, MR, Richards, WN, and Sherlock, JG (1985) Successful abatement of lead exposure from water supplies in the west of Scotland. *Environ Res* 38:67–76.

Otto, D, Robinson, G, Baumann, S, et al. (1985) 5-year follow up study of children with low to moderate lead absorption: Electrophysiological evaluation. *Environ Res* 38:168–186.

Ray, WA and Griffin, MR (1989) Use of Medicaid data for pharmacoepidemiology. *Am J Epidemiol* 129(4):837–849.

Schoenberg, BS (ed) (1978) *Advances in Neurology,* Vol

19. New York: Raven Press [several chapters of this volume are devoted to neuroepidemiology].

Spencer, PS, Nunn, PB, Hugon, J, et al. (1987) Guam amyotrophic lateral sclerosis–parkinsonism–dementia linked to a plant excitant neurotoxin. *Science* 237:517–522.

Valciukas, JA, Lilis, R, Wolff, M, et al. (1979) The neurotoxicity of polybrominated biphenyls: Results of a clinical field study. In *The Scientific Basis for the Public Control of Environmental Health Hazards,* WJ Nicholson and JA Moore (eds) pp. 684–702. New York: The New York Academy of Sciences.

Vimpani, G, McMichael, A, Robertson, E, et al. (1985) The Port Pirie study: A prospective study of pregnancy outcome and early childhood growth and development in a lead-exposed community—protocol and status report. *Environ Res* 38:19–23.

Winneke, G, Beguinn, U, Ewert, T, et al. (1985) Comparing the effects of perinatal and later childhood lead exposure on neuropsychological outcome. *Environ Res* 38:155–167.

SUGGESTED READINGS

Anderson, R, Kasper, J, and Frankel, MR (1979) *Total Survey Error*. San Francisco: Jossey-Bass.

Baker, EL (1985) Epidemiologic issues in neurotoxicity research. *Neurobehav Toxicol Teratol* 7(4):293–297.

Bakir, F, Damluji, SF, Amin-Zaki, L, et al. (1973) Methylmercury poisoning in Iraq: An inter-university report. *Science* 181:230–241.

Bertazzi, PA (1989) Industrial disasters and epidemiology: A review of recent experiences. *Scand J Work Environ Health* 15(2):85–100.

Black, B (1990) Matching evidence about clustered health events with tort law requirements. *Am J Epidemiol* 132 Suppl No. 1:S79–S86.

Black, B and Lilienfeld, DE (1984) Epidemiologic proof in toxic tort litigation. *Fordham Law Rev* 52:732–785.

Bracken, MB (ed)(1984) *Perinatal Epidemiology*. New York: Oxford University Press.

Carter, AO, Millson, ME, and Allen, DE (1989) Epidemiologic study of deaths and injuries due to tornadoes. *Am J Epidemiol* 130(6):1209–1218.

Checkoway, H, Dement, JM, Fowler, DP, et al. (1987) Industrial hygiene involvement in occupational epidemiology. *Am Ind Hyg Assoc J* 48(6):515–523.

Checkoway, H, Pearce, N, and Dement, JM (1989) Design and conduct of occupational epidemiology: I. Design aspects of cohort studies. *Am J Ind Med* 15:363–373.

Checkoway, H, Pearce, N, and Dement, JM (1989) Design and conduct of occupational epidemiology: II. Analysis of cohort data. *Am J Ind Med* 15:375–394.

Checkoway, H, Pearce, N, and Dement, JM (1989) Design and conduct of occupational epidemiology: III. Design aspects of case-control studies. *Am J Ind Med* 15:395–402.

Cook, TD and Campbell, DT (1979) *Quasi Experimentation Design and Analysis Issues for Field Settings*. Chicago: Rand McNally College Publishing Co.

Dukes, WF (1965) $N = 1$. *Psychol Bull* 64:74–79.

Eaton, WW, Holzer, CE, Von Korff, M, et al. (1984) The design of epidemiologic catchment area surveys: The control and measurement of error. *Arch Gen Psychiatry* 41:942–947.

Edlavitch, SA (1989) *Pharmaco-epidemiology*. Boca Raton, FL: Lewis Publishers.

Feinstein, AR (1985) *Clinical Epidemiology: The Architecture of Clinical Research*. Philadelphia: Saunders.

Ferguson, D (1973) A study of neurosis and occupation. *Br J Ind Med* 30:187–198.

Forthofer, RN (1983) Investigation of non-response bias in NHANES II. *Am J Epidemiol* 117:507–514.

Fox, AJ and Collier, PF (1976) Low mortality rates in industry cohort studies due to selection for work and survival in industry. *Br J Prev Soc Med* 30:225–230.

Freeman, DX (1984) Psychiatric epidemiology counts. *Arch Gen Psychiatry* 41:931–933.

Friedman, GD (1980) *Primer of Epidemiology* (2nd ed). New York: McGraw-Hill.

Glass, RI (1986) New prospects for epidemiologic investigations. *Science* 234:951–956.

Goldsmith, JR (1975) What do we expect from an occupational cohort? *J Occup Med* 17:126–131.

Goldsmith, JR (1986) *Environmental Epidemiology: Epidemiological Investigation of Community Environmental Health Problems*. Boca Raton, FL: CRC Press.

Gordis, L (ed)(1988) *Epidemiology and Health Risk Assessment*. New York: Oxford University Press.

Gregersen P (1988) Neurotoxic effects of organic solvents in exposed workers: Two controlled follow-up studies after 5.5 and 10.6 years. *Am J Ind Med* 14:681–701.

Hallenbeck, WH and Cunningham, KM (1986) *Quantative Risk Assessment for Environmental and Occupational Health*. Chelsea, MI: Lewis.

Hersen, M and Barlow, DH (1976) *Single Case Experimental Design*. New York: Collier.

Hoffman, RE (1984) The use of epidemiologic data in the courts. *Am J Epidemiol* 120:190–202.

Howe, GR, Chiarelli, AM, and Lindsay, JP (1988) Components and modifiers of the healthy worker effect: Evidence from three occupational cohorts and implications for industrial compensation. *Am J Epidemiol* 128(6):1364–1375.

Johnson, BL (ed)(1987) *Prevention of Neurotoxic Illness in Working Populations*. New York: John Wiley & Sons.

Johnson, LD, O'Malley, PM, and Bachman, JG (1986) *Drug Use among American High School Students, College Students, and Other Young Adults*. Rockville, MD: National Institute on Drug Abuse.

Juntunen, J, Kinnunen, E, Antti–Poika, M, et al. (1989) Multiple sclerosis and occupational exposure to chemicals: A co-twin control study of a nationwide series of twins. *Brit J Ind Med* 46(6):417–419.

Kahn, HA and Sempos, CT (1989) *Statistical Methods in Epidemiology*. New York: Oxford University Press.

Karvonen, M and Mikheev, MI (eds)(1986) *Epidemiology of Occupational Health*. Copenhagen: WHO.

Kelsey, JL, Thompson, WD, and Evans, AS (1986) *Methods in Observational Epidemiology*. New York: Oxford University Press.

Kish, L (1987) *Statistical Design for Research*. New York: John Wiley & Sons.

Kleinbaum, DG, Kupper, LL, and Morgenstern, H (1982) *Epidemiologic Research: Principles and Quantitative Methods*. Belmont, CA: Lifetime Learning Publications.

Kozel, NJ and Adams, EH (1986) Epidemiology of drug abuse: An overview. *Science* 234:970–974.

Landrigan, PJ (1983) Epidemiologic approaches to persons with exposures to waste chemicals. *Environ Health Perspect* 48:93–97.

Last, JM (1986) Epidemiology and health information. In *Maxcy–Rosenau Public Health and Preventive Medicine*, JM Last (ed) pp. 9–74. Norrwalk, CT: Appleton-Century-Crofts.

Lawson, DH (1984) Pharmacoepidemiology: A new discipline. *Br Med J* 289:940–941.

Lilienfeld, AM and Lilienfeld, DE (1980) *Foundations of Epidemiology*, 2nd ed. New York: Oxford University Press.

Lilienfeld, DE and Black, B (1986) The epidemiology in court: Some comments. *Am J Epidemiol* 123(6):961–964.

McKeown-Eyssem, GE and Ruedy, J (1983) Prevalence of neurological abnormalities in Cree Indians exposed to methylmercury in northern Quebec. *Clin Invest Med* 6:161–169.

Meinert, CL (1986) *Clinical Trials: Design, Conduct, and Analysis*. New York: Oxford University Press.

Meyer, AF and Mitchell, HB (1961) Medicolegal aspects of disaster operations. *Am Ind Hyg Assoc J* 21:223–231.

Miettinen, OS (1982) Design options in epidemiologic research: An update. *Scand J Work Environ Health* 1:7–14.

Miettinen, OS (1985) *Theoretical Epidemiology: Principles of Occurrence Research in Medicine*. New York: John Wiley & Sons.

Millard, SP (1987) Environmental monitoring, statistics and the law: Room for improvement. *Am Stat Assoc* 41(4):249–259.

Mobilia, MA and Rossingol, AM (1983) The role of epidemiology in determining causation in toxic shock syndrome. *Jurimetrics J* Fall, 78–86.

Monson, RR (1985) *Occupational Epidemiology*. Boca Raton, FL: CRC Press.

Mortimer, JA and Shuman, LM (eds)(1981) *The Epidemiology of Dementia*. New York: Oxford University Press.

Myers, JK, Weissman, MM, Tischler, GL, et al. (1984) Six-month prevalence of psychiatric disorders in three communities. *Arch Gen Psychiatry* 41:959–967.

National Institute on Drug Abuse (1983) *National Survey on Drug Abuse: Main Findings 1982*. Rockville, MD: NIDA.

National Institute on Drug Abuse (1984) *Epidemiology of Heroin 1964–1984*. Rockville, MD: NIDA.

Poole, C (1986) Exposure opportunity in case-control studies. *Am J Epidemiol* 123: 352–358.

Poole, C (1987) Critical appraisal of the exposure-potential restriction rule. *Am J Epidemiol* 125:179–183.

Regier, DA, Myers, JK, Kramer, M, et al. (1984) The NIMH epidemiologic catchment area program: Historical context, major objectives, and study population characteristics. *Arch Gen Psychiatry* 41:934–941.

Robins, JM and Greenland, S (1986) The role of model selection in causal inference from nonexperimental data. *Am J Epidemiol* 123:392–402.

Robins, LN (1978) Psychiatric epidemiology. *Arch Gen Psychiatry* 35:697–702.

Robins, LN, Helzer, JE, Croughan, J, et al. (1981) National Institute of Mental Health diagnostic interview schedule: Its history, characteristics, and validity. *Arch Gen Psychiatry* 38:381–389.

Robins, LN, Helzer, JE, Weissma, MM, et al. (1984) Lifetime prevalence of specific psychiatric disorders in three sites. *Arch Gen Psychiatry* 41:949–958.

Rosenman, KD (1988) Use of hospital discharge data in the surveillance of occupational disease. *Am J Ind Med* 13:281–289.

Schlesselman, JJ (1982) *Case-Control Studies: Design, Conduct, Analysis*. New York: Oxford University Press.

Schulte, PA (1985) *Case-Control Studies: Design, Conduct, Analysis*. New York: Oxford University Press.

Schulte, PA, Singal, M, Stringer, WT, et al. (1982) The efficacy of a population-based comparison group in cross-sectional occupational health studies. *Am J Epidemiol* 116:981–989.

Selikoff, IJ (1984) Twenty lessons from asbestos. *EPA J* 10(4):21–24.

Shepherd, M (1978) Epidemiology and clinical psychiatry. *Br J Psychiatry* 133:289–298.

Slovic, P (1987) Perception of risk. *Science* 236:280–285.

Soskolne, CL (1989) Epidemiology: Question of science, ethics, morality and law. *Am J Epidemiol* 129(1):1–18.

Tierney, KJ (1979) *Crisis Intervention Programs for Disarter Victims: A Source Book and Manual for Smaller Communities*. Washington, DC: US Department of Health, Education and Welfare, Public Health Service, Alcohol, Drug Abuse and Mental Health Administration.

Vinni, K and Hakama, M (1980) Healthy worker effect in the total Finnish population. *Br J Ind Med* 37:180–184.

Webb, DB (1989) PBB: An environmental contamination in Michigan. *J Comm Psychol* 17(1):30–46.

Weiss, NS (1986) *Clinical Epidemiology: The Study of the Outcome of Illness*. New York: Oxford University Press.

Weissman, MM and Klerman, GL (1978) Epidemiology of mental disorders. *Arch Gen Psychiatry* 35:705–712.

Wing, JK, Mann, SA, Leff, JP, et al. (1978) The concept of "case" in psychiatric population surveys. *Psychol Med* 8:203–217.

Witts, LJ (ed)(1964) *Medical Surveys and Clinical Trials*. London: Oxford University Press.

13

Surveys

The American Statistical Association describes a *survey* as ". . . a method of gathering information from a number of individuals, a 'sample', in order to learn something about the larger population from which the sample has been drawn." Last (1983) defines a survey as "an investigation in which information is systematically collected but in which the experimental method is not used." When the sample of people being surveyed is obtained at random, about 1500 individuals are needed to define the American national profile of nearly 250 million people.

Surveys are the newest technique to appear in the arsenal of methods aimed at the evaluation and prevention of environmental and occupational health problems. The term "survey" was used in the 19th century to indicate "a supposedly impartial, first-hand investigation of a community or a group" (Turner and Martin 1984). "Social surveys" were first mentioned in the Encyclopedia of Social Sciences *in 1936. In the latter, surveys of poverty, quantitative patterns of life of the working classes, and "straw votes" are given as examples.*

We seem to have been surveyed for generations, but, in truth, scientific surveying has a relatively short history. Survey and polls will forever be as-

sociated with the fiasco used by the Literary Digest *to predict the presidential elections of 1936. Roosevelt ran against Landon, and the* Literary Digest *incorrectly predicted that Landon would win the election (Dillman 1978). Ten million votes were distributed, and close to two million were processed. Reliance on volunteer responses and the bias introduced from the use of telephone directories and automobile registration lists are often cited as the reason for that failure. The episode, however, gave impetus to theoretical work on the concept of probability sampling. The Gallup Poll, which incorporated many of the newly learned statistical principles, was founded in 1936. In the 1940s the United States government began to use survey methods. The Monthly Report on the Labor Force, which still continues today, is one of the most widely known surveys.*

Surveys began to be performed in academic circles after World War II, particularly by social scientists. Public opinion and market research were the major applications. Throughout the 1940s many important centers of research were founded in New York (eg, Bureau of Applied Social Research at Columbia University) and Chicago (eg, the National Opinion Research Center affiliated with the University of Chicago). A comprehensive history of surveys in the United States has been written by Converse (1987).

Medical field surveys of occupational diseases have an even shorter history. Their roots can be traced to epidemiology. Alice Hamilton's "sur-

veys" of occupational diseases, performed in the United States early in this century, are mentioned in the Introduction to this book. More recently, Professor Irving J. Selikoff at the Mount Sinai Medical Center in New York City became known around the world for his surveys on the adverse health effects of exposure to asbestos. In collaboration with Dr. C. Hammond (1912–1986) of the American Cancer Society, the database from which inferences about the deleterious effects of asbestos were drawn exceeded one million cases. The research protocol of the first medical health surveys conducted by Dr. Hammond and his colleagues at the Environmental Sciences Laboratory at Mount Sinai Medical School was very simple, confined to a few variables. Probability sampling in medical field surveys was introduced in the late 1970s. A random sample of the population of the state of Michigan was selected by the Michigan State School of Public Health for the Mount Sinai Medical School team when they were conducting a medical study of the extent of polybrominated biphenyls (PBB)-related disease in that state.

A number of studies in environmental and occupational neurotoxicology have been conducted recently in the context of a medical field survey. A medical field survey involves the transport of an entire medical laboratory and personnel, commonly associated with a permanent setting, to a field location. The site can be a local union, a school, an armory, a local hospital, a gymnasium, etc.

Many groups of people must be made familiar with the objectives and methods of a survey. For example:

- People living near a source of emission of chemical pollutants may request local, state, or federal agencies to conduct a survey of the extent of health problems related to such emissions.
- The potential readership of a survey may need to be involved in the organization of such a survey.
- Managers of a plant suspected of emitting chemical pollutants may be informed that a survey on the premises is planned by an outside group of investigators.

- Health officials may need to know how to interpret the information derived from a survey.

Conducted scientifically—meaning, in particular, free of bias—surveys are one of the most expensive methods of health information gathering.

TYPES OF SURVEYS

There are several types of surveys. Surveys can be classified by their content, size, medium, and method of data collection.

The **content** reflects the objective of the survey: there are monthly U.S. surveys to estimate national unemployment; there are surveys on attitudes about health questions and health care delivery, including some specifically targeted to mental health care of the elderly; and there are medical field surveys aimed at ascertaining the prevalence of occupationally related toxic illness.

Surveys can also be classified by **size** (Table 13.1). The U.S. census, which is performed every 10 years, is aimed at counting every United States citizen. This count is required to make important decisions regarding number of seats in Congress for each state, how much money should be allocated to different national, state, and local districts, etc. The U.S. census is the largest survey in the world.

In certain European countries such as Finland, Sweden, Switzerland, and West Germany, national census information can be and has been utilized in the design of certain neurotoxicological studies. In Finland, for example, every pair of twins can be identified. Thus, important studies on the role of genetic and environmental (including occupational) factors on neurotoxic illness can be performed (H. Hänninen, personal communication).

It needs to be emphasized that the quality of the inferences that can be made is not a function of the size of the sample of people surveyed but rather is a function of how the

Table 13.1. Size of Surveys

Number of Cases	Example
1–10	Case reports, cluster of cases
10–100	Most occupational health studies
100–1000	Many community-based studies
1000–10,000	HANES* studies
10,000–100,000	HANES* Veterans Administration study
100,000–1,000,000	Cancer studies (eg, asbestos)

*HANES, Health and Nutrition Examination Survey.

sampling has been performed. As noted earlier, only 1500 people are needed to probe national attitudes about important national issues provided that the sampling is random—that is, a sample in which every individual in the United States has an equal chance of being a respondent. Complete lists of members of professional organizations (eg, all the psychologists that are members of the American Psychological Association) are one source of participants in taking polls. In occupational neurotoxicology important sources are rosters existing in labor organizations. These rosters are a good source for surveying occupations that traditionally are unionized (eg, insulators, industrial painters).

Surveys can also be classified by the **medium** used to collect data—eg, paper-and-pencil questionnaires, printed forms readable through optical scanners, or computer-based procedures. A poll is intimately related to its medium: the questionnaire. Whether boxes are checked or a computer is used to assist in the data-collection phase of the surveys, the questionnaire is the heart of the survey. A medical health survey is also related to the medium: the research protocol (the plan for the systematic collection of data).

Telephone, mail, and personal interview surveys represent different **methods** of data collection. One type of survey that allows contact with a sample of about 1500 individuals said to be representative of the people of the United States is the telephone survey. A telephone survey conducted 40 years ago would have been a biased source because not many people had telephones then.

Medical Field Surveys, Health Surveys, and Polls

A *medical field survey* is different from a poll. In a poll there is verbal (eg, telephone, face-to-face survey) or written (eg, mail survey) interaction between the respondent and the interviewer. In a medical field survey there is physical contact by health researchers. A physical examination of the subject is performed: blood, urine, hair, nail, or other specimens are collected; chest X-rays are taken; pulmonary function tests, psychometric tests, etc are performed.

A *poll* is usually brief and designed to achieve a narrow objective such as the identification of attitudes toward creating a drug rehabilitation center within a well-established community. A medical survey, on the other hand, is more exhaustive. A medical field survey generates a large data bank. Five hundred to 700 pieces of information for 3000 people might be collected during the course of a medical field survey.

A medical field survey is different from a health survey or a health survey questionnaire. Last (1983) describes a *health survey* as "a survey designed to provide information on the health status of a population." It may be descriptive, exploratory, or explanatory. A health survey is invariably a mail, telephone, or face-to-face interview based on a questionnaire. Signs and symptoms of disease are self-assessed, and the interviewer does not normally intervene physically to verify the respondents' subjective appraisal. Health surveys sometimes provide valuable clinical and epidemiological information on neuro-toxin-induced illness. When psychometric, electrophysiological, and other objective testing procedures are not available, a well-planned health survey is the technique of choice.

The National Health Interview Survey. Health surveys can have wide-ranging objectives. The National Health Interview Survey (NHIS) is a good example. As described by Croner et al. (1985), the

> NHIS is a health survey of the American people that has been conducted since July 1957 by the National Center of Health Statistics (NCHS). The NHIS involves continuous sampling and interviewing of the civilian noninstitutionalized population of the United States. The NHIS provides information on the social, demographic, and economic aspects of illness, disability, and use of medical services. Approximately 42,000 households including 110,000 persons are samples for the survey each year.

Surveys Conducted to Ascertain the Extent of Chemically Induced Neurological Disorders. Health surveys may also have narrow, well-defined objectives. The following is an example.

Freeman and collaborators (1985) have developed an eight-item self-administered questionnaire for assessing signs and symptoms (of peripheral neuropathy, for example). Questions include presence of cramps in muscles of arms or legs, twitching of muscles, need for help getting out of a chair, difficulties in opening screw-top lids, tingling or "pins-and-needles" sensations, numbness in parts of the body, burning sensation in arms and legs, and pain in arms after work when resting. The questionnaire was mailed to 19 persons who had neuropathy confirmed by a neurologist's examination and electrodiagnostic studies and to 37 persons without known neuropathy. For each question, respondents were asked whether the phenomenon occurred 5–7 days per week, 1–4 days per week, less than 1 day a week, or never.

A scoring system was devised so that the greater the frequency of occurrence of the symptom, the greater the score. An arbitrary score of zero was used to predict group membership.

The validation study was performed by means of a statistical procedure called "cross-validation." The results indicated that needing help to get out of a chair one or more days per week was very likely to indicate a case of peripheral neuropathy and that a "case" was also likely to be one with frequent cramps in arms or legs and frequent paresthesias (altered sensations) in arms, hands, legs, or feet.

The self-administered questionnaire had a sensitivity of 76.5% and a specificity of 93.3%. In a screening test, *sensitivity* is the proportion of truly diseased persons in the screened population who are identified as diseased. Thus, sensitivity becomes the probability of making a correct diagnosis. *Specificity* is the proportion of the nondiseased population correctly identified as such. Specificity is then the probability of identifying a healthy individual (Last 1983).

THE RESEARCH PROTOCOL OF A MEDICAL FIELD SURVEY

The research protocol of a medical field survey includes enough information to perform two radically different tasks: 1) to allow a physician to assess the health status of a single individual; and 2) to perform epidemiological research on the extent of occupational diseases or to ascertain whether a dose–response relationship exists between levels of a toxic agent and neuropsychological functioning. In order to accelerate the process of data collection, in a medical field survey the research protocol may contain questionnaires similar to those used in face-to-face or mail surveys. Between one-fourth and one-third of the medical field survey protocols are questionnaires similar to those used in polls.

A medical field survey has well-defined objectives, such as ascertaining the prevalence of lead-related diseases among foundry workers, whether existing levels of methylmercury in local rivers are affecting the health of residents who consumed fish caught in their waters, or the extent of toxin-induced encephalopathy produced by solvents in professional painters. In most cases, all pieces of information collected during the course of a medical field survey are directly or indirectly related to the objectives of the survey.

Sometimes, however, the research carried out during a medical field survey is unrelated to the objectives. Because large numbers of subjects are already there, health investigators may try out new techniques and even carry out ancillary tests. For example, insulation workers examined to ascertain asbestos-related diseases can also serve as a good reference group for psychometric studies of neurotoxic agents among certain types of workers exposed to lead. Insulators are presumably exposed to neurotoxic agents at levels comparable to the rest of the population. Because the medical examinations are free, most workers volunteer to participate in those ancillary studies as long as their purpose is explained to them. However, ancillary studies have to be performed with caution because of the excessive burden they may place on the subjects.

Formal Aspects of the Research Protocol

The external aspects and contents of the research protocol need to be reviewed. These two fundamental aspects of the research protocol vary from institution to institution and from country to country. (The difficulties in unifying medical survey protocols around the world are caused, in the main, by the different circumstances investigators face in different countries. In the Scandinavian countries, for example, environmental sampling is part of the medical survey. In the United States, inspection of the workplace is possible either at the discretion of management or as a result of a warrant.) The formal aspects of the protocol, at least, have been unified in the United

States, consisting in the vast majority of cases of computer-compatible questionnaires.

A research protocol describes how various investigators, cooperating in the medical field survey, plan to collect all the information about a single individual. Since all the data gathered in the survey will be stored in a computer-based data bank, all questionnaires, forms, laboratory reports, etc are designed to be computer compatible. Data-entry technicians punch the codes for subsequent statistical analysis after the research team returns to its home laboratory with all the completed questionnaires. Figure 13.1 is a sample of a page of a computer-compatible form for demographic data.

Data from a form can also be read directly. It is possible to read the information contained in a computer-compatible questionnaire by using an optical scanner or by punching information directly into a personal computer. These procedures are adequate in permanent clinical settings. Forms designed to be read by an optical scanner are acceptable when plenty of time is available to design such forms. However, when computer-compatible questionnaires must be developed in a matter of hours, the use of forms to be read by optical scanners is not recommended.

Personal computers cannot be taken to remote, unknown areas or even to different countries without a considerable measure of risk. Entire data sets can be lost as a result of technical problems that may occur during the data-collection phase, problems about which the technician was unaware. Also, data gathered by inexperienced personnel require extensive proofreading before merging with other information in the data bank. Forms with clearly drawn boxes and clear explanations on the use of valid codes are by far the most reliable method.

All questionnaires are administered by specially trained interviewers. The method of self-administration is less reliable. However, when self-administered questionnaires need to be used because of time limitations, completed forms are reviewed by members of the re-

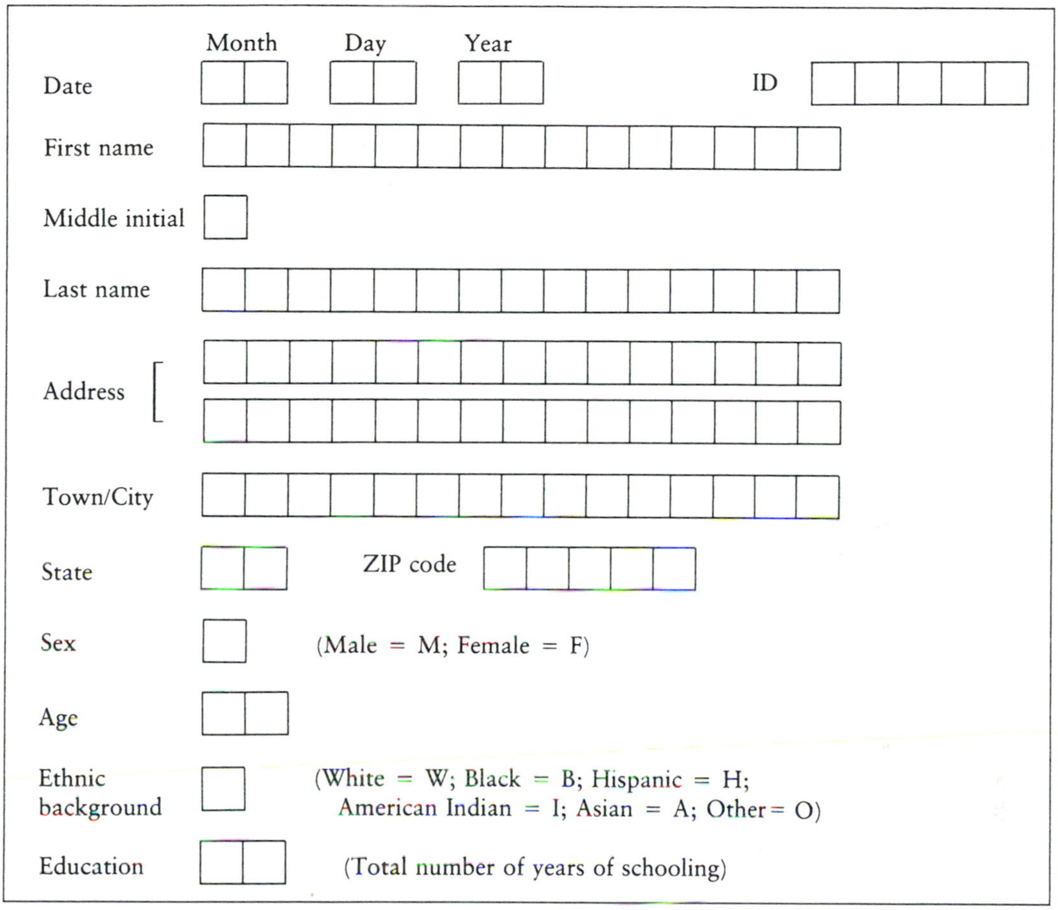
Month Day Year
Date ID
First name
Middle initial
Last name
Address
Town/City
State ZIP code
Sex (Male = M; Female = F)
Age
Ethnic background (White = W; Black = B; Hispanic = H; American Indian = I; Asian = A; Other = O)
Education (Total number of years of schooling)

Fig. 13.1. Sample of a page of a computer-compatible form for collection of demographic data.

search team. The administration of questionnaires such as those concerning use of alcohol and signs of alcoholism seem to be less embarrassing—and probably more accurate—when performed by the subject himself/herself.

Notes or Codes? Most of the computer-compatible questionnaires are menu oriented: physicians and interviewers have all possible codes. A good questionnaire contains cells for coding of unexpected conditions. It is unwise to try to anticipate all possible contingencies by creating a fixed menu. Circumstances change from study to study, and so must the questionnaires change.

The traditional view is to take notes and then hire people to code the written notes. This is still done in the transcription of medical charts, occupational records existing in companies or labor unions, company diaries and log books, etc. Needless to say, difficulties are encountered in the transcription of such notes. These include the inability to read other people's notes, the impossibility of knowing whether the absence of information on a particular point means that the respondent did not have that condition or that the interviewer never asked the question, the need to correlate information provided by several individuals with different professional backgrounds, and the need to control for subjective interpretation of information by allowing two, sometimes three, individuals to code the same information.

Except for workers whose jobs one is very

familiar with, occupational histories of unknown groups should be written.

Contents of the Medical Health Survey Protocol

Protocols vary in content according to needs, but the core protocol for a medical field survey where an environmental or occupational neurotoxic agent is investigated consists of the following types of data.

Demographic data.   These are usually found on the first page of the medical field survey protocol and include the case identification number and the name, address, age, gender, ethnic background, and education of the subject. Figure 13.1 is an illustration of such a form.

Occupational History.   A lifetime working history of each participant is carefully recorded. As discussed in Chapter 11, the occupational history starts with the first job and continues in chronological order to the present job assignment. Interviews are conducted by trained personnel, who gather information on the duration of employment in each job, plant, or department, associated exposures, date of onset of employment, personal habits with regard to food intake and smoking at the worksite, use of protective equipment, etc. Interviewers pay close attention to practices regarding work clothing, storage in appropriate lockers for work and street clothes, and the availability of showers and whether their use is required at the end of the work shift. Sometimes a residence and travel history is recorded with special reference to sources where neurotoxic agents are known to be present.

Medical History.   The medical history is recorded by a trained physician on a form where a code menu is available. The form includes codes for cardiovascular and respiratory diseases, kidney and urinary tract conditions, gastrointestinal, hematologic, neurological,

endocrinologic, metabolic, and connective tissue disorders, etc. Medical histories have biases in reporting and recall which are extensively discussed in the epidemiological literature. Figure 13.2 illustrates the first page of such a form.

The medical history includes smoking, use and abuse of medications, and alcohol intake. Alcohol consumption is given special attention because alcohol use can be a confounding factor in evaluating neurotoxic effects. The average amount of alcoholic beverages consumed at one sitting and weekly intake are recorded separately for beer, wine, and hard liquor. Changes in drinking habits over time are also recorded. In addition to the questionnaire on alcohol consumption, a special questionnaire designed to detect signs of alcoholism can also be included.

Physical Examination.   This examination is conducted by a physician trained in occupational medicine. The form includes information on weight and height, cardiovascular system, and a comprehensive list of codes for neurological signs. Figure 13.3 is the first page of such a form.

Review of Symptoms.   This questionnaire is administered by physicians or experienced interviewers. Different types of questionnaires have been designed by different professionals: occupational physicians, psychologists, psychiatrists, neurologists, epidemiologists, industrial hygienists, etc. The content of these questionnaires often reflects these professional backgrounds. Figure 13.4 is a fragment of a form recommended for the quantitative assessment of signs and symptoms of neurological diseases.

There are literally hundreds of questionnaires on symptoms, but few of them have been validated. An example of a validated symptoms questionnaire is the Minnesota Multiphasic Personality Inventory (MMPI-2). However, a questionnaire such as the MMPI-2 is either too long to be administered under field conditions or does not cover specific symptoms associated with a specific neuro-

SELECTED PAST HISTORY
1. EYES, EARS, NOSE, THROAT
2. glaucoma
3. cataracts
4. impaired hearing
5. tonsils & adenoids
6. laryngeal polyps
7. allergies
8. RESPIRATORY
9. pneumonia
0. pleurisy
1. asthma
2. chronic bronchitis
3. emphysema
4. tuberculosis
5. pneumoconiosis
6. CARDIOVASCULAR
7. heart murmur
8. high blood pressure
9. heart attack
0. vericose veins
1. GASTROINTESTINAL
2. ulcer/told by MD
3. ulcer/dx. UGIS
4. ulcer/bleed
5. rectal bleeding
6. rectal polyps/other Ps
7. H. hernia/dx UGIS
8. gastritis
9. hepatitis
0. jaundice
1. gallstones/no surg.
2. cholecystectomy
33. liver disease
34. enlarged liver
35. cirrhosis
36. ulcerative colitis
37. diverticulitis/dx BE
38. GENITOURINARY
39. kidney disease
40. kidney stones
41. bladder infection
42. BPH/no surg.
43. BPH/surg.
44. vasectomy
45. hysterectomy
46. menometrorrhagia
47. D & C
48. tubal ligation
49. NERVOUS SYSTEM
50. seizure disorder
51. stroke
52. TIA
53. Parkinson's disease
54. migraine headaches
55. psychiatric illness
56. SKIN
57. eczema
58. psoriasis
59. MUSCULOSKELETAL
60. rheumatoid arthritis
61. degen. arthritis
62. disc disease/no surg.
63. disc disease/surg.
64. back injury
65. knee injury/surgical
66. skeletal abnormality
67. BLOOD
68. anemia
69. sickle cell
70. low white count
71. METABOLIC
72. thyroid/goiter
73. diabetes/insulin
74. diabetes/oral
75. gout
76. CANCER
77. skin
78. throat
79. lung
80. stomach
81 bowel
82. rectum
83. prostate
84. breast
85. cervix
86. uterine

HOSPITALIZATION HISTORY

Have you ever been hospitalized? 1 = yes, 2 = no, 3 = don't know

Record information below

Date   Hospital   Reason

_____

_____

_____

_____

Are you currently taking any medication?
1 = yes, 2 = no, 3 = don't know

IF YES: What are they? (use medication code)

01 = Diuretics (water pills)
02 = High Blood Pressure meds (other)
03 = Nitroglycerine
04 = Digitalis
05 = Other cardiac
06 = Antihyperlipidemics
07 = Anticoagulants (blood thinner)
08 = TB medication
09 = Long-term antibiotics
10 = Short-term antibiotics
11 = Steroids-oral
12 = Steroids-topical
13 = Broncho-dilators
14 = Insulin
15 = Oral diabetes meds
16 = Thyroid meds
17 = gout medication
18 = Tranquilizers
19 = Anti-depressants
20 = Anti-psychotics
21 = Sleeping pills daily
22 = Have you ever had radiotherapy?
23 = Anti-convulsants
24 = Anti-inflammatories
25 = Laxatives
26 = Antihistinines
27 = Deocongestants
28 = Analgesics
29 = Antacids
30 = Other (specify)

Are you currently under the care of a physician or being treated for a medical condition?

1 = yes, 2 = no, 3 = don't know

Note key punch operator: copy column 1-5 from previous card

IF YES: List all diseases and year of onset. Use code to left.

Condition comments: _____

_____

Condition comments: _____

_____

Condition comments: _____

_____

Condition comments: _____

_____

Condition comments: _____

_____

Condition comments: _____

_____

55

56

57 58   59 60

61 62   63 64

65 66   67 68

69 70   71 72

73

☐☐☐☐ 0 G
1 2 3 4 5 6

condition   year
7   8   9   10

11 12   13 14

15 16   17 18

19 20   21 22

23 24   25 26

27 28   29 30

Fig. 13.2. A page of a medical history computer-compatible form (reprinted with permission of Dr. Irving J. Selikoff).

ENVIRONMENTAL SCIENCES LABORATORY
MOUNT SINAI SCHOOL OF MEDICINE OF THE CITY UNIVERSITY OF NEW YORK

O J
1 2 3 4 5 6

ADULT PHYSICAL EXAMINATION

INTERVIEWER
IDENTIFICATION

7 8

9 10

11 12 13

Mo   Day   Year

14 15 16 17 18 19

20

21

Height in inches:

Weight in pounds:

Date of birth:

Sex: 1 = male, 2 = female

Race 1 = black, 2 = white, 3 = Oriental, 4 = American Indian, 5 = other

INSTRUCTIONS: Write in code number after each system examined if normal or abnormal (1 = normal, 2 = abnormal). If abnormal, list the code number, in the boxes to the right, of the abnormalities found. Code 74 at end of examination acts as a "flag" to identify that one or more unlisted abnormalities is present. List these on line provided for code 74 abnormalities:

Examination summary: 1 = normal, 2 = abnormal, 3 = referred to LMD

22

1 = normal
2 = abnormal
3 = not performed

Blood Pressure   23   Record Pressure.

24 25 26 / 27 28 29

Pulse   30   Record rate:

31 32 33

Heart regularity: 34

General appearance: 35

Abnormality code:
02 overweight
03 underweight
04 appears ill

other_____

36 37 38 39

Extremities: 40

Abnormality Code: 08 swollen, tender joints/hands
05 clubbing   09 crepitations
06 cyanosis   10 amputation
07 deformed joints/hands 11 ankle edema

other_____

abnormality

41 42 43 44

45 46 47 48

49 50

Fig. 13.3. Organization of a page of a computer-compatible form for further statistical analysis (by permission of Dr. Irving J. Selikoff).

Chronic Symptoms

Below is a list of questions concerning symptoms you may have had. Check the appropriate box if you have been experiencing symptoms *in the past month.* If you have experienced the symptom, please indicate in the space provided:

Have you tired more easily than expected for the amount of activity you do?
☐ not at all   ☐ a little   ☐ moderately   ☐ quite a bit   ☐ extremely
1   2   3   4   5

Have you felt lightheaded or dizzy?
☐ not at all   ☐ a little   ☐ moderately   ☐ quite a bit   ☐ extremely
1   2   3   4   5

Have you had difficulty concentrating?
☐ not at all   ☐ a little   ☐ moderately   ☐ quite a bit   ☐ extremely
1   2   3   4   5

Have you been confused or disoriented?
☐ not at all   ☐ a little   ☐ moderately   ☐ quite a bit   ☐ extremely
1   2   3   4   5

Have you had trouble remembering things?
☐ not at all   ☐ a little   ☐ moderately   ☐ quite a bit   ☐ extremely
1   2   3   4   5

Have your relatives noticed that you have trouble remembering things?
☐ not at all   ☐ a little   ☐ moderately   ☐ quite a bit   ☐ extremely
1   2   3   4   5

Fig. 13.4. A chronic symptoms questionnaire. (From Johnson, 1987, modified from Hogstedt et al. 1985.)

toxic agent. A standardized questionnaire suitable for the study of all neurotoxic agents in unrealistic.

Sometimes the process of validation is impossible. On many occasions we have dealt with epidemic outbreaks, such as the accidental PBB contamination of cattle feed in Michigan, for which no previous human data could be found. Under such circumstances, a flexible questionnaire is an asset.

Theoretically, a questionnaire on symptoms has to be validated every time questions are added or deleted or the phrasing or codes are changed. Attempting to validate a newly designed questionnaire moments after an environmental disaster or occupational acci-

dent has occurred is not possible. Sometimes strict adherence to methodological issues creates unjustified delays in dealing with such tragedies.

Psychometric Tests. These are increasingly being used in medical field surveys. Only the scored data are entered in the data banks. In certain cases, such as when studies are done on the reliability and validity of a test, raw data (eg, times for individual tests) may be necessary. Observations about the details of the subject's behavior during testing are kept by the test administrator, and sometimes these notes are used when issuing individual reports (Fig. 13.5).

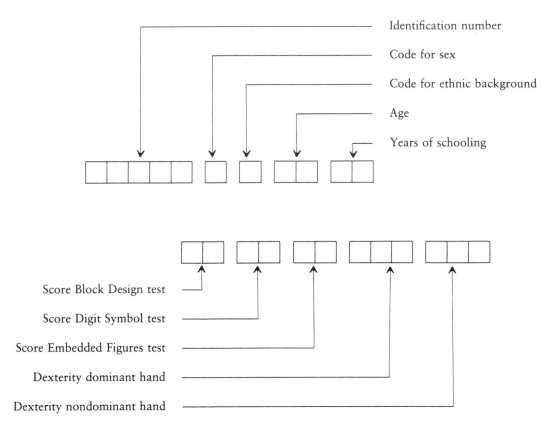

Fig. 13.5. Data entry organization for psychometric tests.

Electrophysiological Procedures. Procedures such as the determination of nerve conduction velocities to evaluate peripheral nervous system function are sometimes used under field conditions. Because these techniques are time consuming and laborious, a subset of the examined population, selected by well-defined criteria, is chosen for examination.

Biological Markers of Exposure. Blood and urine analysis—and sometimes hair, nails, fat, etc—are collected by nurses or specially trained technicians. Absorption of some neurotoxic agents—such as lead—leaves behind "biological indicators of absorption," but others do not. Exposure to some neurotoxic agents can be acute. The absorption and elimination rates can be very fast, and when this happens the personal recollection of the interviewee is the only information available; such is the case with exposure to many industrial solvents.

Professionals Participating in a Survey

Numerous professionals take part in various phases of a medical field survey. The **director of the medical field survey** is usually a physician trained in occupational medicine or preventive medicine. Although different aspects of the survey are under the care and control of various professionals, the director of the medical survey is responsible for the execution of all steps of the survey and the scientific analysis of the data.

The **survey account manager** is the coordinator of the technical aspects of the survey including questionnaire design, data collection, quality control, data proofreading, data management, and report writing. The survey account manager is responsible for the integrity of the data and for assuring privacy of the information collected.

The **epidemiologist,** in cooperation with the **statistician,** is in charge of all aspects of sampling, the effects of the response rates on the quality of data collection, and the analysis of the data. Epidemiologists and statisticians are responsible for conducting validity and reliability studies of the diverse techniques used in the medical survey protocol.

The occupational history, a vital piece of information in a medical field survey, is generally obtained by the **occupational history interviewer,** an individual with a degree in industrial hygiene or public health.

Psychometric and electrophysiological procedures are performed either by a **clinical neuropsychologist** or an **electrophysiologist.**

Environmental samples (eg, pesticides in soil) are collected by **industrial hygienists** and analyzed by **analytical chemists.** Blood, urine, and other specimens are obtained by specially trained **nurses.** Tests for the vast majority of biological indicators of neurotoxic effects (eg, zinc protoporphyrin levels in blood) are carried out by either **biochemists, physical chemists,** or **analytical chemists.**

FACTORS AFFECTING RESPONSE RATES TO SURVEYS

When a study of people at risk of neurotoxic exposure is conducted, the list of participants can be constructed from, for example, the entire work force of a factory where an occupational accident involving a neurotoxic agent has occurred, all dwellings at various distances from a known source of neurotoxic agents, such as a lead-smelting facility, or all the union members of a labor organization.

In medium-based epidemiological investigations—ranging from 100 to 1000 individuals—a database is created with last name, first name, middle initial, junior/senior, address, town, state, zip code, and telephone number. Each individual in the study group under investigation—the sample—is invited to participate in the medical field survey by personal letter of invitation. The letter includes a stamped card to be returned to the laboratory, allowing the subject to decide whether or not to participate in the medical survey. The card contains information regarding the most convenient time the subject is available to participate in the examination. Daily schedules are designed on the basis of this information, and telephone calls are placed to individuals with special needs, such as those on night shifts.

The response rate is defined as:

$$\frac{\text{Number of completed interviews}}{\text{Number of potential respondents}} \times 100$$

The ideal response rate is 100%, but this ideal is rarely achieved in health surveys. A medical field survey of people affected by environmental disasters or occupational accidents may test up to 90% of the affected population. Among public health investigators 70% to 80% is considered a "good" response rate.

Both the numerator and denominator of this ratio can be affected by various factors. The "number of completed interviews" changes with the number of participants in a survey, the number of forms compiled, or the actual data extracted from the forms. In self-administered questionnaires, it is often the case that many questionnaires have to be discarded because respondents failed to include some important information such as demographic data (gender, age, education). The "number of potential respondents" can also change.

Health surveyors differentiate between *nonsample* and *nonresponse.* A nonsample is a person erroneously classified as a potential member of the sample. For example, a mentally incompetent individual is a nonsample. A nonresponse is an individual who refuses to participate in a survey. Changes in the numerator or the denominator can modify the response rates by as much as 25%.

Response rates are indicative of both the overall quality of the survey operation and the respondents' perceived significance of the problem under investigation.

Social Factors

It has been argued that surveys are now more difficult to perform than a generation ago and that the difficulties stem from important changes occurring in our society. These social factors are likely to apply to polls (eg, measurement of attitudes to government policies). However, medical field surveys have also not escaped from these factors. Some of the factors can be changed, particularly through the dogged determination of field coordinators, but some cannot. In the examination of blue-collar workers, for example, a persistent problem is people's attitude toward health and illness. Many people do not want to know their health status and tremble at the thought of undergoing a complete medical examination. Others have a very stoic attitude toward work-related illness and readily accept disease as part of work.

Availability. Individuals fitting the profile of the targeted population may not be available for examination. If workers suspected of being affected by a neurotoxic agent need to be examined, they rarely have the support of management to participate in a medical field survey. As a result, medical field surveys are carried out on Saturdays and Sundays or holidays.

Privacy. People refuse to participate in surveys because they fear that information collected may be misused. This trend has been on the increase for the past quarter century and has been highlighted by the passage of laws that guarantee such privacy. During the course of a medical field survey, people volunteer intimate information about themselves, such as drinking habits, sexual problems, pregnancies and abortions, etc. The perception is that investigators may not be

careful enough in keeping this information from loved ones, the workers' management, or anyone with an interest in such information. There has been little research to ascertain whether this perception is accurate.

Physical Security. Many people, particularly in urban areas, are afraid to open their doors to strangers. The prominent display of identification and letters of introduction helps very little. As part of the environmental sampling of a medical field survey, technicians may have to go door to door, asking people for permission to take soil samples of their gardens or of dust that has accumulated in various rooms. The problem is particularly severe in multiple dwellings such as those existing in major cities of the United States.

Some potential subjects may be threatened for personal reasons. A door-to-door survey in sections of a city where many illegal aliens are known to live can create panic.

Apathy and Distrust. There is also a prevailing feeling that people are oversurveyed. People have developed an apathy to an important research tool—the survey—that is used more often for entertainment or business purposes. People often do not believe that the aims of the survey are the ones stated by the interviewers. Despite the presence of important regulations—such as "truth in testing," to which human research scientists now have to adhere—many people think that there are ulterior motives behind particular questions.

Other reasons are unfortunately justified from experience. Many people think that individuals who come to their doors are salespeople posing as interviewers. However, many people who conduct marketing research are in fact bona fide interviewers.

Demographic Factors

The effects of demographic factors on response rates have been determined by those interested in market research. There are numerous possible interrelationships among these factors.

Gender. Respondent gender has been consistently shown not to be a factor in response rates in polls. In environmental and occupational health surveys, however, there are many situations in which gender may play a role. In many countries of the world, men work and their wives stay home. When an environmental emergency occurs, women are more likely to accept an invitation for a medical examination because the men need to attend to their jobs. In certain cultures where women carry the burden of the daily work, the opposite is true. Also, women live longer than men, and these differences in survival influence response rates in surveys involving all age sectors of a community.

Age. There have been many studies reporting on age as a factor in response rates. Most organizations, such as the Survey Research Center, report that age is a factor in urban communities, where the elderly are afraid to answer questions over the phone or cooperate with interviewers at the door. Andrews and Herzog (1986) published a report on the effects of age on the quality of survey data on the basis of five national surveys of American adults and one survey in a Canadian corporation totaling 7706 respondents in all. They concluded that ". . . older respondents tend to provide a somewhat less precise indication of the attitudes, behaviors, or other characteristics being measured than do . . . younger respondents, but that relationships among survey measures [are] not necessarily weaker." Older people have a less differentiated view about their world.

Educational Level. In general, the higher the educational level, the higher the response rates. However, education is related to age—the older, the less educated—and in some countries gender is related to education.

Income. As a rule, people in the lower income brackets have a lower response rate than those in higher income brackets. However, these trends may also be related to educational level. An individual's socioeconomic status is an arbitrary figure that can be arrived at by multiplying brackets of yearly income by years of schooling.

Other Demographic Factors. In general, inhabitants of rural environments have better response rates than those living in urban areas. Ethnic background is also a factor. It is difficult to quantify race or ethnic background, particularly among Hispanics (McKenney et al. 1985) and American Indians (Passell and Berman 1985). The use of the native language of the respondents not only increases response rates but facilitates rapport during the interviewing process.

Survey Characteristics

There are survey characteristics that are associated with refusal to participate. Most people are willing to participate in one-time, in-person, population surveys. Medical surveys are by definition in-person surveys and in general have the support of communities where there is a need for their performance—particularly if they are not too extensive. Health questionnaires sometimes are administered via the telephone and are associated with response rates as high as 97%.

Repeated interview surveys are performed by many polling services. The selected individuals are often a random sample of the population of the United States. The purpose of maintaining and testing the same group is to observe changes in attitudes or perceptions as a result of social events during the life of the individuals. Follow-up medical surveys are also performed to study the time course of diseases, including many environmental health problems and occupational diseases. Sometimes, during a follow-up survey, a large number of individuals may drop from the survey during the early stages, but others remain "loyal" to the study thereafter.

There are many factors that, to a certain

extent, can be manipulated to maximize the response rates.

Auspices. The reputation of the organization sponsoring the survey, the name of its director, and whether the survey is private or government sponsored are all important factors in obtaining people's cooperation. The Census Bureau, for example, has obtained a "brand name," and its surveys are generally successful. Sometimes, however, when environmental disasters occur or chronic occupational health problems are investigated, government-sponsored surveys are not readily accepted by people.

Monetary Premiums. Cash rewards are well-known incentives for increasing response rates. Monetary premiums can be awarded to all participants in equal amounts or can be applied selectively. A "differential survey treatment" is one that awards cash to targeted groups only. McConochie and Rankin (1985) refer to the example of awarding five dollars to follow-up contacts in black households with males aged 18 to 34 because this particular group was underrepresented in polls designated to measure opinions in the television and radio markets.

Season of the Year. The time of the year in which a medical field survey is conducted is important in the determination of response rate. The season depends, of course, on the geographical location of the site and the local culture. On the one hand, in northern portions of the United States, the response rate for the summer is slightly higher than that for winter. However, in the months of July and August, people coded as "temporarily absent" are more prevalent. On the other hand, in the northern portions of Canada, residents who can afford to do so escape from long winters and take their vacations in the middle of the coldest months of the season.

In medical field surveys, people have to be present at the examination site. Therefore, any contingency related to the weather such as excessive rains, snow, heat wave, etc can be a factor influencing the response rate.

The rates of reported signs and symptoms of disease may be influenced by the season. Experimental designs often call for the examination of a study group and a control. The examination of the study group in the winter during the flu season and the control in the summer will likely be reflected in the differential rate of reporting of many flu-related medical conditions.

Motivation. The participant's perception of the medical field survey is created and modified by many group phenomena known to sociologists and social psychologists. People affected by a chronic environmental problem, such as the presence of a lead smelter in the community, have a strong motivation to participate in a health survey. However, actual participation may be influenced by unexpected factors. As stated above, studies in locations where many illegal immigrants are likely to be present are difficult because aliens may think that their names will be reported to the police. Close cooperation with community leaders and the physical presence of the director of the field survey are necessary to reassure participants of confidentiality of information.

A key motivational factor for attending a medical field survey is the understanding that the subject will receive a complete medical examination followed by an individual report mailed to his/her address and to his/her personal physician if the subject so requests.

Advance Notice. The design, wording, and timing of the advance letters of invitation or brochures are also factors to be considered. The letter of invitation has the letterhead of the sponsoring institution or a special printed letterhead with the name of the survey and contains a stamped, return envelope where the addressee writes down the best day and time for the examination. The letters need to be mailed about a month to 6 weeks prior to the actual testing. People tend to forget commitments made over longer periods of time. On the other hand, letters of invitation sent too close to the time of examination may conflict with people's prior appointments.

More importantly, the institution carrying out the survey must be prepared with adequate equipment and personnel to cope with the hectic times surrounding the reception of mail and scheduling of appointments. The response rate may be influenced by what is perceived as a lack of efficiency in the handling of scheduling of examinations and even the tone of voice of the interviewers in handling people's needs.

Follow-up: Reminders and Offers of Physical Assistance.

Survey participants need to be reminded of their appointments. Sometimes, a phone call the evening before the scheduled examination date is enough. In regions of the country where minorities live, callers should use the prevailing language in the last-minute, reassuring call.

In medical field surveys, the technical personnel need to be prepared for innumerable contingencies such as picking up a participant who lacks means of transportation or babysitting for a participant's children during the examination. A survey having good auspices and efficient organization can be conducted under seemingly trying conditions. At Mount Sinai Medical School, our survey team has participated in medical surveys in which the participants had to travel several hundred miles to the site.

Survey Length and Complexity.

The length of the medical survey affects participation rate. Remember that the participant rarely "discovers" what the medical survey is all about: he or she has already been informed about the content and organizational features by others who have already participated or by local helpers with a good knowledge of the details of the survey. In the letter of invitation, participants need to be informed that the medical field survey may take up to 4 hours.

The actual design of the questionnaire is important. As a rule, self-administered questionnaires need to be simple and easily understood by participants with a minimum of education. Questionnaires designed to be read by optical scanners or computer-based questionnaires must be administered by adequately trained personnel.

Personnel.

Even the most qualified professionals may experience personal shortcomings in the midst of a medical field survey. This is particularly true when teams must reside at distant locations for extended periods of time. The personal discomfort associated with unfamiliar accommodations, diet, meal scheduling, and excessive hours of work may be reflected ultimately in how a particular team member handles a situation. A survey participant may be positively affected by the contact of an efficient and dedicated team and is likely to communicate those feelings of support to others.

Community Support.

A medical field survey needs to be planned allowing for the respondent's participation in many phases of the design, execution, data management, and analysis—but not interpretation—of the data. Ideally, the feeling must be created that the community "owns" the survey as much as the health scientists. In fact, surveys lacking community support are very likely to result in failure. A prompt answer to the extent and possible causes of a health problem—which is often promised during the planning phases of the study—needs to be fulfilled. The presence of a community liaison in the scientific laboratory where the research work is being conducted is sometimes a good recourse in order to avoid possible misinterpretations regarding the generation of reports.

Participation of community members or representatives of workers' organizations—often, their occupational and safety representative—is important in epidemiological studies to enhance response rate. In follow-up studies this participation is essential. Their role is limited to the execution of the technical aspects of the survey and does not include the interpretation of research findings. The vital role of community leaders and labor organizations in the design and execution of medical surveys is often misunderstood as an inherent bias by those who are not familiar with the intricacies of this type of epidemiological research.

Organization and Management.   There is a paucity of information on the reasons why some organizations and research groups are more efficient than others in performing medical surveys. The intrinsic personal and professional merits of their team members is no doubt of importance. Managing practices within these organizations are critical: communities and workers that are surveyed perceive these qualities, and this affects the success of the survey.

The medical field survey is an example of applied research carried out to understand the nature of an environmental or occupational health problem with the goal of eventually doing something about it. If a medical field survey is carried out for the intellectual satisfaction of "pure" science, then it is likely to alienate the potential beneficiaries of that knowledge. Many organizations around the world that carry out medical surveys have been created by people with a commitment to both community health and scientific vision. These health organizations have been able to attract highly qualified individuals who continue to adhere to the ideals of preventive medicine while maintaining essential skills necessary for meaningful scientific research. The intrinsic professional merit of the members of the medical field survey team cannot be easily dissociated from the goals of health and medical organizations.

In spite of numerous difficulties, many organizations and research groups have managed to maintain high management standards for performance of medical field surveys. These standards allow for permanence in a continually changing social environment.

Many medical field surveys that have been scheduled to be performed on a one-time basis have failed.

A health organization can excel academically, and its team can function according to the latest trends in management, and still fail to accomplish a useful purpose because of the lack of an authentic commitment to prevention of human suffering. A "low response rate" may be related to people's perception of such lack of commitment.

REFERENCES

Andrews, FM and Herzog, AR (1986) The quality of survey data as related to age of the respondent. *J Am Statist Assoc* 81:403–410.

Converse, JM (1987) *Survey Research in the United States: Roots and Emergence.* Berkeley, CA: University of California Press.

Croner, CM, Williams, PD, and Hsiung, S (1985) Call back response in the National Health Interview Survey pp. 164–169. In *American Statistical Association 1985 Proceedings of the Section on Survey Research Methods.* Washington, DC: American Statistical Association.

Dillman, DA (1978) *Mail and Telephone Surveys.* New York: John Wiley & Sons.

Freeman, RW, Bleecker, ML, Comstock, GW, et al. (1985) Validation of self-administered questionnaire for study of peripheral neuropathy. *Am J Epidemiol* 121(2):291–300.

Hogstedt, C, Anderson, K, and Kane, M (1984) A questionnaire approach to the monitoring of early disturbances in central nervous functions. In *Biological Monitoring and Surveillance of Workers Exposed to Chemicals.* R Aito, R Riihimaki, and H Vainio (eds). Washington, DC: Hemisphere Publishing.

Johnson, BL (1987) *Preventing of Neurotoxic Illness in the Working Population.* New York: John Wiley & Sons.

Last, J (1983) *A Dictionary of Epidemiology.* New York: Oxford University Press.

McConochie, RM and Rankin, CA (1985) Effects of monetary premium variations on response/ nonresponse bias. In *American Statistical Association 1985 Proceedings of the Section on Survey Research Methods,* pp. 42–44. Washington, DC: American Statistical Association.

McKenney, NR, Fernadez, EW, and Masumara, W (1985) The quality of the race and Spanish origin information reported in the 1980 census. In *American Statistical Association 1985 Proceedings of the Sec-*

tion on *Survey Research Methods,* pp. 46–49. Washington, DC: American Statistical Association.

Passel, JS and Berman, PA (1985) The assessment of the quality of the 1980 census data for American Indians. In *American Statistical Association 1985 Proceedings of the Section on Survey Research Methods,* pp. 50–59. Washington, DC: American Statistical Association.

Turner, CF and Martin, E (eds) (1984) *Surveying Subjective Phenomena, Vols 1 and 2.* New York: Russell Sage Foundation.

SUGGESTED READINGS

Abrahamson, JH (1974) *Survey Methods in Community Medicine,* Edinburgh: Churchill Livingstone.

American Statistical Association (1985) *Proceedings of the Section on Surveys Research Methods.* Washington, DC: American Statistical Association.

Andjelkovich, DA and Levine, RJ (1988) Identification of an industrial cohort and verification of its completeness using a complicated system of plant records. *Am J Ind Med* 13:593–599.

Bernstein, AB and Meyers, SM (1985) Coding of occupational categories: A comparison between expert and survey respondent coders. In *American Statistical Association 1985 Proceedings of the Section on Survey Research Methods,* pp. 497–502. Washington, DC: American Statistical Association.

Bradburn, NM, Rips, LJ, and Shevel, SK (1987) Answering autobiographical questions: The impact of memory and inference on surveys. *Science* 236:157–161.

Bradburn, NM and Sudman, S (1982) *Asking Questions: A Practical Guide to Questionnaire Design.* San Francisco: Jossey-Bass.

Bradburn, NM and Sudman, S (1988) *Polls and Surveys: Understanding What They Tell Us.* San Francisco: Jossey-Bass.

Brambillar, DJ and McKinlay, SM (1987) A comparison of responses to mailed questionnaire and telephone interviews in a mixed mode health survey. *Am J Epidemiol* 126:962–971.

Bryson, MC (1976) The *Literary Digest* poll: Making of a statistical myth. *Am Statist* 30:184–185.

Bull SB, Pederson, LL, Ashley, MJ, et al. (1988) Intensity of follow-up: Effects on estimates in a population telephone survey with an extension of Kish's (1965) approach. *Am J Epidemiol* 127(3):552–561.

Cartwright, A (1983) *Health Survey in Practice and in Potential: A Critical Review of Their Scope and Methods.* New York: Oxford University Press.

Cochran, WG (1977) *Sampling Techniques,* 3rd ed. New York: John Wiley & Sons.

Conway, DA and Roberts, HV (1985) Homogeneous groups, candidate pools, and employment discrimination. In *American Statistical Association 1985 Proceedings of the Section on Survey Research Methods,* pp. 77–86. Washington, DC: American Statistical Association.

Danchick, KM and Drurym, TF (1985) Evaluating the effects of survey design and administration on the measurement of subjective phenomena. In *American Statistical Association 1985 Proceedings of the Section on Survey Research Methods,* pp. 464–469. Washington, DC: American Statistical Association.

Enterline, PE and Marsh, GM (1982) Missing records in occupational disease epidemiology. *J Occup Med* 24:677–680.

Ferber, R, Sheatsley, P, Turner, A, et al. (1980) *What is a Survey?* Washington, DC: American Statistical Association.

Fienberg, SE and Tanur, JM (1989) Combining cognitive and statistical approaches to survey design. *Science* 243:1017–1022.

Fitzgerald, R and Fuller, L (1982) I hear you knocking but you can't come in. *Social Methods Res* 11:3–32.

Fowler, FJ (1984) *Survey Research Methods.* Beverly Hills, CA: Sage.

Frey, JH (1983) *Survey Research by Telephone.* Beverly Hills, CA: Sage.

Gentry, EM (1985) The behavioral risk factor surveys: Designs, methods, and estimates from combined state data. In *American Statistical Association 1985 Proceedings of the Section on Survey Research Methods,* pp. 176–178. Washington, DC: American Statistical Association.

Goodman, RA, Buehler, JW, and Koplan, JP (1990) The epidemiologic field investigation: Science and judgment in public health practice. *Am J Epidemiol* 132(1):9–16.

Gregg, MB (1985) The principles of an epidemic field investigation. In *Oxford Textbook of Public Health,* WW Holland, R Detels, and G Knox (eds) pp. 284–299. New York: Oxford University Press.

Groves, RM, Biemer, P, Lyberg, L, et al. (1988) *Telephone Survey Methodology.* New York: John Wiley & Sons.

Harlow, BL, Rosenthal, and Ziegler, RG (1985) A comparison of computer assisted and hard copy telephone interviewing. *Am J Epidemiol* 122(2):335–340.

Hochstim, JR (1967) A critical comparison of three strategies of collecting data from households. *J Am Statist Assoc* 62:976–989.

Hochstim, JR and Athanasopoulos, DA (1970) Personal follow-up in a mail survey: Its contribution and its cost. *Public Opin Q* 43:43–69.

Hyett, K (1984) Interviewing techniques: Preparing for staff selection. *Nursing Times* 80(3):51–53.

Jabine, T, Straf, M, Tanur, J, et al. (1984) *Cognitive Aspects of Survey Methodology: Building a Bridge between Disciplines*. Washington, DC: National Academy Press.

Kalsbeek, W and Lessler, J (1979) Total survey design: Effect of nonresponse bias and procedures for controlling errors. In *American Statistical Association 1985 Proceedings of the Section on Survey Research Methods*, pp. 19–41. Washington, DC: American Statistical Association.

Kish, L (1965) *Survey Sampling*. New York: John Wiley & Sons.

Labaw, PJ (1980) *Advanced Questionnaire Design*. Cambridge, MA: Abt Books.

Lam, Y-M, Wong, J, and Lee, N (1985) A two-phase sampling plan to identify psychiatric disorders in community. In *American Statistical Association 1985 Proceedings of the Section on Survey Research Methods*, pp. 247–251. Washington, DC: American Statistical Association.

Marsh, GM (1982) Computerized approach to verifying study population data in occupational epidemiology. *J Occup Med* 24:596–601.

Marsh, GM and Enterline, PE (1979) A method for verifying the completeness of cohorts used in occupational mortality studies. *J Occup Med* 21:665–670.

Marquis, KH, Marquis, MS, and Polich, JM (1986) Response bias and reliability in sensitive topic surveys. *J Am Statist Assoc* 81:381–389.

Moss, L and Goldstein, H (eds) (1985) *The Recall Method in Social Surveys*. London: University of London Institute of Education.

National Center for Health Services Research (1979) *Health Survey Research Methods*. Washington, DC: US Department of Health, Education, and Welfare.

National Center for Health Services Research (1977) *Experiments in Interviewing Techniques: Field Experiments in Health Reporting 1971–1977*. Washington, DC: US Department of Health, Education, and Welfare, Public Health Service, Health Resources Administration, DHEW Publication No (HRA) 78-3204.

O'Toole, BI, Battistutta, D, Long, D, et al. (1986) A comparison of costs and data quality of three health

survey methods: Mail, telephone, and personal home interview. *Am J Epidemiol* 124:317–327.

Payne, SL (1951) *The Art of Asking Questions*. Princeton, NJ: Princeton University Press.

Pearson, RW and Boruch, RF (eds) (1986) *Survey Research Designs: Towards a Better Understanding of Their Costs and Benefits*. Berlin: Springer-Verlag.

Rossi, PH, Wright, JD, and Anderson, AB (1985) *Handbook of Survey Research*. New York: Academic Press.

Schultz, BD, and Cox, DC (1985) Sampling designs for verification of cleanup at PCB spill sites. In *American Statistical Association 1985 Proceedings of the Section on Survey Research Methods*, pp. 142–147. Washington, DC: American Statistical Association.

Siemiatycki, J and Campbell, S (1984) Non-response bias and early vs all responders in mail and telephone surveys. *Am J Epidemiol* 120:291–301.

Spry, VM, Hovell, MF, Sallis, JG, et al. (1989) Recruiting survey respondents to mailed surveys: Controlled trials of incentives and prompts. *Am J Epidemiol* 130(1):166–172.

Stinchcombe, AL, Jones, C, and Sheatsley, P (1981) Nonresponse bias for attitude questions. *Public Opin Q* 45:359–375.

Sudman, S and Bradburn, NM (1974) *Response Effects in Surveys: A Review and Synthesis*. Chicago: Aldine.

Tourangeau, J, Lessler, W, and Salter, W (1986) *Cognitive Aspects of Questionnaire Design, Part C (Technical Report)*. Chicago: National Opinion Research Center.

U.S. Department of Health and Human Services (1981) *Health Survey Research Methods*. Washington, DC: USDHHS, Public Health Service, Office of Health Research, Statistics, and Technology, National Center for Health Services Research, DHHS Publication No. (PHS) 81-3268.

Wilcox, JB (1977) The interaction of refusals and not-at-home sources of nonresponse bias. *J Market Res* 14:592–597.

Yates, F (1981) *Sampling Methods for Censuses and Surveys*, 4th ed. New York: Oxford University Press.

14

Data Management

DATA COLLECTION AND CLASSIFICATION

The Individual Record as a Unit of Analysis

A medical field survey generates truckloads of data. Epidemiological studies and statistical analysis of data require the existence of a system for collection and maintenance of masses of different pieces of information.

In epidemiological studies, a *record* is the primary datum of information. A record can be an entry of a birth in a church book, a piece of paper, a 3 × 5 library card, field notes, a computer punched card, etc. A *primary record* is that information collected on the subject, such as height and weight, or the subject's biological samples, such as the concentration of methylmercury in urine or lead in blood. The primary record is also called the raw data.

Different disciplines train scientists in the use of various methods of raw data collection. Examples of primary records include the following:

- The patient's chart for a physician.
- For a psychometrist, the forms where the time, errors, and observations on the sub-

ject's behavior during testing have been recorded.

- For an electrophysiologist who measures nerve conduction velocities, the record paper containing the actual waveforms, electrode settings, distance from stimulating to recording electrode, temperature, etc.
- For a biologist performing field observations, his or her diary and pictures of the conditions observed.
- For a forensic psychologist and for a plaintiff seeking compensation for a neurological illness said to have developed at work, the original documentation presented to the court stating the charges against the employer.

A researcher in the environmental sciences is likely to encounter almost all modes of record-keeping systems now coexisting in the physical, life, and social sciences.

A *secondary record* is the information as it is transcribed to another medium suitable for statistical analysis. A computer file is an example of a secondary record of information.

Because the labors of environmental scientists have often been scrutinized in courts, increasing concern about the accuracy of primary and secondary records has been raised. The accuracy of this information needs to be assured. The existence of a primary record assumes a responsible individual who collected the information or who directed others in their collection. A neurologist who performed a physical examination during the course of a field survey by means of a computer-compatible form initials the form as a sign that he or she is accountable for the quality of the information gathered. The accuracy of the secondary record of information—including proofreading—is the responsibility of the data manager. In health research, the principal investigator is technically responsible for all the information collected and for the accuracy of all the data sets associated with a medical field survey.

Types of Data

In science, Stevens (1948) recognized the presence of four types of data, also known as variables or scales: nominal, ordinal, interval, and ratio.

Nominal scales are those in which numbers are used to label, name, and/or classify characteristics, but no particular order is implied to exist in the attributes so labeled. The identification numbers of three study subjects (eg, 321, 746, and 129) are unrelated to any attribute of those subjects.

Ordinal scales are those in which numbers signify increments in the magnitude of a measurable property of the study subject, but those increments are not equal. If 1 designates "no formal education," 2 "10th year of school," 3 "high school graduate," and so on, 3 indicates a higher level of education than 2. But the distances between 1 and 2 and between 2 and 3 are not equal. During the course of a neurological examination, findings such as "within normal limits," "questionable presence," "slight reduction in activity," "marked decrease in function," etc may be converted into ordinal scales.

The *interval scale* is identical to the ordinal scale except that the increments designated by the number are equal. The amount of time

elapsing between 9:00 A.M. Tuesday and 9:00 A.M. Wednesday is the same as that between Thursday and Friday. An interval scale has no known origin. Almost all psychometric tests whose scores are measures of time—such as Digit Symbol—are interval scales.

A *ratio scale* is an interval scale in which a zero can be established or a value such as a threshold of detection for chemical analytical equipment can be agreed on. The meter of a scale has equal intervals and has zero as its origin. Sound and light are measured on ratio scales.

Figure 14.1 shows various testing techniques and their typical scales of measurement.

These four scales represent a hierarchy in quantification. For example, more powerful statistical techniques can be applied on interval and ratio scales than in ordinal scales. An alert reader seeks a justification when an ordinal scale has been treated as an interval scale. This is why measurement, epidemiology, and statistics are so intimately related. Often, the relative position of a particular discipline is judged on the basis of the nature of the variables with which it deals.

The File Structure

The *file structure* is the way a computer-compatible questionnaire is organized. Table 14.1 is an example of the file structure of demographic data. The entire research protocol of a medical survey may contain up to 1000 variables, of which approximately 80% are derived from questionnaires and 20% from results of the laboratory analysis of samples, results of psychometric testing or electrophysiological procedures, environmental exposure codes, etc.

The Data Manager

Data management is that segment of scientific activity dealing with data record keep-

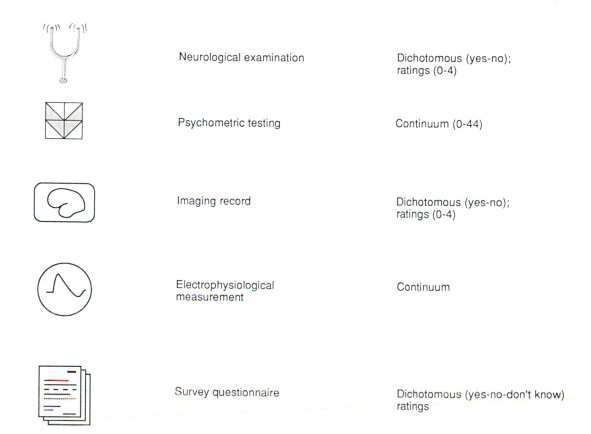

	Neurological examination	Dichotomous (yes-no); ratings (0-4)
	Psychometric testing	Continuum (0-44)
	Imaging record	Dichotomous (yes-no); ratings (0-4)
	Electrophysiological measurement	Continuum
	Survey questionnaire	Dichotomous (yes-no-don't know) ratings

Fig. 14.1. Various tests and their scales of measurement.

Table 14.1. Structure of a File

Field*	Meaning	Type†	Length‡
ID	Identification	N	5
LNAME	Last name	C	25
FNAME	First name	C	15
MI	Middle initial	C	1
MOB	Month of birth	N	2
DOB	Day of birth	N	2
YOB	Year of birth	N	2
DISK	Raw data disk	C	3

*The abbreviations are called "variable names."

†N, numerical; C, character (letter). A variable combining letters and numbers is often called "alphanumeric."

‡Number of characters, letters, or a combination of characters and letters.

ing, data quality control, and accountability of all the data collected in the process of carrying out a research project. Although the concept of data management was implicit in earlier forms of data record keeping—use of diaries, log books, data books, photographs, films, samples, results of laboratory tests, etc—it surfaced as a distinct aspect of research in the early 1960s with the increasing availability of large computers, also called mainframes. Large computers allowed handling of data of an order of magnitude unthinkable 20 years ago. Large data sets require conscious planning for data maintenance and quality.

In recent years, raw data—in the form of original charts, notes, computer cards, tapes, diskettes, etc—have increasingly been requested in litigations. Organizations that need to comply with these legal requirements are confronted with serious problems of maintaining confidentiality of information.

In the environmental sciences, the data manager is the individual in charge of purchasing, maintaining, and updating equipment and maintaining the computer facilities; creating or recommending the use of data-gathering devices (eg, computer-compatible questionnaires, optical scanners, computer-based data entry devices, etc); anticipating all formats of all sources of information originated in surveys so these separated data, when collected, will form a data bank; suggesting systems for physical data storage, data retrieval, and updating of files; dealing with issues of safety, protection from damage, or unauthorized retrieval; preserving the confidentiality of information; and auditing data. Numerous other activities, such as contracting out data-punching services, creating labels that need to be attached to each personal record or specimen, constructing the list of invitees, creating the list of volunteers to participate, keeping the final list of participants who actually participate in the study and the list of participants in follow-up studies, and issuing individual reports are all the responsibility of data managers.

Sometimes data managers need to work in close cooperation with "systems managers" or "electronic office managers" in the development of efficient record-filing systems and library facilities.

For a review of the forces expected to have a major effect on quality control in the future, the benefits of preparation for team auditing, the duties of an audit coordinator in the preaudit, audit, and postaudit phases, methods and procedures, methods of sampling, etc, see Hoover and Baldwin (1984). Although this publication reflects a view from private industry, the needs of quality assurance in data management are clearly outlined.

The technological aspects of data acquisition methods have developed into a rapidly evolving technology. Computers, mainframe and personal, have already changed the organization of procedures for data management and the skills of professional and technical personnel attached to this fundamental aspect of research. However, the principles of data management have remained quite unchanged over the years. This is an important reminder for scientists working in underdeveloped countries, who may equate "computer methods" with "better methods" of record keeping.

THE ART AND SCIENCE OF DESIGNING COMPUTER-COMPATIBLE FORMS

Surveys of populations at risk—described in the last chapter— require an intimate knowledge of form design. Although numerous books exist on the subject, form design has been discussed from a number of different specific angles (eg, wording, format). Form design remains very much an art, difficult to teach. Contrary to most expectations, forms and questionnaires are not designed by following precise rules. Empty formats do not take precedence over substance. Precisely the opposite is true: the objectives of the research and the needs to be fulfilled dictate format shape and form.

The research protocol of a medical field survey is now in most cases a computer-compatible file, but not necessarily a printed form. In most cases, it is a photoduplicated draft containing penciled corrections not affecting the readability of the protocol. Questionnaires need to be extensively field-tested in draft form before they can be used in an actual survey. Printing is both costly and time consuming. Because most professional printers are not expected to be familiar with the substance of a questionnaire, extensive proofreading is needed before the final version is acceptable. Sometimes 20 or more revisions of the complete research protocol are necessary before its final use under field conditions. Personal computers and software for desktop publishing specifically created to design forms have considerably aided the development of forms suitable for data collection.

Context

The kind of questionnaire to be used depends on the size of the population to be tested. The larger the targeted population, the greater the care in the design. Sometimes a medical field survey has to be performed in a small group (between 20 and 100 individuals) where local health officials have detected an environmental health hazard. Under these circumstances one may decide to use an existing modular questionnaire with a few pages attached. These additional pages are aimed, for instance, at obtaining data on specific job practices and health problems existing in the specific facility. No special questionnaires need be created in these circumstances.

A larger study population involves shorter questionnaires, simpler formats, and a reduced number of variables. In the study of middle-sized groups, between 100 and 1000, there are many factors that may adversely affect the quality of the data collection. There

are many interviewers needing to be trained and many unexpected situations that may be encountered. Proofreading and quality control no longer can be performed by a single individual as is the case with a small-scaled medical survey. The agreed-upon design needs to be field tested several times before use.

Large epidemiological studies of cancer—for example, smoking and cancer or asbestosis—have been conducted with populations of over one million people. But these studies are uncommon. Most frequent are studies of large groups of 100,000 people and over (eg, the NHIS survey described in the Chapter 13). An error in format, a wrong wording, or a confounder variable that was not included in the list of questions can create havoc. In order not to lose perspective of the substantive aspects of the subject under investigation, those responsible for large medical surveys try to keep the number of questions to a bare minimum.

Urgency

The urgency of a medical field survey can be classified as "high," "moderate," or "low." An experienced medical survey team can design a questionnaire in a matter of hours. A team rarely starts anew; a large part of the job consists of cutting and pasting existing forms utilized in other medical surveys. Environmental response teams, particularly those needing to work in foreign countries, perform excellent improvisations when few resources are available. The collection of information on 3×5 cards is an example. Until a computer becomes available, data can be sorted by hand in small piles according to variables under investigation (for example, proximity to the toxic source).

Studies of data collection that needs to be carried out periodically on large populations require a great deal of attention to details. The form used by the Internal Revenue Service in tax returns is a good example of bad design. The design is meant to be clear to people who analyze the data once the information is transferred to computer banks. But, as has been amply discussed, tax forms are not clear to people who need to use them. Tax forms are also a good example of the rigidity and lack of common sense often encountered when the same instruments are used over many years.

Available Personnel

Two extremes need to be envisioned in planning questionnaires: the presence of a large number of personnel, and the presence of only a minimal number of personnel. The need for large numbers of individuals using the same questionnaire requires training and periodic refresher courses. Data managers need to perform periodic checks to see whether specific interviewers tend to yield higher-than-the-norm response rates. That is the reason that the complete name (not initials) of the interviewer needs to appear in a prominent place on the questionnaire. Although computer programs to accomplish this are simple, one needs to be prepared to deal cautiously with "culprits." People made conscious of their overreporting or underreporting may shift wildly to opposite trends. When personnel resources are minimal, computer-based procedures are desirable.

Assuming Roles

The art of questionnaire design consists to a great extent in assuming the role of every person involved in the development and use of the medical survey protocol.

The **study subject** sometimes fills out the questionnaire by him or herself. As stated earlier, in medical field surveys, the subject rarely fills out forms unsupervised or without quality verification. The major consideration for a form whose data collection is unsupervised is simplicity and clarity.

The **examiner** is the physician or health worker seeking information about the indi-

vidual or the group. The information contained in an individual's form needs to be comprehensive enough for a physician to write a personal report to the subject or to his or her physician. This evaluation is the main motivating factor for people participating in medical surveys. As a result, the medical information will involve sectors that may or may not be related to the major objectives of the survey. On occasion, for example, an individual participating in a medical survey has been alerted to the presence of cancer, something not anticipated or aimed at in the main purpose of the survey.

People in the **art department** produce the layout of the protocol. In cases of emergency, the "protocol" may be only a collection of 3 × 5 cards in which each card represents an individual. Technical aides and typists usually see the preparation of the research protocol as a nightmare. Word processors and desktop publishing software have improved this perception considerably. As explained above, sometimes 20 or more revisions of the protocol are necessary to reach a workable stage. If a word processor is not available, the most effective way to lay out a protocol is by typing words and drawing boxes separately. Every revision is then a cut-and-paste job. Sending out the protocol for professional printing is not advisable because of the many revisions of the forms required up to the last moment. In addition, professionally printed forms need to be carefully proofread, adding to the load of activities related to the preparation of the medical survey.

The most common problem in the layout of the protocol is omission of variables necessary for statistical analysis, absence of boxes for data entry for a given question, boxes for nonexisting questions, inadequate numbers of boxes pertinent to the question (one box for "year of birth," requiring four), misalignment between questions and the boxes where the data must be entered, absence of required branching, branching to nonexisting questions, etc.

An **engineer** designs on-line data entry devices, or a **computer programmer** is in charge of developing a computer-based system. In various organizations, project directors maintain different relationships with engineers and software developers. These relationships range from dominance of the engineers and systems developers to the (wrong) assumption that theirs is only a lowly technical aspect of the entire project.

The **data manager** creates data banks and maintains quality control of all phases of data entry. The data manager, generally an expert computer programmer as well, needs to be involved early in the development of research protocol. He or she also needs to be informed of changes occurring during all phases of questionnaire design. The data manager needs to format the questionnaire—create the file structure of the database—according to the kinds of variables that are involved (dichotomous, continua, etc), how the data will be entered into the large computers, where the data will be placed, how many records are expected per individual, and who is expected to contribute what pieces during the data-collection phase of the survey. The data manager needs to work very closely with the person in charge of the composition of the forms, the engineer, or the software developer.

The data manager sees the questionnaire from the point of view of the file structure and often has strong views about how the data should be collected. As a rule of thumb, the "simpler" the format of the questionnaire, the easier it is for the subject to understand the question, but the longer it takes the computer programmer to program reading of raw data. The users' wishes sometimes create great difficulty in programming. Weeks need to be spent in programming and computer program proofreading. Computer program proofreading is a lonely and poorly understood task accomplished by computer programmers. Conversely, a thoroughly logical questionnaire with explicit valid codes fitting the programmer's wishes might be rejected by users. Months need to be spent in proofreading and correcting users' errors.

In the United States, the era of the research-institution-based, all-powerful data-processing managers and managers of information systems is rapidly disappearing. The availability of personal computers is the reason for this change. Some of the most commonly used statistical packages—such as SAS, BDMP, and SPSS—are now available in personal computers. Custom-made programs need to be avoided because one needs to be in constant contact with the original developer of the program for necessary changes. The wisdom is that if one cannot make the changes oneself, one should not accept a custom-made program. One is bound to be at the mercy of the computer programmer.

The **interviewer** must fill out the questionnaire. Specially trained personnel can handle complex questionnaire layouts. Sometimes, several days of training and subsequent quality control of training are required to be sure interviewers know how to create an optimum professional rapport with the subject, how the data should be collected, when branching to other questions needs to be done, etc. A good questionnaire design is one that allows for partial memorization. The survey participant needs to be the primary object of the interviewer's attention; the questionnaire should be eventually unnoticeable so that the subject does not have the feeling of being interviewed.

The **data proofreader** is a part of overall quality control. Computer-compatible questionnaires need to facilitate the process of proofreading. There are two types of proofreading: literal and semantic.

Literal proofreading is the reading of the data for completeness and accuracy and occurs at various stages once the forms have been filled. First, a quality controller (generally the data manager) verifies all forms at the time when the subject is about to leave the examination site. Second, before all forms are sent out for punching, every page needs to be identified.

Semantic proofreading is a further check for accuracy and meaning. It is best performed by means of computer programming and only after all the data sets are in the data bank. Many different parts of the protocol may be involved in the process of quality checking. Examples of "findings" during semantic proofreading are that some subjects are found to have symptoms before they were born; two males have had hysterectomies; one subject is 3 inches in height.

Data proofreaders need to have a great deal of space in data printouts to indicate corrections.

The computer-compatible questionnaire is designed in such a manner that the **keypuncher** (or data-entry technician) can transfer the data from the input medium (cards, tape, diskettes) with minimal difficulty. The layout of the boxes needs to be taken into consideration. Keypunchers find it easy to read from top to bottom and from left to right. The boxes are positioned in such a manner to facilitate eye scanning.

Data entry instructions are written so that no misunderstanding in punching occurs. The instructions are usually accompanied by a set of blank forms in which every column number has been appropriately identified. The data manager may add the list of all the variable names per form to this master form. The keypuncher is not expected to understand anything about the subject matter of the questionnaire or how the examinee responded to the question. The keypuncher should never be expected to act as a coder. Coding needs to be done by specially trained individuals familiar with the objective of the survey.

A draft of a computer-compatible questionnaire is shown to a **statistician** very early in its development, as should all subsequent changes. A knowledge of statistics is clearly reflected in the design of the questionnaires. The types of statistical analyses that can be made on the data depend on the type of data collected (yes/no; agreement scales). The ready availability of computers is associated with an increasing lack of attention to the bearing different statistical methods have on the type of tests performed.

People who read a report and need to interpret the information will respond to how a form is designed; this is very much related to its ultimate acceptance by the scientific community. There are different views as to whether the actual method protocol should be presented along with the report of the original findings. Most scientists expect such inclusions, but scientific journals often have space limitations making this impossible. Authors, in such a case, write a note indicating that the protocol is available on request. Some may not be interested in the questionnaire itself but only in the conclusions of the study. In some other cases, copyright restrictions prevent printing a questionnaire along with the report of findings. In addition, instruments such as the Minnesota Multiphasic Personality Inventory (or MMPI-2) do not need to be published, as the test is both lengthy and well known to professionals in the field. Sometimes laboratories do not publish their research protocols as a matter of policy, but they can become available to individuals trained in such facilities.

In conclusion, the art of designing effective computer-compatible questionnaires involves having a clear idea of the needs of everyone involved in the different phases of the process. The design of a questionnaire is never considered a "menial" or "technical" job better left to someone else. Figure 14.2 is a summary of the relations among different people and roles during the planning and composition of a computer-compatible form.

COMPUTER PACKAGES FOR DATA MANAGEMENT

The distinction between a *mainframe* and a *personal computer* is rapidly fading away. A mainframe is a large-volume high-speed computer usually remotely located with respect to the user. The user "talks" to the mainframe via telephone lines or cables. A personal computer—also called miniframe or microframe—is located where the user is.

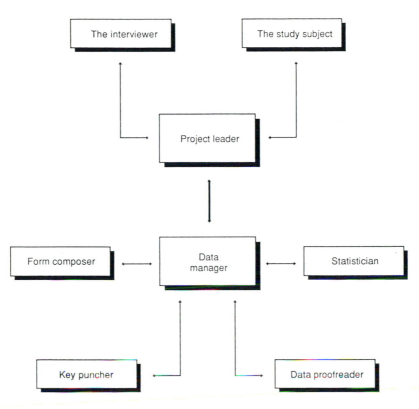

Fig. 14.2. Relationship between different people and roles during the planning and composition of a computer-compatible research protocol for a medical field survey.

Several personal computers can be linked together with many other devices, including mainframes, word processors, facsimiles, electronic mail, etc, via a "network."

In the 1980s personal computers increased the capacity and speed of handling large-volume data to a level unthinkable only a generation ago. Large-scale statistical analysis of data can now be performed on personal computers. In addition, personal computers have already lost the aura of novelty they once had; they have been incorporated into our lives just as the car, radio, telephone, and television have in the past.

The availability of personal computers and the market shift in training toward achieving "computer literacy" have redefined the role of computer programmers. The vast majority of researchers are now their own computer programmers or know how to read outputs generated from computers. A computer programmer is now either a consultant or a superspecialist, familiar with routines and aspects of programming on which investigators cannot be kept abreast.

Multipurpose software has now become readily available. Anybody who has the talent, time, and patience can now develop a computer testing procedure via Advanced BASIC in the IBM or IBM clones. With the Macintosh, one can use MacPaint, MacDraw, and Adobe Illustrator, which are packages that allow one to paint with as much sophistication as one would with pencils or a brush. But even if one is not artistically endowed, there are many software packages containing copyright-free, already drawn "icons" that can be easily edited.

Computer-Supported Data Management Systems

Data management and statistical analysis are now performed almost exclusively via computers. The vast majority of large epidemiological studies—ie, those involving 10,000 or more subjects—are performed via mainframes. But, as stated earlier, as personal computers increase in capacity and speed, the once essential difference between mainframes and personal computers is disappearing rapidly.

Computer literacy in environmental and occupational health research is now essential. It includes an understanding of how data are transferred in computers, how a database is organized (both reviewed above), how computer jobs are planned and executed, and what statistical packages and graphic capabilities are available.

A *software package* is a collection of computer programs that allow data manipulation and statistical analysis with minimal knowledge of computer programming. SAS, SPSS, and BMDP are examples of such software packages.

Job Control Languages

These are languages specifically designed to run computers. Most computer users do not need to know much about how job control languages and computers are run. But a serious investigator needs to know the essentials of job control language (JCL).

JCL is difficult because computers have become more complex, and their possibilities have been widened. When first introduced in the 1960s, JCL created quite a stir. As Brown (1977) stated, "Programmers, who had barely tolerated having to add a few cards to their programs, suddenly found that these control cards had blossomed into a full-blown language—a language more complex and difficult than their programming language" (p. 1).

JCL is a language that guides the computer in what to do and what resources to use. A typical JCL statement consists of estimating the lapse of time and the amount of space needed to accomplish a job. JCL statements are necessary to input information from cards, tapes, disks, and data residing in other computers linked in a network; to create computer-based data sets from such information; to run statistical jobs; and to store information residing in the computer on tapes, disks, and other networked computers.

A person in a leadership position who is not a programmer himself needs to understand that programmers have limited control over a computer system or its configuration and use. Often, computer system managers and programmers are adversarial in their perception of needs. The wide acceptability of personal computers has resulted in part from the need to resolve such chronic conflicts.

Data Management Software

A *database* is all the data generated in the course of the execution of a single project—for example, all the data collected in the course of a medical field survey, all the OSHA inspections for the year 1983, or all the bibliographic references to organochlorine pesticides. There are specifically designed computer languages to assist in the organization, creation, and maintenance of databases. Sometimes these languages are called "editors" because they allow the editing of data, which is not their only function. A current name is "data managers." Data management software packages are available for mainframe and minicomputers. In some cases, such as WYLBUR, to be described below, the same packages are available for both.

Database management software is used to create and update a computer file, to label variables, to update information—delete, add, or replace existing information—and for sorting. Data management software is widely available for personal computers. Some recent databases such as the Hypercard (developed for the Macintosh) link databases to telephones for automatic dialing. In general these take the general features of software that have been in existence for mainframes. Typical minicomputer-based software can store several tens of thousands of cases. Programming is also possible with the aid of so-called "macro" commands.

Considerable epidemiological research can be done with data management software having commands such as "count" and "sum." With the aid of a calculator or the language BASIC, now widely available, most of the statistical calculations can be performed. Experienced teachers consider this the best way to introduce students to the concepts and skills needed in statistics.

Data management software is essential in epidemiological studies. A typical application is the creation of data sets with the names, addresses, and telephone numbers of all members of a particular union. Because data management programs can be linked with mailing software, it may be possible to enter the original information only once.

Cutting Scientific Problems to the Size of Computer Packages

It is a poor philosophy to cut scientific problems to the size of computer packages. A professional investigator goes to manual operations when needed and works the algebra or calculus via a calculator or an easy-to-learn computer language such as BASIC.

However, it is fair to say that statistical packages—particularly SAS, SPSS, and BMDP—have been written with such intelligence and vision that most of the computational needs are satisfied by these software packages.

GRAPHIC REPRESENTATION OF DATA

Graphic representation is a system of visual communication. As Schmid (1986) has stated, the system consists of three primary components: the chart maker, the chart, and the chart user.

Generally, the chart maker is responsible for selecting the particular graphic to be used as well as for designing and constructing the chart. The chart is the medium that embodies the message being transmitted. The chart user is the recipient to whom the message is directed. It is evident that if one or more of the three primary elements in the communication system is in any way inadequate or deficient, the communication process can be seriously flawed.

Scattergrams

A *scattergram* is the visual representation of the relative distribution of two variables such as Y and X. Scattergrams can be drawn by hand or by means of many graphing devices. A $Y–X$ plotter is the simplest form of such a device, but there are many others that have been specifically designed for mainframes and are now available for minicomputers.

Many seasoned investigators consider the plotting of a scattergram to be an essential step in data analysis. For example, the presence of outliers (data away from the normal or expected range, defined below) or clusters of data can readily be observed in a scattergram. Sometimes, whether these outliers result from data generation or data-entry errors on the one hand or have scientific meaning on the other can be decided on the basis of perusing scattergrams. In addition, scattergrams can be very powerful hypothesis-generating devices.

Outliers. An *outlier* is an invalid, unlikely, or impossible data point. If the code for "yes" is Y and the code for "no" is N, and no other codes have been planned, the presence of an S is obviously a mistake. The data manager has to resolve whether the S is truly a Y or an N. If it is truly an S, resulting from an interviewer's use of an invalid option, the datum needs to be translated into a valid code (if possible) or dropped as missing data.

Outliers sometimes are unlikely but not

impossible data points. Only rarely does someone achieve a score of 90 in the Digit Symbol test. Such a score may result from a malfunction of a stopwatch or the fact that the test administrator did not click the stopwatch when 90 seconds had elapsed. Such points need to be checked; a note from the test administrator—lost in the data-entry process—may have indicated that something unusual happened. An expert psychometrist has to decide whether to accept or reject the piece of information.

Outliers sometimes are impossible data. For humans, a visual reaction time measure of 2 msec is impossible. The original data point needs to be checked. Sometimes zeroes are entered in an area beyond the allocated boxes and are not read by the keypuncher. The true value is confirmed to be 250 msec.

Outliers are difficult to detect when data are presented in tabular form. There are many informal studies in which experienced investigators are unable to recognize the degree of disparity of an outlier with respect to the rest of the data. It is the responsibility of the data manager in consultation with the principal investigator to deal with outliers.

There are computer software programs that allow error checking while the data are being entered. Valid codes and likely boundaries are stated for each variable to be entered. The keypuncher is alerted—eg, by a sound—whenever an invalid or unlikely datum has been entered.

An outlier can be present in the independent variable, for example, the blood lead levels (Pb-B). Let's consider the investigation of the hypothetical Dr. Carl Oxford on a new psychometric technique he has proposed for detecting early signs of nervous system dysfunction. Mr. John Doe, one of the subjects in the study, is shown to have a Pb-B level of 120 μg/dL. All other of the 100 workers studied do not exceed 60 μg/dL. There is no data-entry error. In addition, the laboratory where the analysis of lead was made has been contacted, and there is no evidence of a technical error. The performance measures are within normal limits. If Dr. Oxford eliminates this subject from the data set, he can claim that there is correlation between performance measures and neurobehavioral test scores, but if he includes Mr. Doe, whose performance test results are within normal limits, he cannot make that claim.

An outlier should never be removed from a study because it is in the independent variable. If the results change as a result of including or excluding such data, the investigator has the obligation of showing the results both ways.

There are no clearly established rules about how to handle outliers when they occur in the dependent variable. For example, during the tenth consecutive day of an investigation of children exposed to pesticides, the person in charge of quality control is out to lunch, and an assistant not very familiar with the rejection criteria accepts for psychometric testing a subject who does not speak English. The child, called James Smith and thought to be an English speaker, in fact speaks Spanish, as he was born and educated in Venezuela. James Smith is found to have verbal scores consistent with severe mental retardation; his motor performance scores are not that bad. The child is only later discovered not to speak English. Because 200 children were involved, the principal investigator orders a special examination of two scattergrams, one in which the results of James Smith are included and the other in which they are excluded. The main conclusions of the investigation are found not to change as the result of his inclusion or exclusion.

In summary, outliers may mask a correlation when one is present, produce a significant correlation when none is present, or not change the conclusions of a study.

Every data manager develops his or her own way of "flagging" outliers in a computer-generated data bank. One of the simplest procedures is sorting, a procedure available in both mainframes and minicomputers. If blood lead levels together with identification numbers are sorted, "low" and "high" outliers can be easily spotted. Or, one can make use of existing software meant to be used in statistics. For example, if only three codes (1, 2, and 3) have been planned to deal with the intensity of exposure for those engaged in painting operations, the presence of a 4 or a 7 is clearly incorrect. These errors are sometimes caused by data-entry technicians who are unable to tell the difference between numbers written in the computer-compatible protocols.

Outliers and Data Transformation. The "pulling" effect of individual outliers of the group mean sometimes disappears when data are transformed. For example, the distribution pattern of zinc protoporphyrin (ZPP) in a group barely exposed to lead is markedly skewed to the left, reflecting the fact that most people have low levels of this biological indicator of lead absorption. But some individuals may have elevated levels of ZPP. A logarithmic transformation of all levels will reduce the pulling of outliers.

Data analysis is a craft. Students learn from their mentors numerous skills for avoiding many pitfalls in data analysis. Some of these phenomena, known to seasoned investigators, are now being studied scientifically.

Variables on Scatterplots Look More Highly Correlated When Scales Are Increased. Since the early 1980s there has been an explosion in the development of computer-based graphic systems. In the mid-1980s desktop publishing software became available for personal computers. Along with this important development appeared a renewed interest in the study of perceptual factors in the evaluation of graphs (Chambers et al. 1983; Cleveland et al. 1985; Marr 1982).

Cleveland and collaborators, as an example, published an article in 1982 that reported the results of an experimental study on how the judged association between variables depicted in a scatterplot varies as a function of varying the size of the scales. Subjects were students in a university course on statistics, university faculty members, and practicing statisticians in government and industry.

The written instruction to the subjects was as follows:

> This is an experiment to find out how people such as you assess the association of two variables from a scatterplot. We will measure association on a scale of 0 to 100. Zero means no association, and 100 means perfect linear association. We are going to show you scatterplots and ask you to rate on a scale of 0 to 100 what your subjective impression of the association is. There is no right answer. We are interested in what the association appears to be to you.

The investigators varied two factors: amounts of association and point size. There were 10 levels of association, each scatterplot having a value of $1 - (1 - r^2)^{1/2}$ equal to 0, 0.5, 0.1, 0.2, . . . , 0.8. The value $1 - (1 - r)^{1/2}$ was used because it seemed closer to people's subjective impression than r. There were four point-cloud sizes labeled 1 to 4, size 1 being the smallest and 4 the largest. Each scatterplot had 200 points and a fixed square frame of 17.3 cm.

Increasing the scales on the horizontal and vertical axes of a scatterplot so as to increase the point-cloud size increased the judged association.

In an article published in 1985, Cleveland and McGill introduced the intriguing concept of *graphic perception*, defined as ". . . the visual decoding of the quantitative and qualitative information encoded in graphs."

Other Graphic Methods

There are numerous graphic methods that have been available for quite some time but that have not been extensively used in E & O health research. Cleveland and McGill (1985) have described and discussed the visual representational advantage of dot charts, Tukey box plots, graphic on a log base 2 scale, two-tiered error bars, and lowess-smoothing scatterplots.

GENERATION AND MAINTENANCE OF DATA SETS AND DATA ANALYSIS

Computer-Based Data Sets and the Intimacy of the Contact with Raw Data

The advent of computer-based data sets has both facilitated the process of data analysis and alienated scientists from the data that are the source of scientific analysis. How computers have facilitated data analysis hardly merits discussion: simply stated, the computer makes it possible to perform research unthinkable 20 years ago. However, how computers have created a distance between scientists and data remains largely unrecognized. The image of a biologist going to the field with his of her notebook to collect impressions of behavior of animals in the wild—which probably suited Ramazzini and Hamilton—hardly fits that of a scientist conducting E & O health research today.

The pooled data set comprised of all quantitative data derived from a medical field survey is the core from which hypotheses are generated and tested, where causation is first suspected and then demonstrated. As explained in Chapter 13, the complete data set from a medical field survey can amount to close to a million data entries. Sometimes there are dozens of professionals who contribute to the generation of these data sets. The data set of the Noranda field study, completed at Mount Sinai School Of Medicine by this author, in which the health effects of people living close to a copper-smelting facility and copper miners in a community in Canada were collected, was 700 variables for 900 individuals. Schwartz and Otto (1987) published a study linking a reduction of hearing threshold with elevated blood lead level in children and youths. The study was carried out during the Second National Health and Nutrition Survey (NHANES II) on samples to be representative of the civilian noninstitutionalized U.S. population aged from 6 months to 74 years of age. A total of 20,322 people were examined. Blood lead levels were obtained for a subsample of 9932 also chosen to be representative of the U.S. population. Audiometric testing was conducted on a nationally representative subsample of 5717 children and youths aged 4 to 19 years. Of those, blood lead levels were available for 4519.

The Control of Data Sets

Although large data sets, such as that of the U.S. Census, have long been in existence, computer-based data sets in the health sciences can be traced only to the late 1960s. The general public has not heard much about these issues but the question has arisen from time to time to whom these data sets actually belong.

The control of these data sets is a major stumbling block. Professionals who contribute to the pool of data can legitimately claim that they are entitled to other parts of the data they have not collected. For example, a biochemist who contributes data on hemoglobin levels to a large data pool may want to stratify hemoglobin levels among lead workers by race, information that he or she does not have. The biochemist may feel entitled to have access to this information from the data manager for the analysis of the data.

The team leader—under the advice of a statistician—may not agree about how the data on biochemistries have been analyzed and may exert pressure on an individual who tries to publish information without a written consent from other team members. The team leader may feel that the research is not worth publishing even if the source of data is fully acknowledged. Individual research facilities may or may not solve these problems. In recent years, several instances of fabrication of data have been reported in the literature.

Creation of a Computer-Based Data Set for Group Analysis

In the process of creating a large data set, several professionals and technical personnel interact in the clarification of the soundness of the data that eventually lead to judgments on whether or not a given toxic agent may be the cause of a nervous system dysfunction.

The following scenario exemplifies a gray zone that belongs equally to the end of the process of creation of a large data set or to the beginning of data analysis. Since this process is close to an art, it has received little attention in texts where the data set is assumed to already exist.

Before a medical survey is conducted, the data manager may have a vague notion of all the components that will form the final data set. A data set may be created from a rather informal process. A neurologist, for example, may one day contribute to the pool of data with 200 nerve conduction velocity determinations under field conditions, data that have been collected with the help of two technicians. The neurologist, who does not have hands-on experience with computers, may be present the first day of the field study, but the actual quality control of the data is left to the more senior of the two technicians.

Back from the medical field survey, the neurologist instructs the senior technician to go to the research facility where the medical field study was organized, such as a medical school, to help with the data-entry process. Identification numbers, the numerical values of records (printouts from the electromyograph) of nerve conduction velocities and skin temperature, for example, are entered into the large computer-based data bank.

A few days later, the computer programmer—under the instruction from the statistician who acts as a consultant for the study—provides the neurologist with the frequency distributions of median motor, median sensory, peroneal motor, and sural nerves and the distribution of skin temperature (a part of the nerve conduction velocity determination where skin temperature is confounder).

From the examination of frequency distribu-

tions, the neurologist detects 25 data points that are clearly outliers. Would these points be explained on the basis of existing medical conditions at the time of testing? These should not have occurred, as the senior technician left in the field was provided with a checklist that excluded testing people affected by conditions such as traumatic injury to the limbs, diabetes, or excessive alcohol intake.

The neurologist calls the team leader, who in turn instructs the data manager to provide the identification numbers and the names of the 25 outliers. The information is supplied to the neurologist, who instructs the senior technician to pull out individual records and notes taken during the medical field survey. Except for four cases where excessive alcohol intake is suspected (at a level that the senior technician did not judge to be excessive at the time of testing), there is no simple explanation why the other 21 are outliers, that is, exhibit abnormally low values in nerve conduction velocity. As a result of the neurologist's recommendation, the four outliers are kept in the data set at this point.

The neurologist, in conjunction with the team leader and the data manager, suggests a list of possible medical conditions, medications, and laboratory findings—obtained from several sections of the medical field survey protocol—that may explain the abnormally low values. Three individuals are over 60 years of age, and one is found to suffer from hypothyroidism (which condition was missed in the notes of the senior technician who participated in the medical field survey). Two individuals who are under 65 are kept in the data sets, and the examinee who is 68 and the one who suffers from hypothyroidism are deleted from the data set. One of the four people who are thought to consume excessive alcohol is dropped from the data set on the basis of a note taken during the field survey that the subject suffered an automobile accident while driving intoxicated. Thus, only three cases are eliminated, and the data set of nerve conduction velocities now consists of 197 individuals.

In the meantime, investigator A and investigator B, in conjunction with the data manager and the statistician, are looking into the matter of environmental lead exposures, biological indicators of lead absorption, and biological indicators of lead effects. A separate data set, created by investigator A, exists on variables such as occupational codes, environmental ratings of lead exposure on the basis of measures provided by the industrial hygienist participating in the survey, current blood lead levels, historical values of blood lead levels, zinc protoporphyrin (ZPP) levels at the time of examination, and historical values of ZPP.

The data set on environmental and biological indicators of exposure and effects is eventually merged with the large data set encompassing all variables of the medical field survey. The historical values of blood lead levels come from the union members, the current blood lead levels are from the Department of Biochemistry of a major city hospital, and the ZPP levels have been collected with a technician affiliated with investigator B.

The neurologist—an expert clinician with limited expertise in epidemiological research—joins forces with investigator A—an epidemiologist who has a limited knowledge of neurological diseases—in the analysis of the data relating blood lead levels and nerve conduction velocities. The analysis of dose–response relationships between electrophysiological indicators of peripheral nervous system function and biological indicators of lead exposure and effects is performed by a team that includes the team leader, the statistician, and the data manager. A chapter of the scientific report deals with the relationship between lead exposure and nerve conduction velocities. Neurological signs and symptoms—collected from computer-compatible questionnaires from physicians under the direction of the team leader—are not part of this report, since data proofreaders who must check computer files against individual medical folders have not been found yet.

A graduate student in neurophysiology with hands-on training in computer-based analytical techniques has conducted 100 vibratory thresholds with an equipment of her own design among 50 workers who have the highest values of the index of lead exposure proposed by investigator B and among 50 workers of the same pool who have the lowest value of the index of lead exposure. The selection procedure has been suggested by the epidemiologist, who is an expert on study design. The equipment developed by the student is hoped to be eventually proposed as a new screening procedure, and the data collected are part of the requirements for a doctoral dissertation.

The graduate student, with the aid of the neurologist, proofreads the neurological signs and symptoms of the 100 cases who were tested by means of the new vibratory thresholds device. The data set to which the graduate student has access is comprised of the demographic profile of each subject, confounding medical and laboratory findings, the test results of all psychometric testing performed during the medical field survey, neurological signs and symptoms, nerve conduction velocity determinations, and her own data on vibratory thresholds. In her doctoral dissertation the student creates a mathematical model of how endogenous and remote factors lead to changes in nervous system functions among workers exposed to lead. Her proposed "index of neurological handicap" is now a part of the large data set. (However, the data on neurological signs and symptoms of people who have not been tested by her vibratory threshold techniques are never proofread; in the absence of a diary documenting all changes in data sets, years later, someone may assume that the proofreading has been performed for all data.)

An economist from upstate New York, who has joined the research team in order to study how workers are compensated for the occupational diseases, finds the "handicap index" proposed by the graduate student a valuable measure to correlate with potential financial compensation. A scheme is developed by the economist, who is familiar with computer modeling; such a scheme could be useful to lawyers in litigation cases.

An epidemiologist who analyzes the data set several years after its compilation relates cumulative indices of lead exposure, the "handicap index," and risk of coronary diseases in the original 200 workers.

In conclusion, a data set

- cannot always be thoroughly planned beforehand, in terms of its depth and extent of analysis
- is not a dead, archival deposit of data—it is quite "alive" and continuously evolving as a result of the different input from various professionals
- is a valuable source to which many people contribute and from which many people draw

- requires the same familiarity that the field biologist has with his or her notes
- can never be accepted uncritically.

It is unfortunate that no current guidelines exist about responsibilities for generation, proofreading and maintenance of data sets—processes that affect many decision-making policies.

ISSUES SURROUNDING DATA MANAGEMENT

Assurance of Confidentiality

As a rule, a human subject's file contains numerous pieces of personal information that have the potential of being used for purposes for which the subjects may not have volunteered. For example, a subject may admit to a professional collecting data for a medical survey that he or she suffered a mental breakdown that required hospitalization; a segment of the occupational history may indicate that the person was in jail because of a rather serious crime; an employee may admit to use of alcohol, drugs, or both; a worker may volunteer that she tested positive for exposure to the AIDS virus. All these data could be used against the employee who volunteered to participate in a research project.

In human toxicological research there are pieces of individual information—such as a family history of severe forms of degenerative diseases, sexual impotence, severe depression, etc—that sometimes need to be collected, information that may not threaten a job but disclosure of which may be a source of embarrassment for the subject. Heads of laboratories and principal investigators are ultimately responsible for designing adequate data management systems that assure confidentiality of information.

Moreover, there have been many reports on fraudulent data manipulation or data fabrication. These criminal episodes have forced leaders in the academic world, editors of scientific publications, and government institutions to develop strategies to prevent their occurrence or at least to recognize them when present.

Electronic Record Systems and Individual Privacy

The Senate Committee on Governmental Affairs, the House Committee on the Judiciary, Subcommittee on Courts, Civil Liberties, and the Administration of Justice requested from the Office of Technology Assessment an evaluation of the impact of electronic record systems on civil liberties. A Federal Government Information Technology report was published in 1986. This report addressed four important areas: technological developments relevant to government record systems; current and prospective Federal agency use of electronic record systems; the interaction of technology and public law relevant to protection of privacy; and possible policy actions that warrant congressional attention, including the amendment of existing laws such as the Privacy Act of 1974 and establishment of new mechanisms such as a Data Protection Board or Privacy Protection Commission. What follows is taken from the summary of the report:

All governments collect and use personal information in order to govern. Democratic governments moderate this need with the requirements to be open to the people and accountable to the legislature, so as to protect the privacy of individuals. Advances in information technology have greatly facilitated the collection and uses of personal information by the Federal Government, but also have made it more difficult to oversee agency practices and to protect the rights of individuals.

In 1974, Congress passed the Privacy Act to address the tension between the individual's interest in personal information and the Federal Government's collection and use of that information. The Privacy Act codified principles of fair information use that specified the requirements that agencies were to meet in handling personal information as well as rights for individuals who were the subjects of that information. To ensure agency compliance with these principles, the act enabled individuals to bring civil and criminal suits if information was willfully and intentionally handled in violation of the act. In addition, the Office of Management and Budget (OMB) was assigned the responsibility for overseeing agency implementation of the act. At the time the Privacy Act was debated and enacted, there were technological limitations on the use of individual records by Federal agencies. The vast majority of record systems in Federal agencies was manual. Computers were used only to store and retrieve, not to manipulate or exchange information. It was theoretically possible to match personal information from different files, to manually verify information provided on government application forms, and to prepare a profile of a subset of individuals of interest to an agency. However, the number of records involved made such application impractical.

In the 12 years since the Privacy Act was passed, at least two generations of information technology have become available to Federal Agencies. Advances in computer and data communication technology enable agencies to collect, use, store, exchange, and manipulate individual records in electronic form. Microcomputers are now widely used in the Federal Government, vastly increasing the potential points of access to personal record systems and the creation of new systems. Computer matching and computer-assisted front-end verification are becoming routine for many Federal benefit programs, and use of computer profiling for Federal investigations is expanding. [Whereas computer matching involves comparing records after an individual is already receiving government benefits or services, front-end verification is used to certify the accuracy and completeness of personal information at the time an individual applies for government benefits, employment, or services. Like computer matching, any large-scale application of front-end verification is dependent on computers and telecommunications systems.] These technological advances enable agencies to manipulate and exchange entire record systems, as well as individual records, in a way not envisioned in 1974. Moreover, the widespread use of computerized databases, electronic record searches and matches, and computer networking is leading rapidly to the creation of a de facto national database [the term de facto is used to distinguish it from a national database that was created by law] containing personal information on most Americans. And use of the social security number as a de facto electronic national identifier facilitates the development of this database.

These technological advances have opened many new possibilities for improving the efficiency of government record keeping; the detection and prevention of fraud; and law enforcement investigations. At the same time, the opportunities for inappropriate, unauthorized, or illegal access to and use of personal information have expanded. Because of the expanded access to and use of personal information in decisions about individuals, the completeness, accuracy, and relevance of information [are] even more important. Additionally, the expanded access and use make it nearly impossible for individuals to learn about, let alone seek redress for, misuse of their records. Even within agencies, it is often not known what applications of personal information are being used. Nor does the OMB or other relevant congressional committees know whether personal information is being used in conformity with the Privacy Act.

Overall, OTA [the Office of Technology Assessment] has concluded that Federal use of new electronic technologies in processing personal information has eroded the protections of the Privacy Act of 1974. Many of the electronic record applications being used by Federal agencies, eg, computer profiling and front-end verifications, are not explicitly covered by the act or by subsequent OMB guidelines. The rights and remedies available to the individual, as well as agency responsibilities for handling personal information, are not clear. Even where applications are covered by the Privacy Act or related OMB guidelines, there is little oversight to ensure agency compliance. More importantly, neither Congress nor the executive branch is providing a forum in which the conflicts—between privacy interest and management or law enforcement interests—generated by Federal use of new applications or information technology can be debated and resolved. Without such a forum, agencies have little incentive to consider privacy concerns when deciding to establish or expand the use of personal record systems.

The Privacy of Unpublished Data

Environmental scientists have been involved in many unprecedented litigations regarding the public scrutiny of scientific research. One of the early controversies arose with the publication of data on TCDD, a contaminant found in herbicides such as 2,4,5-T and silvex.

Records and scientific truths are different. Scientific "facts"— or truths—are based on the reasoned evaluation of records. But the records by themselves mean little without the trained scientist who studies them. An attorney for the University of Wisconsin, Michael A. Liethen, has stated the following view: ". . . [A] scientist has to be free to take his inquiries where they lead him, and . . . a scientist should not be forced to disclose his research data until he has the results he is willing to stand behind" (Broad 1982).

Dangers in Data Compactness

The trends toward miniaturization of data storage systems has increased the danger of theft. *The New York Times* published an article on Nov. 19, 1986 indicating that personal records of 16 million Canadians—virtually every taxpayer in that nation—were stolen on October 30 from a Government tax office. Although the records were returned within 3 hours after the disclosure, the theft raised concerns that terrorists or criminals may have copied the data to use for obtaining false birth certificates or passports or for filing fraudulent claims for welfare or pensions. The bundle of tax records—described as being about the size of a lunch bucket—were recorded in 2000 acetate microfiche cards,

transparent 4-by-6 inch plastic sheets on which thousands of pages of information were stored.

CONCLUSION

Epidemiological studies of the effects of toxic agents in the environment and the workplace generate large quantities of data. The availability of large and small computers has greatly facilitated the record-keeping aspects of science, but it has generated new problems, both for the scientists who perform research and for the individuals who participate in such studies. Many such problems concern the ethical issues associated with the conflicting need of researchers to perform meaningful research and the rights of individuals to preserve their privacy.

REFERENCES

Broad, WJ (1982) Court upholds privacy of unpublished data. *Science* 216:34–36.

Brown, GD (1977) *System/370 Job Control Language.* New York: John Wiley & Sons.

Chambers, JM, Cleveland, WS, Kleiner, B, et al. (1983) *Graphical Methods for Data Analysis.* Monterey, CA: Wadsworth Advanced Books and Software.

Cleveland, WS, Diaconis, P, and McGill R (1982) Variables on scatterplots look more correlated when the scales are increased. *Science* 216:1138–1141.

Cleveland, WS and McGill, R (1985) Graphical perception and graphical methods for analyzing scientific data. *Science* 229:828–833.

Cleveland, WS, Kleiner, B, and Tukey, A (1985) *The Elements of Graphing Data.* Monterey, CA: Wadsworth Advanced Books and Software.

Federal Government Information Technology (1986) *Electronic Record Systems and Individual Privacy.* Washington, DC: Congress of the United States, Office of Technology Assessment.

Hoover, BK and Baldwin, J (1984) Meeting the quality assurance challenges of the 1980s: Team auditing by toxicologists and QA professionals. *J Am Coll of Toxicol* 3(2):129–139.

Marr, DC (1982) *Vision: A Computational Investigation into the Human Representation and Processing of Visual Information.* San Francisco: Freeman.

New York Times (1986) *New York Times* Nov. 19.

Schmid, CF (1986) Whatever has happened to the semilogarithmic chart? *Am Stat* 40:238–244.

Schwartz, J and Otto, D (1987) Blood lead, hearing thresholds, and neurobehavioral development in children and youth. *Arch Environ Res* 42(2):153–160.

Stevens, SS (1948) On the theory of scales of measurement. *Science* 103:677–680.

SUGGESTED READINGS

Abelson, PH (1989) Editorial: Retrieval of scientific and technical data. *Science* 245:9.

Abramson, JH (1988) *Making Sense of Data.* New York: Oxford University Press.

Atre, S (1980) *Data Base: Structured Techniques for Design, Performance, and Management.* New York: John Wiley & Sons.

Baldwin, JA, Acheson, ED, and Graham, WJ (1987) *Textbook of Medical Record Linkage.* New York: Oxford University Press.

Barnett, V and Lewis T (1978) *Outliers in Statistical Data.* New York: John Wiley & Sons.

Beale, EML and Little, RJA (1975) Missing values in multivariate analysis. *J R Stat Soc* [B]37:129–146.

Beckman, RJ and Cook, RD (1983) Outliers. *Technometrics* 25:119–149.

Berk, KN (1987) Effective microcomputer statistical software. *Am Stat* 41(3):222–228.

Booth, W (1988) The long, lost survey on sex: With data for AIDS epidemiology scarce, a major 1970 Kinsey Institute survey on sexual behavior is still under wraps because of a fight over authorship. *Science* 239:1084–1085.

Bracewell, RN (1990) Numerical transformations. *Science* 248:697–704.

Burditt, GM (1978) Legal implications of documentation. *Clin Toxicol* 12(2):179–187.

Burhman, D (1984) Use of computers for dossiers prompting concern. *The New York Times,* June 10.

Colledge, MF, Johnson, JH, Paré, R, et al. (1978) Large scale imputation of survey data. In *Proceedings of the Survey Research Methods Section,* pp. 431–436. Washington, DC: American Statistical Association.

Daniel, C and Wood, F (1980) *Fitting Equations to Data* 2nd ed. New York: John Wiley & Sons.

Fellegi, IP and Holt, D (1976) A systematic approach to automatic edit and imputation. *J Am Stat Assoc* 71:17–35.

Gad, SC and Weil, CS (1988) *Statistics and Experimental Design for Toxicologists,* 2nd ed. Caldwell, NJ: Telford.

Gosh, SP (1986) *Data Base Organization for Data Management,* 2nd ed. Orlando, FL: Academic Press.

Harlow, SD and Linet, MS (1989) Agreement between questionnaire data and medical records: The evidence for accuracy of recall. *Am J Epidemiol* 129(2):233–248.

Hawkins, DA (1980) *Identification of Outliers.* London: Chapman and Hall.

Hofstadter, DR (1982) Metamagical themas: Number numbness or why innumeracy may be just as dangerous as illiteracy. *Sci Am* 246:20–34.

Holland, WW (ed)(1970) *Data Handling in Epidemiology.* London: Oxford University Press.

Hoover, BK, Baldwin, JK, Uelner, AF et al. (1986) *Managing Quality: Conduct and Data of Toxicology Studies.* Princeton: Princeton Scientific Publishing.

Hosmer, DW and Lemeshow, S (1989) *Applied Logistic Regression.* New York: John Wiley & Sons.

Houts, PL (1977) *The Myth of Measurability.* New York: Hart Publishing.

Kindred, AR (1980) *Data Systems and Management,* 2nd ed. Englewood Cliffs, NJ: Prentice Hall.

Kotz, S and Johnson, NL (eds-in-chief)(1982–1988) *Encyclopedia of Statistical Sciences* (9 vols). New York: John Wiley & Sons.

Lefkowitz, JM (1985) *Introduction to Statistical Computer Packages.* Boston: Duxbury Press.

Liedel, NA and Busch, KA (1985) Statistical design and data analysis requirements. In *Patty's Industrial Hygiene and Toxicology,* Vol III, *Theory and Rational for Industrial Hygiene Practice,* 2nd ed, 3A, *The Work Environment,* LJ Cralley and LV Cralley, (eds) pp. 395–507. New York: John Wiley & Sons.

Little, RJA And Rubin, DB (1987) *Statistical Analysis with Missing Data.* New York: John Wiley & Sons.

Little, RJA and Smith, PJ (1987) Editing and imputation for quantitative survey data. *J Am Stat Assoc* 82:58–68.

Luce, RD and Narensm, L (1987) Measurement scales on the continuum. *Science* 236:1527–1532.

Marshall, E (1988) The scourge of computer viruses. *Science* 240:133–134.

Newcombe, HB (1988) *Handbook of Record Linkage: Methods of Health and Statistical Studies, Administration and Business.* New York: Oxford University Press.

Nixon, WJ and Brown, MB (eds) (1979) *BMDP-79, Biomedical Computer Programs, P-Series,* Berkeley: University of California Press.

Oppenheim, AN (1968) *Questionnaire Design and Attitude Measurement.* London: Heinemann Education Books.

Paredaens, J (ed)(1987) *Databases.* Orlando, FL: Academic Press.

Peter, R (1988) An average reader finishes this article in about 2 1/2 minutes [about an idea of alerting tax form preparers about the paper burden estimates]. *The New York Times,* March 8.

Sande, IG (1982) Imputation in surveys: Coping and reality. *Am Stat* 36:145–152.

SAS (1985) *SAS® User's Guide: Statistics, Version 5 Edition.* Cary, NC: SAS Institute.

SAS 1982) *SAS® User's Guide: Basics.* Cary, NC: SAS Institute.

Schmid, CF (1983) *Statistical Graphics: Design Principles and Practices.* New York: John Wiley & Sons.

Schmid, CF and Schmid, SE (1979) *Handbook of Graphic Presentation.* New York: John Wiley & Sons.

Shayne, G and Weil, C (1986) *Statistics and Experimental Design for Toxicologists.* Caldwell, NJ: The Teldfor Press.

SPSS Inc (1983) *SPSS X: User's Guide.* New York: McGraw-Hill Co.

Stellman, SD (1989) The case of the missing eights: An object lesson in data quality assurance. *Am J Epidemiol* 129(4):857–860.

Tuckey, JW (1977) *Exploratory Data Analysis.* Reading, MA: Addison-Wesley.

Tufte, ER (1983) *The Visual Display of Quantitative Information.* Cheshire, CT: Graphics.

Wainer, H (1984) How to display data badly. *Am Stat* 38:137–147.

Walter, RK (1986) *Introduction to Data Management and Design.* Englewood Cliffs, NJ: Prentice Hall.

Wilcox, KR, Baynes, TE, Crable JV, et al. (1978) *Quality Assurance Practices for Health Laboratories.* Washington, DC: American Public Health Association.

Young, ML (1979) Legal responsibility of the scientist in handling data. *Clin Toxicol* 15(5):605–611.

15

Introduction to Data Analysis

Webster's dictionary defines *analysis* as the act of separating or breaking up any whole into its parts so as to find out their nature, proportion, function, and relationships, and, importantly, a statement of the results of this process. In this chapter we examine in detail the process by which neurological causation is established, that is, the link between the human absorption of a chemical compound and neuropsychological function. It is assumed that the rationale and uses of the chi-square test, *t*-test, regression equations, correlation coefficients, and the notions of association and causality are understood. Those who are not familiar with these concepts are urged to consult the many available textbooks included among this chapter's Suggested Readings. Those interested in statistics as it pertains to animal research—which is not discussed here—are directed to the book by Gad and Weil, *Statistics and Experimental Design for Toxicologists,* published in 1986.

DATA ANALYSIS AND STATISTICS

Teaching data analysis shares a lot with teaching painting. In both cases a mentor places himself or herself as a role model in a creative process in which the tools—and sometimes the tricks—of an art are taught in order to accomplish specific objectives (ie, the "vision" of an artist or the "truth" of a scientist). The comparison is appropriate: data analysis requires intuition, a sort of "knowing" that results from many years of contact and familiarity with data, any sort of data.

Science teaching is experiencing a revolution in that the intuitive process that is at the core of scientific analysis is finally being recognized as important. It is not a coincidence that as the rote part of science—such as computation, which once occupied a major part of the training in data analysis—is now taken up by electronic calculators and by personal computers, the role of imagination is now placed in the fore.

An alert reader may wonder why I choose to designate this series of chapters as "data analysis" rather than "statistics." This is because statistics provides only one of several possible models of data analysis. Granted, probably 95% of all reports in environmental health sciences involve some sort of statistical analysis. But, as will be seen later, this may change in the future.

The Evolution of Procedures for Data Analysis in Health Research

Data-analytical methods in epidemiology and toxicology evolved from case observations to an increasing reliance on quantitative methods and statistics. Ramazzini, the father of modern occupational medicine, was both a physician and an epidemiologist. In his book *Diseases of Workers* (1713), Ramazzini who probably knew all there was to be known about medicine and epidemiology in his time, used almost no quantitative information in describing the diseases of workers.

═══════════════════════

When epidemiology—a quantitative discipline since its beginning—developed as an independent endeavor in the 19th century, little overlap existed between epidemiology and occupational medicine. Hamilton's early publications, for example, relied on case presentations. A case presentation is a discussion of a "typical" example that reveals a larger truth. A report on a case of lead poisoning, for example, is indicative of the health hazards of lead in general. (The importance of case presentations as sentinel events is discussed in Chapter 19.) When a cluster of cases were discussed, percentages were, in the early 1900s, the most rigorous and most generally accepted form of quantitative expression. In clinical medicine, they still are.

Both Ramazzini and Hamilton established causation between occupational exposures and health effects on the basis of case presentations and subjectively perceived associations. The bases of these inferences were rarely questioned. The notion that the observers were "experts" in the field was enough proof. Importantly, in most cases, they did not ask why or how this association existed. It is only recently that dose–response relationships and mechanism of action are expected to complement a claim of toxic causation.

The changes in data-analytical strategies are the reflection of the increasing demands for "causation" and "mechanisms of action" that researchers in the field are expected to address. Thus, environmental and occupational health scientists today need to rely increasingly on the methods that are commonplace in mathematics and in pharmacological studies of drugs carried out in experimental animals.

Health researchers most probably improved their methods as a result of criticisms by those who created the health problem in the first place. Among the few positive things that can be said about the health hazards of smoking, asbestos, lead, pesticides, etc is that the process of trying to understand their health effects, assessing human risks, and extrapolating laboratory results to human populations stimulated vigorous efforts on the part of statisticians hired by industry who criticized these studies. Statisticians and epidemiologists are now routinely consulted by people in industry, both to improve their own standards of data analysis and to seek and discover weaknesses and mistakes by their colleagues on the other side of a controversy. Long complacent, E & O toxicologists were forced into the development of a stronger science.

═══════════════════════

Variables

One of the first data-analytical steps in almost all kinds of research is the recognition of variables. In the previous chapter on data management, a variable was defined as any attribute or property that varies, that is, can have different values. The following are examples of variables commonly encountered in epidemiological research:

- Gender—ie, either male or female
- Age in years
- Level of lead exposure in job category—ie, "low," "medium," or "high"
- Use of respirator ("Yes" or "No")
- Involvement in a litigation concerning occupation-induced illness ("Yes" or "No")
- Results of blood and urinalysis
- Presence or absence of signs and symptoms of peripheral nervous system dysfunction
- Voltages from a study of somatic sensory cortical potentials
- Results of psychometric tests

The *nature* and the *position* of the variables in theoretical models describing how environmental and occupational toxic agents affect neuropsychological functioning are two important attributes that need to be reviewed because they determine—along with the study design—the selection of appropriate statistical tests.

The nature of the variables was discussed in the previous chapter, namely, that four types of data are encountered: nominal, ordinal, interval, and ratio. It is also important to recognize the position of variables in models.

The Position of Variables in Models

The "position" of a variable means whether the variable is dependent, independent, or a confounder, as defined below. In experimental toxicology, the *independent variable* is the treatment variable, the quantity that is under the control of the experimenter. For example, in the experimental study of the chronic effects of inhaling a given solvent, the concentration of solvents (in parts per million) is the independent variable.

In epidemiology, the independent variable is *not* under the control of the investigator. The concentration of pesticides found in the blood of chemical operators, for example, is dependent on the laborers' daily contact with this chemical compound, the method of pesticide application, the use of protective equipment, and the observance of hygiene practices, just to name the most obvious factors.

The independent variable is often thought of as the cause of a change. For example, the level of solvent in the exposure chamber where a laboratory rat is housed and the level of pesticides in the environment where people work are thought to be potential determinants of adverse health effects. However, as we saw in Chapter 9, scientists rarely think in terms of these simplistic models. Rather, they consider both the environmental level and the biological indicators of absorption as potential causes of health problems.

When independent variables are placed in a model for statistical analysis, similar statistical procedures are followed regardless of whether the independent variables are under the investigator's control.

A *dependent variable* is always defined in relation to independent variables. Dependent variables are those thought to vary as a result of introducing the independent variable. Thus, they are thought to be, in experimental toxicology, the effect of an experimental treatment; in human epidemiology, the dependent variable is often called an *outcome*.

In a theoretical model, the position of a variable may act as a *confounder*—a factor that distorts the apparent magnitude of the relationship between two other variables (see Chapter 18). Gender, race, age, ethnic background, income, and education are well-recognized confounders in the analysis of neurotoxic effects in human epidemiological studies. If any of these factors are present, the investigator is expected to explain how he or she has dealt with them. In experimental animal studies, body weight and gender—or their interaction, because a male mouse, for example, usually weighs more than a female mouse—are common confounders.

The same variable may be either an independent, a dependent, or a confounding variable depending on the objective of the research. Alcohol intake is an example. In a study on the effect of alcohol on performance, alcohol is an independent variable—the investigator wants to know whether and how alcohol impairs performance. In a study on the effect of occupational stress on alcohol intake, alcohol is a dependent variable—stress is hypothesized to lead people to drink. In a study on the effect of lead among laborers, alcohol intake needs to be taken into account as a confounder—lead may be a problem, but alcohol is as well. Figure 15.1 is a block diagram illustrating the relationships among independent, dependent, and confounding variables.

In Chapter 19, additional variables (sometimes called factors or causes) will also be identified, namely, direct and indirect, proximal and remote. These types of variables are important in forensic sciences. In addition, the reader will be introduced to seemingly

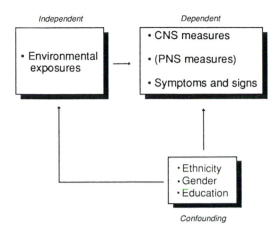

Independent

Dependent

• Environmental
 exposures

• CNS measures

• (PNS measures)

• Symptoms and signs

• Ethnicity
• Gender
• Education

Confounding

Fig. 15.1 Relationships among independent, dependent, and confounding variables. CNS, central nervous system; PNS, peripheral nervous system.

perplexing data-analytical strategies in which a construct (a hypothetical factor) is said to be the reason the data look the way they do. These are factor-analysis and latent-variable models.

Although a review of common and different features of statistical methodology as used in experimental science (eg, the study of neurotoxic agents in animals and humans under laboratory conditions) and nonexperimental science (eg, epidemiological studies of children exposed to various levels of lead) is relevant, such a review is beyond the scope of the present chapter. Here and in the following three chapters, only methodology as used in the epidemiological study of neurotoxic effects in humans is discussed.

STATISTICS AS A SCIENTIFIC FIELD

It is commonly accepted that the convergence between statistics and toxicology occurred in the 1960s as scientists were confronted with problems of increasing difficulty and as a result began to be questioned, often within legal contexts (Gad and Weill 1986).

Until recently, analytic chemists and toxicologists were rarely trained in quantitative thinking and statistical methodology beyond the use of the chi-square test, t-test, linear regression, and sometimes analysis of variance. Now, among toxicologists and human health scientists, computer-based statistical skills are considered essential.

It was not until the late 1970s that statisticians began to make important contributions to the methodology of the environmental and occupational health sciences. But even today, dual training in statistics and biological sciences is the exception rather than the rule.

Last (1983) defines statistics as "the science and art of dealing with variation in data through collection, classification, and analysis in such a way as to obtain reliable results." ("Statistics" is also the name reserved for the data themselves, a term widely used in journalism that will not be favored here.) Statistics encompasses several branches.

Statistics is both a theoretical and an applied discipline. In its theoretical aspects, statisticians are involved in the creation and validation of new analytical and evaluative procedures and the ascertainment of limits of applicability of well-established methods. In the 1980s this "pure" aspect of the discipline appears to have bloomed as the foundation for essential concepts in epidemiology such as risk analysis and the applicability of animal data to human populations. Many articles that have appeared in recent years in the *American Journal of Statistics* and *The American Statistician* deal with the adequacy of statistical procedures for environmental and occupational health matters.

Descriptive statistics is one of the simplest forms of applied statistics involving the quantitative characterization of exposures—the independent variables—and health effects—the dependent variables. Traditionally, in epidemiological and toxicological research, descriptive statistics has been, to a large extent, univariate statistics.

Inferential statistics is the use of statistical concepts for scientific research in general and for hypothesis testing in particular. Inferential statistics is closely linked to modeling.

Univariate statistics is a collection of concepts and methods dealing with the description of the quantitative and statistical variables taken one at a time. For example, the contrast in age, education, gender, and ethnic background between two populations exposed to welding fumes is an example of univariate statistics. Often, univariate statistics also involve the relationship between two variables at a time, for example, a cross tabulation of education and age in two groups exposed to toxic agents.

Multivariate statistics is a collection of concepts and methods for dealing with the quantitative and statistical description of the relationships of more than two variables at a time. There are procedures that deal with several independent variables and one dependent variable and others—less frequently used in toxicology and epidemiology—dealing with the description of several independent and several dependent variables. Today, E & O neurotoxicology is relying increasingly on the use of multivariate statistics in the description of relationships between toxic exposures and health effects.

STATISTICS AS A SCIENTIFIC METHOD

Statistics provides an agreed-upon methodology for data analysis, one of the most important of which is modeling.

Modeling

A model is the physical or conceptual reproduction of the essential aspects of a system necessary to predict the behavior of the system or to explain why the system works in the manner it does. In Chapter 24 we will see how Békésy was able to discover the traveling wave when he reproduced the essential human cochlea in a rubber model and thus could predict and explain how sounds were translated into neural messages. Békésy's is an example of a physical model; in toxicology, models are generally less tangible. Figure 15.1 is a generalized model of toxic causation

that is probably true for the effects of the vast majority of environmental neurotoxic agents.

Models are used in E & O neurotoxicology essentially for the same purposes: to predict and to explain. Until recently, toxicologists and epidemiologists gave justifiable emphasis to the use of statistical concepts to predict the levels of toxic agents in the environment that might be harmful to human health. For example, the level of lead in blood considered harmful to the adult—40 µg/dL of blood—is a prediction that resulted from numerous studies on the relationship between blood lead levels and changes in various targets such as the blood-forming system, the nervous system, and the kidney.

As the association between toxic dose and health effects became firmly established, the need arose to explain why the toxic agents cause the effect. There is an intimate relationship between statistical models used to predict and models used to explain. Once the mechanism of action of lead in the brain of children was understood, for example, this information was often applied to refine the prediction of the statistical models.

The Use of Statistical Models in Toxicology

Statistical models were once feared in toxicology. Among other things, it was thought that statistical models would replace the painful procedures of data collection requiring hands-on experience with various in vitro and in vivo techniques, which pharmacologists and toxicologists alike use to study the drug effects in living systems. It was thought that statistical modeling might create a further distance between raw data and the inferences that can be made from these data.

Both the gathering and organization of data as well as sometimes piercing and imaginative uses of statistical models are essential. We have gone from a period where the question to ask was "show me the data," into one in which the question was "show me the way the data have been analyzed," into an even more exciting one in which novel analytical strategies such as the use of computer-intensive methods and computer-generated graphics (described below) are being increasingly proposed.

Decision-System Approach

The most recent approach in teaching data-analytical techniques is the decision-system approach. A decision system is a semiformalized statement of how and where to proceed on the basis of the available information. Figure 15.2 illustrates the concept of a decision system in which all possible branches of the decision-making process are shown at the same time. This approach is important in that it is based on what experienced analysts think and do when confronted with data.

Andrews et al. (1981) have published a valuable small book titled *A Guide for Selecting Statistical Techniques for Analyzing Social Science Data* using this approach.

The following is a highly schematic decision system that health scientists confront and resolve vis-à-vis their data.

1. Dependent variables
    a) Does one have information on environmental (chemical) exposures?
    b) Does one have information on indirect measures of neurotoxic exposure?
    c) Does one have information on biological indicators of neurotoxic effects?
2. Dependent variables
    a) Are clinical (neurological, psychiatric, neuropsychological) evaluations performed by trained observers available?
    b) Is there any other information gathered in a systematic, quantitative form (eg, questionnaires) available?
    c) Are there results of objective examining or testing procedures (eg, imaging, psychometric or neurophysiological tests) available?

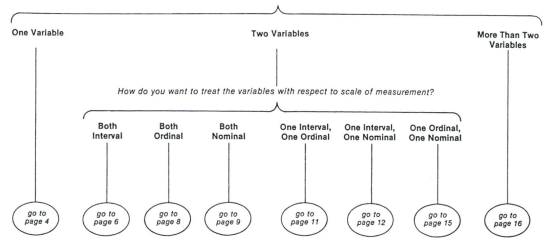

Fig. 15.2. An example of a decision system for analysis of statistical data. (From Institute of Social Research, University of Michigan, and Andrews et al. 1981.)

3. Confounding variables
   a) Have demographic variables of the subjects (eg, age, gender, ethnic background, education) been properly obtained?
   b) Are there any other confounding variables unique to the study population suspected?
4. Assessment of dose–response relationships and cause
   a) The judgment of adverse health effects attributed to a suspected toxic agent is based on observed group differences (eg, the difference in prevalence rate of neurological signs and symptoms of a study group compared with control populations).
   b) The judgment of adverse health effects attributed to the suspected toxic agent is based on an association between levels of the toxic agent and the levels of outcome.
   c. There is one single toxic agent in the environment that is suspected (eg, lead, pesticide), but there is information available on several outcomes (eg, results of biochemical tests, neurological signs and symptoms, results of psychometric testing).
   d) There are several agents having a neurotoxic potential and some confounding variables, but there is a single measure of outcome (eg, psychometric tests only).
5. Assessment of cause and underlying mechanisms by means of multivariate analysis
   a) The analysis of group differences in neuropsychological functioning.
   b) The study of contrasts.
   c) Correlational analysis.
   d) Threshold determinations.
   e) Multiregression analysis.
   f) Larger perspectives of causation.

The following four chapters contain a detailed analysis of the branches this decision tree leads to. However, alternative data-analytical strategies will also be quickly reviewed.

ALTERNATIVE DATA-ANALYTICAL STRATEGIES

Bayesian statistics (described below), computer-intensive methods, and graphics are increasingly being used as alternative data-analytical strategies in environmental health sciences.

Bayesian Statistics

Bayesian statistics is rapidly being assimilated into epidemiology but is literally absent in toxicology (Neutra and Drolette 1978). Bayesian statistics differs from statistical methods in that the former is not based on the notion of frequency distribution. It was proposed by Thomas Bayes (1702–1761), an English clergyman and mathematician, author of *Essay Toward Solving a Problem of the Doctrine of Chance*. This book contains the Bayes theorem.

The Bayes theorem is a theorem in probability theory. According to Last (1983), it is used in epidemiology ". . . to obtain the probability of disease in a group of people with some characteristics on the basis of the overall rate of that disease (the prior probability of disease) and of the likelihood of those characteristics [appearing] in healthy and disabled individuals." The Bayes theorem is supported by the clinical intuition that, given a symptom, the probability of a disease depends not only on how characteristic the symptom is of the disease but also on how frequently the disease occurs in the population studied.

Bayesian statistics is different from frequency-distribution-based statistics in three major ways: the use of prior information to ascertain probabilities, the notion of subjective probability, and the notion of conditional probability.

Computer-Intensive Procedures

Although computers have long been recognized as having had a profound impact on statistics, the extent of this impact has not been adequately reviewed in standard textbooks of statistics. Computer-intensive procedures are often alternatives to well-known standard statistical techniques. Four examples are discussed: sorting, bootstrapping, and classic and computer graphics.

Sorting. Some applications of computer-intensive procedures have resolved some of the problems associated with graphing a bivariate versus a continuum variable. For example, in a recent work (Lilis and Valciukas 1985), this author suggested a method of plotting values relating blood lead levels and neurological symptoms that relies on the ease with which computers perform sorting. The study group was comprised of 680 active copper smelter workers exposed to lead and arsenic. (For the purpose of illustrating this point, arsenic will be ignored.) Blood lead levels were low in general. If the usual approach of establishing subgroups splitting the range of blood lead levels had been chosen (less than 40 μg/dL; between 40 and 59 μg/dL; and equal to or greater than 60 μg/dL), the means would have represented groups of highly different sizes. This is a reflection of the fact that most people had low blood lead and few had high blood lead levels, and therefore the distribution is highly skewed.

The following procedure was used to give each data point of the independent variable (blood levels) an equal weight. First, the 680 currently active copper smelter workers were sorted by increasing levels of lead in blood. Second, the median for each subgroup of 50 subjects was calculated. Thus, 14 data points (representing the median of each ascending subgroup) were obtained (Fig. 15.3). The dependent variable (prevalence of individual neurological symptoms) was computed by dividing the number of subjects reporting the symptom by the total number of subjects in

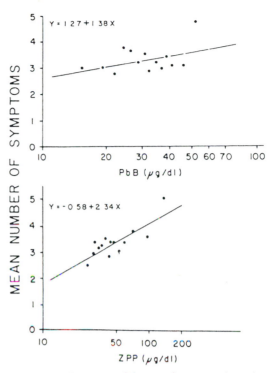

Fig. 15.3. Illustration of the use of computer-intensive methods for the study of the relationships between blood lead levels and neurological symptoms (see text). Number of reported symptoms as a function of levels of blood lead (Pb-B) and zinc protoporphyrin (ZPP) in active copper smelter workers ($N = 678$ for Pb-B and $N = 673$ for ZPP). (From Lilis, R. et al. 1985.)

each subgroup as defined above. As a result, each point now represents 50 individuals and therefore has an identical "weight" when the dose–response relationship is studied.

In this report, it was concluded that central nervous system symptoms—such as fatigue, sleep disturbances, weakness, paresthesia, and joint pain—are related to both blood lead and zinc protoporphyrin (an indicator of lead effects) levels. The regression line of the latter consistently exhibited a steeper slope with symptoms, indicating a comparatively higher sensitivity than blood lead. Most important, there was no evidence of a threshold for lead effects.

Bootstrapping. Diasconis and Efron (1983) argued that most statistical methods in common use today were developed between 1880 and 1930, when computation was slow and expensive. With the advent of computers with larger and larger memory and faster speeds, billions of operations can now be performed in a few seconds. The payoff for such intensive computation, these investigators argue, is freedom from two limiting factors that have dominated statistical theory since its beginnings: the assumption that the data conform to a bell-shaped curve and the need to focus on statistical measures whose theoretical properties can be analyzed mathematically. The bootstrap method is one example.

The bootstrap method was developed in 1977 by Efron. The name derives from the proverbial man who wanted to go up in the air by pulling on his bootstraps. It is a method for estimating the accuracy of statistics from data on a single sample. A sample contains a lot of information on the frequency distribution of the statistics for the universe. "It is as if statisticians had discovered the statistical analogue of the hologram, a pattern of light wave that is preserved on a surface. The scene from which the light waves are emitted can be reconstructed in great detail from the whole surface of the hologram, but, if pieces of the surface are broken off, the entire scene can still be reconstructed from each piece" (Diaconis and Efron 1983, p. 122).

For example, the bootstrapping method for calculating the frequency distribution of the correlation coefficient r from data on two tests of 15 schools involves copying the data from each school a billion times. The resulting 15 billion copies are thoroughly mixed, 1000 samples of size 15 are then selected at random, and the correlation coefficient is calculated for each sample. Copying, mixing, and selecting are done via computers. The distribution of the correlation coefficients for the bootstrap samples can be treated as if it were a distribution for real samples. The width of the interval is the measure of accuracy of the statistics for the sample. There have been applications of bootstrap methods in envi-

ronmental sciences (eg, estimates of distribution patterns of acid rain).

Classic Graphic Methods. Ronnie D. Horner of the Department of Family Medicine, East Carolina University School of Medicine, Greenville, North Carolina, argued that clues to the relative importance of possible etiological factors for dementia of the Alzheimer's type may be gained by examining the fit of cases of Sartwell's model of the distribution of incubation periods. Sartwell demonstrated that the natural variation in the incubation period of many infectious diseases conforms to a distribution of the logarithmic/normal type, also called the lognormal curve. In the lognormal curve, the ordinate is the cumulative percentage of cases, and the abscissa is the logarithm, in this case, of age at onset in years.

In a paper published in 1987, Horner published the results of a secondary analysis of data on the age of onset of cases of Alzheimer's disease of four case series available from the published literature. If age at disease onset is used as the incubation period of the disease, a genetic or environmental factor acting during the prenatal period is suggested if the distribution of these ages fits the lognormal curve; otherwise, environmental factors acting after birth are thought to be implicated.

The distribution of age at disease onset for each series was graphically and statistically assessed for fit to the lognormal distribution. Each case series fit the lognormal curve well. To Horner, this suggested that research into the etiology of dementia of the Alzheimer's type should focus on the prenatal experiences of patients with this disease.

Computer Graphics. Computer graphics have now come into use in statistics. It has been mentioned at the beginning of this chapter that statistics never attempted to replace intuition and "the uniquely human ability to recognize meaningful patterns in data" (Kolata 1982). Recently developed computer software allows the visualization of data in manners depicted from standard statistical techniques. In particular, the depiction of color-coded, multidimensional data on computer screens, data that can be rotated along various axes at various speeds, allows statisticians to find relationships never thought possible.

Some investigators resent the excessive reliance on graphs. Gladen and Bogan (1983), for example, stated: "If a graph is considered to be merely the alternative to a table (a list of numbers), then almost any format [for graphs] will be acceptable. However, we think that the function of a graph is to convey an immediate impression of the relationship among these numbers, and thus the format becomes critical." On these grounds, they suggest that "graphs of rate ratios often fail to give an adequate visual impression of the information because the scale of the graph does not correspond to the scale of the data."

REFERENCES

Andrews, FM, Klem, L, Davidson, TN, et al. (1981) *A Guide for Selecting Statistical Techniques for Analyzing Social Science Data.* Ann Arbor: Survey Research Center, The University of Michigan.

Diaconis, P and Efron B (1983) Computer intensive methods in statistics. *Scient Am* 248(5):116–130.

Gad, S and Weil, CS (1986) *Statistics and Experimental Design for Toxicologists.* Caldwell, NJ: Telford Press.

Gladen, BC and Bogan, WJ (1983) On graphing rate ratios. *Am J Epidemiol* 118:905–908.

Horner, RD (1987) Age of onset of Alzheimer's disease: Clue to the relative importance of etiologic factors? *Am J Epidemiol* 126(3):409–414.

Kolata, G (1982) Computer graphics comes to statistics. *Science* 217:919–920.

Last, JM (1983) *A Dictionary of Epidemiology.* New York: Oxford University Press.

Lilis, R, Valciukas, JA, Malkin, J, et al. (1985) Effect of low-level lead and arsenic exposure on copper smelter workers. *Arch Environ Health* 40:38–47.

Neutra, RR and Drolette, ME (1978) Estimating exposure-specific disease rates from case-control studies using Bayes's theorem. *Am J Epidemiol* 108:214–222.

Ramazzini, B (1713) *De Morbis Artificum Diatriba* (translated as *Diseases of Workers*). New York: New York Academy of Medicine.

SUGGESTED READINGS

Ad Hoc Committee on Professional Ethics (1983) Ethical guidelines for statistical practice. *Am Stat* 37:1–20.

Aigner, DJ and Goldberger, AS (eds) (1977) *Latent Variables in Socioeconomic Models.* Amsterdam: North Holland.

Alwin, DF and Tessler, RC (1974) Causal models, unobservable variables, and experimental data. *Am J Sociol* 80:58–86.

Anderson, AJB (1988) *Interpreting Data.* New York: Chapman and Hall.

Asher, HB (1976) *Causal Modeling.* Beverly Hills: Sage.

Baggaley, AR (1964) *Intermediate Correlational Methods.* New York: John Wiley & Sons.

Baka, D (1966) The test of significance in psychological research. *Psychol Bull* 66:432–437.

Blalock, HM (ed) (1971) *Causal Models in the Social Sciences.* Chicago: Aldine-Atherton.

Bolton, S (1984) *Pharmaceutical Statistics: Practical and Clinical Applications.* New York: Marcel Dekker.

Broemeling, LD (1985) *Bayesian Analysis of Linear Models.* New York: Marcel Dekker.

Brook, RJ and Arnold, G (1985) *Applied Regression Analysis and Experimental Design.* New York: Marcel Dekker.

Cattell, RB (1978): *The Scientific Use of Factor Analysis in Behavioral and Life Sciences.* New York: Plenum Press.

Cowles, M and Davis, C (1982) On the origins of the .05 level of statistical significance. *Am Psychol* 5:553–558.

Cox, DR (1970) *Analysis of Binary Data.* London: Methuen.

Darby, WP and Cohaga, JK (1988) Analysis of bioassay data drawn from several sources. *J Am Coll Toxicol* 7(5):591–601.

DeGroot, M, Fienberg, S, and Kadane, JB (eds) (1986) *Statistics and the Law.* New York: John Wiley & Sons.

Denby, L and Pregibon, D (1987) An example of the use of graphics in regression. *Am Stat* 41:33–38.

Drapper, NR and Smith, H (1981) *Applied Regression Analysis,* 2nd ed. New York: John Wiley & Sons.

Eaton, WW (1975) Causal models for the study of prevalence. *Soc Forces* 54:415–426.

Feinberg, SE and Straf, ML (1982) Statistical assessments as evidence. *J R Stat Soc [A]* 145:410–421.

Finkelstein, MO (1980) The judicial reception of multiple regression studies in race and sex discrimination cases. *Columbia Law Rev* 80:737–754.

Fisher, FM (1980) Multiregression in legal proceedings. *Columbia Law Rev* 80:702–736.

Fisher, FM (1986) Statisticians, econometricians, and adversary proceedings. *Am Stat Assoc* 81:277–286.

Freeman, DH (1987) *Applied Categorical Data Analysis.* New York: Marcel Dekker.

Gad, SC and Weil, CS (1988) *Statistics and Experimental Design for Toxicologists,* 2nd ed. Caldwell, NJ: Telford.

Gibbons, JD (1973) A question of ethics. *Am Stat* 27:72–76.

Gnanadesikan, R and Kettenring, JR (1984) A pragmatic review of multivariate methods in applications. In *Statistics: An Appraisal: Proceedings of the 50th Anniversary Conference of the Iowa State University Statistics Laboratory,* pp. 309–337. Ames, IA: Iowa State University Press.

Haber, A, Runyon, RP, and Badia, P (eds) (1970) *Readings in Statistics.* Reading, MA: Addison-Wesley.

Hacking, I (1984) Trial by number: Karl Pearson's chi-square test measured the fit between theory and reality, ushering in a new sort of decision making. *Science '84* November, pp. 69–70.

Hamilton, A (1925) *Industrial Poisons in the United States.* New York: Macmillan.

Hartly, HO (1980) Statistics as a science and as profession. *J Am Stat Assoc* 75:1–7.

Hedges, LV and Olkin, I (1985) *Statistical Methods for Meta-Analysis.* New York: Academic Press.

Heise, DR (1975) *Causal Analysis.* New York: John Wiley & Sons.

Hellevik, O (1988) *Introduction to Causal Analysis: Exploring Survey Data by Cross-Tabulation.* New York: Oxford University Press.

Hill, AB (1965) The environment and disease: Association or causation? *Proc R Soc Med* 58:295–300.

Hofstadter, DR (1982) Metamagical themas: Number numbness or why innumeracy may be just as dangerous as illiteracy. *Sci Am* 246:20–34.

Huff, D (1973) *How to Lie with Statistics.* Middlesex: Penguin Books.

James, IR and Knuiman, MW (1987) An application of Bayes methodology to the analysis of diary records from water use study. *J Am Stat Assoc* 82:705–711.

Kelsey, JL, Thompson, WD, and Evans, AS (1986) *Methods in Observational Epidemiology.* New York: Oxford University Press.

Kenny, DA (1979) *Correlation and Causality.* New York: John Wiley & Sons.

Levi, E (1948) *An Introduction to Legal Reasoning.* Chicago: Phoenix Books (reprinted by University of Chicago Press, 1962).

Marquart, DW (1987) The importance of statisticians. *J Am Stat Assoc* 82(397):1–7.

Marshall, E (1983) EPA faults classic lead poisoning study. *Science* 222:906–907.

Meier, P (1986) Damned liars and expert witness. *J Am Stat Assoc* 81:269–276.

Muller, KE, Barton, CN, and Benignus, VA (1984) Recommendations for appropriate statistical practice in toxicological experiments. *Neurotoxicology* 5(2):113–126.

Newell, D (1982) The role of the statistician as an expert witness. *J R Stat Soc* [A] 145:403–409.

Owen, DB (Ed) (1976) *On the History of Statistics and Probability.* New York: Marcel Dekker.

Peterson, DW (1983) Statistical inference in litigation. *Law Contemp Prob* 46(4):1–303.

Proceedings of the Biopharmaceutical Section (1986) Alexandria, VA: American Statistical Association.

Tukey, JW (1977) *Exploratory Data Analysis.* Reading, MA: Addison-Wesley.

Vandernbroucke, JP (1987) Should we abandon statistical modeling altogether? *Am J Epidemiol* 126:10–13.

Walker, HM (1929) *Studies in the History of Statistical Method.* Baltimore, MD: Williams & Wilkins.

Wallenstein, S (1986) *Pharmaceutical Statistics: Practical and Clinical Applications* by S Bolton (book review). *J Am Stat Assoc* 81:576–577.

Walter, SD, Feinstein, AR, and Wells, CK (1987) Coding ordinal independent variables in multiple regression analysis. *Am J Epidemiol* 125:319–323.

Weed, DL (1986) On the logic of causal inference. *Am J Epidemiol* 123:965–979.

16

Assessment of Human Exposure and Dose

In the following two chapters we examine the process of transformation of data obtained from data-gathering devices into variables. This chapter deals with the independent variables: environmental levels of chemical compounds and/or levels of bio logical indicators of exposure and absorption. The next chapter deals with the de pendent variables: measures of nervous system function as ascertained by clinical (observational) methods, psychometric procedures and/or electrophysiological techniques.

The topics of air, soil, and water sampling and the analytical methods used to characterize these substances chemically are beyond the scope of this book. The book edited by O'Donoghue, *Neurotoxicity of Industrial and Commercial Chemicals,* published in 1985, and the book by Lauwerys, *Industrial Chemical Exposure: Guidelines for Biological Monitoring,* published in 1983, are good introductions to this topic.

In Chapter 10, the notion was introduced that in epidemiological studies of neurotoxic illnesses, human dose can rarely be fully characterized as is sometimes possible in laboratory-based experimental toxicology. In human epidemiological studies, it can only be estimated. In recent years, there has been an increasing interaction among industrial hygienists, analytical chemists, pharmacologists, epidemiologists, and statisticians to define human dose. Figure 16.1 shows in an oversimplified view the key phases that can be identified between the environmental presence of a neurotoxicant, exposures, absorption, and, ultimately, neuropsychological effect.

From the data-analytical point of view, it should be noted that in a study of environmental levels, the focus of the study (usually an industrial hygiene study) is the substance present in the environment or the workplace; these levels are measured in units that are appropriate for each chemical compound—eg, parts per million (ppm). On the other hand, in the assessment of exposures and human dose, the individual is the focus of the investigation. How high is the exposure to mercury at the workplace? How much mercury has been absorbed by each of the 120 workers who presently work at the plant? These levels are assessed by several strategies, some of which are reviewed in this chapter, and the units of measurement take several factors into consideration—eg, modes of application, protective equipment, hygienic

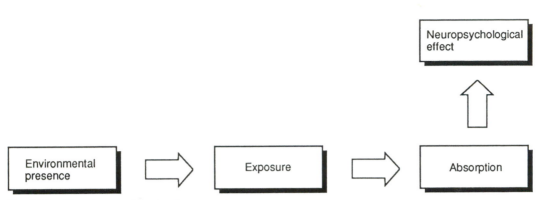

Fig. 16.1. The pharmacokinesis of neurotoxic compounds in humans.

practices, hours per day, days per week, weeks per year.

Although it is not always possible, under ideal circumstances the first step of an environmental and occupational study is the characterization of the environment in which people live or workers work. A great deal of sophistication has been achieved in the identification, measurement, and quantitative study of chemical compounds in the environment and the workplace that can be harmful to the nervous system. Figure 16.2, for example, is

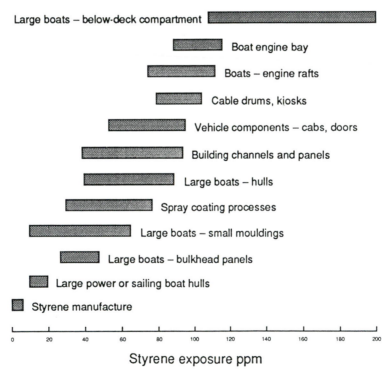

Styrene exposure ppm

Fig. 16.2. Environmental levels of styrene (in ppm) as measured in various occupational environments. [From Morris, DG. Hygiene strategies and regulatory aspects. In *Organic Solvents and the Central Nervous System*. WHO Regional Office for Europe, Copenhagen, 1985, p. 272 (Environmental Health Series, No. 5).]

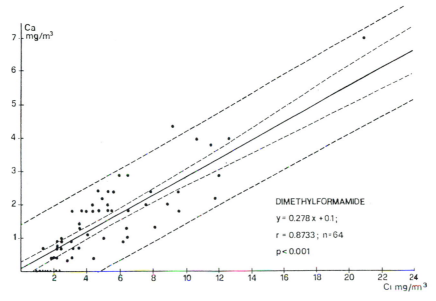

Fig. 16.3. Dose–response relationship between alveolar (Ca) and airborne (Ci) concentrations of demethylformamide under laboratory conditions. [From Brugone, F. and Perbillini, L. Biological monitoring of occupational exposure to solvents by analysis of alveolar air and blood. In *Organic Solvents and the Central Nervous System*. WHO Regional Office for Europe, Copenhagen, 1985, p. 60 (Environmental Health Series, No. 5).]

an illustration of ranges of environmental levels of styrene to which different occupational groups are exposed. Note that nothing is said about how styrene is absorbed and ultimately affects—either acutely or chronically—nervous system function. These measurements help to characterize the relative risk of such neurotoxic exposure—in this case, styrene—in various occupations. These measures are essential for the monitoring and controlling of harmful substances in the environment and the workplace.

The second step is the description of dose–response relationships between environmental levels of chemical exposure and biological indicators of human exposure, such as blood lead levels or levels of mandelic acid, a biological marker of styrene exposure. Figure 16.3, for example, is a study of such relationships obtained in humans under laboratory conditions. By mathematical extrapolation from these data, it is possible to ascertain from these experimental studies the buildup of concentration levels in the human body and the time it takes to excrete them.

Epidemiological studies sometimes take advantage of natural experiments—eg, environmental health problems existing in a community—to study dose–response relationships between environmental levels of

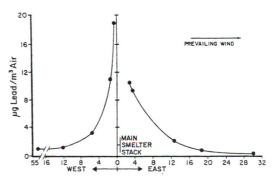

Fig. 16.4. Particulate lead concentration in air as a function of distance from a source of environmental lead. (From Landrigan et al., 1976, reprinted by permission of Mosby.)

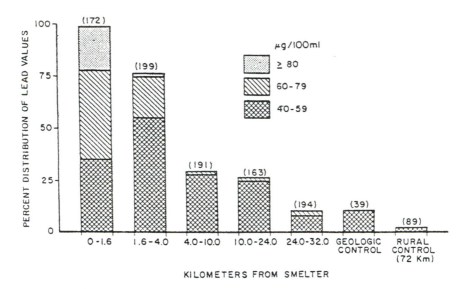

Fig. 16.5. Blood lead levels as a function of the distance from the source of environmental lead. (From Landrigan et al., 1976, reprinted by permission of Mosby.)

chemical compounds and levels of biological indicators of absorption. Figure 16.4 shows concentration levels in air of particulate lead in relation to the proximity of a lead-smelting facility. Figure 16.5 contains the distribution patterns of values of blood lead as a function of the distance from the source of lead contamination.

Sometimes, information on environmental levels of chemical exposure is not available or cannot be obtained—eg, because access to the offending facility is denied. Workers may carry in their own bodies the acute or cumulative history of their occupational exposures. Figure 16.6, for example, shows the distribution patterns of blood lead levels and zinc protoporphyrin (ZPP)—a marker of lead effect—in a nonexposed group and three groups with increasing levels of occupational exposure.

In recent years, there have been many efforts that have helped characterize human exposure. The important contributions by Checkoway (1986) and Smith (1987) toward the definition of human toxic dose and three examples of environmental measures of

exposures—the "hygienic effect," the "time-weighted average" (TWA), and a quantitative method for assessment of solvent exposure (the solvent index) by Fiedler and collaborators are reviewed here.

EXPOSURE DATA IN OCCUPATIONAL EPIDEMIOLOGY

Checkoway (1986) argues that schemes for toxic assessment in occupational epidemiology have evolved from crude classification systems to sophisticated quantitative assessment of dose. Six exposure classification schemes are recognized:

1. Ever versus never employed in industry.
2. Duration of employment in industry.
3. Job categories by process division or task duties—eg, custodians, pipe fitters, painters, mechanics, office workers.
4. Job categories ranked ordinally by exposure—eg, lead smelters (heaviest exposure to lead), packers and workers in the unloading deck carrying batteries to

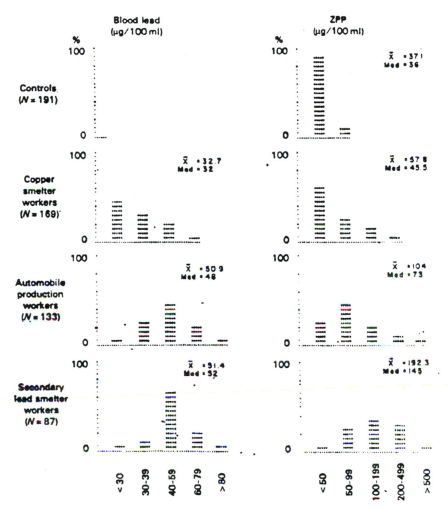

Fig. 16.6. Distribution of blood lead levels and zinc protoporphyrin (ZPP) in a control group and three occupational groups with increasing exposure levels to lead. (From Valciukas and Lilis, 1982.)

the smelter (intermediate exposure), and workers in the shipping department (minimal exposure).

5. Quantitative exposure—eg, intensity categories ascertained by industrial hygienists who obtain samples in representative environments.

6. Quantitative dose estimates—eg, levels of lead in blood, or levels of metabolites known to be associated with toxic agents (ie, mandelic acid as a result of exposure to styrene).

The following are examples for each exposure category; categories 4 and 5 are combined, since it is not always possible to make such fine distinctions.

Ever versus Never Employed in Industry

The most general classification scheme of "exposure" relies on the question of whether people work at a facility where neurotoxic exposure is known to be present. People's occupations are the proxy for exposure. In epidemiological studies of neurotoxic illness, the design of these studies is called case–control (see Chapter 12). For example, the mean urinary mercury levels of people employed in a facility in which mercury has been found as a pollutant are contrasted with the mean urinary levels from other facilities not as contaminated.

In computer-based data sets, the variable ever versus never employed is generally coded as a dichotomous variable. For example, the variable "employed" has either a numerical code ("1" for "ever employed" and "2" for "never employed") or a character (letter) code ("Yes" or "No").

The major difficulty with this classification is that "toxic exposure" is equated with "industry"; ie, industry X makes its workers sick. Thus, "ever versus never employed" is one of the weakest sources of information on occupational exposures, particularly when not accompanied by assessment of environmental exposures or biological markers of toxic absorption. However, when no other source of information is available, "ever versus never employed" may provide important leads to a more refined assessment of toxic exposure.

Duration of Employment in Industry

When no other information on exposure is available, sometimes the variable "duration of employment" (sometimes called "duration of exposure") can be utilized to assess occupational dose. For some toxic agents with delayed toxicity extending many years, such as asbestos, certain investigators differentiate the variables "duration of employment" from "duration from onset of employment." The latter is a variable that includes the time elapsed since the worker was ever exposed to the toxic agent, regardless of whether employment was continuous or not.

Checkoway argues that length of employment can be used as a surrogate for dose only when the following four conditions are met:

(1) the intensity levels of exposure are relatively constant throughout work areas of the plant; (2) intensity levels have not varied substantially over time; (3) work assignments into higher- and lower-intensity job categories are unrelated to employment tenure; and (4) nonoccupational risk factors do not vary systematically with employment duration.

In computer-based data sets, the variable "duration of exposure" ranges from zero to as many years as the longest-employed worker has worked in the facility. The analysis of the distribution pattern of "duration of exposure" reveals that such a distribution is rarely normal (bell-shaped). In some cases the distribution may be skewed to the left, revealing a relatively new work force where most of the workers have a relatively short time of employment. The distribution may be skewed to the right, indicating the presence of a relatively stable work force where most of the workers have had a relatively long-term employment. The distribution may be bimodal (two-peaked) indicating the presence of two distinctive groups, "old-timers" and "newcomers."

In epidemiological studies of neurotoxic illness, "duration of employment" is often found to be a "noisy" variable (subjected to spurious effects not related to occupational exposures). The major difficulties are that most psychometric and neurophysiological tests of nervous system function are sensitive to normal aging effects, and the variable "age" and "duration of employment" are often highly correlated. Thus, if one attempts to remove effects related to "age" from the effects related to "duration of employment," any possible effects that might be associated with "duration of employment" are lost when "age" is removed.

Job Categories by Process Division or Task Duties

This is among the most common systems of exposure classification in which "occupation" or "task duty" is the surrogate of "exposure." Job categories are identified from the occupational history, in which the individual is asked about the first job ever held (not necessarily in the present company) and jobs and exposure in the present work facility.

In computer-based data sets, job categories are assigned a number (1, welder; 2, sweeper; 3, maintenance worker; 4, electrician; etc). Sometimes it is possible to combine the variables "job category" with "duration of employment in that specific job category." This classification system assumes that workers have only one job, that a "job" can be clearly described, and that movement among job categories is uncommon.

Job Categories Ranked by Exposure

This involves identification of the variation of specific exposures (eg, lead) among subgroups of the work force classified as mutually exclusive categories. Table 16.1, for example, shows the median and mean blood lead levels in different job categories of copper smelter employees (Lilis et al. 1984). Like the previous classification system, this classification assumes that workers have only one job and that movement among job categories is uncommon.

The ranking by exposure of specific job categories can provide useful criteria for grouping according to severity of exposure. For instance, during the phase of data analysis, all workers can be classified into four groups: "no indication of exposure," in which a given biological indicator of exposure (such as blood lead levels) is found to be within normal levels, and "low," "intermediate," and "high" levels of exposure.

These stratifications can be performed as a result of industrial hygiene data indicating the presence of a given toxic agent at certain locations of a given environmental or industrial facility. Thus, jobs are ranked ordinally (using ordinal scales) in which "intermedi-

Table 16.1. Median and Mean of Blood Lead Levels in Different Job Categories of Copper Smelter Employees

Job Category	Median	Mean
Rigger	27	39.60
Reactor feeder	47	38.30
Dust collector	20	36.10
Furnace maintenance	84	32.50
Converter	72	31.30
Sample mill	32	31.20
Concentrator unloading site	26	30.10
Pipefitter or plumber	23	29.60
Heavy equipment maintenance	46	29.00
Welder	18	28.90
Roaster or mixer	16	28.20
Machine shop	28	25.60
Electrical shop	36	25.30
Powerhouse boiler	15	25.20
Carpenter	22	25.00
Laborer (outside)	21	24.50
Concentrator	25	23.20
Railroad construction yard	24	22.10

From Lilis et al. (1984).

ate" is always higher than "low" and "high" is always higher than "intermediate," but there are not equal steps between each level.

We have mentioned that ordinal scales are those in which numbers mean increments in the magnitude of a measureable property of the study subject, although those increments are not equal. The proper identification of scales is necessary for the proper use of statistical tests in the analysis of data, a topic that is beyond the scope of the present work.

There are no rules as to which numerical values are to be taken to designate these categories, but, when possible, this categorization is established on the basis of maximum recommended levels of exposure. For example, workers in a secondary lead smelter could be placed into the three categories "low" (less than 40 µg/dL), "intermediate" (between 40 and 60 µg/dL), and "high" (more than 60 µg/dL), exposure, where 60 µg/dL is the maximum recommended level of exposure.

The variable "blood lead levels" is an example of the use of an interval scale in the rating of exposures (an interval scale is similar to an ordinal scale except that the increments designated by the numbers are, for all practical purposes, equal).

Quantitative Dose Estimates

Quantitative dose estimates in occupational epidemiology dealing with problems of mortality have been available for some time now. Examples are the use of "million particles of asbestos per cubic feet per year" or "cumulative rems of ionizing radiation" to estimate cancer risks.

In occupational epidemiology dealing with morbidity problems, such as neurotoxicology, quantitative dose estimates have appeared more recently. How the variables "hygienic effect," "time-weighted average," and "index of solvent exposure" are calculated is reviewed below.

INDICES OF EXPOSURE

The following are just three examples of proposed environmental indices of exposure; some, such as the hygienic effect and the time-weighted average, are widely accepted by the scientific community. Some others, such as the integrative index of solvent exposure, are new and have not been challenged by critics.

The Hygienic Effect

Swedish investigators (eg, Gregersen et al. 1984; Ørbæck et al. 1985) report solvent exposure levels in relation to current occupational standards (OS) for each solvent. The hygienic effect (HE) for a mixture of solvents is defined as:

$$HE = C_1/OS_1 + C_2/OS_2 + \cdots + C_n/OS_n$$

where C_1 is the observed atmospheric concentration of solvent 1 and OS_1 is the occupational standard for the same solvent.

The following is an example of the calculation of HE for styrene and acetone derived from figures reported by Gregersen et al. (1984).

$$HE = \frac{C_{styrene}}{TLV_{styrene}} + \frac{C_{acetone}}{TLV_{acetone}} = \frac{261}{210} + \frac{176}{1200}$$

$$= 1.24 + 0.15 = 1.39$$

where TLV is the threshold limit value, which functions as the occupational standard in this case.

The hygienic effect can be expressed as a summation:

$$HE = \Sigma \frac{C_i}{TLV_i}$$

Time-Weighted Average

Sometimes it is possible to express exposures in time-weighted averages (TWAs).

$$\text{TWA}_{\text{B-Pb}} = \sum_{i=1}^{n-1} \frac{0.5 \times (P_{i+1} + P_i) \times (t_{i+1} - t_i)}{t_n - t_1}$$

The TWA is a measure of exposure averaged over time. In the formula, t_i is the time of measurement i, and P_i is the blood lead level (B-Pb) at measurement i; $i + 1$ is the measurement following i, and t_n is the time of the last measurement. To multiply by 0.5 is the same as to divide by 2; division by two is necessary because two measurements are taken at the time to calculate TWA, where C_i is the concentration level of any given solvent and TLV_i is the threshold limit value for that particular solvent.

An Index of Solvent Inhalation

Fiedler et al. (1987) performed one of the most comprehensive treatments for the development of a solvent exposure index (EI).

$$\text{EI}_j = \sum_i \sum_r \sum_m (T_j F_{mrij})(R_{mj} E_m) \, [(1 - R_r) \, V_i]$$

where EI is the exposure index; j is the jth individual; i is outdoor/indoor (1 = indoor; 2 = outdoor); r is respirator type (1 = none or dust; 2 = cartridge; 3 = airline); m is the method of paint application (1 = spray; 2 = roll; 3 = brush); T is the time spent painting (hours); F is the fraction of time in spraying, rolling, or brushing; R is paint application rate (gallons per hour); E is the relative vapor emission factor for each method of paint application (2.5, 1.25, and 1, respectively); P is the protection factor for each type of respirator (none or dust = 0; cartridge = 0.65; airline = 0.90); and V is the ventilation factor relative to outdoors (1, 5, respectively). Thus, this time-weighted average provides time components (T and F); an estimation of strength of the emission source (R and E); and an estimation of emission source modifiers (P and V).

A report published in 1987 describes a detailed attempt to derive an estimate of airborne solvent exposure using questionnaire responses from a population of construction workers and maintenance painters. The authors conclude that the exposure index provides a useful relative estimate of airborne exposure to organic solvent mixtures that may by used as a dose surrogate in epidemiological investigations.

The breathing zone concentration depends on numerous factors such as the surface where evaporation occurs, temperature, ventilation, air currents, configuration of the industrial operations, etc.

Distribution Patterns of Exposure and Dose

A *distribution pattern* is the manner in which a variable can be characterized statistically. It is important to know the characteristics of the distribution, such as kurtosis (describing a distribution that is symmetrical, or bell-shaped, or that contains data accumulated either to the right or to the left side of the distribution) and skewness (describing a distribution with peaked or flattened characteristics) beause this type of analysis helps one to decide whether raw or transformed values of the variables should be used in the actual performance of statistical tests and in making predictions on the basis of mathematical equations. Once the type of distribution is established, the appropriate descriptive statistics for values of central tendency—mean, median, geometric mean—and spread—range, standard deviation—can be selected. For example, if the distribution is skewed, the median is a better descriptive statistic than the mean.

Further, variables that are normally distributed are analyzed by parametric statistical tests. Variables that are not so distributed are sometimes analyzed by nonparametric tests. Some statistical tests are so robust that whether the variables are normally distributed or not has little bearing on their use (such as the t-test).

There are only a few studies in which the distribution patterns of quantitative estimates of exposures and dose are offered. For example, Fiedler et al. (1987) have shown that the distribution pattern of their "index of solvent exposure" is skewed to the left, an indication of the fact that, in the group of workers they studied, most people have low exposure and few people have had high exposures (Fig. 16.7).

The characteristic of the distribution patterns of dose is important. When it is excessively skewed, for example, the mean level of exposure is an inadequate describer of exposure among a specific occupational group. In addition, when correlational studies between exposures and health effects are performed, the presence of normally distributed data or skewed data dictates the kind of correlation coefficient to be used. In normally distributed data, for example, the computation of Pearson's correlation coefficient r will be justified; in a nonnormal distribution, Spearman's correlation coefficient will be more appropriate since this coefficient does not assume normality. Finally, if a logarithmic transformation of essentially skewed data normalizes the distribution, Pearson's correlation may be applicable.

Pharmacological Characterization of Exposures in E & O Neurotoxicology

In recent years, there has been an increasing interest in relating occupational exposures (as derived from industrial hygiene) to dose (as ascertained by pharmacological–toxicological thinking). This comprehensive view is deemed necessary since several steps separate the environmental presence of a chemical compound that can be neurotoxic and the ultimate neural effect. The effect is thought to be related to the magnitude of the absorption occurring at specific neural targets.

Dr. Thomas J. Smith of the University of Massachusetts Medical School at Worcester has summarized a general approach com-

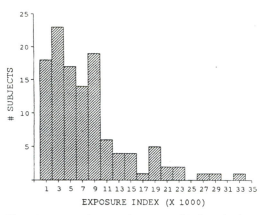

Fig. 16.7.   Distribution of a proposed index of solvent exposure. (Courtesy of Dr. A. T. Fiedler.)

prising six steps. Although this line of thinking has been derived from several studies of pulmonary effects produced from exposure to insoluble dusts containing silicon carbide particles, it might have a greater applicability including the evaluation of neurotoxic agents at the workplace. The following is a brief review of his thoughts are they appear in Smith (1987), with examples applicable to neurotoxic agents.

Smith's six-step procedure consists of the following:

1. Identification of target tissues and a route of entry
2. Identification of possible agents and mode of exposure
3. Development of a toxicokinetic model
4. Development of a pharmacodynamic model
5. Development of an exposure assessment strategy and collection of the data
6. Data analysis.

Strategies for the analysis of human dose based on toxicokinesis and pharmacokinesis have already been applied and validated for other target systems, most notably the lung. For instance, there are several independent measures against which a new dose index for, for example, a fibrous element such as asbestos that ultimately alters pulmonary function can be compared. Radiological findings obtained by physicians who read the X-rays blindly (not knowing the details of the medical history of the subject), pulmonary function tests, and even the result of lung biopsy while the patient is still alive are all available as measures against which the validity of the new proposed index can be tested.

Formidable obstacles are found when similar strategies are translated for the assessment of chronic or "nervous system" dose. (Measurement of acute dose is simple by comparison.) Only a partial list of difficulties is presented here.

- The nervous system is not a homogeneous structure; all areas of the nervous system simply do not function in the same way. For example, the very notion of a "brain dose" for a solvent does not take into consideration that solvents also affect the peripheral nervous system, sometimes affecting the nerves directly (ie, without being absorbed into the bloodstream first).
- The targets of the vast majority of environmental and occupational neurotoxic agents are not known. More importantly, as pointed out in Chapter 2, the notion of target is sometimes ambiguous; a "target" may be a relatively large gross morphological structure of the brain (eg, the cerebellum, the hypothalamus), one type of neuron (eg, Purkinje cells), portions of neurons (eg, the axons of the neuron), or a molecular site within the cell defined pharmacologically (eg, a receptor site in the postsynaptic membrane).
- "Nervous system dose" cannot be independently measured with our current technology and within the framework of ethical restrictions on research. One of the most exciting possibilities of the new imaging techniques is that in the future they might become likely candidates for these badly needed independent measures of exposure and dose. But unless we take these imaging techniques to the field or expose a subject to hazardous levels of

neurotoxic agents under controlled laboratory conditions—which is morally unacceptable—the imaging techniques are limited to validating chronic human dose assessment.

- The proposed index of exposure for complex mixtures such as solvents is expected to account for the differential toxicity of each neurotoxic agent and the likely possibility that solvents may interact with each other in a synergistic or antagonistic fashion.
- A cumulative index that takes into account exposure to a given solvent over a number of years must assume that neurotoxic agents were always present in the environment in the same form (as, for example, solvents in paints and paint systems were similar over a span of 20 years).

REFERENCES

Brugone, F and Perbellini, L (1985) Biological monitoring of occupational exposure to solvents by analysis of alveolar air and blood. In *Organic Solvents and the Central Nervous System* (Environmental Health Series, No. 5) p. 60. Copenhagen: WHO Regional Office for Europe.

Checkoway, H (1986) Methods of treatment of exposure data in occupational epidemiology. *Med Lav* 77:48–73.

Fiedler, AT, Baker, EL, and Letz, RE (1987) Estimation of long term exposure to mixed solvents from questionnaire data: A tool for epidemiological investigations. *Br J Ind Med* 44:133–141.

Gregersen, P, Angelsø, B, Nielsen, TE, et al. (1984) Neurotoxic effects of organic solvents in exposed workers: An occupational, neuropsychological, and neurological investigation. *Am J Ind Med* 5:210–225.

Landrigan, PJ, Baker, EL, Feldman, RG, et al. (1976) Increased lead absorption with anemia and slowed nerve conduction in children near a lead smelter. *J Pediat* 89(6):904–910.

Lauwerys, RR (1983) *Industrial Chemical Exposure: Guidelines for Biological Monitoring.* Davis, CA: Biomedical Publications.

Lilis, R, Valciukas, JA, Malkin, J, et al. (1985) Effects of low-level lead and arsenic exposure on copper smelter workers. *Arch Environ Health* 40(1):38–47.

Morris, DG (1985) Hygiene strategies and regulatory aspects. In *Organic Solvents and the Central Ner-*

vous System (Environmental Health Series, No. 5) p. 272. Copenhagen: WHO, Regional Office for Europe.

O'Donoghue, JL (ed) (1985) *Neurotoxicity of Industrial and Commercial Chemicals.* Boca Raton, FL: CRC Press.

Ørbaeck, P, Risberg J, Rosén, I, et al. (1985) Effects of long-term exposure to solvents in the paint industry. *Scand J Work Environ Health* 11(Suppl 2):1–28.

Smith, TJ (1987) Exposure assessment for occupational epidemiology. *Am J Ind Med* 12:249–268.

Valciukas, JA and Lilis, R (1982) A composite index of lead effects: Comparative study of four occupational groups with different levels of lead absorption. *Int Arch Occup Environ Health* 51:1–14.

SUGGESTED READINGS

Atkinson, AC (1986) *Plots, Transformations, and Regression: Introduction to Graphical Methods of Diagnostic Regression Analysis.* New York: Oxford University Press.

Checkoway, H, Dement, JM, Fowler, DP, et al. (1987) Industrial hygiene involvement in occupational epidemiology. *Am Ind Hyg Assoc J* 48(6):515–523.

Committee on Methods for the In Vivo Toxicity Testing of Complex Mixtures (1988) *Complex Mixtures: Methods for In Vivo Toxicity Testing.* Washington, DC: National Academy Press.

Corn, M and Esmen, NA (1979) Workplace exposure zones for classification of employee exposures to physical and chemical agents. *Am Ind Hyg Assoc J* 40:47–57.

Falco, J (1983) Exposure assessment techniques used by EPA. *J Toxicol* 21:27–38.

Frazier, T (1983) NIOSH occupational health and hazard surveillance systems. *J Toxicol* 21:201–209.

Gerin, M, Siemiatycki, J, Kemper, H, et al. (1985) Obtaining occupational histories in epidemiologic case-control studies. *J Occup Med* 27:420–426.

Hoar, S (1983) Job exposure matrix methodology. *J Toxicol* 21:9–26.

Jedrychowski, W (1976) Hierarchic analysis of variance in the classification of industrial environments hazards. *Int Arch Occup Environ Health* 38:61–67.

Kromhout, H, Oostendorp, Y, Heederik, D, et al. (1987) Agreement between qualitative exposure estimates and quantitative exposure measurements. *Am J Ind Med* 12:551–562.

Ott, MG, Teta, MJ, and Greenberg, HL (1989) Assessment of exposure to chemicals in a complex work environment. *Am J Ind Med* 16:617–630.

Riordan, C (1983) Human exposure to environmental pollutants. *J Toxicol* 21:1–8.

Seixas, NS, Robins, TG, and Moulton, LH (1988) The use of geometric and arithmetic mean exposures in occupational epidemiology. *Am J Ind Med* 14:465–477.

Siemiatycki, J, Dewar, R, and Richardson, L (1989) Costs and statistical power associated with five methods of collecting occupational exposure information for population-based case-control studies. *Am J Epidemiol* 130(6):1236–1246.

Socha, GE, Langner, RR, Olson, RD, et al. (1979) Computer handling of occupational exposure data. *Am Ind Hyg Assoc J* 40:553–561.

Weiss, NS (1981) Inferring causal relationships: Elaboration of the criterion on "dose–response." *Am J Epidemiol* 113:487–490.

17

Assessment of Nervous System Functions in Groups

Science cannot exist without an observer. Although the discussion of the observer applies both to the ascertainment of environmental exposure and to the calculation of dose—an industrial hygienist or a chemical analyst is also a trained observer—a discussion of the data-analytical aspects of the assessment of nervous system function in human groups must address the inescapable fact that human behavior is assessed by other humans. There are at least four types of professionals who perform such assessments of behavior and nervous system function, namely, neurologists, psychiatrists, neuropsychologists, and sometimes electrophysiologists.

When such professionals are asked to become members of a medical field survey, they act both as professionals in their own fields and as scientists in the specific aspect of data collection and, later, the data-analytical aspects of the research. To accomplish the latter, some working habits and thinking need to be modified somewhat. For example, a neurologist may examine 50 or more individuals per day over several consecutive days with the aid of a computer-compatible questionnaire; in certain critical surveys, epidemiologists insist that the medical or occupational histories should not be available to the examining physicians to prevent bias in the assessment of critical symptoms, a requirement that can be quite taxing to a physician; similarly, a neuropsychologist may examine large numbers of individuals per day with a screening psychometric battery that includes little or nothing on personality or IQ assessment.

In this chapter it will be shown how data obtained from three different sources—neurological signs and symptoms, psychometric test scores, and neurophysiological measures—are transformed into variables suitable for further toxic dose–neural response analysis.

DATA ANALYSIS OF NEUROLOGICAL SIGNS AND SYMPTOMS

Questionnaire Design

At present in clinical neurotoxicology research empirical approaches to symptom questionnaire designs coexist with time-honored symptoms inventories. Descriptions of single cases or clusters of cases where no quantification is attempted are also present in contemporary neurotoxicology literature.

However, it is noteworthy that there is an increasing degree of quantification in symptom questionnaire designs. The trend has been from Yes–No types of classification (dichotomies such as "Do you have a headache now?" to which the subject can only respond "Yes" or "No") to statements indicating a range. The latter are illustrated by statements indicating range of feeling in the Beck inventory:

0. I do not feel sad.
1. I feel sad.
2. I am sad all the time, and I can't snap out of it.
3. I am so sad or unhappy that I can't stand it.

Currently, most symptom questionnaires are rating scales. The rationale for this is that rating scales allow the use of more powerful statistics than simple dichotomies; simple statements regarding the frequency of occurrence of a given symptom can be recorded by hand and therefore are favored by those who do not have access to large-memory computers; and data generated from scales allow analysis of many of the respondent's characteristics that cannot be analyzed by the use of dichotomies. Some of the rating scales are "frequency" scales:

"I need my wife (partner) to remind me of things I have to do."

_____ Constantly
_____ Almost every day
_____ Sometimes
_____ Rarely

Others are "agreement" scales:

"I am afraid my friends notice that I am not the person I used to be."

_____ Strongly agree
_____ Moderately agree
_____ Moderately disagree
_____ Strongly disagree

The Prevalence and Incidence of Sign and Symptoms

Before performing a statistical analysis of neurological signs and symptoms vis-à-vis toxic exposure (the topic of Chapter 19), health researchers are expected to be familiar with quantitative properties of neurological signs and symptoms. Thus, the prevalence of each individual sign or symptom in a group suspected to be exposed is computed and, when the information is available, compared to the prevalence in control populations. In Chapter 12 I referred to the "occupational link fallacy," in which the prevalence of the toxic effect typical of the community in which workers live is attached causally to the workers' occupation.

The *prevalence* of a sign or symptom is defined as the number of instances in which these signs or symptoms appear in a given population at a given time. The concept of point prevalence is sometimes used to emphasize that the prevalence is calculated for a given point in time. As will be shown in Chapter 19, comparison of the prevalence rates of two populations—the study group and the control—is the first indication of a possible toxic causation.

The prevalence is reported either in table form or in a bar diagram. The researcher makes his or her own decision regarding the best way to report data on prevalences. Most expert health researchers have both available in laboratory reports as data are analyzed. But because of page limits, most journals cannot accept both when the reports are formally published.

The *incidence* is the number of new cases that occur in a fixed period of time—eg, the number of new diagnosed cases of lead poisoning that occur each year. The study of the incidence of diseases is important in environmental health sciences as they provide, for example, a good measure of the time course of environmental and occupational diseases and the efficacy of current regulatory measures.

Assessment of the Time Course of Neurological Signs and Symptoms in a Population Exposed to Polybrominated Biphenyls

In 1979, the author and collaborators published a comparative neurobehavioral study of a polybrominated-biphenyl-exposed population in Michigan and a nonexposed group in Wisconsin. Figure 17.1 shows the proportion of cases exhibiting neurological symptoms in Michigan and Wisconsin—retrospectively for a 5-year period—in a subsample of the study population examined by means of performance tests. The bar diagram is preferred here because of the complexity of the data reported. The total number of individuals examined in Michigan and Wisconsin was 170 and 93, respectively. Although in the Wisconsin group the number of reported symptoms during the period 1972 to 1976 was stable, there was a marked increase in these symptoms in the Michigan group over the same period.

Figure 17.2 shows the method used to calculate the time of onset of symptoms in the Michigan population. Proportions of persons with and without symptoms in the Michigan and Wisconsin populations were compared for each year (1972 through 1976) by the chi-square test. The value of the chi-square was plotted against time, and the statistical significance at the 0.05 and 0.01 levels was indicated by the two parallel horizontal lines. The points at which these lines intersect with the curve resulting from successive chi-square values indicate the times at which a symptom became significantly more prevalent in the Michigan population. By this method it is possible to determine the approximate time

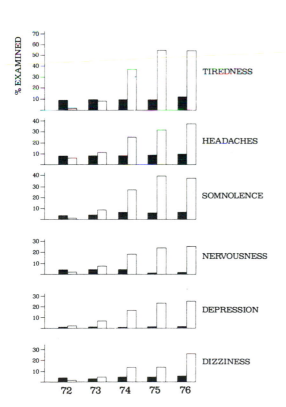

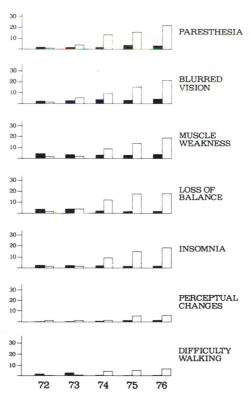

Fig. 17.1. Comparison of the prevalence of neurological symptoms in a group exposed to polybrominated biphenyls (PBBs) (white bars) and a nonexposed group (black bars). (From Valciukas et al. 1979.)

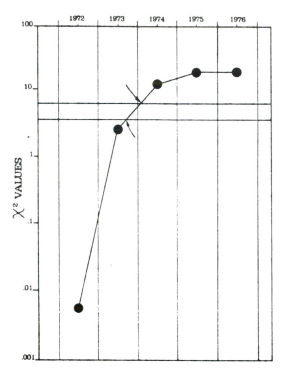

Fig. 17.2. Illustration of the method used to calculate the time of onset of symptoms in a population affected by polybrominated biphenyls (PBBs) (see text). (From Valciukas et al. 1979.)

of onset of the various neurological signs and symptoms in the group at the 5% and 1% level of significance.

Figure 17.3 shows changes in chi-square values over time for individuals according to this method. All symptoms in which there was a significant difference between the Michigan and Wisconsin population in 1976 are represented. As can be observed, neurological symptoms were dominant. All seemed to reach a plateau, but none decreased over the years studied.

Figure 17.4 shows the time course of onset of all significant symptoms in the Michigan population. The upper scale indicates months as relative units. Although no attempt was made to determine the precise time of onset of the symptoms, their onset could be ascertained with respect to each other. Significance at the 5% and 1% levels is indicated by white

and dashed bars, respectively, and the arrangement is made according to the 1% level of significance.

Integrative Indices of Neurological Signs and Symptoms

In a study of shipyard painters exposed to solvents, this author and his colleagues ascertained the prevalence of neuropsychological symptoms using integrative indices of signs and symptoms (Valciukas et al. 1985). The questionnaire included symptoms transitory in nature and known to occur with significant solvent exposure and to disappear after cessation of exposure. Acute symptoms such as dizziness, lightheadedness, nausea, headache, exhilaration, loss of balance, and loss of consciousness were coded in terms of frequency of appearance. Chronic nervous system symptoms were those that persisted on weekends and vacations. These included fatigability, sleep disturbances, irritability, lack of concentration, memory problems, instability of mood, decreased libido or potency, and diminished alcohol tolerance.

For each group of shipyard painters, the total number of acute and chronic symptoms was computed as an additive score. The additive score for eight acute symptoms was computed as follows:

$$ACUTE = \sum_{1}^{8} X_i$$

where X is the symptom and i the frequency code of its occurrence (1 for monthly, 2 for monthly to weekly, 3 for weekly, and 5 for daily). Since chronic symptoms were recorded as yes/no variables (ie, the symptom was either "present" or "absent"), the additive score for 16 chronic symptoms was computed as follows:

$$CHRONIC = \sum_{1}^{16} X$$

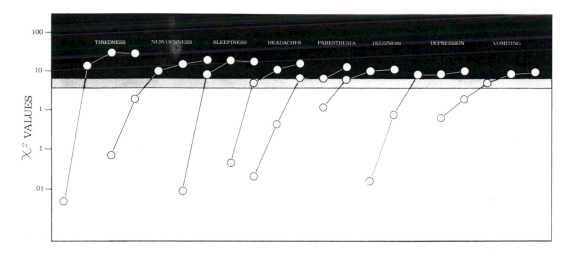

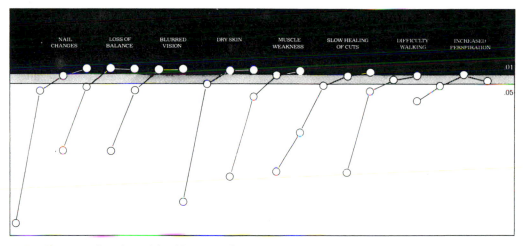

Fig. 17.3. Changes in the values of the chi-square value over time (see text).

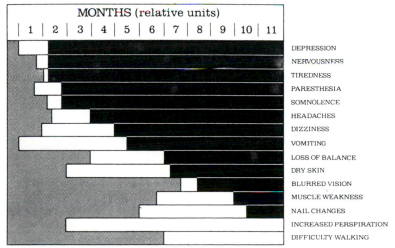

Fig. 17.4. Time of onset of significant neurological symptoms in a population affected by PBBs (see text). (From Valciukas et al. 1979.)

The Pros and Cons of Data Lumping

In data analysis, "lumping" refers to a data-analytical strategy that consists of creating new variables out of groups of single variables. Lumping is necessary because there are sometimes several dozens of variables dealing with nervous system function alone. For example, in a questionnaire about neurological signs, the investigator may decide to lump all the variables dealing with peripheral nervous system (PNS) function in a single variable called PNS. However, this cannot be performed without a thorough understanding of how the component variables of the lumped variable behave or the neurological principles of disease causation.

For example, in an early study on lead-induced neurobehavioral changes, "symptomatic" individuals were compared with "asymptomatic" individuals. The variables that entered into the definition of "symptomatic"—irritability, memory problems, sleep problems, etc—were dictated by what was known about the toxicity of lead.

But sometimes, this knowledge is not available; the investigator sometimes "discovers" or "uncovers" these correlations. With the aid of a computer, for example, the investigator searches for significant correlations (in both the statistical and clinical sense) between neurological signs and symptoms themselves. There are no rules about how this process should be performed. A matrix of intercorrelations is sometimes helpful. This author sometimes pastes such large matrices of correlations on the walls of his office and spends several days examining them and marking significant correlations with pencils of different colors.

The Distribution Patterns of Proposed Integrative Indices Should Be Carefully Studied

In the previous chapter, dealing with data-analytical aspects of the assessment of human dose, I stressed the importance of knowing the characteristics of the distribution patterns of dose before attempting further analysis of data. Similar statements can be made regarding newly defined integrative indices of nervous system function or additive scores of neurological signs and symptoms.

Additive scores such as *ACUTE* or *CHRONIC* are markedly skewed to the left, an expression of the fact that most people have few neurological signs and symptoms and few people have a large number of signs and symptoms. When a distribution is excessively skewed to the left, for example, the mean of the additive scores is an inadequate descriptor of the symptoms among a specific occupational group.

SCORING AND DATA ANALYSIS OF PSYCHOMETRIC TESTS

In epidemiological research, scoring is only the beginning of the data-analytical process. The process that is described here for the analysis of psychometric test scores is essentially the same as that for any continuous variables when confounding variables (eg, age, education) are present. For example, in the analysis of nerve conduction velocity—in which temperature and age are confounders—the "scoring" (which the observer performs with automatic readouts) and data transformation are essentially identical to those used for psychometric tests.

Thus, for purposes of brevity, only the data-analytical phase of psychometric test scores are explained in detail below.

Scoring of Individual Neuropsychological Tests

Score generation from the tests of our screening battery is illustrated. Description of these and other psychometric tests under this heading are found in Chapter 4. In the **Block Design** test, the task involves arranging the cubes in such a way that the top surfaces of four (or nine) cubes reproduce a design displayed by the test administrator. In the first six trials, only four cubes are used, and the designs are relatively simple. In the last four trials, nine cubes are used, and the designs are more complex. The time for each pattern is read against a table in which time is converted to a number. The total score for the test is the sum of the scores achieved for the individual patterns correctly duplicated.

In a data set accessed by the neuropsychologist in charge of testing, for example, investigators may choose to enter the time it took to complete each test and perform the scoring by computer programs. This is important in order to decide which individual components of the test are most sensitive to neurotoxin-induced brain dysfunction. In data sets of entire medical field surveys, however, neuropsychologists are expected to provide only the total score of the Block Design tests as well as demographic confounders—such as ethnic background, age, education—that may influence the interpretation of test results.

In the **Digit Symbol** test the subject is given a list in which digits from 1 to 9 are associated with symbols and is asked to enter the symbols into the blank spaces next to a list of random digits on a form. Subjects are instructed to fill the blanks with the symbols that correspond to each number. The test provides only one score, which is entered in large data sets (ie, the number of correct symbols completed in 90 seconds).

In the **Embedded Figures** test the subject is shown four sets of 10 superimposed outline drawings of common objects and is required to identify as many objects as possible. During test development, neuropsychologists may opt for entering the successful completion of each outline into their private data set in order, for example, to develop indices that attach more weight to outlines that are rarely detected. Others may keep a record of responses to separate outlines. In data sets meant to be used in epidemiological studies, however, the score is the total number of correctly identified outlines minus "confabulation"

(outlines that are statistically rare and generally result from combining features of two or more outlines).

In the **Grooved Pegboard Dexterity** test subjects are instructed to insert key-shaped pieces of metal into grooved metal holes. Holes are cut in such a manner that the subject has to rotate the metal piece in several positions to match the grooves cut in the metal sheet. Subjects are instructed to perform the task with both the preferred and the nonpreferred hand. The score is the time in seconds that the subject takes to complete the task.

The group analysis of motor coordination needs to be done separately for the preferred hand, the nonpreferred hand, and for both hands. Thus, the data set contains data fields allocated for each of these measures. The analysis of data for the right hand and the left hand is incorrect in that it does not take into account the fact that most people exhibit hand preference, a performance characteristic that is related to brain dominance.

The fundamentals of reaction testing are described in Chapter 27. In general, the shorter the reaction time, measured in milliseconds, the "better" the score. However, what constitutes the score is not always easy to ascertain.

Each individual has his or her own statistical distribution of measures of reaction time. The distribution of, let's say, 20 sample measures of John Doe's reaction time may or may not be statistically "normal." Whether to take John Doe's shortest time value, the mean, the median, or a given quartile—a fourth of the entire distribution of reaction time measures—is always an issue. In general, scientists take the position that the individual value needs to be the one that best summarizes the behavior of the individual. Thus, quartiles, which are not affected by the shape of the statistical distribution of data derived from a single individual, are favored.

In large data sets comprised of all the variables derived from a medical field survey, sometimes amounting to thousands, data managers do not expect individual team members to contribute with all the reaction time measures collected from one

Table 17.1. Transformation of Raw Scores into Standardized Scores (Z)

Test	Raw Score				Standardized Score
Block Design (BD)	Pattern	Time	Individual Score		
	1	t_1	bd_1	$\text{BD score} = \sum_{1}^{10} bd$	$Z_{BD} = (BD - \overline{X}_{BD})/SD_{BD}$
	.	.	.		
	.	.	.		
	10	t_{10}	bd_{10}		
Digit Symbol (DS)	Correct symbols in 90 seconds			$\text{DS score} = \text{no. of symbols}$	$Z_{DS} = (DS - \overline{X}_{DS})/SD_{DS}$
Embedded Figure (EF)	Plate	Individual Score			
	1	$ef_1 = \text{correct} - \text{incorrect}$		$\text{EF score} = \sum_{1}^{4} ef$	$Z_{EF} = (EF - \overline{X}_{EF})/SD_{EF}$
	2	$ef_2 = \text{correct} - \text{incorrect}$			
	3	$ef_3 = \text{correct} - \text{incorrect}$			
	4	$ef_4 = \text{correct} - \text{incorrect}$			

$\overline{X}$, Mean score; SD, standard deviation.

individual during the testing session. If a reaction-testing device generates 20 measures, for example, 20 variables for each subject would have been allocated for this test alone. The team leader, and the data manager, expect that the neurotoxicologist has already performed initial research in his or her data set and has already selected the measure(s) that are likely to describe best the performance of an individual (such as the median and a given quartile).

Test Score Transformation

Z scores are one of the simplest, most versatile, and widely used forms of expressing results from tests scores. A Z score, or standard score as it is often called, is expressed as the departure of the raw scores from the mean in terms of standard deviation units (Table 17.1).

$$Z = (\text{raw score} - \text{mean score})/\text{standard deviation}$$

Standard scores are useful in psychometry and in the analysis of psychometric data in neurotoxicology because they allow a comparison of tests of different ranges along a common denominator, the degree of departure from the group mean of a control (a non-neurotoxin-exposed group). For example, in the Block Design test scores vary from 0 to 44 (in our scoring system); in the Digit Symbol test, from 0 to 90; in the Embedded Figures test, from 0 to 40.

Age Trends for Psychometric Test Scores

A performance test that may be sensitive to a neurotoxically induced nervous system change may also reflect the effects of normal aging. Thus, to assess nervous system changes associated with neurotoxic absorption, it is necessary to study the effect of normal aging on psychometric test scores. (In the next chapter, the procedure by which age trends are mathematically removed from data for further analysis is explained.)

Figure 17.5 shows age trends for means

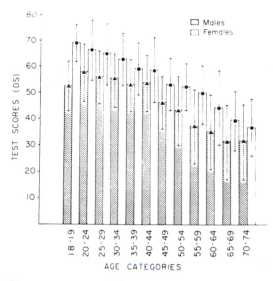

Fig. 17.5. Age trends for the Digit Symbol test. (From Valciukas and Lilis 1980.)

and standard deviations for the Digit Symbol test. Males and females of different age categories are represented in the form of bar diagrams. These data, which have been obtained cross-sectionally, show reductions in test scores as a function of age. As a rule, these trends are less marked when data are obtained prospectively, ie, in follow-up studies of the same individuals.

Figure 17.6 shows age trends of psychometric test scores versus age in the form of a scattergram. Age-related trends in the study group can be markedly influenced by the fact that the entire group, or a subset of the group, shows a deterioration in performance as a result of the effects of the neurotoxic agent under study. It is apparent from the scattergram that the correlation coefficient r, which describes the degree of association between test score and age, is reduced as a result of a group being selectively affected by a neurotoxic agent. The figure illustrates the case of negative trends—ie, the older, the poorer performance.

It is shown that:

- The selective effect of a neurotoxic agent on scores of a young group will be associated with a reduction in the magni-

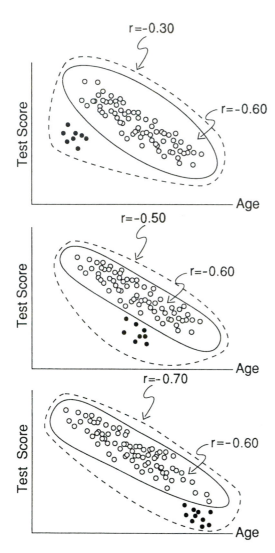

Fig. 17.6. Scattergrams showing the relationship between test scores and age, illustrating the selective effects of a neurotoxic agent on three age groups: young (top panel), middle age (middle panel), and old (bottom panel). Black circles represent affected individuals. (See text.)

cated at the center of the scattergram where people of middle age are plotted.

- The selective effects on the older group enhance the slope of the function, and as a result the correlation coefficient becomes more negative.

Figure 17.7 shows the results of an unpublished study by the author in which the quantitative changes in the constants of the linear regression equations and correlation equations change as a result of introducing computer-generated "impairments" of three increasing levels of severity in three age groups: young, middle age, and old.

The differential effect of a neurotoxic agent on the relationship between test score and age in various age groups is the reason why test scores need to be age-corrected on the basis of trends observed in nonexposed groups. This correction needs to be performed before the data are prepared for analysis. Certain statistical procedures, such as multiregression analysis, calculate the constants of the regression equations of the affected groups. These computer-generated models are shown to demonstrate that age-correcting trends should be based on trends observed in the nonexposed rather than the toxically exposed population.

DATA-ANALYTICAL ASPECTS OF ELECTROPHYSIOLOGICAL MEASURES

To a great extent, the analysis of electrophysiological measures such as nerve conduction velocities—particularly those obtained under medical field conditions—accounts for and controls the confounding factors that are known to affect these measurements. The next chapter is devoted to a review of some confounders that play roles in the assessment of nervous system function by means of psychometric techniques. The following is a brief account of the analysis of nerve conduction velocities (NCVs) when age and temperature are taken into account.

tude of the correlation coefficient. The reduced scores of the young pull down data points, creating a concave-downward curvilinear trend.

- The selective effects on the middle age group do not influence the magnitude of the correlation coefficient very much because the mean of all data points is lo-

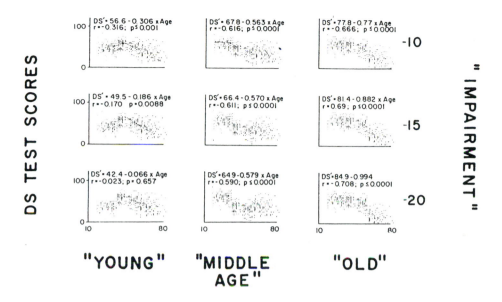

DS TEST SCORES

"IMPAIRMENT"

"YOUNG"   "MIDDLE AGE"   "OLD"

Fig. 17.7. Model of quantative changes in the constants of linear regression equations and correlation coefficients describing the association between a performance test score and age as a result of introducing a computer-generated "impairment" of three levels of severity in the age groups "young," "middle age," and "old" (JA Valciukas, unpublished studies).

In Chapter 5 I reviewed part of the work by Buchthal, Behse, and Rosenfalck from the Institute of Neurophysiology, University of Copenhagen and the Rigshopital in Copenhagen, Denmark. These researchers have performed the most exhaustive NCV studies in large unexposed groups to date. These investigators have provided data on NCV of numerous nerves under various sets of stimulation and recording conditions among people not exposed to neurotoxic agents.

An important piece of information derived from this monumental effort is how NCVs change cross-sectionally, that is, when individuals of different ages are studied at one point in time. The numerical values of the constants of the linear regression equations are valuable for calculating discrepancies between expected and actual values for a given individual.

I have also stated that when extensive data exist on NCVs for nonexposed people, NCVs are useful for the assessment of dose–response relationships between toxic agents and the status of the peripheral nervous system. The expected value of the NCV of an individual is obtained from his/her age and limb temperature. A ratio between the measured value of NCV and the expected value of NCV for the individual's age and skin temperature is then calculated.

$$Z = \frac{\text{observed velocity} - \text{expected velocity}}{\text{standard error of the estimate}}$$

Sometimes the disparity between the measured and the expected value of NCV is assessed by means of statistical procedures, namely, the use of standardized scores (or Z scores). Thus, the strategy is very similar to the evaluation of an individual by means of any standardized psychometric test.

Nerve conduction velocity declines with age at the approximate rate of 1.5 m/sec per decade depending on the nerve examined (Singer et al. 1982). In epidemiological studies, it is conceivable to match each subject with an appropriate control of approximately the same age, but this procedure is impractical, as it is sometimes difficult to find the appropriate match for each study subject.

Limb temperature also affects nerve conduction velocity: the lower the temperature the lower the conduction velocity of the nerves. The reduction in conduction velocity is approximately at the rate of 2 m/sec per degree centigrade (Singer et al. 1982). Limb temperature is affected by various factors including room (or outdoor) temperature, amount of clothing worn, blood circulation, and the subject's age.

In the clinic, where room temperature can be assumed to be constant, the need to account for limb temperature in the assessment of nerve conduction velocity rarely arises. However, when these electrophysiological measurements are performed under field conditions, sometimes in various places, the need to account for this factor is essential.

The effect of temperature on nerve conduction can be controlled by warming the limbs to a standard temperature. However, in medical field surveys this procedure is impractical, as many subjects need to be examined in a short period of time.

A current approach is the mathematical adjustment of all velocities to those expected at a standard temperature. The equations to make these adjustments are derived from experimental manipulation of limb temperatures in the laboratory. Rosenfalck (1975) reported norms based on the heating of limbs to 35 to 37°C.

REFERENCES

Rosenfalck, P (1975) Electromyography—Sensory and Motor Conduction Findings in Normal Subjects.

Technical Report, Laboratory of Clinical Neurophysiology, Rigshospitalet, Copenhagen.

Singer, R, Moses, M, Valciukas, JA, et al. (1982) Nerve conduction velocity studies of workers employed in the manufacture of phenoxy herbicides. Environ Res 29:297–311.

Valciukas, JA and Lilis, R (1980) Psychometric techniques in environmental research. Environ Res 21:275–297.

Valciukas, JA, Lilis, R, Anderson, HA, et al. (1979) The neurotoxicity of polybrominated biphenyls: Results of a medical field survey. In Health Effects of Aromatic Hydrocarbons, WJ Nicholson and John A Moore (eds) pp. 337–367. New York: The New York Academy of Sciences.

Valciukas, JA, Lilis, R, Singer, RM, et al. (1985) Neurobehavioral changes among shipyard painters exposed to solvents. Arch Environ Health 40(1):47–52.

SUGGESTED READINGS

Aiken, M, Anderson, D, Francis, B, et al. (1989) Statistical Modelling in GLIM. New York: Oxford University Press.

Anastasi, A (1982) Psychological Testing, 5th ed. New York: Macmillan.

Amstrong, BG and Sloan, M (1989) Ordinal regression models for epidemiological data. Am J Epidemiol 129(1):191–204.

Belsley, D, Kih, E, and Welsch, RE (1980) Regression Diagnostics. New York: John Wiley & Sons.

Cook, N (1982) Residuals and Influence in Regression. New York: Chapman and Hall.

Fleiss, JL (1981) Statistical Methods for Rates and Proportions, 2nd ed. New York: John Wiley & Sons.

Ley, P (1973) Quantitative Aspects of Psychological Assessment. New York: Harper & Row.

Roderick, J, Little, JA, and Rubin, DB (1987) Statistical Analysis with Missing Data. New York: John Wiley & Sons.

Valciukas, JA, Lilis, R, and Petrocci, M (1981) An integrative index of biological effects of lead. Am J Ind Med 2:261–272.

Valciukas, JA and Lilis, R (1982) A composite index of lead effects: Comparative study of four occupational groups with different levels of lead absorption. Int Arch Environ Occup Health 51:1–14.

Waternaux, C, Laird, NM, and Ware, JH (1989) Methods for analysis of longitudinal data: Blood lead concentrations and cognitive development. J Am Stat Assoc 84:33–41.

18

Control of Demographic Confounders

In epidemiological studies of the potential adverse health effects associated with chemical compounds in the environment and the workplace, an increased level of sophistication is now possible in order to control confounding factors such as gender, ethnic background, education, and age.

What is a confounding factor? A *confounding factor* or *confounding variable* is that factor or variable that distorts the apparent magnitude of the relationship between two variables. Ethnic background, for example, is a confounding factor in the study of the association between neurotoxic agents and neuropsychological function among groups of people.

Consider the following situation. As a group, blacks score lower than whites in certain psychometric tests. (Why this is so is still a matter of controversy.) Let's assume that we are comparing two groups: group A is comprised of 30% blacks, and group B 45% blacks. If we use a psychometric test for which blacks tend to score lower than whites, we might observe that group B scored significantly lower than A. If group B is the study group—the group known to be exposed to neurotoxic agents—then most probably one would conclude that chemical compound X is adversely affecting group B. The fact is that

compound X probably has nothing to do with the difference in test results: we have not been careful enough in the selection of the tests and have underestimated the importance of accounting and correcting for confounding variables. This is the reason that group differences should never be taken by themselves as the only basis for a judgment of neurotoxicity.

The distortion that the confounding factor causes in the magnitude of the relationship between the independent and the dependent variables can result from either (1) the creation of a false relationship between toxic absorption and neuropsychological functioning, a relationship that disappears when the confounding factor is successfully controlled, or (2) the obscuring of an existing relationship between toxic absorption and neuropsychological functioning, a relationship that becomes apparent only when the confounder is removed.

Confounders can be controlled in essentially three ways:

1. **By selection before testing is performed.** For example, during a medical field survey, measurements of nerve conduction velocities may not be made in participants who have a history of diabetes,

excessive alcohol consumption, or limb trauma. (This is sometimes problematic and unwarranted. For example, by not testing all participants who suffer from alcoholism, we miss the chance of studying the synergistic effects of alcohol and occupational exposures to neurotoxic agents.)

2. **By correcting for their effects before variables are placed into models.** This is the procedure favored by this author. As explained in the previous chapter, the demographic trends of neurotoxically affected groups of people, such as age trends, cannot be taken as identical to those of nonexposed individuals.

3. **By correcting for their effects once the variables are placed into models.** This procedure is followed in most multivariate techniques such as multiregression analysis, analysis of covariance, factor analysis, and path analysis.

The analysis of confounders is a complex research topic. An experienced research neurotoxicologist knows possible confounders that might affect the results of a study and knows how to control these confounders. The most important factors affecting the interpretations of the effect of environmental chemicals on neuropsychological functions are **gender, ethnic background, education, age,** and **medical conditions.** In the next chapter we will see that social scientists also consider remote factors, such as mother's behavior in childhood lead poisoning, as confounding factors.

GENDER

In the context of neurotoxicological research, gender differences in performance test scores and neurophysiological measures have not been studied as much as they should. The lack of information on gender differences sometimes results from the fact that the need to contrast the performance or neurophysiological measures of males to females is just not present in certain male-dominated occupations. In the United States, for example, it can be said that the neurotoxicology of metals such as lead in the working adult is the neurotoxicology of the male adult.

Some gender differences are assumed not to exist, or, if they were present, they would be difficult to explain. For example, there is very little information on how males differ from females in nerve conduction velocity. Physical factors such as body mass would be the most likely factor accounting for such differences, if there were such differences.

Some gender differences arise from prejudices or preconceptions about how males and females are supposed to behave, prejudices that even scientists embrace. Personality assessment is the most striking example. Clinical studies derived from in-depth observations of a few individuals provide data about prevalence of personality traits that sometimes cannot be substantiated in large-scale studies of populations. For example, the notion that females are more "sensitive" than males or that males are more "aggressive" than females is not supported by epidemiological studies. How much of this performance results from genetic factors and how much from environmental factors has been the subject of research for several generations of psychologists, with no resolution.

Gender differences in neurological signs and symptoms, results of psychometric tests, or results derived from neurophysiological procedures are important considerations because neurotoxic agents may have different effects on males and females. Some gender differences are related to dose, the independent variable. In Chapter 9 I mentioned that there are physical, pharmacological and even cultural factors determining the differential exposures, absorption, and storage of neurotoxic agents among males and females. Some of the sexual differences are typical of the dependent variable. For example, when large numbers of people are studied, such as in epidemiological surveys, there are gender differences in performance even when no neurotoxic agent is suspected. In the last chapter

(Fig. 17.7), for example, we saw that females perform consistently better than males in the Digit Symbol test across all ages.

From a data-analytical point of view, gender is coded in a nominal scale. For example, 1 for males or 2 for females. Sometimes, for expediency, a separate entry for designating male or female exists in the research protocol of a medical field survey; the interviewer checks the appropriate entry with a check mark. Thus, if a check mark exists for male, the computer programmer sees male = 1 (it is a male) or male = 0 (it is not male), following the general rule that what is most expedient for the interviewer might not make the most sense to the computer programmer. The computer programmer eventually defines gender as a nominal scale with either a numerical (1 or 2) or a character code (M or F). (In computer sciences, "character" is a letter; an alphanumeric variable is a combination of characters and letters.)

Stratification for Gender

When data from epidemiological studies are analyzed separately for males and females, data are said to be "stratified for gender." The origin of this strange expression is not known, but it probably refers to the appearance of tables containing large quantities of numerical information. Strata (such as that of rocks) are observed in the columns of the data sheets. Gender stratification is characteristic of univariate analysis of data in which the effects of variables are analyzed one at a time. Almost without exception, all norms for scoring psychometric test are stratified by gender.

In a multivariate analysis of data, the variable "gender" is placed along with other independent variables. Table 18.1 is an example of such an analysis. It is shown that, to the greatest extent, the variable "gender" explains the performance in such a test. In the multivariate analysis some investigators look for interactions between gender and other variables that may be associated with gender.

Table 18.1. Multiregression Analysis of Age- and Education-corrected DS Test Scores and Demographic Variables (Best Subset Method)

Model	r^2	t
One variable		
Gender	0.132	−10.49
Two variables		
Gender		−10.69
Race	0.183	−6.77
Three variables		
Gender		−10.67
Race		−6.71
Age	0.186	−1.26
Four variables		
Gender		−10.66
Race		−6.69
Age		−1.28
Education	0.186	−0.22

$N = 725$ (Valciukas, unpublished data)

In epidemiological studies of cancer, for example, investigators need to take into account the fact that females live longer than males.

RACE AND ETHNIC BACKGROUND

When one analyzes the contribution of demographic confounding factors such as race or ethnic background in making judgments of neurotoxicity, subtle factors may be overlooked. Unfortunately, job discrimination is still with us in unexpected ways. For example, blacks are often assigned dirtier jobs than whites. As a result, biological indicators of neurotoxic exposure or absorption may be observed in greater proportion among blacks than whites. Without a careful examination of occupational histories, one may conclude that blacks are genetically "more sensitive" to neurotoxic exposure than whites.

The original developers of behavioral toxicology were Scandinavians. Since the populations studied for suspected neurotoxic exposure were by and large genetically and culturally homogeneous, there was little thought on how to deal with the question of race or ethnic background as a possible confounder in the interpretations of scientific reports. The issue simply was never addressed because it was not relevant.

A researcher based in a large city of the United States, however, is normally challenged with the task of looking for toxic causation among people who, in cases such as New York, literally represent a sample of all people of the world. The issue of race or ethnicity is inescapable. How race or ethnicity is to be coded and how data need to be analyzed represents one of the most difficult challenges in data analysis in environmental and occupational health sciences today.

Traditional popular anthropology maintained that there were four races of people: white, black, yellow (Asians), and red (American Indians). However, from the beginning of this century, generations of scholars working in such diverse disciplines as biology, psychology, ethnography, cultural anthropology, and comparative linguistics broke the mold of this traditional thinking. In Chapter 31, we discuss how biological determinants of personality—genetic, hormonal, neural, and pharmacological—and cultural and educational factors are all interwoven in the determination of the individual personality.

In epidemiological research, there has been increasing awareness of the role race or ethnic background plays in the determination of nervous system function. But the use of the terms "race" and "ethnic background" interchangeably is unwarranted. In environmental and occupational health research, "race" is normally used to indicate only the physical makeup of the individual, namely, how the individual looks before us without moving or talking. The genetic and biological components of the physical makeup are essential in the study of important health problems such as Tay–Sachs disease, sickle cell anemia, and hypertension. The codes for race are based on biological and anthropometric considerations and include a reduced number of manageable categories such as "Caucasian," "Negroid," "American Indian," etc.

This coding of race is sometimes surprising. For example, most Indians from India—some of them deeply dark-skinned—are Caucasians, a term that for the layman is associated with "white." For the expert, many "whites" have so many negroid features such as bushy hair, flat and wide nose, prognathism (protuding jaw), and receding front that some individuals are more aptly classified as "blacks" than "whites." It is fair to say that few of the psychometric test scores presently used for the assessment of neurotoxicity depend very much on this biological component.

"Ethnic background" is an assessment of "race" giving emphasis to the cultural and linguistic aspects of the individual personality. For example: a "Caribbean" person is someone born in the Caribbean region, regardless of whether he or she is "black" or "white"—for an E & O neurotoxicologist, the performance of a "black" from Cuba cannot be compared with the performance of a "black" from Liberia; in spite of their Asian appearance, a Philippine person has many features in common with Hispanics because the Philippines were once a Spanish colony; also, an "Asian" from the Philippines cannot be compared with an "Asian" from Korea.

The codes for ethnic backgrounds are based on cultural and linguistic considerations and include a large number of categories. When a medium-sized group of, let's say, 200 individuals is stratified by gender and ethnic background, the number of individuals per cell is greatly reduced, making data analysis impossible.

Many language-based psychometric tests presently used for the assessment of neurotoxicity, such as tests of memory based on the recollection of a story read by the test administrator to the survey participant, depend on this cultural and linguistic component of personality and behavior.

Stratification for Ethnic Background

In univariate analysis of data, ethnic background is a stratifying variable. There are statistical as well as other practical considerations in the selection of the number of categories. Among the statistical considerations, for example, are the number of individuals per cell needed to fulfill the requirement for statistical analysis (as a rule of thumb, no less than 5 for chi-square analysis; no less than 20 for t-tests). Therefore, a code for ethnic background that allows finer gradations of culture is to be avoided when the total number of individuals in the study group is small (less than 200).

Among the additional practical considerations is a classification of ethnic background that makes sense for the group of people under study. For example, in a study of the neurotoxicity of pesticides among vegetable pickers in California where most workers are Hispanics, a simple classification of "Hispanics" and "Others" would suffice.

Ethnic Background as a "Dummy" Variable

There have been many unsuccessful attempts to give "dummy" variables another name, but the term is now so widely used that attempts to change it may create confusion. For example, Last (1983) defines them as "indicator variables." A *dummy variable* is one artificially created by the investigator in order to understand the nature of the relationship between two or more variables. The best example is that of trying to understand how different regions of the United States contribute to an explanation of the prevalence of a given disease. We can use the familiar procedure of stratifying the data by region. In this case, there is an inherent limitation on how much analysis can be performed on the data because the variable "region" is categorical; that is, it designates mutually exclusive regions.

A categorical variable can be upgraded in order to perform further analysis of the data. To upgrade the variable "region" we first divide regions of the United States into "Northeast," "Southeast," "Southwest," and so on. Then, we further compare "Northeast" versus "Rest of the Country" (in which Northeast is not included), "Southeast" versus "Rest of the Country" (in which "Northeast" is now included but "Southeast" is not), and so forth.

Computationally this is done as follows. A dummy variable "Northeast" is created having two values: either 1, indicating an individual from that region, or 0, indicating an individual who lives anywhere else except the Northeast. The dummy variable "Southeast" is similarly created. So, each region of the country will have two values, 1 and 0, indicating area of the country. Now, instead of the single variable "region" we have as many variables as there are regions of the country we decide to designate. Dummy variables are very useful because they allow analysis of data in a manner that transcends the confining mold of the data-analytical strategies of stratification; dummy variables can be used, for example, in multiregression analysis.

From the data-analytical point of view, the variable "ethnic background" can be similarly treated as "region." Each ethnic group is designated as "white" with either 1 or 0, "black" with either 1 or 0, "Hispanic" with either 1 or 0, and so forth. In a multiregressional analysis of data, the inclusion of the variable "ethnic background" would then be meaningless because "ethnic background" designates mutually exclusive categories. Instead, ethnic background variables redefined as multiple dummy variables having values of 1 and 0 can be used to study the role ethnicity plays—by itself or in combination with other variables—in the determination of psychometric test scores.

There are no a priori rules regarding confounding variables and when transformation to dummy variables is indicated. In the neurotoxicological literature, an increasing number of studies include medical conditions (eg, diabetes, chronic alcoholism, head concussion, epilepsy) as confounding dummy variables. This is a valid and desirable trend in data-analytical procedures. As explained above, the need to transform a categorical variable into a dummy arises when the variable that one wishes to study must be placed in a multiregressional model as an independent variable.

EDUCATION

Literally, education amounts to the schooling one has. Conceptually, in the data-analytical phase of an epidemiological study, coding for the variable "education" is complex in both format and meaning.

Education is most frequently coded as the number of years of school, including grammar, high school, college, and graduate school. Thus conceived, the variable "education" is a rating scale in which a number can designate years of schooling. When defined as "years of schooling," the variable "education" can be analyzed by all available statistical tests in which ordinal scales are acceptable.

Why is education an ordinal scale and not an interval scale? Because, even if it is true that we can assume that all calendar years are equal (a requirement for classifying a scale as "interval"), 1 year in grammar school is not equivalent to 1 year in college. Thus, years are differentially weighted as one progresses toward advanced education.

With number of years of schooling taken as an estimate of the variable "education," there is not much room for questioning the quality of information one obtains. Consider the following examples: subjects sometimes claim to have "advanced degrees" through mail-order courses—in several parts of the country a Doctor of Divinity degree, for example, is easily obtained by almost anyone; sometimes it is necessary to examine people who received their education in foreign countries—in many countries of the world, a child knows how to read and write quite fluently in grammar school; finally, some subjects may fail to report several years of formal training while serving in the Armed Forces, special trade school, or continuing education for adults.

At Mount Sinai Medical School in New York City we use the following rating scale to assess education:

1.0—Never went to school
1.1—1st grade
1.2—2nd grade
1.3—3rd grade
1.4—4th grade
1.5—5th grade
1.6—6th grade
1.7—7th grade
2.0—8th grade
2.2—9th grade
2.4—10th grade
2.5—High school equivalent
2.6—11th grade
2.8—12th grade
3.0—Finished high school or trade school
4.0—Associate degree in a junior college
5.0—Finished college with Bachelor's degree
6.0—Finished college with Master's degree
7.0—Finished university with doctoral degree
8.0—Doctoral working in field

Psychometricians are instructed to circle the number that is closest to the interviewer's estimation—not the subject's estimation—of formal education and to use decimal points (eg, 3.4) when necessary.

Interaction of Education with Other Demographic Variables

Almost all demographic variables interact with the variable of education.

In the United States, age and education are closely (negatively) correlated: in epidemiological community-based studies, the older the individual, the less education he or she is likely to have. In studies in which the variable of age has been statistically removed as a confounder before a formal analysis of toxic causation can be performed, the variable education is also removed because of this close association. However, this correlation between age and education should never be assumed for all study groups: the degree of association between the variables "age" and "education" has to be examined in each group under study.

Education is closely related to ethnic background. In the United States, for example, whites as a group have consistently higher levels of education than nonwhites. When other factors are controlled, such as socioeconomic status, the degree of association between education and ethnic background is not as marked, however.

The correlation between the variable of education and the variable of gender is complex and usually is an expression of socioeconomic and cultural factors typical of the community under study. For example, even after significant advances in world education, in many cultures the role of women has been traditionally viewed as that of a housewife, and therefore women are not expected to have a higher education.

In epidemiological studies in which demographic confounders need to be accounted for, it is not uncommon to find a three-way interaction among ethnic background, gender, and education, an expression of their close interrelationships.

Is Education a Cause or an Effect of Neuropsychological Functioning?

In epidemiological studies of the possible toxic effects of environmental and occupational toxic agents, the role of the variable education in multivariate models of causation is not clear. The variable education is sometimes conceived of as a factor that explains psychometric scores in direct proportion to the level of education, thus providing the reason why test scores are either high or low.

Education can also be legitimately viewed as an expression of innate intelligence. In this view, the greater the innate intelligence, the higher the education for which the individual would strive. Based on this assumption, the level of education achieved by the subject is sometimes used as an estimate of "premorbid intelligence," the intelligence the individual had before being chronically affected by a neurotoxic agent.

Education can be viewed in certain cases as unrelated to performance. This view has gained credence among some in selecting personnel through psychometric testing not directly related to the occupation the individual is expected to fill.

AGE

We need to differentiate between chronological age—ie, the age the calendar says we are—and functional age—ie, the age our physiological systems most resemble. Chronological age is not always a predictor of functional age. In Chapter 32 I discuss the mismatch between chronological and functional age in more detail.

Age is recorded as the age of the survey participant or the clinic patient at his or her nearest birthday. Thus, an individual can be artificially coded as being younger or older than he or she is. In studies of adults, the differences in rounding off age to the closest birthday are trivial; in the neonate, however, an accurate assessment of age—sometimes in weeks—is essential for assessment of normal behavioral development.

Corrections for Age Trends in Psychometric Data

As indicated in the previous chapter, performance tests that may be sensitive to a neurotoxically induced nervous system change may also reflect the effects of normal aging. Thus, to assess nervous system changes associated with neurotoxic absorption, it is necessary to control for the confounding effect of age.

It was also indicated that age-related trends

in the study group can be markedly influenced by the fact that the entire group—or a subset of the group—shows deterioration in performance as a result of the effects of the neurotoxic agent under study.

The procedure to be described here for removing age effects is preferred to that of partial correlation or covariance analysis, in which age effects are corrected on the basis of trends observed in the affected populations.

In a study of the effects of lead on neuropsychological function in adult males, Valciukas and collaborators (1981; Valciukas and Lilis, 1982) employed the following procedure. Each performance test score in the Block Design (BD), Digit Symbol (DS), and Embedded Figures (EF) tests was first transformed into a Z score: the expected value of each test score (BD', DS', and EF') was calculated on the basis of the linear age trends observed in the control group, and then the ratios S.BD, S.DS, and S.EF were computed as

$$S.BD = BD/BD'; \quad S.DS = DS/DS'; \quad S.EF = EF/EF'$$

If BD is identical to BD', it follows that S.BD is equal to 1.

The distribution of S.BD, S.DS, and S.EF can be studied. In a normal population, if the age-correction procedure is appropriate, the mean value of an age-corrected test score is 1 or close to 1 depending on the precision of the figures. The mean and standard deviation can then be used to calculate Z scores. For example, $Z.BD = (BD/BD' - 1)/SD$.

Therefore, Z.BD (or Z.DS or Z.EF) is a departure from 1 in terms of the empirical values of the standard deviations for each test. In a control group, the three standardized performance tests (Z.BD, Z.DS, and Z.EF) have an expected value of zero. Ley (1972), Anastasi (1982), and Valciukas and Lilis (1980) have referred to the statistical basis for and the use of these standardized indices.

Age-corrected performance test scores can be combined in a composite index, since individual test scores correlate highly among themselves. In a study by Valciukas et al.

(1978), it was shown that in secondary lead smelter workers, a composite index of performance test scores showed a higher correlation with zinc protoporphyrin than with blood lead, and the composite index of performance exhibited a higher correlation with zinc protoporphyrin than each of the individual performance tests.

A measure of central nervous system function can then be calculated as CNS = (Z.BD + Z.DS + Z.EF)/3. In the next chapter we will see how scattergrams of CNS can be plotted versus zinc protoporphyrin levels for groups with increased levels of lead absorption.

Correction for Age Trends in Neurophysiological Data

We have referred in Chapter 5 to the work by Buchthal, Rosenfalck, and Behse (1975) from the Institute of Neurophysiology, University of Copenhagen in Denmark and the Rigshopital in Copenhagen. They have performed the most exhaustive nerve conduction velocity (NCV) studies in a large unexposed group to date, providing information on NCV of numerous nerves under various sets of stimulation and recording conditions.

An important piece of information derived from this effort is that NCVs decrease with age. These trends are observed cross-sectionally; that is, individuals of different ages are studied at one point in time. The numerical values of the constants of the linear regression equations are valuable for calculating discrepancies between expected and actual values for a given individual.

Age and temperature adjustments are now possible because of the availability of this base-line information. It is important to note that most measurements of NCV and the study of the effects of neurotoxic agents on NCV have not adopted this rigorous treatment of the data.

We have also stated that when extensive data exist on NCVs for nonexposed people,

NCVs are useful for the assessment of dose–response relationships between toxic agent and the status of the peripheral nervous system. The expected value of the NCV of an individual is obtained from both his/her age and limb temperature. A ratio between the measured value of NCV and the expected value of NCV for the age and the skin temperature of the individual is then calculated. Sometimes the disparity between measured and expected value of NCV is assessed by means of statistical procures, namely, the use of standardized scores (Z scores). Thus, the strategy is very similar for the evaluation of an individual by means of psychometric tests.

DEMOGRAPHIC VARIABLES AND THEIR INTERRELATIONSHIPS

In epidemiological studies of neurotoxic agents, interactions between demographic variables such as gender and education, gender and race, and gender and age should be thoroughly understood. A competent investigator performs a multivariate analysis for each neurological sign or symptom, for each test score, and for each physiological measurement **before** engaging in higher-order statistical analysis when searching for possible neurotoxic causation. When epidemiological data are presented in a court, it has been customary to dismiss toxic causation on the basis of such interactions. Needless to say, investigators performing health research that is likely to end up in court need to perform a thorough analysis of these interactions and be fully prepared to discuss the role of these interactions in explaining the findings.

Primarily because publication space is always at a premium, investigators are now forced to make painful decisions about which information dealing with demographic interactions to submit for publication and which to retain as a laboratory record. There is no rule of thumb about when and whether to share this information with the reader.

There are three possible circumstances:

1. The most frequent case is that the study of the role of demographic confounders has not been performed. Peer reviewers of health reports submitted for publication sometimes recommend that the authors perform such an analysis before the manuscript can be accepted into the scientific literature.
2. The author of the publication can inform the reader that such an analysis has been performed and then include the major findings. Because of publication space limitations, it has become customary for an author to invite the reader to write to the author for information that has not been published.
3. Sometimes the interaction between demographic variables becomes the major focus of the research. For example, Bornschein et al. (1985) published a study on the influence of social and environmental factors on dust lead, hand lead, and blood lead in young children.

In the next chapter a more thorough discussion of the latter circumstance is presented.

Computer-Based Testing Procedures Accounting for Demographic Confounding Factors

We have the technology available for the development of a new generation of computer-based psychometric, psychophysical, and perhaps electrophysiological data-gathering devices. In Chapter 4 we saw that some computer-based procedures are already in use in environmental and occupational neurotoxicology. I also have mentioned that computer-based procedures occupy an important niche among psychometric techniques in eliminating some laborious procedures such as scoring. Current misgivings regarding the use of computers as "interpreters" of the results of psychometric testing have also been discussed.

Environmental and occupational health investigators continue to strive for good control of possible demographic factors in our search for possible toxic causation. Computer-based procedures, for example, can help us in "memorizing" some trends—such as age and education—to make quick assessments of individual or group neuropsychological functions in the presence of confounders. As large-scale epidemiological studies are conducted—such as the National Health and Nutrition Survey (NHANES), involving tens of thousands of individuals who are "normal" in the sense that they are not known to be exposed to neurotoxic chemical agents—quantitative information about demographic and other confounding factors can be obtained.

Computer-based procedures can, at the same time, be dangerous in creating a false sense of quality when none is there. For example, the variables "age" and "education" are correlated. This correlation may be a temporary trend that may disappear someday as a result of better (or worse) schooling, the presence of more foreigners in specific communities, etc. Would somebody familiar with the workings of a given model of computer (which may or may not then be obsolete) or software (which may or may not then be discarded) be ready to enter the new numerical values of equations that predict test scores on the basis of demographic and other confounders?

REFERENCES

Anastasi, A (1982) *Psychological Testing,* 5th ed. New York: Macmillan.

Bornschein, RL, Succop, P, Dietrich, KN, et al. (1985) The influence of social and environmental factors in dust lead, hand lead, and blood lead levels in young children. *Environ Res* 38:108–118.

Buchthal, F, Rosenfalck, A, and Behse, F (1975) Sensory potentials of normal and diseased nerves. In *Peripheral Neuropathy,* Vol. 1, PJ Dyck, PK Thomas, and EH Lambert (eds) pp. 442–464. Philadelphia: WB Saunders.

Last, JM (1983) *A Dictionary of Epidemiology.* New York: Oxford University Press.

Ley, P (1972) *Quantitative Aspects of Psychological Assessment.* New York: Harper & Row.

Valciukas, JA and Lilis, R (1980) Psychometric techniques in environmental research. *Environ Res* 21:275–297.

Valciukas, JA and Lilis, R (1982) A composite index of lead effects. Comparative study of four occupational groups with different levels of lead absorption. *Int Arch Environ Health* 51:1–14.

Valciukas, JA, Lilis, R, Eisinger, J, et al. (1978) Behavioral indicators of lead neurotoxicity: Results of a clinical field survey. *Int Arch Occup Environ Health* 41:217–236.

Valciukas, JA, Lilis, R, and Petrocci, M (1981) An integrative index of biological effects of lead. *Am J Ind Med* 2:261–272.

SUGGESTED READINGS

Amante, D, Van Houten, WW, and Griever, JH (1977) Neuropsychological deficit, ethnicity, and socioeconomic status. *J Consult Clini Psychol* 45:524–535.

Andrews, FM, Klem, L, and Davidson, TN (1981) *A Guide for Selecting Statistical Techniques for Analyzing Social Science Data.* Ann Arbor: Survey Research Center, Institute for Social Research, The University of Michigan.

Birren, JE and Morrison, DF (1961) Analysis of the WAIS subsets in relation to age and education. *J Gerontol* 16:363–369.

Draper, N and Smith, H (1981) *Applied Regression Analysis,* 2nd ed. New York: John Wiley & Sons.

Finlayson, MAJ, Johnson, KA, and Reitan, RM (1977) Relationship of level of education to neuropsychological measures in brain-damaged and non-brain-damaged adults. *J Consult Clini Psychol* 45:536–542.

Fitzhugh, KB, Fitzhugh, LC, and Reitan, RM (1964) Influence of age upon measures of problem solving and experiential background in subjects with long-standing cerebral dysfunction. *J Gerontol* 19:132–134.

Hollingshead, AB and Redlich, FC (1958) *Social Class and Mental Illness: A Community Study.* New York: John Wiley & Sons.

Johnson, S and Garzon, SR (1978) Alcoholism and women. *Am J Drug Alcohol Abuse* 5:107–122.

Kosten, TR, Gawin, FH, Rounsaville, BJ, et al. (1986) Cocaine abusers among opioid addicts: Demographic and diagnostic factors in treatments. *Am J Drug Alcohol Abuse* 12:1–16.

Marvel, GA, Golden, CJ, Hammeke, T, et al. (1979) Relationship of age and education to performance on a standardized version of Luria's neuropsychological tests in different patient populations. *Int J Neurosci* 9:63–70.

Prigatano, GP and Parsons, OA (1976) The relationship of age and education to Halstead test performance in different patient populations. *J Consult Clini Psychol* 44:527–533.

Reed, HB and Reitan, RM (1963) Changes in psychological test performance associated with the normal aging process. *J Gerontol* 18:271–274.

Scarr, S (1981) *Race, Social Class and Individual Differences in IQ.* Hillsdale, NJ: Lawrence Erlbaum.

Scarr, S (1988) Race and gender as psychological variables. *Am Psychol* 43:56–59.

Valciukas, JA (1985) Control of confounding demographic factors in the analysis of neurotoxicological data. In *2nd International Symposium on Neurobehavioral Methods in Occupational and Environmental Health,* pp. 49–53. Copenhagen: World Health Organization, Environmental Health, Document 3.

19

Determining Toxic Causation

How does one make a judgment that a toxic compound in the environment or the workplace is or is not neurotoxic? Are there formalized steps that health scientists follow to reach such conclusions? This chapter is devoted to scientific methodology in human health research. It deals with multiple perspectives for viewing toxic causation and the diversity of strategies that investigators follow to establish or negate a link between absorption of a chemical compound and neuropsychological deficits in humans.

CLINICAL AND PHARMACOLOGICAL PERSPECTIVES

Sentinel Events

Toxic causation sometimes is established on the basis of observation of single cases even when little documentation is available to support facts. For example, probably no epidemiological study has ever been conducted to support the fact that hemlock is toxic to humans; it is likely that many thousands of years ago, perhaps somewhere in the Mediterranean sea region, someone ate the seeds of this plant and died,

and someone else witnessed the event. It is also likely that for hundreds of generations, people shared verbal information about the toxic properties of the plant.

Thus, the search for toxic causation may start with one observation of a *sentinel event* (Rutstein et al. 1983). According to Webster's dictionary, a sentinel is "a person or animal that guards a group against surprise." A sentinel event is an event that warns us of danger. The presence of a single confirmed case of bubonic disease, polyomyelitis, typhus fever, etc in a given community is enough to put dozens or hundreds of health officials on the alert. The term "sentinel event" originated in the health sciences, and its original meaning was confined to the presence of highly infectious diseases that might spread quickly into the community at large.

There are also sentinel events involving chemical compounds in the environment and the workplace. For example, the presence of a single case of highly elevated blood lead levels in a child living in a decaying region of a large city, a single fatality from pesticide poisoning, or a worker who suffers paralysis soon after a new solvent is introduced in the production of shoes, each send health officials quickly to find the source of the problem. Lead is found in the old house; one learns that workers were allowed to go into the lettuce fields immediately after pesticides were applied; methyl butyl ketone (an industrial solvent) was found to be used for the first time by workers unable to read labels written in English. These are all cases in which the importance of sentinel events is clear. This recognition is possible because we now know how to assess blood lead levels; the health problems associated with pesticide exposure are now well recognized; and we know that certain solvents can cause paralysis.

Environmental and occupational toxicologists are prepared to recognize sentinel events. This is a basic form of epidemiology, where $N = 1$ (N is the statistical notation for "number of cases" in a study). The intuition, knowledge, and experience that are required to recognize, understand, and take appropriate action after a sentinel event has occurred cannot be easily taught. Toxic causation can then be legitimately established as a result of a human observer perceiving a logical connection between two events— presence of a chemical compound and a subsequent neuropsychological effect—that are often not closely related in time. Although it might seem a truism, an epidemiological study always starts with the first case.

Health scientists going to the scene where a sentinel event has occurred engage in detective work that can be appreciated as one observes them at work—ie, the questions they ask, or the personal exploration they make. As a health scientist observes a cluster of cases, his or her view is constantly modified, new ideas are considered and old strategies are abandoned.

A scientific paper rarely catches the excitement of this detective work. It is fair to say that when a disease is studied with the rigor of science, "a lot of water has flowed under the bridges." For example, a health report of a study involving 500 people, in which a multivariate analysis is performed with many dependent and independent variables identified and important confounders detected and controlled, may take 2 to 3 years. The preparation of the data set itself may take 1 year. An additional 1 or 2 years sometimes elapses before the research is published.

Thus, the first evidence of possible toxic effects of a chemical compound may result from the observation of a single case or a cluster of cases. A cluster of cases is usually first presented in a clinical report, by a qualified and reputable professional, of a number of individuals having a disease of common etiology. In Chapter 3, we saw that professionals perform three types of examination— the symptomatic, the anatomic, and the etiological examination—establishing the differential diagnosis of an illness. In human toxicology, a cluster of cases are sentinel events indicative of a larger truth; the truth of an association between toxic agents and neuropsychological dysfunction may be validly expressed with little quantitative information and no statistical analysis of any kind.

Pharmacological Perspective of Causation

Toxic causation can also be established when a dose–response relationship between the environmental chemical compound and the neuropsychological function is found. The vast majority of reports in E & O neurotoxicology can be judged primarily by their success or failure to meet this widely accepted paradigm. The demonstration of a dose–response relationship is a fundamental concept on which both laboratory-based animal researchers and human health scientists agree.

In Chapter 9 we examined important tenets underlying pharmacological research. A receptor has been defined as a place where any biologically active agent is capable of producing a physiological, structural, or molecular change. We also discussed the idea that there is a dose–response relationship between dose and the receptor effect. Finally, we also mentioned that the concept of "dose" has been established in the context of experimental science—such as in animal studies— where the "dose" is under the control of the experimenter.

A dose–response curve describes the changes in pharmacological action in relation to the concentration of the agent present in the receptor. At low doses, few receptors are involved, and the pharmacological effects are minimal. As the dose is increased, more and more receptors become involved. The pharmacological effects eventually reach a saturation point after which a further increase in the dose no longer leads to any increased pharmacological effect.

In epidemiological studies of large numbers of people, it is now widely accepted that mathematics, statistics, and—more recently—computer-intensive methods have provided data-analytical strategies by means of which investigators search for possible toxic causation between toxic compounds in the environment and the workplace and neuropsychological changes.

Data-Analytical Strategies

Although there are no currently agreed-upon data-analytical criteria for studying toxic causation, in the vast majority of cases in the reported literature the link between the absorption of a chemical compound and the neuropsychological deficit in a group of people is established by one or more of the following time-honored strategies:

- The analysis of group differences in neuropsychological functioning
- The study of contrasts
- Correlational analysis
- Threshold determinations
- Multiregression analysis
- Larger perspectives of causation.

This review is not exhaustive. There are many other data-analytical strategies that are used in clinical, experimental, and epidemiological studies, such as the models of the analysis of variance (ANOVA) or analysis of covariance (ANCOVA), which have also been widely used in human neurotoxicology.

THE CASE–CONTROL STUDY

Last (1983) defines a *case–control study* as a "study that starts with the identification of persons with the disease (the outcome variable) of interest, and a suitable control group [namely] of persons without the disease." The relationship of an attribute to the disease is examined by comparing diseased and nondiseased persons with regard to how frequently the attribute is present or the levels in which the attribute is found in each of the groups. In the case of E & O neurotoxicology, the "diseased" individuals are individuals whose health has been adversely affected by exposure to and absorption of neurotoxic agents in the environment or the workplace. In Chapter 12 I mentioned that such studies are often called "retrospective" because the postulated causal factors are sought by looking back in time after the onset of the disease.

The book by Schlesselman, *Case–Control Studies,* published in 1982, is a good introduction to this topic.

Neurobehavioral Changes among Shipyard Painters Exposed to Solvents

Valciukas et al. (1985) studied painters and other workers in three shipyards exposed to a wide variety of solvents. A short battery of performance tests, a detailed occupational history, and a special questionnaire were administered to assess acute and chronic symptoms. The prevalence of the reported acute neurological symptoms among shipyard painters was found to be significantly greater than that in other occupational groups in the same yards; for chronic, persistent symptoms the difference was not statistically significant.

In this study, *one-to-one matching* was performed by means of an editor language available in a mainframe (WYLBUR). One-to-one matching is an alternative to controlling confounding variables in that confounders are not allowed to be present in the data set. An initial pool of 412 males who had been tested around the continental United States and who were not known to have been exposed to neurotoxic agents served as controls. The demographic profiles of the study subjects—eg, gender, ethnic background, age, and education—were brought to the computer screen one by one, and adequate matches in the available pool of painters were sought. Ethnic background was matched first (eg, black with black, white with white). A "window" was selected for the variables age and education. Thus, controls were selected if they fell within 5 years of the age of the individual from the study group. The variable "education," derived from a rating scale, was allowed to vary 0.5 points. Table 19.1 shows the successful matching for these variables; the means and standard deviations for the two groups are almost identical, and the t-tests are not significant.

The result of this study indicated that painters showed decrements in central nervous system function, as revealed by neuropsychological testing, when compared with controls matched for age, gender, race, and education. But were these changes related to exposure to solvents or to something else? On the basis of information on occupational history and symptoms, the authors concluded that differential solvent exposure might be the plausible explanation.

The case–control paradigm is the strategy of choice when no other environmental or biological indicator of neurotoxic exposure is available. As discussed in Chapter 16, this represents the simplest form of dose assessment, by comparing employees ever versus never employed in a given industry. Considering the fact that for the vast majority of neurotoxic chemical compounds, no objective biological indicators of exposure are available (or if they are, their half-life is too short to be of any practical value), the case–control paradigm is a widely accepted strategy for the assessment of toxic causation.

CONTRASTS

A widely used data-analytical strategy among health scientists is the study of *contrasts*. Briefly, it can be said that a contrast study is a case–control study performed within the study population itself. Let's assume that we want to know whether the subjective symptom "fatigue" is in any way related to lead. We identify all individuals who at the moment of the examination said they were "fatigued" at the time and code them as "1"; then, we look for all individuals who said they were not "fatigued" and code them as "0." The values of blood lead (Pb-B) and zinc protoporphyrin (ZPP) are available for each

Table 19.1. Controls versus Solvent-Exposed Painters: Mean and Standard Deviation of Demographic Variables, Performance Test Scores, and an Integrative Index of Performance

	Controls (N = 55)		Painters (N = 55)		t^*	p
	Mean	(SD)	Mean	(SD)		
Age	58.3	(8.7)	58.2	(8.8)	n.s.	
Education	2.41	(0.64)	2.37	(0.58)	n.s.	
BD	20.5	(11.2)	14.5	(8.1)	4.43	0.0001
DS	31.9	(12.9)	29.6	(10.2)	1.65	0.104
EF	27.3	(6.5)	23.8	(8.1)	2.99	0.004
Z.CNS	−0.001	(1.07)	−0.60	(0.91)	4.24	0.0001

n.s., not significant; *p*, probability level.
*t-tests for matched pairs.
From Valciukas et al. (1985).

Table 19.2. Blood Lead Levels in Active Copper Smelter Workers ($N = 678$): Comparison between Those Who Reported Symptoms and Those Who Did Not Report Symptoms

Symptoms	Blood Lead Levels (μg/L)							
	Symptom Reported			Symptom Not Reported				
	N	$\overline{X} \pm SD$	Median	N	$\overline{X} \pm SD$	Median	t	p
Irritability	159	318.5 $\pm$ 102.8	308	516	308.8 $\pm$ 95.1	304.5	0.90	.37
Fatigue	232	326.1 $\pm$ 102.4	312	442	303.4 $\pm$ 93.2	303	2.61	.0092
Weakness	77	321.3 $\pm$ 101.2	295	595	309.4 $\pm$ 96.5	306	1.03	.30
Sleep disturbances	280	314.6 $\pm$ 102.5	307.5	394	308.3 $\pm$ 93.1	304	0.42	.67
Depression	62	311.9 $\pm$ 113.0	296.5	613	310.7 $\pm$ 95.4	306	0.30	.77
Memory problems	122	308.9 $\pm$ 101.2	292	552	311.4 $\pm$ 96.2	310	0.29	.77

f, probability level.
From Lilis et al. (1985).

subject who did or did not experience the symptom.

A contrast study is performed to determine whether the mean levels of Pb-B (or ZPP) in people who are "fatigued" is significantly different from those who are not "fatigued." Should we find that the mean levels of Pb-B among symptomatic workers are statistically significantly different from asymptomatic individuals, we would conclude that the symptom "fatigue" is probably linked to lead exposure; *t*-tests for significant differences of two means are usually used for a study of contrasts (Tables 19.2 and 19.3). The so-called point-biserial correlation coefficient can be calculated for exactly the same purpose, except for the fact that the procedure for the calculation of the *t*-test is widely known and

that for the point-biserial correlation coefficient is not.

Contrasts have been extensively used for validity studies of psychometric techniques. For example, we can ask the question whether people who exhibit a given syndrome or individual symptom are likely to show significant changes in neuropsychological functions. This is very important in neuropsychological assessment: the fact that what the neurologist sees during the course of the clinical examination is confirmed with the aid of special testing. In Table 19.4 neuropsychological testing shows the performance test scores of PBB-exposed males exhibiting the most prominent symptom (tiredness) as compared with males without this symptom.

Studies of contrasts have also been used

Table 19.3. Zinc Protoporphyrin Levels in Active Copper Smelter Workers ($N = 673$): Comparison between Those Who Reported Symptoms and Those Who Did Not Report Symptoms

Symptoms	Zinc Protoporphyrin Levels (μg/L)							
	Symptom Reported			Symptom Not Reported				
	N	$\overline{X} \pm SD$	Median	N	$\overline{X} \pm SD$	Median	t	p
Irritability	157	49.7 $\pm$ 27.7	42.5	513	49.7 $\pm$ 26.5	41.5	0.26	.80
Fatigue	230	54.5 $\pm$ 30.6	42.25	439	41.1 $\pm$ 24.3	40	3.47	.0006
Weakness	76	56.5 $\pm$ 29.0	46.25	591	48.7 $\pm$ 26.4	41	2.89	.004
Sleep disturbances	278	52.3 $\pm$ 29.0	43.5	391	47.8 $\pm$ 25.0	40.5	2.22	.027
Depression	61	52.2 $\pm$ 29.2	41	609	49.4 $\pm$ 26.6	41.5	0.73	.47
Memory problems	120	52.1 $\pm$ 29.1	40.75	549	49.1 $\pm$ 26.3	41.5	0.95	.35

f, probability level.
From Lilis et al. (1985).

Table 19.4. Performance Test Scores in PBB-Exposed Males Exhibiting the Most Prominent Neurologic Symptom (Tiredness) and Males Without the Most Prominent Neurologic Symptom ($N = 102$)

		Tiredness	
		−	+
Age	$\overline{X}$	36.5	38.2
	SD	15.1	11.9
	t	−0.58	
BD*	$\overline{X}$	30.5	25.3
	SD	9.3	8.6
	t	2.52**	
DS	$\overline{X}$	47.1	41.0
	SD	14.8	12.2
	t	1.96*	
EF	$\overline{X}$	31.8	30.0
	SD	7.54	5.55
	t	1.22	
INDEX	$\overline{X}$	0.29	−0.14
	SD	1.03	0.83
	t	2.03*	

Adapted from Valciukas et al. (1979).
*$t \geq 1.697$; $p \leq 0.05$; **$t \geq 2.45$; $p \leq 0.01$.

for the assessment of the important truth that psychometric techniques sometimes provide subclinical evidence of neuropsychological dysfunction (neuropsychological impairment in asymptomatic individuals). Table 19.5 shows the correlation coefficients between test scores and ZPP levels in secondary lead smelter workers with neurological symptoms (CNS$^+$) and without neurological symptoms (CNS$^-$). It can be demonstrated that even in asymp-tomatic individuals, there is a significant correlation between neuropsychological functions and levels of ZPP.

CORRELATIONAL ANALYSIS

A *correlational analysis* is a data-analytical technique in which correlations—that is, changes in two or more variables as a function of each other—are sought or established. Correlational analysis among dose or absorption of chemical compounds, neuropsychological functions, and neurophysiological measures is by far the most widely accepted methodology for the assessment of possible toxic causation. This data-analytical strategy is used by both experimental scientists working under controlled laboratory conditions and epidemiologists studying large groups of people.

The correlation coefficient r, by now a familiar concept, represents the degree of association between two variables. Regression equations can be fitted to the data describing the association between biological indicators of neurotoxin absorption and objective changes in behavior or neurophysiological function. These regression equations can be used to predict potential risks associated with specific levels or patterns of exposure. Regression equations are one of the bases used to recommend standards for maximum allowable exposure levels.

A correlation coefficient is not necessarily an expression of causality. Two variables may

Table 19.5. Performance Test Mean Scores of Lead Workers With and Without CNS Symptoms

	CNS$^+$		CNS$^-$		
	Mean	SD	Mean	SD	t
BD	12.7	(9.9)	13.2	(9.3)	0.25 (n.s.)
DS	31.6	(13.3)	31.6	(13.1)	0.00 (n.s.)
EF	26.6	(5.6)	25.3	(7.4)	0.92 (n.s.)
DH	18.7	(3.9)	19.1	(4.1)	0.39 (n.s.)
BH	10.9	(3.4)	11.9	(3.2)	1.31 (n.s.)

n.s., not significant.
From Valciukas et al. (1978).

be correlated as a result of confounding variables that have to be identified and controlled by using more advanced methods such as multivariate techniques (to be reviewed below).

"Correlation" is a term that does not necessarily imply the computation of a correlation coefficient. A correlation can be established using a variety of different statistical procedures. The chi-square paradigm, for example, is also a measure of correlation, in this case between two categorical variables.

A good introductory book on correlational analysis, with examples drawn from the behavioral sciences, is that by Baggaley (1964).

Psychological Performance of People with Low (Safe) Exposures to Lead

In 1978, Hänninen and co-workers from the Institute of Occupational Health in Helsinki published a study concluding that impairment in neuropsychological function among lead workers was observed to occur below 70 µg/dL, at that time the accepted maximal recommended lead level for Finland. The major conclusion of this important study is that the (then) current Finnish standard for lead was probably not stringent enough.

These authors had examined their data in a number of ways including case–control, correlational analysis, an analysis of the matrix of intercorrelations of performance test scores within exposed and control groups, and a factor-analytical study of the intercorrelation matrix of the exposed and control groups. Only the correlational strategy is reviewed here.

The group consisted of 49 workers occupationally exposed to lead, 36 of whom worked in one of two storage battery plants and 13 of whom worked in a machine shop on the Finnish State Railroad. Ten of the storage battery workers were women. The exposure period ranged from 2 to 9 years, and blood lead levels were regularly recorded during the entire exposure period. Only sub-

jects whose blood lead levels had never exceeded 70 µg/dL were included in the study.

The control group included 24 workers with no history of occupational lead exposure. Eleven were new employees of one of the storage battery plants, and 13 were employed by an electronics plant and worked in a section of the plant where no exposure to chemicals occurred.

The psychological examination consisted of a short interview, a performance test battery, and a personality inventory.

Blood lead (Pb-B) levels were recorded for all subjects at the time of examination. In addition, the highest blood lead level ever recorded (max Pb-B) for each subject and the time-weighted average of the Pb-B levels (TWA Pb-B) were used as indicators of lead uptake in the exposed group. The TWA was calculated as the total lead uptake during the exposure time divided by the duration of exposure (ie, the time between the first and the last Pb-B recording). (The formula is described in Chapter 16.) None of these measurements correlated with age. If they did, a different research strategy would have been required in which age would have been treated as a confounding variable.

In the Hänninen and co-worker's study, all the correlations between measures of neuropsychological function and the actual, maximal, and TWA Pb-B levels were computed. Significant negative correlations with one or more variables of lead dose were observed. Of all the measures of dose, neuropsychological measures correlated best with TWA and least with actual Pb-B, that is, the last value of blood lead available.

The investigators also plotted test scores for various psychometric tests, such as the score for the preferred hand in the Santa Ana Dexterity test, against the maximal exposure value of the exposed group (Fig. 19.1) As the levels of Pb-B increased, the performance test scores for the Santa Ana Dexterity test decreased. In other publications, Hänninen repeatedly found that dexterity test scores decreased with increased levels of lead in blood, which is the basis for Hänninen's contention

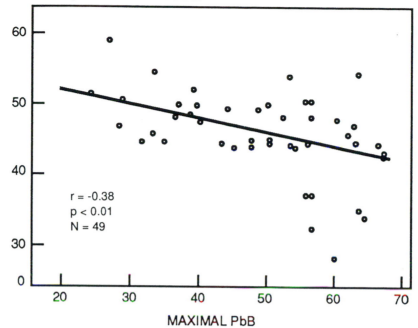

SANTA ANA, PREFERRED HAND

r = -0.38
p < 0.01
N = 49

MAXIMAL PbB

Fig. 19.1. Correlation between maximal blood lead levels and scores for the Santa Ana Dexterity test (From Hänninen et al. 1978, reproduced by permission of Dr. Helena Hänninen.)

that dexterity tests of this kind should be included among psychometric batteries designed for screening purposes.

The conclusion of this study is that at blood lead levels generally considered safe in Finland at that time (70 µg/dL), it was still possible to observe a dose–response relationship between lead and neuropsychological function, meaning that lead was adversely affecting neuropsychological functioning. Since that time and until recently, investigators around the world were still trying to determine the true safe blood lead levels at which no adverse neuropsychological function could be observed.

Correlational Analysis of Adult Neuropsychological Function with Lead Absorption and Effects

One approach followed by this author and his colleagues at Mount Sinai School of Medicine in New York City has been to use a correlational strategy relating both measures of lead absorption (such as blood lead levels) and measures of lead effects (such as zinc protoporphyrin levels) in studies of dose–response relationships.

Central nervous system dysfunction in workers occupationally exposed to lead was investigated by means of performance tests. The test scores of lead-exposed workers were then compared with those of control groups (steel workers, papermill workers, and farmers)(Fig. 19.2). We found that secondary lead smelter workers showed significantly poorer performance test scores than nonexposed control groups. The group differences between steel workers and lead workers in test scores were not attributable to differences in age and education because these were removed by means of mathematical procedures described in the last chapter.

In lead-exposed workers, correlations between test scores and indicators of lead absorption (blood lead) and lead effects (zinc protoporphyrin, or ZPP) were analyzed. In-

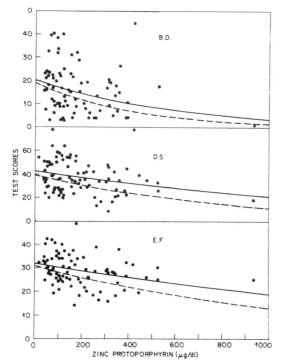

Fig. 19.2. Relationships between performance test scores and ZPP, a biological indicator of lead absorption, in lead-exposed workers. BD, Block Design test; DS Digit Symbol test; EF Embedded Figures test. (From Valciukas et al. 1978. © 1978 by American Association for the Advancement of Sciences.)

creases in ZPP levels were found to be highly correlated with decreases in test scores. Table 19.6 shows the correlation coefficients between test scores and ZPP, which were, as a rule, higher than those relating test scores to Pb-B levels.

These data added support to the (then) new contention that psychometric tests could be used for the study of subclinical nervous system function resulting from lead toxicity or other chemical compounds. In addition, significant correlations between ZPP levels and behavioral test scores are consistent with the etiological relationship between decrements in performance and lead effects on the central nervous system.

An Integrative Index of Central Nervous System Effects of Lead

From the data-analytical point of view, the test-by-test correlational analysis in relation to biological indicators of toxic effects is cumbersome if not misleading; cumbersome because the correlational coefficients of each test (and sometimes the number of psychometric tests reaches 20 or more) need to be examined vis-à-vis the biological indicators of toxicity.

In the early 1970s there were no agreed upon criteria for displaying results of E & O neurotoxicological studies. At that time, authors felt that they were expected to report details of their analytical strategies close to the literal reporting of raw data. Since the early 1980s there have been attempts at synthesis (or "data lumping"), such as the construction of integrative indices of nervous system function on the basis of combining

Table 19.6. Controls versus Lead-Exposed Workers: Correlations between Individual Performance Test Scores, Integrative Index of Performance (INDEX), and Two Biological Indicators of Exposure (Linear Relationships)

	Blood Lead (N = 72)		ZPP (N = 89)	
	r	p	r	p
BD	−0.17	n.s.	−0.36	<0.0005
DS	+0.07	n.s.	−0.35	<0.0005
EF	−0.13	n.s.	−0.39	<0.0005
INDEX	−0.21	<0.05	−0.46	<0.0005

n.s., not significant.
From Valciukas and Lilis (1980).

the results of several test scores described in Chapter 17.

The test-by-test approach can also be misleading. One fundamental tenet of psychometric theory is that several tests—eg, a battery of tests of IQ assessment—are more likely to provide a more realistic assessment of the cognitive status of an individual than a single test.

Another fundamental tenet is that tests that measure the same cognitive function are more correlated among each other than those that test different functions. For example, it has been known for a number of years that measures of cognitive function and motor performance are weakly correlated. Should we need to "lump" individual test results into more manageable categories, integrative indices for motor and for cognitive functions need to be created separately. In Chapter 18, the details of construction of these indices are explained.

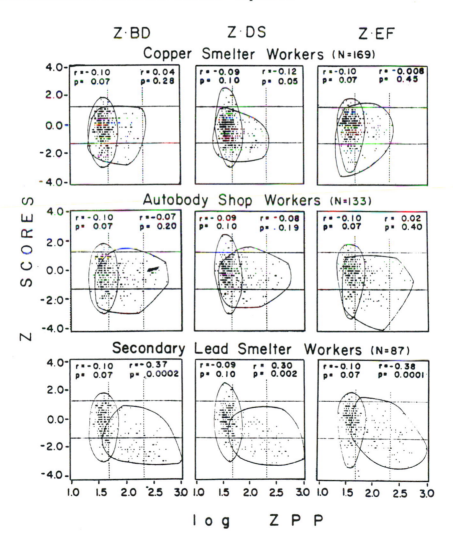

Fig. 19.3. Scattergrams of standardized performance test scores (Z.BD, Z.DS, and Z.EF) and the logarithmic value of ZPP, a biological indicator of lead absorption. (From Valciukas and Lilis 1982.)

In 1981, this author and his colleagues at Mount Sinai School of Medicine constructed an integrative index of central nervous system function—called "CNS index"—by combining the results of three psychometric tests of our screening battery. The CNS index was then studied vis-à-vis biological indicators of lead absorption in three populations with increased levels of lead absorption.

The control group consisted of 191 males examined during three medical surveys conducted by the Environmental Sciences Laboratory on populations without any known exposure to lead. They were selected as controls on the basis of good health status, as determined by a comprehensive medical examination, and the absence of exposure to neurotoxic agents, as determined by occupational and medical history.

The study group with the lowest level of lead exposure consisted of 169 copper smelter workers. The group was comprised of active smelter workers; lead, cadmium, and arsenic were known to be present as contaminants of the copper ore and concentrate.

The study group with an intermediate level of lead exposure was 133 auto body shop workers who were examined as part of a cross-sectional medical examination. Lead exposure in the body shop resulted from the use of lead for retouching body panel defects.

The study group with the highest level of lead exposure was 87 secondary lead smelter workers who engaged in recovering lead from scrap storage batteries and casting of the metal for reuse.

Figure 16.6 shows the distribution of blood lead and ZPP levels in the controls and in these three occupational groups exposed to different incremental levels of lead. This figure illustrates trends of the independent variable, that is, the "cause" of diminished test results.

Individual psychometric tests and the integrative CNS index were then studied for their ability to discriminate lead groups with such increased levels of absorption. For that purpose, scattergrams of values for the in-

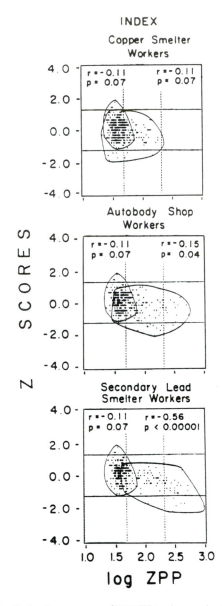

Fig. 19.4.   Scattergram of INDEX (an integrative index of central nervous system function) and the logarithmic value of ZPP, a biological indicator of lead absorption. (From Valciukas and Lilis 1982.)

dividual were plotted against ZPP measurements (Fig. 19.3). Figure 19.4 shows scattergrams of CNS indices with the outlines of clusters of data for the three groups occupationally exposed to incremental levels of lead.

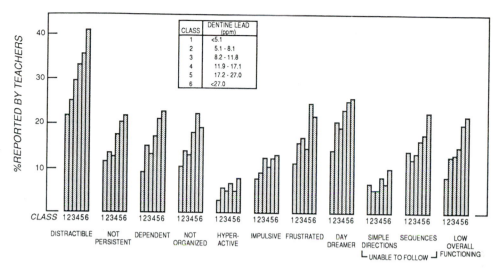

Fig. 19.5. Correlation between dentine levels (as indicated in the window) and percentage of teachers' report of behavioral characteristics of students. (From Needleman et al. 1979, reproduced by permission of the author).

Dentine Lead Level and Students' Performance

Lead has been established as a powerful neurotoxic agent on the basis of numerous studies of dose–response relationships between biological indicators of lead absorption and neuropsychological functions of the type reviewed above. However, dose–response relationships have also been observed employing other techniques of behavioral assessment and with the use of little statistical methodology.

Figure 19.5 shows the results of a large-scale epidemiological study conducted by Needleman et al. and described in more detail in Chapter 20. A dose–response relationship between dentine lead levels and teachers' ratings of student performance in the classroom was observed. This is an excellent example of the increasing use of graphic methods of data-analytical strategies in the search for possible toxic causation.

THRESHOLD DETERMINATIONS

The procedure for making threshold determinations and the correlational strategy of data analysis are closely related. Figure 19.6 shows the highlights of the procedure called "split windowing."

Figure 19.6a represents the usual analytical strategy of focusing on the entire range of available data. A dose–response relationship is found when measures of biological indicators of lead effects (eg, ZPP) and objective measures of CNS functions are contrasted. For example, two windows (a left and a right window) can be created at the limit of the 25th percentile; 100 and 300 data points can be carefully analyzed in the left and right windows, respectively. This is demonstrated in Figure 19.6b. At the 50th percentile, 200 data points at each window are available for study. This is demonstrated in Figure 19.6c. Finally, at the 75th percentile, 300 and 100 data points are available (Fig. 19.6d).

If a correlation coefficient computed in the left window at the 25th percentile is significant, that indicates that lead might have a lower threshold value or no threshold at all for neuropsychological effects. Thus, a further splitting can be performed at lower percentiles (ie, at the 20th, 15th, and 10th percentiles, etc). But, as the sample size is reduced, so is the power of the correlation coefficient

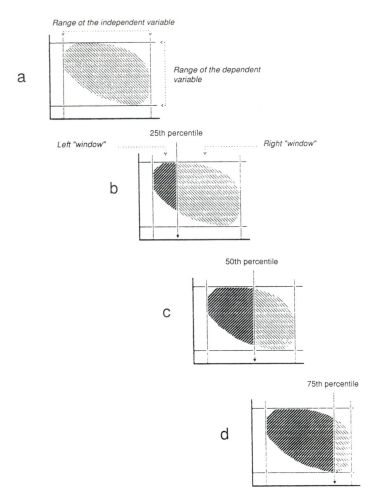

Fig. 19.6. The search for the threshold between a biological indicator of exposure and performance test scores by split-windowing (JA Valciukas, unpublished study). For explanation, see text.

found between dose and response. Hypotheses such as that lead has no threshold for its effects in humans can be effectively tested only in large-scale epidemiological studies.

This analytical strategy was first used by Seppäläinen in Hernberg (1972) to demonstrate that nerve conduction velocity changes could be observed among lead-exposed individuals at lead levels previously considered "safe" in Finland (70 µg/dL). The same strategy was again used in the studies of Hänninen and co-workers on neuropsychological function among lead workers exposed to "safe" levels. Dr. Ruth Lilis and her colleagues in 1977 used a similar strategy to show a dose–response relationship between biological indicators of lead exposure (blood lead levels) and effects (ZPP) at "safe" levels of lead exposure (Lilis et al. 1977).

MULTIREGRESSION ANALYSIS

Multiregression analysis is the name attached to a family of multivariate statistical techniques based on the concept of correlation. As its name implies, a multiregression technique is one that searches for and tests one or many independent variables and one or many dependent variables.

A *canonical correlation* is a technique specifically aimed at studying several independent variables vis-à-vis several dependent variables. Although widely accepted in such disciplines as econometrics and sociological research, it has rarely been used in environmental and occupational toxicology research. Computer software for handling computational problems of these techniques is now widely available. However, models that handle multiple independent and multiple dependent variables have not been extensively used in environmental health sciences and will not be reviewed further.

The typical application of a multiregression model is to explain a single dependent variable—for example, scores on a particular psychometric test—on the basis of several independent variables—such as lead in blood, age, and education. Multiregression analysis can be considered statistical procedures that facilitate the interpretation of numerical data displayed in the form of a matrix of intercorrelations, where a hint of these multiple causations is almost always first perceived.

Matrices of Intercorrelations

A matrix of intercorrelations is a way of describing data by providing the actual numerical values of correlation coefficients for each variable with every other variable. For example, if we study the intercorrelations among five variables, such a matrix will look like a square containing 25 correlation coefficients.

Actually, a matrix of intercorrelations will contain redundant information. The correlation coefficient between age and the score for a particular test is the same as that of the score and age. The correlation coefficient of each variable with itself is exactly 1 and is of little empirical interest. Thus, only 10 correlation coefficients in a matrix of 25 variables are of any potential interest. Table 19.7 shows a typical matrix of intercorrelations for three tests related to the demographic variables age and education.

There are no a priori restrictions about what kinds of variables can be shown in such a matrix. A simple table of intercorrelations among performance tests or nerve conduction velocities in arms and legs can be shown, for example. But a more elaborate matrix describing the intercorrelations among certain environmental data (such as lead in air), a variety of biological indicators of neurotoxic exposure (such as blood lead levels and zinc protoporphyrin), information on demographic variables (such as age and education level), and performance test scores can all be reported in a single matrix. In fact, a package of statistical computer programs will produce such matrices routinely. A dense matrix of intercorrelations is very close to a summary of an entire study.

How a matrix of intercorrelations is calculated is of little consequence. A simple matrix of correlations can be constructed by hand by calculating the correlation coefficients among all the variables in either the upper

Table 19.7. A Typical Matrix of Intercorrelations among Age, Education, and Performance Test Scores

| | Papermill Workers ($N = 99$) | | | | |
	EF	DS	BD	Education	Age
Age	−0.66	−0.79	−0.71	−0.69	1.00
Education	0.54	0.73	0.59	1.00	
BD	0.67	0.72	1.00		
DS	0.62	1.00			
EF	1.00				

For $r = 0.16$, $p \leq 0.05$; for $r = 0.23$, $p \leq 0.01$.
From Valciukas and Lilis (1980).

or the lower part of the diagonal of the matrix containing the nonredundant information.

Many multivariate statistical techniques have as their foundations a matrix of intercorrelations. Most of these multivariate procedures are designed to overcome the formidable task of interpreting the data contained in a large matrix. However, it must be emphasized that because a matrix of intercorrelations is by itself a summary of data, such data must be studied carefully before the analysis is continued with higher-order statistics. The study of a matrix of intercorrelations is to multivariate analysis what the "eyeballing" of raw data is to their subsequent analysis.

A necessary prerequisite for interpreting a matrix of intercorrelations is the intuitive understanding of how possible direct or indirect effects among independent, dependent, and confounding variables takes place. Results of a multivariate analysis can only occasionally surprise an investigator who has closely studied a matrix of intercorrelations. The surprise is almost certainly the result of overlooking patterns of intercorrelations that were present in the matrix of intercorrelations in the first place.

Although it is true that multiregression analyses are now very rarely performed by hand, no one who lacks access to computer routines should feel that he or she is behind the current state of the art. A matrix of intercorrelations can be sent to a laboratory where computer facilities exist, the matrix being the "data" from which multiregression analysis can be performed.

How Multiregression Analysis Works

The best way to explain multiregression analysis is to use a simple example. Let us pretend that we need to know whether the many cases of neurological disorders that have appeared in a community are or are not the result of exposure to lead in the environment. As a result of a health survey, environmental levels of lead, blood lead levels, biological indicators of lead exposure and absorption, the results of physical examinations, and special psychological and neurophysiological test results are available. To make a judgment whether several dependent variables are related to several independent variables, and rule out a number of confounding factors, a multiregression approach is appropriate.

A *stepwise correlational analysis* is a good example of a multiregression analysis. A stepwise correlational analysis is an aid to thinking, and it is only recommended if a computer is available because of the intense mathematical calculations it requires.

In this example, let us replace the variables by letters: A, B, and C for the dependent variables, X, Y, and Z for the independent, and P and Q for the confounding variables. A stepwise correlational analysis is a procedure by which the correlation of A (alone) is studied vis-à-vis X, Y, Z, P, and Q, taking the latter set one at a time, two at a time, and so on. Certain procedures will produce the best set of variables that maximize the multiregression coefficients. *Mallow's Cp criterion* and the *r-square criterion* (Draper and Smith 1981) are the two most common for ranking the significance of the contribution of each variable or a set of variables to the determination of A. The technique is invaluable in that confounding variables sometimes may appear to explain most of the correlations with the dependent variable! This finding may or may not be obvious from visual inspection of a matrix of intercorrelations. The procedure can be repeated for B alone and for C alone. In turn, A, B, and C can be combined into a single dependent variable.

Effect of Low-Level Lead and Arsenic Exposure on Copper Smelter Workers

Lilis and collaborators (1985) performed an analysis of reported symptoms and their relationships with indicators of lead absorption [blood lead (Pb-B) and zinc protoporphyrin

(ZPP)] and arsenic absorption [urinary arsenic (As-U)] among 680 active copper smelter workers. Lead, cadmium, and arsenic emissions from a large Canadian copper smelter were found to result in environmental contamination and significant absorption of these metals in segments of the population living in the area immediately surrounding the smelter. This study has been chosen to illustrate various data-analytical steps that sometimes are necessary before subjecting data to multiregression analysis.

Statistical Analysis of Data.   The prevalence of individual symptoms was computed by dividing the number of subjects who reported the symptoms by the total number of subjects for each subgroup of 50, as defined below. The symptoms were then treated as categorical variables ("yes"/"no" type). The variable "total number of symptoms" ("Total" for short) was a continuous variable that resulted from adding "yes" responses to questions relating to individual symptoms. Thus, "Total" = 0 indicated that the subject had no symptoms, whereas "Total" = 5 meant that there had been a positive response to five questions referring to separate symptoms. The variable "Total" (number of symptoms) varied from 0 to 14. The distribution of "Total" was not normal; it was highly skewed to the left, which indicated that most of the subjects had only a few symptoms. Although a logarithmic transformation slightly improved the distribution, no attempt was made to normalize the distribution of this variable. Because of the nonnormal distribution of "Total," all correlation coefficients where this variable intervened were computed using nonparametric techniques (Spearman's correlation coefficient r).

For each symptom, mean Pb-B, mean ZPP, and mean As-U in subjects who reported a symptom were compared with the corresponding mean values in subjects who had not reported the symptom. The significance of the difference between metal absorption among symptomatic and asymptomatic individuals was tested by means of t-tests.

Graphic Representation of Data.   Graphs illustrating the relationship between "Total" and indicators of lead and arsenic absorption (Pb-B, ZPP, and As-U) were then constructed. In addition, graphs illustrating the relationship between prevalence rates of individual symptoms and indicators of lead and arsenic absorption were prepared. The following procedure was used.

First, the 680 currently active copper smelter workers were sorted by increasing levels of the biological indicator of exposure (eg, Pb-B). Second, the median level of Pb-B for each subgroup of 50 subjects was calculated. For Pb-B and ZPP, 14 such points (representing the median value of 14 subgroups as defined above) were thus determined. For As-U, only 12 such points were calculated because a number of As-U values were missing.

By using this approach, we attempted to minimize the effect of the fact that there were many more subjects with relatively lower Pb-B, ZPP, and As-U than there were individuals with more elevated levels. If the usual approach of establishing subgroups according to the range—for example, of Pb less than 40, 40 to 59, or equal to or greater than 60 µg/dL—had been chosen, the points on the graph would have represented groups of highly different size. Thus, we attempted to minimize the differential "weight" associated with each point as we calculated the constants a (the Y-intercept) and b (the slope) of regression equations.

Logarithmic values of the median Pb-B, ZPP, or As-U were plotted against the abscissae. As indicated, the logarithmic transformation of Pb-B, ZPP, and As-U approximated the normal distribution better than did the raw values. Moreover, median values of raw data (ie, not logarithmically transformed) produced graphs where most of the points were clustered to the left, a reflection of the fact that many subjects had relatively low levels of Pb-B, ZPP, and As-U.

Graphs were constructed by plotting prevalence rates of individual symptoms on the ordinate for each subgroup of 50 subjects. Prevalence is a percentage computed as

Yes/(Yes + No), where Yes is a subject who reported the symptom and No is a subject who did not report the symptom. In addition, graphs were constructed with the total number of symptoms on the ordinate for each subgroup of 50 subjects. The total number of symptoms was, as indicated above, the mean value of the number of symptoms reported by subjects in the subgroups. Ordering the subjects by levels of biological indicators of metal absorption and calculating the constants of the linear regression equation was accomplished by means of the SAS statistical package.

An intercorrelation matrix was constructed showing the correlation coefficients of the total number of symptoms, age, duration of employment in the copper smelter, log ZPP, log Pb-B, and log As-U. Data from this intercorrelation matrix provided the hypothesis on which the multiregression analysis was based.

Multiregression Analysis of Data. Stepwise multiregression analysis was used to explore the relationships between independent variables—age, duration from onset of exposure, duration of employment, Pb-B, ZPP, and As-U—and the dependent variable "Total" (number of symptoms). For that purpose, the SAS computer package PROC STEPWISE with maximum R^2 was used. Several independent variables were added and removed in these exploratory analyses to determine their individual and joint effects on the dependent variable (ie, "Total").

We looked at two characteristics of the multivariate model: that model which produced the largest R^2; and the changes in the probability level associated with the F test in the analysis of the variance as single variables or combinations of variables were added or subtracted.

When it was stated that a variable, such as age, was significant, we meant that the probability of F was significant when the variable was considered by itself and remained significant when other variables were added to the model.

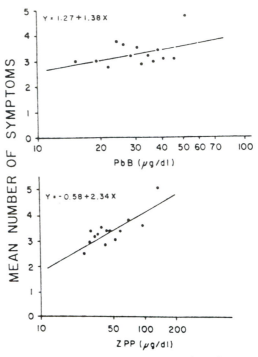

Fig. 19.7. Relationship between number of reported symptoms and levels of blood lead and ZPP in active smelter workers ($N = 678$ for lead; $N = 673$ for ZPP) (From Lilis et al. 1985.)

Figure 19.7 shows the relationship between mean number of reported symptoms and Pb-B and ZPP levels. It was observed that with increasing ZPP levels, there was an increase in the prevalence of the mean total symptoms; the relationship between mean number of symptoms and Pb-B was less marked. Thus, this method of data analysis revealed the comparatively greater sensitivity of ZPP as a measure of lead effect to predict symptoms, a feature of the data that previously needed to be inferred from visual analysis of numerical tables. In addition, when symptoms are considered, ZPP does not seem to have a threshold effect. The increase in levels of symptoms seems to be continuous, from the lowest to the highest ZPP level. This strategy thus illustrates once more the importance of graphic methods as a data-analytical technique.

Table 19.8 shows the results of the multiregression analysis. According to the crite-

Table 19.8. Multiregression Analysis of Total Number of Symptoms versus Age, Duration of Exposure, Pb-B, ZPP, and As-U in Active Copper Smelter Employees

Number of Variables	Best Model	Individual Variables		Aggregation of Variables	
		F	p	F	p
One	log ZPP	10.78	0.0011†	10.78	0.0001‡
Two	Age	6.50	0.0110*	8.69	0.0002‡
	log ZPP	9.41	0.0023†		
Three	Age	6.18	0.0132*	6.05	0.0006†
	log ZPP	8.36	0.0040†		
	log As-U	0.77	0.3800		
Four	Age	4.74	0.0298*	4.53	0.0013†
	log ZPP	8.37	0.0040†		
	log As-U	0.76	0.3836		
	Duration	0.02	0.8884		
Five	Age	4.53	0.0338*	3.62	0.0032†
	log Pb-B	0.00	0.9887		
	log ZPP	6.14	0.0135*		
	log As-U	0.73	0.3919		
	Duration	0.02	0.8880		

*$p \leq 0.05$.
†$p \leq 0.01$.
‡$p \leq 0.001$.
From Lilis et al. (1985).

ria stated above (R^2 and F), ZPP was found to make the most important contribution in the determination of mean number of symptoms, age being the second most important factor. No significant contributions of the other independent variables, either singly or in combination, were found.

LARGER PERSPECTIVES OF CAUSATION

Proximal versus Remote and Direct versus Indirect Causes

In Chapter 15 we reviewed the familiar concepts of independent, dependent, and confounding variables. Briefly, in E & O neurotoxicology: the independent variable is conceived of as the neurotoxic agent—measured by environmental levels and/or absorbed dose—or other factor causing a neuropsychological change; the dependent variable is a quantitative value of neurolog-

ical signs or symptoms, test scores derived from psychometric testing, and/or data obtained from electrophysiological or imaging procedures; and the confounding variables are those properties of the subject's physical or demographic profile—eg, age, gender, ethnic background, education—whose effect may resemble those of the independent variable.

In the 1980s, there was increasing interest among environmental health research workers in the identification of other types of variables to deal with the matter of causation within a wider framework including social factors. Figure 19.8 reviews the concept of both direct and indirect and proximal and remote. *Path analysis* is a data-displaying technique to explain how proximal and remote, direct and indirect factors explain a single variable (eg, blood lead levels) or more complex functions (eg, a child's intelligence).

Path Analysis. The task of displaying, studying, interpreting, and verbalizing findings derived from the study of a matrix of

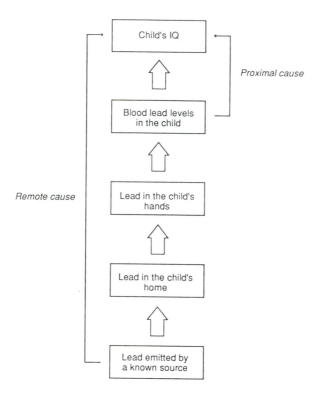

Fig. 19.8. Concept of proximal and remote causes in the relationship between lead and IQ.

intercorrelations among many variables sometimes is formidable. As indicated in Chapter 15, scientists have long recognized the need for better media for data display and communication. Path analysis is such a medium.

Path analysis is both a statistical technique for data analysis and a medium of information display. Its name is derived from the appearance of the illustrations resulting from such an analysis: weak and strong, direct and indirect relations among a set of variables are indicated by means of boxes and arrows. The thickness of arrows sometimes is also used as a visual code to indicate the strength of a relationship. Path analysis, like LISREL, discussed below, deals with intercorrelated sets of dependent, independent, and endogenous variables. An *endogenous variable* is one that can be placed either as a dependent variable in some models or as an independent variable in others.

There is a close relationship between a path display and a matrix of intercorrelations. This relationship is best expressed with an analogy. Path analysis is to the visual examination of a matrix of intercorrelations what a coefficient of correlation r is to the visual examination of a scattergram. Through both, the investigator verifies hunches felt while examining data. Path analysis, like the coefficient of correlation, is a quantitative description of that "hunch." An experienced investigator is able to estimate the correlation coefficient from the visual examination of a scattergram; he or she also can plot a path diagram from a matrix of intercorrelations. Path analysis provides rules for drawing such illustrations.

A single path analysis diagram contains all the elements relevant to a specific problem. It also contains a quantitative estimate of causation. Path analysis looks like a printed circuit of the network of interactions. It is a powerful medium of data reduction and a synthetic visual mode of expression.

Social Factors Determining Environmental and Blood Lead Levels.

R. L. Bornschein and collaborators (1986) at the Department of Environmental Health at the University of Cincinnati Medical Center reported a study of the role of social and environmental factors on dust lead, hand lead, and blood lead levels in a cohort of young children. The subjects were observed at 3-month intervals from birth to 24 months of age. A qualitative rating of the residence and of the socioeconomic status of the family was obtained. Interviews and direct observations of parent and child at home were used to evaluate various aspects of caretaker–child interactions.

This study is interesting in that the role of proximal and remote factors in the determination of levels of toxic agents was ascertained and in that the data were analyzed via statistical techniques of increasing complexity, ranging from simple regression analysis to structural equation analysis.

Figure 19.9 shows a simplified version of the model linking remote and proximal factors in the determination of blood lead levels in the child. To this author's knowledge, this was the first time concepts derived from path analysis and modeling based on structural equations have been used in the field of environmental neurotoxicology.

Multivariate Analysis with Latent Variables

Epidemiology and toxicology are empirical and inductive sciences, and thus the methods of deductive science have yet to be used as tools of the trade by epidemiologists and human toxicologists. There are historical reasons for this: "hard data" is necessary when environmental and occupational toxic limits are proposed and when litigation occurs. In the past 15 years, however, a revolutionary change has taken place in data-analytical techniques which favors the use of latent variables with unique applications in the field.

Latent variables (LV) are constructs, and therefore cannot be measured. Investigators using latent variables take an imaginative look at the data: the statistical properties of the measured variables are explained in terms of the hypothesized variables. As Bentler (1980) has indicated, latent variable models represent the convergence of relatively independent research traditions in psychometrics, econometrics, and biometrics, where this imaginative approach has made important contributions. Many econometric models, for example, are LV models.

Latent variable modeling is intimately related to path analysis as reviewed above. The novelty of this approach is fully understood when one is reminded that in path analysis, the path coefficients linking variables are calculated one by one, and the path picture is

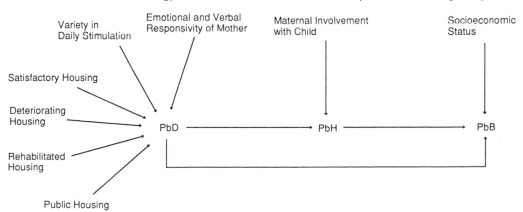

Fig. 19.9. A path-analytical study of the relationships between environmental factors and lead in children. PbD, lead content of surface dust; PbH, lead content of hand; PbB, blood lead levels. (Modified from Borschein et al. 1986.)

assembled as one would a puzzle for which no "right" figure is available. Latent variable modeling is possible thanks to the mathematical work of the Swedish scientist K.G. Jöreskog (1973), who proposed a method for simultaneously resolving a set of equations now called structural equations. LISREL is a LV modeling technique based on those equations. In LISREL, for example, the model or models are proposed by the investigator; LV computer programs containing structural equations determine the relative plausibility of the various models. Latent variables have an important but as yet unexplored role in the understanding of mechanisms of toxic action in humans.

Factor Analysis

Factor analysis is one of the most widely used of the major multivariate techniques. We have mentioned earlier that whereas a matrix of intercorrelations as an expression of scientific results is a widely accepted means of communication, multivariate techniques derived from the analysis of such a matrix have had their ups and downs in scientists' esteem. Factor analysis is a powerful method of data analysis, and it is one of the fundamental methodological pillars of psychometric thinking. However, understanding what factor-analytical techniques can accomplish and how results can be interpreted has been the subject of controversy since their creation by Charles Spearman in 1904.

Factor analysis is a technique of data reduction designed to help one understand the clusters of intercorrelations in an intercorrelation matrix. Higher-order, abstract variables are created as a synthesis of these clusters. These are called factors.

Since Spearman, several schools of thought have developed about the adequate computational and (sometimes) geometric procedures used to extract those factors. Computational procedures range from relatively simple calculations that can be performed by hand to elaborate mathematical procedures that are accomplished via a fairly powerful computer.

In the final stages of analysis, when these clusters are reduced to factors, each variable of the matrix of intercorrelations is tested. The purpose of this test is to determine how much weight each variable has in this abstract factor. As a result of this weighting procedure, some apparent patterns emerge. The irrepressible tendency to associate a factor with a specific brain function results from the analysis of how a group of variables behaves in concert with a factor. Factor analysis of large data banks, where hundreds of variables are involved, is sometimes indispensible. Further, factor analysis of subsets of variables—such as specific sections of a research protocol—is often necessary.

Factor analysis is an extremely useful technique in test selection and battery development. When space and time are constraints, factor analysis is a technique that can be of help in deciding which tests to keep and which to drop without losing a firm statistical footing in the assessment of neurotoxicity.

One of the greatest dangers of factor analysis, however, is to take factors too seriously and to treat them as "brain functions." Factors are very flimsy. They vary drastically as variables are introduced or removed from the original set of variables that must be factor-analyzed. If factors are functions, then an entirely different picture of how the brain works is obtained, depending on which variables are fed into the basic paradigm to begin with. One of the greatest contributions of computers is that factor analysis can now be performed as a matter of routine. Computers have indeed facilitated the intuitive understanding of the powerful features and limitations of this multivariate technique.

Theoretically, there is nothing fundamentally wrong with interpreting factors as brain functions, provided those functions can be anchored with well-established facts of neuropsychological research. The total schism that exists between factor analysts and neuroscientists is certainly not a healthy trend. Health experts who must read and interpret research reports where factor analysis is used must be aware of these shortcomings.

Factor analysis and discriminant analysis (to be reviewed below) have both aided in the clarification of possible toxic causation only peripherally. When these are used according to the classical tenets of psychometric thinking—as illustrated in the following example—it looks as if investigators have tried to identify the "personality of the lead worker" or the "personality of the solvent-exposed worker."

The book by Stephen J. Gould, *The Mismeasure of Man* (1981) contains one of the most lucid explanations of factor analysis ever written for the layperson.

Multivariate Study of Neuropsychological Changes Linked to Occupational Exposure to Neurotoxic Agents.

Hänninen (1971) used factor analysis in an attempt to understand how carbon disulfide affects nervous system function. In particular, she was interested in knowing whether multivariate analysis of the results of intelligence tests and ability tests, motor behavior, personality, and subjective symptoms could be helpful in revealing regions of the nervous system that serve as a primary target of carbon disulfide. Three groups of workers were evaluated: workers admitted to a clinic for carbon disulfide poisoning, a group who had experienced subclinical effects resulting from carbon disulfide exposure, and an "unexposed" group (of workers who had been exposed but showed no manifest symptoms).

The factor-analytical study consisted of three separate analyses of each group. Six factors were extracted: visual intelligence; general intelligence; motor speed and dexterity; a "neuroticism" factor; introverted behavior; and personal tempo.

Important information on details of how the factor analysis was performed are missing from this report; these details are often considered "technical" but now are seen as essential for the understanding of findings. For example, Hänninen did not report on the nature of data involved in the factor-analytical study or the criteria followed to select those factors. In retrospect, there is not enough justification to include continuous variables derived from psychometric testing alongside those from subjective symptoms and neurophysiological data such as information obtained from electromyographic studies. In addition, there are objective criteria as to the number of factors that can reasonably be proposed. These criteria are whether the magnitude of the eigenvalue is 1 or greater than 1 (the eigenvalue being a numerical value associated with the statistical plausibility of the existence of a factor), or the rule-of-thumb criteria of no more than one factor per 10 variables. Hänninen extracted six factors from 28 variables obtained in 50 individuals. It is not surprising that she found factors close to the dimensions of the tests used to assess cognitive ability, personality, and symptoms.

In Hänninen's opinion, the results of the factor-analytical study did not yield a simple factor structure for all three groups. This was explained by the fact that the tests did not measure pure factors but rather detected mental disturbances, which are of a complex nature. In the group of workers who suffered carbon disulfide poisoning, she encountered the following prominent factors: deterioration (as showed by a slowing of speed), rigidity, emotional disturbance, and neurasthenia syndrome. A factor of "spontaneous creativity" revealed in the Rorschach tests of inkblots did not seem to have a connection with the other tests.

Discriminant Analysis

The basic paradigm of discriminant analysis can be illustrated as follows. We know certain facts—ie, that certain demographic variables and performance test scores belong to controls or to the study group. On the basis of one or more variables, appropriately called *discriminant variables,* we can create a model that will predict the likelihood that each of the individuals examined belongs to either the control or the study group.

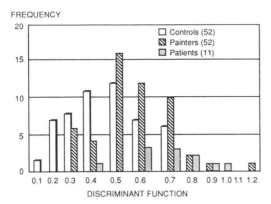

Fig. 19.10. Distribution of the discriminant function of the control of painters, controls, and a small sample of workers with clinical signs of brain dysfunction. (From Hane et al. 1977, reproduced by permission of the author.)

A study by Hane et al. (1977) will be used as an example. These investigators used discriminant functions to ascertain how the results of neuropsychological tests would discriminate among three groups: controls not exposed to solvents, house painters occupationally exposed to solvents, and patients admitted to the clinic for solvent poisoning. Figure 19.10 shows the distribution of the discriminant functions among the three groups. This is a good graphic way to describe peaks and overlaps that occur in the three groups.

The ability of discriminant variables to show whether an individual has been correctly classified is associated with the concept of hit rate. The *hit rate* is the proportion of cases who have been correctly classified as "control" or "study." The greater the sum of these two correct classifications, the greater the hit rate. The hit rate is a measure of success in classifying groups in terms of a variety of sets of variables.

Discriminant analysis can be used as a test of the adequacy of matching because if one can demonstrate that a significant proportion of cases can be predicted to be controls or studies on the basis of demographics alone, then the matching process is poor. But, if by using the identical procedure the matching demographic is acceptable and scores or neu-

rophysiological findings are different in controls and studies, then these findings cannot be considered spurious.

Group differences in neurological symptoms, psychological test scores, and neurophysiological measures are not to be considered "proofs" but rather "suggestions" of neurotoxic effects. But since reliable indicators of exposure and absorption are not available for most neurotoxic agents, group differences are sometimes the only "evidence" of an effect. In an ideal world (which is not the world of occupational health workers and environmental scientists), incontrovertible proof of a neurotoxic effect is the one that results from demonstrating statistically significant correlations between dependent and independent variables and ruling out confounding factors.

FALLACIES IN THE SEARCH FOR POSSIBLE TOXIC CAUSATION

Dr. Herbert L. Needleman from the Children's Hospital of Pittsburgh has argued vehemently of the dangers of adhering too strictly to classical statistical thinking in studies performed to ascertain possible toxic causation in environmental chemicals. The following material is abstracted from a paper presented at the International Workshop on the Effects of Lead Exposure on Neurobehavioral Development in Edinburgh, Scotland in 1986.

In reviewing the literature on the effect of lead on child development, Needleman applauds the increasing sophistication and rigor of studies. But he also observes that

> Making causal connections in the real world is not a pure, value-free enterprise . . . It seem clear that differences in style exist among investigators and interpreters of the same database. These stylistic, value-laden differences in interpreting the data seem to be rather stable traits. It would be of considerable interest to determine whether they segregate with differences in training, discipline, or other variables. (Needleman and Bellinger 1989, p. 303)

Needleman and Bellinger (1989) cite examples of errors in judgment leading to the rejection of valid associations (between potential neurotoxic agents and their effects) as spurious. A detailed review and supporting documentation for such cases—which the authors call "type II fallacies"—are beyond the scope of this chapter. They involve the following:

- A rigid view of the probability level of 0.05 as a cutting point for attributing statistical and biological significance.
- A reliance on phantom covariates whose incorporation into statistical models guarantees the reduction of the effect produced by the toxic agents, or building nonveridical causal models incorporating variable models that overcontrol or minimize the effects of toxic agents.
- Accepting the "null hypothesis"—the hypothesis that no association exists—from studies with inadequate power (that are caused when too many covariates are used in multiregression analysis of very few cases).
- Underestimating the biological significance of a demonstrated difference in (statistical) size—eg, dismissing as trivial a reduction of IQ in children's intelligence.
- Wrong expectations of proof of causality—eg, holding corrective action until the "perfect health study" is performed.
- Seeking toxic causation by concensus though balloting reported studies.

REFERENCES

Baggaley, AR (1964) *Intermediate Correlational Methods*. New York: John Wiley & Sons.

Bentler, PM (1980) Multivariate analysis with latent variables: Causal modelling. *Ann Rev Psychol* 31:419–456.

Bornschein, RL, Succop, PA and Krafft KM (1986) Exterior surface dust, interior house dust lead and childhood lead exposure in an urban environment. In *Trace Substances in Environmental Health: A symposium*, DD Hemphill (ed) pp. 322–332. Columbia, MO: University of Missouri at Columbia.

Draper, NR and Smith, H (1981) *Applied Regression Analysis*, 2nd ed. New York: John Wiley & Sons.

Gould, SJ (1981) *The Mismeasure of Man*. New York: WW Norton.

Hane, M, Axelson, O, Blume, J, et al. (1977) Psychological function changes among house painters. *Scand J Work Environ Health* 3:91–99.

Hänninen, H. (1971) Psychological picture of manifest and latent carbon disulfide poisoning. *Br J Ind Med* 28:374–381.

Hänninen, H, Hernberg, S, Mantere, P (1978) Psychological performance of subjects with low exposure to lead. *J Occup Med* 20:683–689.

Hayes, AW (1982) *Principles and Methods of Toxicology*. New York: Raven Press.

Jöreskog, KG (1973) A general method for estimating a linear structural equation system. In *Structural Equation Models in the Social Sciences*, AS Goldberg and OD Duncan (eds). New York: Seminar Press.

Last, JM (1983) *A Dictionary of Epidemiology*. New York: Oxford University Press.

Lilis, R, Blumberg, WE, Eisinger, J, et al. (1977) Lead effects among secondary lead smelter workers with lead levels below 80 micrograms/100 ml. *Arch Environ Health* 32:256–266.

Lilis, R, Valciukas, JA, Weber, J-P. et al. (1985) Effects of low level lead and arsenic exposure on copper smelter workers. *Arch Environ Health* 40:38–47.

Needleman, HL and Bellinger DC (1989) Type II fallacies in the study of childhood exposure to lead at low dose: A critical and quantitative review. In *Lead Exposure and Child Development: An International Assessment*. MA Smith, LD Grant, and AI Sors (eds) pp. 293–304. Washington, DC: Environmental Protection Agency.

Needleman, HL, Gunnoe, CE, Leviton, A, et al. (1979) Deficits in psychologic and classroom performance of children with elevated lead levels. *N Engl J Med* 300:689–695.

Rutstein, DD, Mullan, RJ, and Frazier, TM (1983) Sentinel health events (occupational): A basis for physician recognition and public health surveillance. *Am J Public Health* 73:1054.

Schlesselman, JJ (1982) *Case-Control Studies: Design, Conduct, Analysis*. New York: Oxford University Press.

Seppäläinen, AM and Hernberg, S (1972) Sensitive technique for detecting subclinical lead neuropathy. *Br J Ind Med* 29:443–449.

Valciukas, JA and Lilis, R (1980) Psychometric techniques in environmental research. *Environ Res* 21:275–297.

Valciukas, JA and Lilis, R (1982) A composite index of lead effects: Comparative study of four occupational groups with different levels of lead absorption. *Int Arch Environ Health* 51:1–14.

Valciukas, JA, Lilis, R, Fischbein, A et al. (1978) Central nervous system dysfunction due to lead exposure. *Science* 201:465–467.

Valciukas, JA, Lilis, R, Anderson, HA et al. (1979) The neurotoxicity of polybrominated biphenyls. Results of a medical field survey. *Ann NY Acad Sci* 320:337–367.

Valciukas, JA, Lilis, R and Petrocci, M (1981) An integrative index of biological effects of lead. *Am J Ind Med* 2:261–272.

Valciukas, JA, Lilis, R, Singer, RM, et al. (1985) Neurobehavioral changes among shipyard painters exposed to solvents. *Arch Environ Health* 40(1):47–52.

SUGGESTED READINGS

Abercrombie, MLJ (1989) *The Anatomy of Judgment: An Investigation into the Process of Perception and Reasoning*. New York: Columbia University Press.

Albert, A and Harris, EK (1987) *Multivariate Interpretation of Clinical Laboratory Data*. New York: Marcel Dekker.

Albert, DA, Munson, R, and Resnik, MD (1988) *Reasoning in Medicine: An Introduction to Clinical Inference*. Baltimore, MD: Johns Hopkins University Press.

Bartholomew, DJ (1987) *Latent Variable Models and Factor Analysis*. New York: Oxford University Press.

Bender, AP, Williams, AN, Johnson, RA, et al. (1990) Appropriate public health responses to clusters. The art of being responsibly responsive. *Am J Epidemiol* 132(1):48–52.

Bernstein, IH (1988) *Applied Multivariate Analysis*. New York: Springer-Verlag.

Black, B (1988) Evolving legal standards for the admissibility of scientific evidence. *Science* 239:1508–1512.

Bogen, DK (1989) Software review: Simulation software for the Macintosh. *Science* 246:138–142.

Bunge, M (1979) *Causality and Modern Science,* 3rd rev ed. New York: Dover Publications.

Burchfiel, JL, Duffy, FH, Bartels, PH, et al. (1980) The combined discrimination power of quantitative electroencephalography and neuropsychologic measures in evaluating central nervous system effects of lead at low levels. In *Low-Level Lead Exposure: The Clinical Implications of Current Research,* HL Needleman (ed) pp. 75–89. New York: Raven Press.

Checkoway, H, Pearce, N, Hickey, JLS, et al. (1990) Latency analysis in occupational epidemiology. *Arch Environ Health* 45(2):95–100.

Culhane, PJ, Friesma, HP, and Beecher, JA (eds) (1987) *The Content and Predictive Accuracy of Environmental Impact Statement*. Boulder, CO: Westview.

Curran, WJ, McGarry, AL, and Petty, CS (eds) (1980) *Modern Legal Medicine, Psychiatry and Forensic Science*. Philadelphia: FA Davis.

Dawes, RM, Faust, D, and Meehl, PE (1989) Clinical versus actuarial judgment. *Science* 243:1668–1674.

Delaunois, AL (ed) (1973) *Biostatistics in Pharmacology, International Encyclopedia of Pharmacology and Therapeutics*. New York: Pergamon Press.

Elwood, JM (1988) *Causal Relationships in Medicine: A Practical System for Critical Appraisal*. New York: Oxford University Press.

Evans, GW and Campbell, JM (1983) Psychological perspectives on air pollution and health. *Basic Appl Soc Psychol* 4(2):137–169.

Everitt, BS (1984) *An Introduction to Latent Variable Models*. New York: Chapman and Hall.

Feinstein, AR (1988) Scientific standards in epidemiologic studies of the menace of daily life. *Science* 242:1257–1263.

Frauenthal, JC (1980) *Mathematical Models in Epidemiology*. New York: Springer-Verlag.

Gray-Donald, K and Kramer, MS (1988) Causality inference in observational vs experimental studies: An empirical comparison. *Am J Epidemiol* 127:885–892.

Harrold, GC (1960) The expert witness. *Am Ind Hyg Assoc J* 21:330–333.

Hayduk, LA (1987) *Structural Equation Modeling with LISREL*. Baltimore: The Johns Hopkins University Press.

Hellevik, O (1988) *Introduction to Causal Analysis: Exploring Survey Data by Cross-Tabulation*. New York: Oxford University Press.

Lorr, M (1983) *Cluster Analysis for Social Scientists: Techniques for Analyzing and Simplifying Complex Blocks of Data*. San Francisco: Jossey-Bass.

McHovec, FJ (1987) *The Expert Witness Survival Manual*. Springfield, IL: Charles C Thomas.

Merret, JD (1966) Discriminant function analysis as an aid to the diagnosis of flax byssinosis. *Br J Ind Med* 23:58–61.

Mottet, NK (1985) *Environmental Pathology*. New York: Oxford University Press.

Ramsey, JD (1975) Causal factors research: Valuable tool. *Int J Occup Health Safety* 44:26–28.

Robins, JM, Landrigan, PJ, Robins, TG, et al. (1985) Decision making under uncertainty in the setting of environmental health regulations. *J Public Health Pol* 3:322–328.

Rodgers, JL and Nicewander, WA (1988) Thirteen ways to look at the correlation coefficient. *Am Statist* 42(2):59–66.

Rothman KJ (1978) Occam's razor pares the choice among statistical models. *Am J Epidemiol* 108:347–349.

Rothman, KJ (ed) (1988) *Causal Inference*. Chestnut, MA: Epidemiology Resources.

Schartz, S and Giffin, T (1986) *Medical Thinking: The Psychology of Medical Judgment and Decision Making*. New York: Springer-Verlag.

Selikoff, IJ (1984) Twenty lessons from asbestos: A bitter harvest of scientific information. *EPA J* 10(4):21–24.

Slovik, P (1987) Perception of risk. *Science* 236:280–285.

Symons, NS (1960) What is expected of the professional person in litigation? *Am Ind Hyg Assoc J* 21:502–509.

Tardiff, RG and Rodricks, JV (eds) (1987) *Principles of Data Interpretation*. New York: Plenum Press.

Walter, SD and Holford, TR (1978) Additive, muliplicative and other models for disease risk. *Am J Epidemiol* 108:341–346.

Zechhauser, RJ and Viscusi, WK (1990) Risk within reason. *Science* 248:559–564.

Part V

The Targets of Neurotoxicity

20

Neurotoxic Agents and Brain Development

The developing nervous system of the embryo, fetus, and child is a vulnerable target of many neurotoxic agents. Two disciplines deal with the study of neurotoxic diseases at these early stages of human and animal development: neuroteratology and pediatric neurotoxicology. These will be discussed in this chapter.

DEVELOPMENT OF THE NERVOUS SYSTEM

The effects of neurotoxic agents on the developing nervous system are best understood if the phases of nervous system development and organogenesis—the development of organs—are reviewed.

Three fundamental regions of the embryo are recognized at the earliest stages of its development: the *endoderm* ("internal skin"), the *mesoderm* ("medial skin"), and the *ectoderm* ("outer skin"). The endoderm and mesoderm give rise to the internal lining of the organs and to bony and muscle structures. These are not further reviewed since the nervous system—the focus of this work—develops from the ectoderm.

The nervous system includes sensory receptors, nerves, and effectors strategically located in almost every region of the body except for "dead" tissues such as hair, nails, the outer layers of the skin, and tooth dentine. Even in the adult, the fundamental features of metamerism—the fact that we are built of a series of building blocks (the metamerae) characteristic of all vertebrates—is readily recognized. Examples of metamerism are the symmetrical positioning of the vertebrae, the manner in which nerves enter and leave the spinal cord, and the configuration of the rib cage in the adult.

The nervous system develops from a thickened area of the ectoderm of the early embryo called the neural plate. *The neural crest develops from the neural plate to form the* neural tube *through a process of inward folding best understood when seen in a motion picture. The anterior portion of the neural plate soon shows a marked enlargement called the* brain vesicles, *the first sign of the origin of the two brain hemispheres.*

Human embryos 4 weeks old show three well-differentiated regions of the brain vesicles: the forebrain, midbrain, and hindbrain. By the fifth week the three vesicles divide: the forebrain becomes the telencephalon and the diencephalon; the midbrain becomes the mesencephalon; and the hindbrain differentiates into the metencephalon and myelencephalon.

Each of these five divisions then gives rise to specific areas of the brain and sense organs during development. Humans ultimately develop 12 cranial nerves—a bare increment of two over their distant relatives, the fish. Some of the nerves are associated with highly specialized sensory systems—for example, the olfactory nerve with olfaction, the optic nerves with vision, and the auditory nerves with audition. The spinal nerves originate at the caudal (tail) region of the neural crest.

The histogenesis (cell formation) of the spinal cord provides a good illustration of the variety of neural cells derived from primitive cells of the neural crest. The cells of the neural tube appear to be relatively similar, but these cells proliferate quickly and become differentiated. By the time the neural crest evolves into the neural tube, three layers of differentiated cells can be observed: marginal, mantle, and ependymal.

From this point onward, cells continue to develop individual characteristics. Of the three layers, the cells of the mantle layer show the most marked differentiation, becoming spongioblasts or neuroblasts. The spongioblasts give rise to supporting tissue, the neuroglia; the neuroblasts develop into the neurons, the basic nerve cell of the differentiated nervous system. (In Chapter 2, the significance of these cells is discussed.)

As a result of attempts to develop guidelines for risk assessment and regulation of potential defect-causing agents, particularly in drug manufacture, critical phases in embryo/fetus (conceptus) development have now been recognized. Phase I, called the *fertility stage,* covers the period before conception and throughout gestation. Phase II, the *teratology stage,* is the period of embryonic development when the conceptus is most vulnerable to toxin-induced malformations—that is, when the most active phase of organogenesis occurs. Phase III, the *perinatal stage,* is the period after fetal organs are fully formed, up to and including lactation (Vorhees and Buchter 1982).

At present there is extensive evidence from morphological, electrophysiological, and pharmacological studies that the process of maturation of the nervous system is that of "restricted malleability" (Purves and Lichtman 1980). Neural development is not necessarily associated with an increment of neural units. For example, synapsis elimination can be observed in the neuromuscular junction, neuron-to-neuron contacts in autonomic ganglia, and in certain areas of the cerebral cortex such as the developing visual cortex. It seems likely that competition for trophic (nutrient) factors, not yet completely understood, is the basis of neuronal death. In brief, muscles and neurons seem to be oversupplied by synapses (the places where neurons connect with each other) at the time of the development of the nervous system.

Critical Periods of Organogenesis

These were described by Stockad in 1921. But the fine details of the manner in which neurotoxic agents in the environment and/or the workplace affect the structural and functional maturation of the human conceptus are largely unknown. For some, specific syndromes have been described: for example, Minamata disease and fetal alcohol syndrome (FAS) (both discussed later in this chapter).

Abnormal embryogenesis (development of the embryo) is initiated by defect-causing agents, or *teratogens,* acting on the developing tissues and cells. It was generally thought that teratological defects are "agent specific," ie, that each agent has the capacity of producing specific defects. However, as a result of increasing information about the mechanisms of action of many teratogenic agents, this view has been changed.

Among the possible ways a teratogen might influence developmental pathogenesis are gene mutation, chromosomal aberrations, mitotic interference, altered nucleic acid integrity or function, altered energy sources, changed membrane characteristics, and enzyme inhibition. (These are terms applied to molecular mechanisms that occur in the neural cell; some of these mechanisms are described in Chapter 2.) A causative agent might initiate one or more of these varied mechanisms. As Wilson (1973) states, the ". . . majority of developmental defects . . . . involve deficiencies in tissue elements or of their biochemical products."

The final manifestation of abnormal development is death, malformation, growth retardation, or functional disorder. Before differentiation begins, the embryo has a high threshold (or tolerance) to most teratogens, but when the threshold is exceeded, death can ensue. Malformations are more likely to occur during the period of organ formation, but death is always possible if high dosages of teratogens are encountered. Growth retardation is characteristic of the fetal period (a period normally characterized by growth). Functional disorders—particularly behavioral disorders, the study of which gave rise to "behavioral toxicology" as a discipline—are more difficult to explain because there is no single explanation of how behavior occurs.

NEUROTERATOLOGY

Teratology is the study of the abnormal development of the embryo, fetus, and child. A *teratogen* (or teratogenic agent) is any chemical substance or physical condition that can produce such abnormalities. Ethanol and X-rays, for example, are known teratogens.

The abnormal development might be expressed—in decreasing order of severity—by death, malformation, growth retardation, and functional disorder. Until recently, studies of teratogenesis were restricted to structural malformations occurring during the gestational stage of development. The definition of teratogenesis has since been expanded to include alterations of structure, growth, and function, whether caused by genetically determined factors, by environmental factors, or by an interaction between genetic and environmental factors in fetus and child.

Studies on experimental teratology, the production of abnormal development in animal models under laboratory conditions, were carried out first in the late 1930s. But observation of single malformations, conjoined twins, and the explanations of these occurrences have a long and fascinating history (Warkany 1977). Observations of malformations in children as the result of maternal pelvic irradiation began to appear in the late 1920s (Goldstein and Murphy 1929). At present, there exists an extensive body of scientific literature on the action of mutagenic agents, the effects of radiation and other physical agents, infectious diseases, nutritional deficiencies and excesses, and the effects of drugs and environmental agents on growth and development of the child (Wilson and Fraser 1977; Scharden 1985).

Teratology was born as a result of changing views of protective placental mechanisms. A commonly held belief was that the "in utero," meaning "in the womb," development was protected by the placenta. Early observations of human and experimental teratogenesis were not readily accepted until the tragic episode of thalidomide in Europe in the late 1950s (Lenz 1961). When ingested by the mother during pregnancy, thalidomide (a tranquilizer) was found to be associated with limb and face malformations in the fetus and newborn.

The effects of drugs and other chemical and physical agents on in utero development were not routinely tested in toxicological studies during drug manufacture until the thalidomide episode shocked the world and focused attention on these potential hazards. The field of teratology—until then an obscure discipline—achieved prominence as a direct result of the thalidomide tragedy. Minamata disease in Japan occurred about a decade later, and it also contributed support to the notion that the embryo and fetus were highly vulnerable to the effects of environmental neurotoxic agents. Minamata disease is a profound nervous system malformation of the fetus and unborn accompanied by severe mental retardation produced by consumption of fish contaminated with methylmercury during pregnancy (Smith and Smith 1975).

Since these two tragic accidental neurotoxin exposures occurred, there has been increasing concern as to whether other toxic agents may also cause changes in the development of the central nervous system either in utero or in the growing child. The most obvious question is whether these structural changes in the nervous system are in turn associated with developmental deficits or mental retardation. The concern has given rise to a new discipline: neuroteratology (sometimes called behavioral teratology or psychoteratology).

Neuroteratology is a discipline that studies the nervous system and behavioral changes occurring as a result of toxic exposure in utero or during the perinatal period of human development. Current research integrates morphological, electrophysiological, and neuropharmacological studies within a development framework.

There is growing evidence of the devastating effects of a number of neurotoxic agents in the embryo or developing child. In the United States, for example, some states now post warning signs in bars—or wherever alcoholic beverages are consumed—alerting women to the damaging effects to the unborn of alcohol consumption during pregnancy.

Neuroteratology and pediatric neurotoxicology are relevant to the field of environmental and occupational health because pregnant women might be exposed to neurotoxic agents at the workplace, thus affecting the unborn; children might live in the proximity of sources releasing neurotoxic agents into the environment, such as lead-smelting plants; children might suffer bystander exposure to neurotoxic agents as a result of their parents' occupation, as in the presence of lead or pesticides on parents' clothing; and because child labor is still common in the United States and in many countries of the world.

Routes of Entry

Environmental teratogens can reach the developing tissue in several ways: directly, via the placenta, in the perinatal period of development through breast feeding, and as a result of the infant's own ingestion.

Placenta. Because of the design of the amniotic sac, the conceptus (embryo/fetus) is well protected against most physical trauma and the action of physical agents. But some agents, such as ionizing radiation, certain microwaves, and ultrasound can penetrate through the womb to affect the conceptus.

The placenta is no longer thought of as an effective protection mechanism against foreign chemicals. According to Wilson (1973), "the question . . . is not whether a given molecule or ion crosses the placenta but at what rate, as determined by its size, charge, lipid solubility, affinity to complex with other chemicals, etc. . . . The embryo probably has a threshold of effect for most chemical agents, that is, a dose below which no effects occur and above which persistent changes may be induced." But these thresholds, particularly in humans, are unknown; and even the very concept of "threshold" is questioned.

Breast Feeding. Until recently, breast feeding was rarely mentioned in the literature as a possible route of entry for teratogens in the perinatal period. Most of what is now known about excretion of toxic chemicals through the mother's milk is very recent. In certain cases of environmental disasters, such as the PBB episode that occurred in Michigan in the early 1970s, infants were known to have ingested contaminated milk from multiple sources, for example, mother's milk and contaminated cow's milk bought in local stores.

Infant's Own Intake. The child can become intoxicated as a result of his or her own intake of harmful chemical compounds. In Chapter 7, "the neurotoxic world of the child" is described, and the manner in which children can become exposed is discussed.

An important route of entry in the child is *pica*. Pica is a child's tendency to carry objects in the mouth, or the actual consumption of nonedible substances such as soil (also called geophagy). Pica is very common source of acute and chronic toxic exposure among chil-

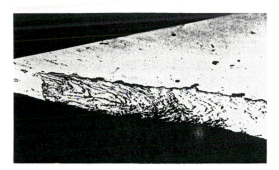

Fig. 20.1.   Chewed bookcase (lead content 11.6%) resulting from an episode of childhood pica. (From Bicknell 1975.)

dren. Urban children living in impoverished areas develop lead poisoning as a result of eating lead-containing paint chips easily removed from the walls of old houses. Figure 20.1 is a dramatic illustration of a piece of furniture painted with lead-containing paint eaten by a young child during a pica episode.

Many features of neurotoxic agents' pharmacokinesis described in Chapter 9 have recently been investigated in experimental laboratory animals. Very little information is available in human infants, primarily because of the ethical constraints on performing research on infants.

Principles of Neuroteratological Research

The number of environmental agents that have been shown to be teratogens is extensive. The list includes natural substances—such as products from plants, fungi, bacteria, and venoms—as well as herbicides, fungicides, insecticides, metals and related elements, solvents, detergents, and other chemical agents derived from industrial, agricultural, and household use (Wilson 1977; Abel 1985).

Wilson has provided teratological generalizations "sufficiently well defined to justify being called principles." These principles can readily be extended to neuroteratologic agents, as Vorhees and Buchter showed in 1982. What follows is based on the lucid review written by Wilson in 1977.

Susceptibility to teratogenesis depends on the individual's genotype (genetic makeup) and the manner in which this genotype interacts with environmental factors. For example, in humans and higher primates, in utero ingestion of thalidomide leads to the development of defects of limbs and face; rabbits and mice require much larger dosages to produce similar defects; other mammalian forms never develop the syndrome.

Susceptibility to teratogenic agents varies with the developmental stage of the species at the time of exposure. The more immature the developing organism, the greater its susceptibility to the effects of a neurotoxic agent.

Within a specific organ, neurotoxic agents are more likely to produce effects during the early stages of organ formation than at later stages; as the basic organization of the organ is completed, abnormal development becomes more unlikely. However, functional disturbances can occur at later stages, even in the fully developed organism. Structural and functional maturation continues in the nervous system after birth; myelinization and glia proliferation are observed up to 2 years after birth. The number of synapses, as stated above, is reduced. Neuroendocrine maturity, particularly sexual and somatic growth, is not completed until puberty.

In addition to Wilson's principles reviewed above, Vorhees and Buchter add an important one: not all agents that are capable of producing malformations are psychoteratogenic (affecting behavior). Thalidomide is a case in point: thalidomide is a very potent teratogen in humans, affecting limbs and face, but it is not primarily a neuroteratogen. Many agents possess a high degree of target specificity affecting systems other than the nervous system, thus not affecting behavior.

Dose–Response Relationships for Teratogenic Agents.   Manifestations of deviant development increase in degree as dose increases from no effect to lethal. When the safety of chemicals or drugs is evaluated for potential teratogenic effects, the main question is whether there is a dose level at which an adverse effect occurs. But sometimes the meaning of "adverse" is not clear, and how and where this information has been gathered is questionable.

Dose–response relationships for teratogenic agents and for most chemicals are at present unknown in humans, although dose–response relationships have been established on the basis of animal studies and then extrapolated to humans. Essential teratological studies of drugs and chemical agents involving a good model of humans—the subhuman primates, for example—are carried out with small numbers of animals in the "treatment" and "control" groups. The reduced number reflects the high cost of monkeys, their availability, and the high emotions that are generated in experimental work with primates.

As we have seen in Chapter 10, knowledge of how pharmacological effects are related to dose is essential for understanding the pharmacokinetics of toxic agents. But the term "dose–response" relationships is not easily extended to teratology. One needs to be reminded that "teratogenesis" can mean either death, malformation, growth retardation, or functional disorder.

It might be conceivable to require from each chemical and drug manufacturer information on dose–response relationships for each of these four aspects of teratogenesis. In the United States, this information is now requested for most drugs but is not available for most environmental and occupational neurotoxic agents. Psychoteratological testing is not required by law. Guidelines for testing these functional disorders are vague even in countries that require psychoteratological defects testing, such as Japan and Great Britain (Vorhees and Buchter 1982).

Human and Animal Studies.   The vast literature on neuroteratology is sharply divided into animal and human studies; animal research is frequently divided into research on subhuman primates and lower species. These

differentiations are sometimes justified and sometimes not. Neuroteratologists, for example, share with clinical and epidemiological neurotoxicologists the common problem of what functions should be tested for which neurotoxic agents and how these functions should be tested. Vorhees and Buchter (1982) wisely observed that "... specifying tests might inhibit the diversity that would otherwise operate to allow the best methods to rise to the top by a process akin to natural selection." (A similar plea has been made against the use of a unifying battery of neurobehavioral tests in humans.)

An interesting concept that neuroteratologists use as a guideline for test selection and development is that of *apical behavior* (from "apex," the top). Apical behavior is in fact an expression derived from a theory of intelligence: intelligence has a common "general intelligence factor," which Spearman, a British psychologist, called *factor g,* on which many other specific motor and cognitive skills depend.

Fetal Alcohol Syndrome.   Although the deleterious effects of alcohol ingestion during pregnancy have been known for many years, the combination of facial dysmorphology (alterations of form and shape of the face), growth retardation, and central nervous system involvement that characterize the fetal alcohol syndrome (FAS) were not described until the early 1970s. The Fetal Alcohol Study Group of the Research Society on Alcoholism has established that the diagnosis FAS should be made on the basis of each of the following categories:

1. Prenatal and/or postnatal growth retardation: weight, length, and/or head circumference below the 10th percentile when corrected for gestational age. (A percentile is the measure of how one individual scores when compared with a group ranked from 1 to 100.)
2. Central nervous system involvement: signs

of neurological abnormality, developmental delay, or intellectual impairment.

3. Characteristic facial dysmorphology with at least two of these three signs:
   a. Microcephalia (head circumference below the third percentile).
   b. Microophthalmia and/or short eyelid fissures.
   c. Poorly developed philtrum (the groove at the median line of the upper lip), thin upper lip, and/or flattening of the maxillary area.

The combination of these three signs is also observed in children of epileptic women who take anticonvulsant drugs, children born from mothers affected by a genetic disease called phenylketonuria, and many other diseases such as congenital heart disease. The diagnosis of FAS cannot be made without a positive history of maternal alcoholism. The book by Rossett and Weiner, *Alcohol and the Fetus: A Clinical Perspective* (1984), contains a comprehensive treatment of FAS.

PEDIATRIC NEUROTOXICOLOGY

Pediatric neurotoxicology is the study of the effects of neurotoxic agents on the infant, the child, and the adolescent. Its scope is wide, covering factors such as the genetic makeup of the child's parents as well as circumstantial events around the time of the child's neurological and psychological examination. Pediatric neurotoxicology is intimately related to neuroteratology, both disciplines lacking clear boundaries. In the main, experimental neuroteratology has been confined to animals, whereas pediatric neurotoxicology is based on clinical observations of children.

The effects of neurotoxic agents from around the time the child is born—studied by a discipline called perinatal toxicology—can be viewed from three intimately related perspectives: from the parent's point of view, studying factors as a fertility/reproduction problem (a family history of mental retardation, malnutrition, alcohol or drug use during pregnancy, breast feeding, etc is taken into consideration); from the conceptus' point of view while in utero or during the earliest phases of perinatal development (the nervous system is not fully mature at the time of birth); and from the child's point of view during the last stages of perinatal development, passing through infancy, childhood, and adolescence (for epidemiological purposes, most investigators around the world consider an 18-year-old person an adult).

Clinical, laboratory-based, and epidemiological studies of the effects of neurotoxic agents on brain and behavioral development are particularly difficult because all three of the abovementioned factors and stages need to be taken into consideration.

Various categories of studies need to be identified; some of them are related to each other, and some are not. The following are listed in progressive order of methodological and technical degree of sophistication:

- Case reports and clinical observations, typical of the early years of environmental and occupational neurotoxicology. Here, the emphasis is placed on the individual case, although the implication is that the findings have a greater applicability. In the majority of cases, no objective measures of nervous system function—such as psychometric testing—are available. The case report relies on clinical observations by pediatric neurologists or child psychologists.
- Studies on fairly large groups of children—including laboratory studies with infants—where often only measures of biological indicators of neurotoxic exposure (blood lead levels, for example) are available.
- Clinical and/or laboratory-based studies of large numbers of children where both indicators of neurotoxic exposure and/or absorption are available and some measurement of neurobehavioral function has been attempted (but with some disregard

for epidemiological considerations of study design and possible sources of bias).

- Epidemiological studies where databases have been obtained in groups of children following well-established rules of sampling and control of biases and where both neurotoxic exposures and measures of nervous system dysfunction are available. Needless to say, these are rare, particularly cases in which the parents' demographic profile—and sometimes the parents' IQ—are available. The study of Needleman and his collaborators in Boston children showing an association between dentine lead and child's IQ—to be reviewed below—is an example of this type of study.

A good deal of information has been accumulated in the context of environmental health research—for example, studies of the health of children living in close proximity to lead-smelting plants. To a lesser extent, a number of studies have dealt with problems of children whose parents work in occupational environments where the father or the mother is exposed to neurotoxic agents—for example, lead brought home on the parents' clothing.

Almost absent from the neurotoxicological literature are studies on neurotoxic exposure among children who work. Child labor has been outlawed in most parts of the world, but, as the world population increases and poverty reaches epidemic proportions in several regions of the world, the proportion of children who work remains high. To a large extent, the need to respond to pressing problems of adults has taken precedence among investigators and health officials. However, lack of awareness on the part of developed countries is possibly a simpler explanation.

Nervous System Development in Infancy and Childhood

The nervous system evolves throughout life. Earlier, simplistic conceptions of cell differ-entiation during early periods of development and cell loss during aging have been replaced by newer concepts arising from a molecular approach in neurobiological research.

The nervous system is not fully mature at birth. In particular, the evolution of motor learning is possible only when motor neural pathways become ensheathed with myelin. Neuroendocrine changes occur, particularly in puberty, in both males and females.

Child psychologists and pediatric neurologists have developed numerous tests and scales to assess child development, many of which are directly or indirectly based on the voluminous work by A. L. Gesell (1880–1961) and collaborators at Yale University. Many have been used for the assessment of the brain-damaged child (see Fig. 20.2).

However, a unifying battery of psychological tests that could be used among children exposed or suspected to be exposed to neurotoxic agents in the environment has yet to be agreed upon. (Some of the testing techniques for children are reviewed in Chapter 4.)

REPRESENTATIVE RESEARCH

Studies on the effects of specific neurotoxic agents on the developing nervous system and behavior have been performed on animals under experimental conditions as well as in clinical studies on children. The vast majority of such studies have been performed to assess the neurotoxic effects of lead.

The suspicion that undue absorption of lead might be associated with mental retardation was raised at the beginning of the last century (Tanquerel des Planches 1839), but the first clinical evidence began to be accumulated in the 1920s. The problem of childhood lead poisoning gained public attention again in the late 1960s and since then it has remained a prominent public health concern. Lead poisoning appears to be discovered as a health problem in each generation.

Lin-Fu (1980) has reviewed the historical back-

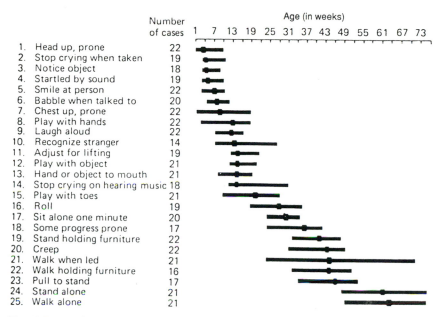

		Number of cases
1.	Head up, prone	22
2.	Stop crying when taken	19
3.	Notice object	18
4.	Startled by sound	19
5.	Smile at person	22
6.	Babble when talked to	20
7.	Chest up, prone	22
8.	Play with hands	22
9.	Laugh aloud	22
10.	Recognize stranger	14
11.	Adjust for lifting	19
12.	Play with object	21
13.	Hand or object to mouth	21
14.	Stop crying on hearing music	18
15.	Play with toes	21
16.	Roll	19
17.	Sit alone one minute	20
18.	Some progress prone	17
19.	Stand holding furniture	22
20.	Creep	22
21.	Walk when led	21
22.	Walk holding furniture	16
23.	Pull to stand	17
24.	Stand alone	21
25.	Walk alone	21

Fig. 20.2. A schedule of motor development in the child. (From Shirley 1931.)

ground surrounding lead poisoning in childhood. Byers and Lord (1943) are generally credited for their clinical observations on the effect of acute lead exposure on neuropsychological functioning. The problem of lead poisoning was first recognized in the clinic; laws for prevention of toxic exposures were passed, and the need to determine the maximum allowable limits was recognized.

Several epidemiological studies in the late 1960s and early 1970s were aimed at resolving the question of what is the maximal allowable level of lead in blood among children. As a result of these investigations, maximum allowable exposure levels to lead have decreased; 30 μg/dL of blood is the presently recommended standard (U.S. Department of Health, Education, and Welfare, Center for Disease Control, 1978). (At this writing, there is much converging evidence that lead may not have a threshold for its effects—ie, there is no lower limit of exposure levels under which effects are not seen.)

Epidemiological Studies

El Paso, Texas. The source of lead in this study by Landrigan and collaborators was a large smelter, which, between the years 1969 and 1971, emitted over 1000 metric tons of inorganic lead along with other metals. Surveys were conducted along three concentric rings with the smelter as their center; the radial distances from the smelter were 1.6, 4.2, and 6.1 km. Interviews were conducted in 670 (80.4%) of the 833 selected occupied households. Blood samples were obtained in all persons ranging from 1 to 19 years of age.

Neuropsychological evaluation was performed in all children between the ages of 3 years 9 months and 15 years 11 months who had lived within 6.6 km of the El Paso smelter for at least 12 of the preceding 24 months. The tests included the Wechsler Intelligence Scale for children (WISC) and the Wechsler Pre-School and Primary Scale of Intelligence (WPPSI), a modification of the WISC. All children 5 years old and older were given special neurological tests to assess motor functioning.

The highest blood lead levels were found in the area closest to the smelter, and the levels decreased in proportion to the distance from the source of lead. No significant differences were found between the groups in the full-scale and verbal IQs. However, significant statistical differences were found in the performance IQ test of both the WISC and WPPSI. Among the subtests that comprised the IQ scales, differences between lead-exposed and control children were maximal in the WISC coding subtest. Finger–wrist tapping was significantly slowed in the dominant hand of children of all ages.

The El Paso smelter area was the subject of numerous reports and follow-ups. A report published in 1979 by Landrigan and his collaborators showed that blood lead levels significantly decreased as compared with the initial period (1969 to 1971), primarily as a result of installation of pollution-control devices at the smelter (Landrigan et al. 1975a,b, 1976, 1979, 1980, 1981).

Kellogg, Idaho.   Landrigan et al. also conducted clinical and epidemiological studies in Idaho, aimed at establishing "safe" levels of lead absorption among children. The levels were determined by studying dose–response relationships. The source of lead was a smelter located in northern Idaho. Between 1955 and 1973, the average emission of lead amounted to 10 metric tons per month, but in September of 1973 there was a sudden increase to 35.3 tons per month as a result of a fire in the filtration unit.

Following the epidemiological study design of the El Paso study, the area around the smelter was divided into five concentric areas: a circle with the smelter at its center and four adjacent rings. Two additional control areas where lead was found to occur naturally in the environment were also included. Peak levels in soil and vegetation were high: 9000 ppm and 3418 ppm, respectively. Complete surveys were carried out in 558 (86%) of the 868 occupied houses. As in the El Paso study, there was a proportional increase in blood lead levels as a function of the proximity to the smelter.

There were two noted improvements in the Idaho study over the El Paso study: (1) the inclusion of a dose–response relationship approach to study the effects of lead and (2) the measurement of nerve conduction veloc-

ities. In the Kellogg, Idaho study, a significant association among blood lead levels, erythrocyte protoporphyrin (EP), and peripheral nerve conduction velocities in the right peroneal nerve was found. The magnitude of the correlation coefficient between EP and nerve conduction velocities was higher than between blood lead levels and nerve conduction velocities.

Suburban Boston, Massachusetts. Although in the last decade several medium-sized and large-scale studies on the association between lead absorption and neuropsychological functioning have been performed, one study that received most of the world's attention was that conducted by Needleman et al. (1979). Several features make this study unique: the very large population from which the study group was drawn, the unusual biological indicator of lead absorption, and the elegance of the study design and logic.

The sample was drawn from 3229 children attending first and second grade in the period between 1975 and 1978 in Chelsea and Somerville, Massachusetts. Children were asked to submit their shed baby teeth to their teachers; the tooth dentine was then analyzed for lead content. A cumulative frequency distribution of dentine lead concentrations was drawn, and subjects were classified as having high or low blood lead levels if they ranked in the highest 10 or the lowest 10 percentiles, respectively.

In the evaluation of the children's neuropsychological functions three sources of data were considered: data from parents, the child's performance in standardized tests of intelligence, and the teachers' rating of child performance in the classroom.

After each child was screened and found not to meet several criteria for exclusion—such as bilingualism, low birth weight, a history of head injury, lead poisoning, etc—parents were asked to participate. Once the parents were in the testing location they received a medical and social history, a questionnaire on attitudes—presumably to assess potential biases against or in favor of the study—and a simplified form of an IQ test.

The children were tested with the Wechsler Intelligence Scale for Children and tests of concrete intelligence, school achievement, auditory and language processing, attentional performance, and motor coordination. Teachers were asked to rate the behavior and performance of each child in the classroom.

The final study group consisted of 58 children with high and 100 with low lead levels; 39 control variables entered in the analysis of covariance (a statistical procedure to control for possible confounding factors such as the parents' IQ).

The study yielded several important results. Children with high lead levels in dentine had significantly lower scores in the IQ test than those with low lead levels. They performed less well in various tests in addition to the IQ test. When the teacher ratings were compared with levels of lead in dentine, there was a remarkable dose–response relationship between dentine lead levels and negative rating of children's behavior—such as distractibility, lack of persistence, and dependency.

Numerous papers were written commenting on the potential flaws of this study. Needleman responded to all of them, even 10 years after the study was published. Today, it represents one of the most important studies in the field of pediatric neurotoxicology.

Glasgow, Scotland. Several other studies have been conducted, adding further proof to the association between increased lead absorption and decreased neuropsychological functioning in children. Moore et al. (1977) performed a retrospective analysis of blood lead in mentally retarded children. Blood lead concentrations were measured in the blood contained in cards used for testing for the genetic disease phenylketonuria in the first 2 weeks of life. Cards from 77 mentally retarded children were then compared with cards belonging to 77 controls. The former had statistically significant higher blood lead levels than controls with normal mental abilities. Moreover, water lead concentration in the maternal homes—an endemic problem in Scotland—during pregnancy correlated with blood lead concentrations in the mentally retarded children.

Electrophysiological Studies

The electrophysiological correlates of a variety of nervous system functions such as conditioning, learning, memory, cognition, etc have been applied to the study of the effects of neurotoxic agents in children. Otto and collaborators (1981), for example, have used slow cortical potentials elicited during sensory conditioning as a neurophysiological indicator of lead intoxication in young children. Several features of this study are noteworthy: (1) the computer-based procedure for measuring sensory-evoked potentials; (2) the manner in which stimuli were presented; (3) the statistical analysis of data; and (4) one of the earliest statements in the literature that lead seems to have no threshold, or lower limit, for producing its biological effects.

The effects of lead, as measured in blood, on slow cortical potentials were studied in 63 children aged 13 to 75 months. The amplitude and the latency of the sensory-evoked potentials were digitized on line (ie, as the data were generated). Two stimulus paradigms were employed. (In the psychological literature, a stimulus paradigm is the manner in which the stimulus is presented to the subject.) The first consisted of the presentation of auditory signals of 1000 Hz at frequent intervals. Then, the signals were replaced in a semirandom fashion by a stimulus of 200 Hz. Physiologically, the amplitude of the frequent tone diminished as a result of habituation; the amplitude of the "rare" tone is preserved. This is called the "frequent–rare" (FR) paradigm. The second—the "tone-shutter" paradigm—consisted of the presentation of a 2000-Hz tone paired with the blackout of a cartoon being watched by the child. After successive pairing, the auditory signal becomes the signal of a blackout in the cartoon presentation.

The effects of lead levels and age on changes in the slow cortical potentials associated with the stimuli paradigms described above were analyzed in a multiregression model. (In statistics, a multiregression model is one that attempts to explain an effect—in this case, slowing of the nerve conduction velocity—resulting from the simultaneous presence of many factors.)

One may or may not agree with the authors' conclusions that measurable slow electrical cortical events are related to lead absorption. It is recognized that blood lead levels "reveal very little above the exposure history of the individual" but are likely to be "an accurate measure of the amount of lead circulating in the body at the time of sampling" (Otto et al. 1981).

CONCLUSIONS

Neuroteratological studies in humans and pediatric neurotoxicological research are two of the most difficult areas of research in environmental and occupational neurotoxicology. A child's behavior depends on numerous genetic and environmental factors such as ethnic background, nutrition, culture, language, and socioeconomic status, to name a few. A scientist who investigates whether an environmental exposure has caused neuropsychological damage in an infant or child has to account for all these factors. Even when these are recognized, there is no agreement among different investigators on how to rule out confounding factors in the assessment of neurotoxic effects. As a result, neuroteratology and pediatric neurotoxicology have been plagued by heated controversies on methodological issues leading to alternative interpretation of findings—for example, in the proper statistical evaluation of alcohol, smoking, and drug use during pregnancy.

The controversies are paradoxical in that, compared to methodological problems encountered in the neurotoxic evaluation of adults, children are relatively "easy" to study. From the assessment point of view, there are many dozens of validated batteries available; from the epidemiological point of view, their behavior and intellectual development can be followed for many years through the school system. Most often, no such possibilities exist in the adult. Once the teenager leaves school, it becomes very difficult to conduct follow-up studies; the interpretations of IQ testing in the adult is always difficult.

Another important controversy centers on the problem of using animal models for the study of human neuroteratological agents and then extrapolating the finding to humans. As shown in the thalidomide tragedy, certain animal species might be insensitive to powerful human neuroteratogens. A predictive neuroteratology based entirely on animal studies can be dangerous.

REFERENCES

Abel, EL (1985) *Behavioral Teratology: A Bibliography to the Study of Birth Defects of the Mind.* Westport, CT: Greenwood Press.

Bicknell, J (1975) *Pica: A Childhood Symptom.* Surrey, UK: Butterworth.

Byers, RK, and Lord, EE (1943) Late effects of lead poisoning on mental development. *Am J Dis Child* 66(5):471–494.

Goldstein, L and Murphy, DP (1929) Etiology of ill-health in children born after maternal pelvic irradiation. II. Defective children born after postception pelvic irradiation. *Am J Roentgen Radium Ther Nucl Med* 22:322–331.

Landrigan, PJ and Baker, EL (1981) Exposure of children to heavy metals from smelters: Epidemiology and toxic consequences. *Environ Res* 25:204–224.

Landrigan, PJ, Gehlbach, SH, Rosenblum, BF, et al. (1975a) Epidemic lead absorption near an ore smelter. *New Engl J Med* 292:123–129.

Landrigan, PJ, Whitworth, RH, Baloh, RW, et al. (1975b) Neuropsychological dysfunction in children with chronic low-level lead absorption. *Lancet* 1:708–712.

Landrigan, PJ, Baker, EL, Feldman, RG, et al. (1976) Increased lead absorption with anemia and slowed nerve conduction in children near a lead smelter. *J Pediatr* 89(6):904–910.

Landrigan, PJ, Baker, EL, Feldman, RG et al. (1976) Increased lead absorption with anaemia and slowed nerve conduction in children near a lead smelter. *J Pediatr* 89:904–910.

Landrigan, PJ, Baker, EL, Whitworth, RH et al. (1980) Neuroepidemiologic evolutions of children with chronic increased lead absorption. In *Low Lead Level Exposure*, HL Needleman (ed) pp. 17–33. New York: Raven Press.

Lenz, W (1961) Kindliche Missbildungen nach Medikament wahrend der Gravidität? *Deut Med Wochenschr* 86:2555–2556.

Lin-Fu, JS (1980) Lead poisoning and undue lead exposure in children. In *Low Level Lead Exposure: The Clinical Implications of Current Research*, HL Needleman (ed) pp. 5–16. New York: Raven Press.

Moore, MR, Meredith, PA, and Goldberg, A (1977) A retrospective analysis of blood lead in mentally retarded children. *Lancet* 1:717–719.

Needleman, HL, Gunnoe, CE, Leviton, A, et al. (1979) Deficits in psychologic and classroom performance of children with elevated blood levels. *N Engl J Med* 300:689–695.

Otto, DA, Beningus, VA, Muller, KE, et al. (1981) Effects of age and body lead burden on CNS function in young children. I. Slow cortical potentials. *Electroencephalogr Clin Neurophysiol* 52:229–239.

Purves, D and Lichtman, JW (1980) Elimination of synapsis in the developing nervous system. *Science* 210:1530–1537.

Rossett, HK and Weiner, L (1984) *Alcohol and the Fetus: A Clinical Perspective*. New York: Oxford University Press.

Scharden, JL (ed) (1985) *Chemically Induced Birth Defects*. New York: Marcel Dekker.

Shirley, MM (1931) *The First Two Years, Vol 1: Postural and Locomotor Developments*. Minneapolis: University of Minnesota Press.

Smith, WE and Smith, AM (1975) *Minamata*. New York: Holt Rinehart and Winston.

Stockad, CR (1921) Developmental rate and structural expression: An experimental study of twins, "double monsters" and single deformites, and the interaction among embryonic organs during their origin and development. *Am J Anat* 28:115–227.

Tanquerel des Planches, L (1839) *Traité des Maladies de Plomb ou Saturnisnes*. Paris.

US Department of Health, Education and Welfare, Center for Disease Control (1978) *Preventing Lead Poisoning in Young Children, A Statement by the Center for Disease Control*. Atlanta: DHEW, PHS, CDC (00-2629).

Vorhees, CV and Buchter, RE (1982) Behavioral teratogenicity. In *Developmental Toxicology*, K. Sneill (ed) pp. 249–297. New York: Praeger.

Warkany, K (1977) History of teratology. In *Handbook of Teratology, Vol. 1, General Principles and Etiology*. JC Wilson and FC Frazier (eds). New York: Plenum Press.

Wilson, JG (1973) *Environmental and Birth Defects*. New York: Academic Press.

Wilson, JG (1977) Feasibility and design of suburban primate studies. In *Handbook of Teratology, Vol. 4, Research Procedures and Data Analysis*, JG Wilson and FC Fraser (eds). pp. 255–273. New York: Plenum Press.

Wilson, JG and Fraser, FC (eds) (1977) *Handbook of Teratology*. New York: Plenum Press.

SUGGESTED READINGS

Abel, EL (1980) Smoking during pregnancy: A review of effects on growth and development of offsprings. *Hum Dev* 52:593–625.

Abel, EL (1981) Behavioral teratology of alcohol. *Psychol Bull* 90:564–581.

Abel, EL (1987) *Fetal Alcohol Syndrome and Fetal Alcohol Effects*. New York: Plenum Press.

Abel, EL (1982) Consumption of alcohol during pregnancy: A review of effects on growth and development of offspring. *Hum Biol* 54:421–453.

Abrams, JH (1979) Development assessment of human infants through 12 weeks of age following chronic prenatal exposure to marijuana. *Dis Abstr Int* 39:3495–B.

Alexander, FW and Delves, HT (1981) Blood lead levels during pregnancy. *Int Arch Occup Environ Health* 48:35–39.

Aman, MG and Singh, NN (1988) *Psychopharmacology of the Developmental Disabilities*. New York: Springer-Verlag.

American Psychological Association (1989) Children and their development: Knowledge base, research agenda, and social policy application. *Am Psychol* 44(2) (special issue).

Angle, CR and McIntire, MS (1979) Environmental lead and children: The Omaha study. *J Toxicol Environ Health* 5:855–870.

Apple, RD (1988) *Mothers and Medicine: A Social History of Infant Feeding, 1890–1950*. Madison, WI: University of Wisconsin Press.

Aronson, M, Kyllerman, M, Sabel, KG, et al. (1985) Children of alcoholic mothers: Developmental, perceptual and behavioral characteristics as compared to matched controls. *Acta Paediat Scand* 74:27–35.

Aub, JC, Fairhall, LT, Minot, AS, et al. (1925) Lead poisoning. *Medicine* 4:1–250.

Ayd, FJ (1964) Children born to mothers treated with chlorpromazine during pregnancy. *Clin Med* 71:1758–1763.

Baghurst, PA, Robertson, EF, McMichael, AJ, et al. (1987) The Port Pirie cohort study: Lead effects on pregnancy outcome and early childhood development. *Neurotoxicol* 8:395–402.

Baker, EL, Folland, DS, Taylor, TA, et al. (1977) Lead poisoning in children of lead workers: Home contamination with industrial dust. *N Engl J Med* 296:260–261.

Barlow, SM and Sullivan, FM (1982) *Reproductive Hazards of Industrial Chemicals: An Evaluation of Animal and Human Data*. London: Academic Press.

Barr, M (1980) Pediatric aspects of the Michigan polybrominated biphenyl contamination. *Environ Res* 21:255–274.

Bayley, N (1969) *The Bayley Scale of Infant Development*. New York: Psychological Corporation.

Bellinger, DC, Needleman, HL, Leviton, A, et al. (1984) Early sensory–motor development and prenatal exposure to lead. *Neurobehav Toxicol Teratol* 6:387–402.

Bellinger, DC, Leviton, A, Waternaux, C, et al. (1987) Longitudinal analysis of prenatal and postnatal lead exposure and early cognitive development. *N Engl J Med* 316(7):1037–1043.

Benignus, VA, Otto, DA, Muller, KE, et al. (1981) Effects of age and body lead burden on CNS function in young children. II. EEG spectra. *Electroenceph Clin Neurophysiol* 52:240–248.

Berkowitz, CS, Holford, TR, and Berkowitz, RL (1982) Effects of cigarette smoking, alcohol, coffee and tea consumption on preterm delivery. *Early Hum Dev* 7:239–250.

Berndt, WO (1989) Renal excretory process in the neonate. *J Am Coll Toxicol* 8(5):963–970.

Biswas, M (1985) *Nutrition and Development*. New York: Oxford University Press.

Bjorklund, DF (1988) *Children's Thinking: Developmental Functions and Individual Differences*. Pacific Grove, CA: Brooks/Cole.

Borella, P, Picco, P, and Masellis, G (1986) Lead content in aborption material from urban women in early pregnancy. *Int Arch Occup Environ Health* 57:93–99.

Boreus, LO (1972) *Fetal Pharmacology*. New York: Raven Press.

Bornschein, R, Pearson, D, and Reiter, L (1980) Behavioral effects of moderate lead exposure in children and animal models, Part I: Clinical Studies. *CRC Crit Rev Toxicol* 8:43–99.

Bracken, MB (ed) (1984) *Perinatal Epidemiology*. New York: Oxford University Press.

Brazelton, TB (1973) *Neonatal Behavioral Assessment Scale*. Philadelphia: Lippincott.

Brenne, W, Edelman, D, and Hendricks, CA (1976) A standard of fetal growth for the United States of America. *Am J Obstet Gynecol* 126:555–564.

Bridbord, K (1978) Occupational lead exposure and women. *Prev Med* 7:311–321.

Briggs, GG, Freeman, RK, and Yaffe, SJ (1986) *Drugs in Pregnancy and Lactation: A Reference Guide to Fetal and Neonatal Risk*. Baltimore: Williams & Wilkins.

Bryce-Smith, D, Matthews, J, and Stephens, R (1978) Mental health effects of lead on children. *Ambio* 7(5–6):192–302.

Buffer, PA and Aase, JM (1982) Genetic risks and environmental surveillance: Epidemiologic aspects of monitoring industrial populations for environmental mutagens. *J Occup Med* 24:305–314.

Bull, RJ, McCauley, PT, Taylor, DH, et al. (1983) The effects of lead on the developing central nervous system. *Neurotoxicology* 4:1–18.

Bushnell, PJ and Bowman, RE (1979) Effects of chronic lead ingestion on social development in infant rhesus monkeys. *Neurobehav Teratol* 1:207–219.

Carpenter, SJ (1974) Placental permeability of lead. *Environ Health Perspect* 1:129–132.

Cawte, J (1985) Psychiatric sequelae of manganese exposure in the adult, foetal, and neonatal nervous systems. *Aust NZ J Psychiatry* 19(3):211–217.

Chasnoff, IJ and Burns, WJ (1984) The Moro reaction: A scoring system for neonatal narcotic withdrawal. *Dev Med Child Neurol* 26:484–489.

Chasnoff, IJ, Burns, WJ, Schnoff, SH, et al. (1985) Cocaine use in pregnancy. *N Engl J Med* 313:666–669.

Chisolm, JJ (1984) The continuing hazard of lead exposure and its effects in children. *Neurotoxicology* 5(3):23–42.

Clark, ARL (1977) Placental transfer of lead and its effects on newborn. *Postgrad Med J* 53(625):674–678.

Clarkson, TW, Nordberg, GF, and Sager, PR (1985) Reproductive and developmental toxicity of metals. *Scand J Work Environ Health* 11:145–154.

Clarren, SK and Smith, DW (1978) The fetal alcohol syndrome. *N Engl J Med* 298:1063–1067.

Clausing, P, Brunekreef, B, and Van Wijnen, JH (1987) A method for estimating soil ingestion by children. *Int Arch Occup Environ Health* 59:73–82.

Committee to Study the Prevention of Low Birth Weight (1985) *Preventing Low Birth Weight*. Washington, DC: National Academy Press.

Conner, C (1969) A teacher rating scale for use in drug studies with children. *Am J Psychiatry* 126:152–156.

Courville, CB (1971) *Birth and Brain Damage*. Pasadena, CA: MF Courville.

Cox, C, Clarkson, TW, Marsh, DO, et al. (1989) Dose–response analysis of infants prenatally exposed to methyl mercury: An application of a single compartment model to single-strand hair analysis. *Environ Res* 49:318–332.

Cratty, BJ (1979) *Perceptual and Motor Development in Infants and Children*, 2nd ed. Englewood Cliffs, NJ: Prentice-Hall.

David, JM and Svendsgaard, DJ (1987) Lead and child development. *Nature* 32(6137):297–300.

David, OI, Clark, J, and Hoffman, S (1979) Childhood poisoning: A re-evaluation. *Arch Environ Health* 34:106–110.

David, O, Clark, J, and Voeller, K (1972) Lead and hyperactivity. *Lancet* 2:900–903.

Davis, JM and Svendsgaard, DJ (1987) Lead and child development. *Nature* 329:297–300.

Day, NL, Wagener, KK, and Taylor, PM (1985) Measurement of substance use during pregnancy: Methodologic issues. In *Current Research on the Consequences of Maternal Drug Use (National Institute on Drug Abuse Research Monographs 59)*, TM Pinkert (ed) pp. 36–47. Washington, DC: US Government Printing Office.

De la Burde, B and Choate, MS (1972) Does asymptomatic lead exposure in children have latent sequelae? *J Pediatr* 81:1088–1091.

De Vellis, J, Ciment, G, and Lauder, J (eds) (1989) *Neuroembryology: Cellular and Molecular Approaches.* New York: Alan R Liss.

Dietrich, KN, Krafft, KM, Bier, M, et al. (1986) Early effects of fetal lead exposure: Neurobehavioral findings at 6 months. *Int J Biosoc Res* 8(2):151–168.

Dine, MS and McGovern, ME (1982) Intentional poisoning of children, an overlooked category of child abuse: Report of seven cases and review of the literature. *Pediatrics* 70(1):32–35.

Dinges, DF, Davis, MM, and Glass, P (1980) Fetal exposure to narcotics: Neonatal sleep as a measure of nervous system disturbance. *Science* 209:619–621.

Dobbing, J (1974) Human brain development and its vulnerability. *Mead Johnson Symp Perinat Dev Med* 6:3–12.

Dodge, PR and Volpe, JJ (1983) Neurologic history and examination. In *Pediatric Neurology,* 3rd ed, TW Farmer (ed) pp. 1–41. Philadelphia: Harper & Row.

Drillien, CM (1964) *The Growth and Development of the Prematurely Born Infant.* Edinburgh: Livingstone.

Dubowitz, L, Dubowitz, A, and Goldberg, G (1970) Clinical assessment of gestational age in the newborn infant. *J Pediatr* 77:1–10.

Edmonds, LD, Anderson, CE, Flynt, JW, et al. (1978) Congenital central nervous system malformations and vinyl chloride monomer exposure: A community exposure. *Teratology* 17:137–142.

Egan, T (1989) A worried liquor industry readies for birth-defect suit. *New York Times,* April 21.

Epstein, W (ed) (1987) *The Ontogenesis of Perception.* Washington, DC: American Psychological Association.

Erhardt, CL, Joshi, GB, Nelson, FG, et al. (1964) Influence of weight and gestation on perinatal and neonatal mortality by ethnic groups. *Am J Public Health* 54:1941–1955.

Eriksson, M, Larsson G, Winbladh et al (1979) Accidental poisoning in pre-school children in the Stockholm area. *Acta Paediatr Scand [Suppl]* 275:96–101.

Ernhart, CB, Landa, B, and Chell, NB (1981) Subclinical levels of lead and development deficits: A multivariated follow-up reassessment. *Pediatrics* 67:911–919.

Ernhart, CB, Wolff, AW, Kennard, MJ, et al. (1986) Intrauterine exposure to low levels of lead: The status of the neonate. *Arch Environ Health* 41(5):287–291.

Eskenazi, B, Gaylord, L, Bracken, MB, et al. (1988) In utero exposure to organic solvents and human neurodevelopment. *Dev Med Child Neurol* 30:492–501.

Eskenazi, B and Pearson, K (1988) Validation of a self-administered questionnaire for assessing occupational and environmental exposures of pregnant women. *Am J Epidemiol* 128(5):1117–1129.

Ethridge, JE (1983) Birth defects and developmental disorders. In *Pediatric Neurology,* 3rd ed, TW Farmer (ed) pp. 61–115. Philadelphia: Harper & Row.

Ewers, U, Brockhaus, A, Winneke, G, et al. (1982) Lead in deciduous teeth of children living in a non-ferrous smelter area and a rural area of the Federal Republic of Germany. *Int Arch Occup Environ Health* 50:139–151.

Fedrick J, Alberman, ED, and Goldstein, H (1971) Possible teratogenic effect of cigarette smoking. *Nature* 231:529–530.

Fein, GG, Schwartz, PM, Jacobson, SW, et al. (1983) Environmental toxins and behavioral development: A new role for psychological research. *Am Psychol* 38:1188–1197.

Feldman, RG, Hayes, MK, Younes, R, et al. (1977) Lead and neuropathy in adults and children. *Arch Neurol* 34:481–488.

Fergusson, DM, Fergusson, JE, Horwood, LJ, et al. (1988) A longitudinal study of dentine lead levels, intelligence, school performance and behavior: I. Dentine lead levels and exposure to environmental risk factors. *J Child Psychol Psychiatr Allied Discip* 29(6):781–792.

Fergusson, DM, Fergusson, JE, Horwood, LJ, et al. (1988) A longitudinal study of dentine lead levels, intelligence, school performance and behaviour: II. Dentine lead and cognitive ability. *J Child Psychol Psychiatr Allied Disc* 29(6):793–809.

Fergusson, DM, Fergusson, JE, Horwood, LJ, et al. (1988) A longitudinal study of dentine lead levels, intelligence, school performance and behaviour: III. Dentine levels and attention/activity. *J Child Psychol Psychiatr Allied Discip* 29(6):811–824.

Fergusson, HB, Rapoport, JL, and Weingartner, HJ (1981) Food dyes and impairment of performance in hyperactive children. *Science* 21:410–411.

Ferm, VH (1972) Teratogenic effects of metals on mammalian embryos. *Adv Teratol* 6:51–75.

Field TM (1979) *Infants Born at Risk*. New York: SP Medical Scientific Books.

Fildes, VA (1986) *Breasts, Bottles and Babies: A History of Infant Feeding*. Edinburgh: Edinburgh University Press (US distributor Columbia University Press).

Finberg, L (1977) PBB's: The ladies' milk is not for burning. *J Pediatr* 90:511–512.

Finney, J, Russo, D, and Cataldo, MF (1982) Reduction of pica in young children with lead poisoning. *J Pediatr Psychol* 7(2):197–207.

Flagler, SL and Wright, L (1987) Recurrent poisoning in children. A review. *J Pediatr Psychol* 12(4):631–641.

Foldspang, A and Hansen, JC (1990) Dietary intake of methylmercury as a correlate of gestational length and birth weight among newborns in Greenland. *Am J Epidemiol* 132(2):310–317.

Fried, P (1980) Marijuana use by pregnant women: Neurobehavioral effects in neonates. *Drug Alcohol Depend* 6:415–424.

Fried, P (1982) Marijuana use by pregnant women and effects on offspring: An update. *Neurobehav Toxicol Teratol* 4:451–454.

Gesell, A (1952) *Infant Development: The Embryology of the Early Human Behavior*. Westport, CT: Greenwood Press.

Gesell, A, Ilg, FI, and Ames, LB (1977) *The Child from Five to Seven*. New York: Harper & Row.

Goldhaber, MK, Polen, MR, and Hiatt, RA (1988) The risk of miscarriage and birth defects among women who use visual display terminals during pregnancy. *Am J Ind Med* 13:695–706.

Goldstein, GW and Betz, AL (1986) The blood–brain barrier. *Sci Am* 255(3):74–83.

Gotelli CA, Astolif, E, Cox, C, et al. (1985) Early biochemical effects of organic mercury fungicide on infants, "Dose makes the poison." *Science* 227:638–640.

Gottlieb, G (ed) (1973) *Behavioral Embryology*. New York: Academic Press.

Gottlieb, G (1978) *Studies on the Development of Behavior and the Nervous System*. London: Academic Press.

Grant, L (1976) Research strategies for behavioral teratology studies. *Environ Health Perspect* 18:85–94.

Green, M and Suffet, F (1981) The neonatal narcotic withdrawal index: A device for the improvement of care in the abstinence syndrome. *Am J Drug Alcohol Abuse* 8:203–213.

Greenberg, RS and Osterhout, SK (1982) Reported multiple victim poisoning of children. *J Toxicol* 19(10):1073–1080.

Greenought, WT and Juraska, M (eds) (1986) *Development Neuro-Psychobiology*. Orlando, FL: Academic Press.

Greenwood, MR, Clarckson, TW, Doherty, RA, et al. (1978) Blood clearance half-times in lactating and non-lactating mothers of a population exposed to methyl mercury. *Environ Res* 16:48–54.

Haas, JF and Schottenfeld, D (1979) Risks of the offspring from parental occupational exposures. *J Occup Med* 21:607–613.

Hachter, SL (1982) The psychological experience of nursing mothers upon learning of a toxic substance in their breast milk. *Psychiatry* 45(2):172–181.

Hall, BK and Hörstadius, S (1988) *The Neural Crest*. New York: Oxford University Press.

Hammond, PB, Clark, CS, Gartside, PS, et al. (1980) Fecal lead excretion in young children as related to sources of lead in their environments. *Int Arch Occup Environ Health* 46:191–202.

Hansen, JC, Christensen, RB, Allermand, H, et al. (1984) Concentrations of mercury, selenium and lead in blood samples from mothers and their newborn babies in four Greenlandic hunting districts. *Meddelelser om Grønland: Man and Society* 6:1–19.

Harwerth, RS, Smith, EL, Duncan, GC, et al (1986) Multiple sensitive periods in the development of the primate visual system. *Science* 235:238.

Hatch, EE and Bracken, MB (1986) Effect of marijuana use in pregnancy on fetal growth. *Am J Epidemiol* 124(6):986–993.

Heber, R (1970) *Epidemiology of Mental Retardation*. Springfield, IL: Charles C Thomas.

Heinonenm OP (1977) *Birth Defects and Drugs in Pregnancy*. Littleton, MA: Publishing Sciences Group.

Hemminki, K (1980) Occupational chemicals tested for teratogenicity. *Int Arch Occup Environ Health* 47:191–207.

Herbert, RFM, Wibowo, AA, Das, HA, et al. (1983) Trace element levels in hair of eight-year-old children. *Int Arch Occup Environ Health* 53:127–137.

Hewson, D and Bennett, A (1987) Childbirth research data: Medical records or women's reports? *Am J Epidemiol* 125:484–491.

Hingson, R, Alpert, J, Day, N, et al. (1982) Effects of maternal drinking and marijuana use on fetal growth and development. *Pediatrics* 70:539–546.

Holmberg, P (1979) Central-nervous-system defects in children born to mothers exposed to organic solvents during pregnancy. *Lancet* 2:177–179.

Householder, J, Hatcher, R, Burns, W, et al. (1982) Infants born to narcotic addicted mothers. *Psychol Bull* 92:453–468.

Householder, S (1989) *Women, Work and Fertility, 1900–1986*. New York: New York University Press.

Hrbek, A, Karlberg, P, Kjellmer, I, et al. (1977) Clinical application of evoked electroencephalographic responses in newborn infants, I. Perinatal asphyxia. *Dev Med Child Neurol* 19:34–44.

Hubermont, G, Buchet, JP, Roels, H, et al. (1978) Placental transfer of lead, mercury and cadmium in women living in a rural area: Importance of drinking water in lead exposure. *Int Arch Occup Environ Health* 41:117–124.

Hunt, VR (1979) *Work and the Health of Women*. Boca Raton, FL: CRC Press.

Hunter, J, Uranowicz, A, Yule, W, et al. (1985) Automated testing of reaction time and its association with lead in children. *Int Arch Occup Environ Health* 57:27–34.

Hutchings, DE (1987) Drug abuse during pregnancy: Embryopathic and neurobehavioral effects. In *Genetic and Perinatal Effects of Abused Substances*, MC Brand and AM Zimmerman (eds) pp. 131–151. New York: Raven Press.

Hutchings, DE (ed) (1989) *Prenatal Abuse of Licit and Illicit Drugs*. New York: New York Academy of Sciences.

Illingworth, RS (1987) *The Development of the Infant and Young Child, Normal and Abnormal,* 9th ed. Edinburgh: Churchill Livingstone.

International Labor Office (1986) *Child Labor: A Briefing Manual*. Washington, DC: ILO.

Jackson, R, Walker, J, and Wynne, N (1968) Circumstances of accidental poisoning in childhood. *Br Med J* 4:245.

Jacobson, JL, Jacobson, SW, and Fein, GG (1986) Intrauterine exposure to environmental toxins: The significance of subtle behavioral effects. *Prev Hum Serv* 4(1–2):125–137.

Jacobson, J, Schwartz, PM, Fein, GG, et al. (1984) Prenatal exposure to an environmental toxin: A test of the multiple effects model. *Dev Psychol* 20(4):523–532.

Jacobson, SW, Fein, GG, Jacobson, JL, et al. (1985) The effect of intauterine PCB exposure on visual recognition memory. *Child Dev* 56:853–860.

Jensen, G and Wilson, W (1960) Preventive implications of a study of 100 poisonings in children. *Pediatrics* 25:490.

Johnson, CC, Annegers, JF, Frankowski, RF, et al. (1987) Childhood nervous system tumors—An evaluation of the association with paternal occupational exposure to hydrocarbons. *Am J Epidemiol* 126(4):605–613.

Johnson, EM and Christina, MS (1984) When is a teratology study not an evaluation of teratogenicity? *Am Coll Toxicol* 3(6):431–434.

Jones, KL and Smith, DW (1975) The fetal alcohol syndrome. *Teratology* 12:1–10.

Juchau, MR (1982) The role of the placenta in development toxicology. In *Developmental Toxicology,* K Snell (ed) pp. 189–209. New York: Praeger.

Kallen, B (1988) *Epidemiology of Human Reproduction*. Boca Raton, FL: CRC Press.

Kaltenbach, K and Finnegan, LP (1984) Developmental outcome of children born to methadone maintained women: A review of longitudinal studies. *Neurobehav Toxicol Teratol* 6:271–275.

Kalter, H (1968) *Teratology of the Central Nervous System*. Chicago: University of Chicago Press.

Kane, DN (1977) Bad air for children. *Environment* 18(9):26–34.

Kane, DN (1985) *Environmental Hazards to Young Children*. Phoenix, AZ: Orynx Press.

Katagiri, Y, Toriumi, H, and Kawai, M (1983) Lead exposure among 3-year-old children and their mothers living in a pottery-producing area. *Int Arch Occup Environ Health* 52:223–229.

Kawai, M, Toriumi, H, Katagiri, Y, et al. (1983) Home lead work as a potential source of lead exposure for children. *Int Arch Occup Environ Health* 53:37–46.

Kawai, M, Okamoto, Y, and Katagiri, Y (1987) Variation of blood-lead levels with age in childhood. *Int Arch Occup Environ Health* 59:91–94.

Kaye, WE, Novotny, TE, and Tucker M (1987) New ceramics-related industry implicated in elevated lead levels in children. *Arch Environ Health* 42:161–164.

Khoury, MJ, Flanders, ED, James, LM, et al. (1989) Human teratogenesis, prenatal mortality and selection bias. *Am J Epidemiol* 130:361–369.

Kimmel, CA and Buelke-Sam, J (1981) *Developmental Toxicology*. New York: Raven Press.

Kline, J, Stein, Z, Strobino, B, et al. (1977) Surveillance of spontaneous abortions: Power in environmental monitoring. *Am J Epidemiol* 106:345–350.

Knowles, JA (1974) Breast milk: A source of more than nutrition for the neonate. *Clin Toxicol* 7(1):69–82.

Kolata, GB (1978) Behavioral teratology: Birth defects of the mind. *Science* 202:732–734.

Kotok, D (1972) Development of children with elevated blood levels: A controlled study. *J Pediatr* 80:57–61.

Krigman, MR and Hogan, EL (1974) Effect of lead intoxication on the postnatal growth of the rat nervous system. *Environ Health Perspect* 1:187–200.

Kuratsune, M, Yoshimura, T, Matsuzaka, J, et al. (1971) Yusho, a poisoning caused by rice oil contaminated with polychlorinated biphenyls. *HSMHA Health Rep* 86:1083–1091.

Kuruvilla, A and Bergeson, PS (1975) Arsenic poisoning in childhood: A unusual case report with special notes on therapy with penicillamine. *Clin Toxicol* 8(5):535–540.

Kuwabara, K, Yakushiiji, T, Watanabe, J, et al. (1979) Levels of polychlorinated biphenyls in blood of breastfed children whose mothers are non-occupationally exposed to PCBs. *Bull Environ Contam Toxicol* 21:458–462.

Kuzma, JW and Kissinger, DG (1981) Patterns of alcohol and cigarette use in pregnancy. *Neurobehav Toxicol Teratol* 3:211–221.

Lacoius-Petrocelli, A (1987) *Perinatal Asphyxia.* New York: Plenum Press.

Lamb, JC (1985) Reproductive toxicity testing: Evaluating and developing new testing systems. *J Am Coll Toxicol* 4(2):163–171.

Landesman-Dwyer, S and Emanuel, I (1979) Smoking during pregnancy. *Teratology* 19:119–126.

Landrigan, PJ, Gehlbach, SH, Rosenblum, BF, et al. (1985) Epidemic lead absorption near an ore smelter: The role of particulate lead. *N Engl J Med* 292(3):123–129.

Landsdown, R, Yule, W, Urabanowicz, M-A, et al. (1986) The relationship between blood-lead concentrations, intelligence, attainment and behavior in a school population: The second London study. *Int Arch Occup Environ Health* 57:225–235.

Langman, J (1975) *Medical Embryology: Human Development—Normal and Abnormal,* 3rd ed. Baltimore: Williams & Wilkins.

Lasch, E and el Shawa, R (1981) Multiple cases of cyanide poisoning by apricot kernels in children from Gaza. *Pediatrics* 68:5.

Laughlin, NK, Bowman, RE, Levin, ED, et al. (1983) Neurobehavioral consequence of early exposure to lead in rhesus monkeys: Effects on cognitive behaviors. In *Reproductive and Development Toxicity of Metals,* TW Clarkson, GF Nordberg, and PR Sager (eds) pp. 497–515. New York: Plenum Press.

Lawless, HT, Hammer, LD, and Corina, MD (1982) Aversion to bitterness and accidental poisonings among preschool children. *J Toxicol* 19(9):951–964.

Levine, R (1988) More infants showing signs of narcotics: Withdrawal symptoms surge in New York City. *New York Times,* April 1.

Little, R (1977) Alcohol consumption during pregnancy and decreased birthweight. *Am J Publ Health* 67:1154–1156.

Lombroso, CT (1982) Some aspects of EEG polygraphy in newborns at risk for neurological disorders. In *Kyoto Symposia,* PA Buser, WC Cobb, and T Okuman (eds) pp. 652–663. Amsterdam: Elsevier.

Lourie, RS, Layman, M, and Millican, FK (1963) Why children eat things that are not food. *Children* 10:143–146.

Lubchenco, LO (1976) *The High Risk Infant.* Philadelphia: WB Saunders.

Lund, RD (1978) *Development and Plasticity of the Brain: An Introduction.* New York: Oxford University Press.

Lyngbye, T, Hansel, ON, and Grandjean, P (1988) Neurological deficits in children: Medical risk factors and lead exposure. *Neurotoxicol Teratol* 10(6):531–537.

Madden, NA, Russo, DC, and Cataldo, MF (1980) Behavioral treatment of pica in children with lead poisoning. *Child Behav Ther* 2(4):67–81.

Madden, NA, Russo, DC, and Cataldo, MF (1980) Environmental influences on mouthing in children with lead intoxication. *J Pediatr Psychol* 5(2):207–216.

Mamelle, N, Laumon, B, and Lazar, P (1984) Prematurity and occupational activity during pregnancy. *Am J Epidemiol* 119(3):309–322.

Marlowe, M, Errera, J, and Jacobs, J (1983) Increased lead and cadmium burdens among mentally retarded children and children with borderline intelligence. *Am J Ment Def* 87(5):477–483.

Marlowe, M, Moon, CE, Errera, J, et al. (1986) Low mercury levels and childhood intelligence. *J Orthomol Med* 1(1):43–49.

Martin, TR, and Bracken, MB (1987) The association between low birth weight and caffeine consumption during pregnancy. *Am J Epidemiol* 126:813–821.

Masuda, Y, Kagawa, R, Kuroki, H, et al. (1978) Transfer of polychlorinated biphenyls from mothers to fetuses and infants. *Bull Environ Contam Toxicol* 16:543–546.

Mattes, J and Gittelman, R (1981) Effects of artificial food coloring in children with hyperactive symptoms: A critical review and results of a controlled study. *Arch Gen Psychiatry* 38(6):714–718.

May, PA, Hymbaught, KJ, Aase, JM, et al. (1983) Epidemiology of fetal alcohol syndrome among American Indians of the Southwest. *Soc Biol* 30(4):374–387.

McBride, WG, Black, BP, and English, BJ (1982) Blood lead levels and behavior of 400 preschool children. *Med J Aust* 2:26–29.

McDonald, AD (1988) Work and pregnancy. *Br J IndMed* 45(9):577–580.

McDonald, AD and McDonald, JC (1986) Outcome of pregnancy in leather workers. *Br Med J* 292:979–981.

McDonald, AD, McDonald, JC, Amstrong, B, et al. (1987) Occupation and pregnancy outcome. *Br J Ind Med* 44:521–526.

McDonald, AD, McDonald, JC, Amstrong, B, et al. (1988) Congenital defects and work in pregnancy. *Br J Ind Med* 45(9):581–588.

McDonald, AD, McDonald, JC, Amstrong, B, et al. (1988) Prematurity and work in pregnancy. *Br J Ind Med* 45:56–62.

McIntire, M, Angle, CR, Ekins, BR, et al. (1983) Trends in childhood poisoning: A collaborative study 1970, 1975, 1980. *J Toxicol* 21:321–331.

McLaughlin, MC (1956) Lead poisoning in children in New York City 1950–1954. *NY State J Med* 56:3711.

Meisami (1988) *Handbook of Human Growth and Developmental Biology* (3 vols). Boca Raton, FL: CRC Press.

Milar, C, Schroeder, SR, Mushak, P, et al. (1981) Failure to find hyperactivity in preschool children with moderately elevated lead burden. *J Pediatr Psychol* 6(1):85–95.

Miller, HC and Merritt, TA (1982) *Fetal Growth in Humans*. Chicago: Year Book Medical Publishers.

Miller, RK (1983) Perinatal toxicology: Its recognition and fundamentals. *Am J Ind Med* 4:205–244.

Miller, RK, Kellog, CK, and Saltzman, RA (1987) Reproductive and perinatal toxicology. In *Handbook of Toxicology*, TJ Haley and WO Berndt (eds) pp. 195–309. Washington, DC: Hemisphere.

Millichap, JA, Lewellin, KR, and Roxburgh, RC (1952) Lead paint: A hazard to children. *Lancet* 2:360.

Ministry of Health (1964) *Deformities Caused by Thalidomide*. London: Her Majesty's Stationery Office.

Mirkin, BL (1976) *Perinatal Pharmacology and Therapeutics*. New York: Academic Press.

Mirkin, BL (1976) Editorial: Drug therapy and the developing human: Who cares? *Clin Toxicol* 9(1):93–106.

Mofenson, HC, Greensher, J, and Horowitz, R (1974) Hazards of maternally administered drugs. *Clin Toxicol* 7(1):59–68.

Moore, MR, Goldberg, A, Bushnell, IWR, et al. (1982) A prospective study of the neurological effects of lead in children. *Neurobehav Toxicol Teratol* 4:739–743.

Mori, T and Nagasawa, H (1988) *Toxicity of Hormones in Perinatal Life*. Boca Raton, FL: CRC Press.

Morrissey, RE and Mottet, NK (1980) Neural tube defects and brain anomalies: A review of selected teratogens and their possible modes of action. *Neurotoxicology* 2:125–162.

Morse, DL, Landrigan, PJ, Rosenblum, BF, et al. (1970) El Paso revisited: Epidemiologic follow-up of an environmental lead problem. *JAMA* 242(4):739–741.

Morton, DE, Saah, AJ, Silberg, SL, et al. (1982) Lead absorption in children of employees in a lead-related industry. *Am J Epidemiol* 115(4):549–555.

Mulvihill, JJ (1973) Caffeine as teratogen and mutagen. *Teratology* 8:68–72.

Mushak, P, Davis, M, Crocetti, AF, et al. (1989) Prenatal and postnatal effects of low-level lead exposure: Integrated summary of a report to the US Congress on childhood lead poisoning. *Environ Res* 50:11–36.

Mussen, PH (ed) (1983) *Handbook of Child Psychology* 4th ed, Vol. 2, *History, Theory and Methods*, W Kessen (ed). New York: John Wiley & Sons.

Nasca, PC, Baptiste, MS, MacCubbin, PA, et al. (1988) An epidemiology case-control study of central nervous system tumors in children and parental occupational exposures. *Am J Epidemiol* 128(6):1256–1265.

Needleman, HL (1982) The neurobehavioral consequences of low lead exposure in children. *Neurobehav Toxicol Teratol* 4:729–732.

Needleman, HL and Bellinger, DC (1981) The epidemiology of low-level lead exposure in childhood. *J Am Acad Child Psychol* 20:496–512.

Needleman, HL, Gunnow, C, Leviton, A, et al. (1970) Deficits in psychologic and classroom performance in children with elevated lead levels. *N Engl J Med* 300(13):689–695.

Needleman, HL, Rabinowitz, M, Leviton, A, et al. (1984) The relationship between prenatal exposure to lead and congenital anomalies. *JAMA* 25(22):2956–2959.

New York Times (1989) Mother charged after her baby dies of cocaine. May 10.

Nicol, AR (ed) (1985) *Longitudinal Studies in Child Psychology and Psychiatry, Practical Lessons from Research Experience*. Chichester: John Wiley & Sons.

Obrzut, JE, and Hynd, GW (eds) (1986) *Child Neuropsychology: Vol. 1, Theory and Research; Vol. 2, Clinical Practice*. New York: Academic Press.

Office of Technology Assessment (1985) *Reproductive Health Hazards in the Workplace*. Washington, DC: US Government Printing Office.

Olegård, R, Sabel, G, Aronsson, M, et al. (1979) Effects on the child of alcohol abuse during pregnancy: Retrospective and prospective studies. *Acta Paediatr Scand Suppl* 275:112–121.

Orvaschel, H, Sholomskas, D, and Weissman, MM (1980) *The Assessment of Psychopathology and Behavioral Problems in Children: A Review of Scales Suitable for Epidemiological and Clinical Research (1967–1979)*. Rockville, MD: US Department of Health and Human Resources, Public Health Service, Alcohol, Drug Abuse, and Mental Health Administration, National Institute of Mental Health, Division of Biometry and Epidemiology.

Orvaschel, H, and Walsh, G (1984) *The Assessment of Adoptive Functioning in Children: A Review of Existing Measures Suitable for Epidemiologic and Clinical Research*. Rockville, MD: US Department of Health and Human Resources, Public Health Service, Alcohol, Drug Abuse, and Mental Health Administration, National Institute of Mental Health, Division of Biometry and Epidemiology.

Otto, DA, Benignus, VA, Muller, KE, et al. (1983) Electrophysiological evidence of changes in CNS function at low-to-moderate blood lead levels in children. In *Lead versus Health*, M Rutter and RR Jones (eds) pp. 319–331. New York: John Wiley & Sons.

O'Tuama, LA and Kim, CS (1983) Intoxications of the nervous system. In *Pediatric Neurology*, 3rd ed, TW Farmer (ed) pp. 421–457. Philadelphia: Harper & Row.

Overmann, SR, Kostas, J, Wilson, LR, et al. (1987) Neurobehavioral and somatic effects of perinatal PCB exposure in rats. *Environ Res* 44:56–70.

Palmisano, PA, Sneed, RC, and Cassady, G (1969) Untaxed whiskey and fetal lead exposure. *J Pediatr* 75:869–871.

Patten, BM (1976) *Human Embryology,* 4th ed. New York: McGraw-Hill.

Pearson, DT and Dietrich, KM (1985) The behavioral toxicology and teratology of childhood: Models, methods and implications for intervention. *Neurotoxicology* 6(3):165–182.

Persaud, TVN (1990) *Environmental Causes of Human Birth Defects.* Springfield, IL: Charles C. Thomas.

Peterson, J (1979) Pb: Advances in research on effects of lead on children's behavior and intelligence. *Ambio* 8(5):223–226.

Rakic, P (1985) Limits of neurogenesis in primates. *Science* 227:1054–1056.

Rakik, P, Bourgeois, J-P, Eckenhoff, MF, et al. (1986) Concurrent overproduction of synapsis in diverse regions of the primate cerebral cortex. *Science* 232:232–238.

Rappoport, SI (1976) *Blood–Brain Barrier in Physiology and Medicine.* New York: Raven Press.

Rauber, A (1975) Poisoning in children under 12 months of age. *Clin Toxicol* 8(4):391–397.

Reuhl, KR and Chang, LW (1979) Effects of methylmercury on the development of the nervous system: A review. *Neurotoxicology* 1:21–25.

Reuhl, KB and Cranmer, JM (1984) Developmental neuropathology of organotin compounds. *Neurotoxicology* 5(2):187–204.

Rie, HE and Rie, ED (eds) (1980) *Handbook of Minimal Brain Dysfunction: A Critical View.* New York: John Wiley & Sons.

Riley, EP and Vorhees, CV (1986) *Handbook of Behavioral Teratology.* New York: Plenum Press.

Roan, CC, Matonoski, GE, McIlnay, CQ, et al. (1984) Spontaneous abortions, stillbirths, and birth defects in families of agricultural pilots. *Arch Environ Health* 39:56–60.

Rockway, SW, Weber, CW, Lei, KY, et al. (1984) Lead concentrations of milk, blood, and hair in lactating women. *Int Arch Occup Environ Health* 53:181–187.

Rodier, PM (1978) Behavioral teratology. In *Handbook of Teratology, Vol 4, Research Procedures and Data Analysis,* JG Wilson and FC Fraser (eds) pp. 397–428. New York: Plenum Press.

Roel, H, Hubermont, G, Buchet, JP, et al. (1978) Placental transfer of lead, mercury, cadmium, and carbon monoxide in women: III. Factors influencing the accumulation of heavy metals in the placenta and the relationship between metal concentration in the placenta and in maternal and cord blood. *Environ Res* 16:236–247.

Rom, WN (1976) Effects of lead on the female and reproduction. A review. *Mount Sinai J Med* 43(5):542–552.

Rosenberg, MJ, Feldblum, PJ, and Marshall, EG (1987) Occupational influences on reproduction: A review of recent literature. *J Occup Med* 29:584–591.

Savits, DA, Whelan, EA, and Kleckne, RC (1989) Effect of parent's occupational exposures on risk of stillbirth, preterm delivery and small-for-gestational-age infants. *Am J Epidemiol* 129(6):1201–1218.

Sayre, JW and Kaymakealan, S (1964) Cyanide poisoning from apricot seeds among children in Central Turkey. *N Engl J Med* 270:1113.

Scarpelli, DG and Migaki, G (eds) (1987) *Transplacental Effects on Fetal Health.* New York: Alan R Liss.

Scarr, S (1981) Testing for children: Assessment and the many determinants of intellectual competence. *Am Psychol* 36(10):1159–1166.

Schaller, KH, Schiele, R, Weltle, D, et al. (1976) Der Blutbleispiegel von Mutter und Kind under der Bleigehalt der menschelichen Plancenta in Aghängigkeit vom Lebensraum. *Int Arch Occup Environ Health* 37:265–276.

Schroeder, SR (1987) *Toxic Substances and Mental Retardation: Neurobehavioral Toxicology and Teratology.* Washington, DC: American Association for Mental Deficiency.

Sever, JL and Brent, RL (periodical) *Teratogen Update: Environmentally Induced Birth Defects Risk.* New York: Alan R Liss.

Shapiro, IM, Dobkin, B, Tunca, OC, et al. (1973) Lead levels in dentine and circumpulped dentine of deciduous teeth of normal and lead poisoned children. *Clin Chem Acta* 46:119.

Shaw, M (1977) Accidental poisoning in children: A psychosocial study. *NZ Med J* 85:269.

Sheick, K (1979) Teratogenic effects of organic solvents. *Lancet* 2:963.

Sheppard, TH (1983) *Catalog of Teratogenic Agents.* Baltimore: The Johns Hopkins University Press.

Smith, M (1985) Recent work on low level lead exposure and its impact on behavior, intelligence and learning. *J Am Acad Child Psychiatry* 24(1):24–32.

Smith, MA, Grant, LD, and Sors, AI (eds) (1989) *Lead Exposure and Child Development: An International Assessment.* Norwell, MA: Kluver.

Smith, SW (1982) *Recognizable Patterns of Human Malformation,* 3rd ed. Philadelphia: WB Saunders.

Smith, TS, Temple, AR, and Reading, JC (1976) Cadmium, lead and copper blood levels in normal children. *Clin Toxicol* 9(1):75–87.

Sokol, RJ, Miller, SI, and Reed, G (1980) Alcohol abuse during pregnancy: An epidemiologic study. *Alcoholism Clin Exp Res* 4(2):135–145.

Spear, LP and Campbell, BA (eds) (1978) *Ontogeny of Learning and Memory.* Hillsdale, NJ: Lawrence Erlbaum Associates.

Spitz, MR and Cole Johnson, C (1985) Neuroblastoma and paternal occupation: A case-control analysis. *Am J Epidemiol* 121:427–435.

Spyker, JM (1972) Behavioral teratology and toxicology. In *Behavioral Toxicology,* B Weiss and VG Laties (eds) pp. 311–344. New York: Plenum Press.

Spyker, JM and Chang, LW (1974) Delayed effects of prenatal exposure to methylmercury—brain ultrastructure and behavior. *Teratology* 9:A–37.

Spyker, JM, Sparber, SB, and Goldberg, AM (1972) Subtle consequences of methylmercury exposure: Behavioral deviations in offspring of treated mothers. *Science* 77:621–623.

Stein, Z, Susser, M, Warburton, D, et al. (1975) Spontaneous abortion as a screening device: The effect of fetal survival on the incidence of birth defects. *Am J Epidemiol* 102:275–290.

Steinhausen, HC, Nestler, V, and Sppohr, HL (1982) Development and pathology of children with the fetal alcohol syndrome. *Dev Behav Pediatr* 3(2):49–54.

Stoddart, C and Knights, RM (1986) Neuropsychological assessment of children. In *Child Neuropsychology*, JE Obrzut and GW Hynd (eds) pp. 229–243. New York: Academic Press.

Streissguth, AP, Barr, HM, Martin, DC, et al. (1980) Effects of maternal alcohol, nicotine, and caffeine use during pregnancy on infant metal and motor development at eight months. *Alcohol Clin Exp Res* 4:152–164.

Streissguth, AP, Clarren, SK, and Jones, KL (1985) Natural history of the fetal alcohol syndrome: A ten-year follow up of eleven patients. *Lancet* 2:85–92.

Streissguth, AP, Ladesman-Dyer, S, Martin, JC et al (1980) Teratogenic effects of alcohol in humans and laboratory animals. *Science* 209:353–381.

Strobino, BR, Kline, J, and Stein, Z (1978) Chemical and physical exposures of parents: Effects on human reproduction and offspring. *Early Hum Dev* 1:371–399.

Subcommittee on Reproductive and Neurodevelopmental Toxicology (1989) *Biological Markers in Reproductive Toxicology*. Washington, DC: National Academy Press.

Surgeon General of the United States (1971) Medical aspects of childhood lead poisoning. *Pediatrics* 48:464–468.

Swain, KF (1988) *Pediatric Neurology: Principles and Practice*. Boca Raton, FL: CRC Press.

Swann, JW and Messer, A (eds) (1988) *Disorders of the Developing Nervous System: Changing Views of Their Origins, Diagnoses and Treatments*. New York: Alan R Liss.

Tanaka, T (1934) So-called breast milk intoxication. *Am J Dis Child* 37:1286.

Taskinen, H, Anttila, A, Lindbohm, M-I, et al. (1989) Spontaneous abortions and congenital malformations among the wives of men occupationally exposed to solvents. *Scand J Work Environ Health* 15(5):345–352.

Taylor, PR, Lawrence, CE, Hwang, HL, et al. (1984) Polychlorinate byphenyls influence on birthweight and gestation. *Am J Public Health* 74:1153–1154.

Taylor, PR, Stelma, JM, and Lawrence, CE (1989) The relation of polychlorinated biphenyls to birth weight and gestational age in the offspring of occupationally exposed mothers. *Am J Epidemiol* 129(2):395–406.

Teeter, PA (1986) Standard neuropsychological batteries for children. In *Child Neuropsychology*, JE Obrzut and GW Hynd (eds) pp. 187–227. New York: Academic Press.

Temple, AR and Streeming, K (1975) Taste as a deterrent in pediatric poisoning. *Clin Toxicol* 8(5):541–546.

Tharp, BR, Cukier, F, and Monod, N (1981) The prognostic value of the electroencephalogram in premature infants. *Electroencephalogr Clin Neurophysiol* 51:219–236.

Thatcher, RW, Lester, ML, McAlaster, R, et al. (1963) Intelligence and lead toxins in rural children. *J Learn Dis* 16(5):355–359.

Thomas, JA (1989) Pharmacologic and toxicologic responses in the neonate. *J Am Coll Toxicol* 8(5):957–962.

Tilley, BC, Barnes, AB, Bergstrahl, E, et al. (1985) A comparison of pregnancy history recall and medical records: Implications for retrospective studies. *Am J Epidemiol* 121(2):269–281.

Toutant, C, and Lippmann, S (1979) Fetal solvents syndrome. *Lancet* 1:1356.

Trattner, WI (1970) *Crusade for the Children: A History of the National Child Labor Committee and Child Labor Reform in America*. Chicago: Quadrangle Books.

Tsuchiya, K, Okubo, T, Nagasaki, M, et al. (1977) Biological effects of lead on school children of urban and suburban Tokyo. *Int Arch Occup Environ Health* 38:247–257.

Tuchmann-Duplesis, H (1984) Drugs and other xenobiotics as teratogens. *Pharmacol Ther* 26:273–344.

Tupper, DE (1986) Neuropsychological screening and soft signs. In *Child Neuropsychology*, JE Obrzut and GW Hynd (eds) pp. 139–186. New York: Academic Press.

US Federal Register (1986) §795250, Developmental neurotoxicity screen, Vol. 51, no. 94. May 15, pp. 17,890–17,892.

Vitéz, M, Korány, G, Gonczy, E, et al. (1984) A semiquantitative score system for epidemiology studies of fetal alcohol syndrome. *Am J Epidemiol* 119:301–308.

Volpe, JJ (1983) Perinatal disorders. In *Pediatric Neurology*, 3rd ed, TW Farmer (ed) pp. 117–151. Philadelphia: Harper & Row.

Vorhees, CV, Brunner, RL, and Butcher, RE (1979) Psychotropic drugs as behavioral teratogens. *Science* 205:1220–1225.

Wagner, RH and Rosettt, HL (1975) The effects of drinking on offspring: An historical survey of the

American and British literature. *J Stud Alcohol* 36:1395–1420.

Wang, J-D, Shy, W-Y, Chen, J-S, et al. (1989) Parental occupational lead exposure and lead concentration of newborn cord blood. *Am J Ind Med* 15:111–115.

Weathersbee, PS and Lodge, JR (1979) Alcohol, caffeine, and nicotine as factors in pregnancy. *Postgrad Med* 66:165–169.

Werboff, J and Gottliev, JS (1983) Drugs in pregnancy: Behavioral teratology. *Obstet Gynecol Surv* 18:420–423.

West, JR (ed) (1986) *Alcohol and Brain Development.* New York: Oxford University Press.

Widdowson, EM (1981) Growth of creatures great and small. *Symp Zool Soc Lond* 46:5–17.

Wilson, D, Esterman, A, Lewis, M, et al. (1986) Children's blood levels in the lead smelting town of Port Pirier, South Australia. *Arch Environ Health* 41(4):245–250.

Wilson, JG (1973) *Environment and Birth Defects.* New York: Academic Press.

Winneke, G, Hrdina, K-G, and Brockhaus, A (1983) Neuropsychological studies in children with elevated tooth lead concentrations. Part I. A pilot study. *Int Arch Occup Environ Health* 51:169–183.

Wisniewska, K, Dambska, M, Sher, JH, et al. (1983) A clinical neuropathological study of the fetal alcohol syndrome. *Neuropediatrics* 14:197–201.

Wolff, PH, and Ferber, R (1979) The development of behavior in human infants, premature and newborn. *Annu Rev Neurosci* 2:291–307.

Woody, RC, Kearns, GL, Brewster, MA, et al. (1986) The neurotoxicity of cyclotrimethylenetrinitramine (RDX) in a child: A clinical and pharmacokinetic evaluation. *Clin Toxicol* 24(4):305–319.

Yanai, J (ed) (1984) *Neurobehavioral Teratology.* Amsterdam: Elsevier.

Yoshimura, T and Ikeda, M (1978) Growth of school children with polychlorinate biphenyl poisoning or Yusho. *Environ Res* 17:416–425.

Yuke, W, Landsdown, R, Millar, IB, et al. (1981) the relationship between blood lead concentrations, intelligence and attainment in a school population: A pilot study. *Dev Med Child Neurol* 23:567–576.

Zielhuis, RL, Del Castillo, P, Herber, RFM, et al. (1979) Concentrations of lead and other metals in blood of two and three-year-old children living near a secondary smelter. *Int Arch Occup Environ Health* 42:213–239.

21

Levels of Consciousness

There are many environmental and occupational neurotoxic agents and drugs that produce alterations in consciousness and the sleep–wakefulness cycle. Acute and chronic occupational exposure to organic carbon monoxide, for example, has been known since the 19th century to be associated with clouding of consciousness, confusion, lack of concentration, and even death.

Consciousness has long been recognized as a basic psychological function without which other psychological processes cannot occur. In the clinic, for example, before any evaluation of mental status is attempted, the examiner first assesses the patient's level of consciousness and orientation in space and time. The examiner then adjusts the level of the interview on the basis of the patient's ability to understand, to concentrate, and to pay attention to simple commands.

An integration of the psychological, biological, neural, electrophysiological, and neuropharmacological bases of the daily cycle of sleep and wakefulness was first attempted only a decade ago. It is not surprising, then, that clinical and epidemiological studies of the effects of neurotoxic agents in humans based on an integrative view of wakefulness and sleep are scant.

Many clinical and experimental pharmacological studies have focused on the effects of drugs for the amelioration of sleep disorders—primarily insomnia and narcolepsy. (Narcolepsy is a neurological disorder in which the afflicted person falls asleep suddenly while carrying out normal daily activity.) However, there have been few studies on the effects of environmental and occupational neurotoxic agents on levels of consciousness and the sleep–wake cycle.

CONSCIOUSNESS

From a clinical point of view, it is customary to describe the range of consciousness along a continuum of attention, alertness, mental relaxation, drowsiness, sleep, and coma. Neurophysiological research performed in the 1950s and 1960s seemed to support the notion that a neural center—the *ascending reticular activating system* (ARAS)—determined these levels of consciousness. The ARAS was conceived as an energizer that "lit up" the activity of the nervous system.

Current research does not support either the existence of this continuum or the neural explanation of several levels of consciousness. Sleep and coma, for example, are now considered different phenomena entirely. Sleep is an active and complex neurophysiological and neurochemical process. Coma differs from sleep both behaviorally and neuropathologically. Behaviorally, coma has a much higher arousal threshold than sleep; lethargy, loss of sensation, stupor, and coma are defined by increasing levels of arousal threshold. In addition, coma is—as a rule—the result of pathological conditions such as a mass or destructive brain lesion, altered metabolic conditions, or, less frequently, psychiatric disorders.

Attention evolved from a primative behavioral pattern: the orienting reflex. This reflex consists of the sudden turning of the head in the general direction of a new and sudden sensory stimulus. Orienting reflexes can be induced in the dog or cat by a sudden noise; the ear—and sometimes the head—will be turned in the general direction of the source of the stimulus. Attention is the capacity to focus on a single or reduced number of objects. Concentration, a closely related phenomenon, is the ability to maintain that focus for extended periods of time while excluding other competing stimuli.

Attention Deficit Disorder

Attention deficit disorder (ADD) is a disorder first evident in infancy or childhood, usually diagnosed at the time the child enters school. This syndrome may or may not be the result of acute or chronic neurotoxic exposure. The essential features of ADD are inattention, impulsivity, and hyperactivity. Two broad categories are recognized: attention disorder with hyperactivity and attention disorders without hyperactivity. The *Diagnostic and Statistical Manual of Mental Disorders* (DMS-III-R) published by the American Psychiatric Association (1987) includes diagnostic criteria for the diagnosis of ADD.

Inattention is a descriptive label used when at least three of the following conditions exist:

- The child often fails to finish things he or she starts.
- The child often does not seem to listen.
- The child is easily distracted.
- The child has difficulty concentrating on schoolwork or other tasks requiring sustained attention.
- The child has difficulty sticking to play activity.

Impulsivity is a term used when the child presents at least three of the following:

- Often acts before thinking.
- Shifts excessively from one activity to another.
- Has difficulty organizing work (when this inability does not depend on cognitive factors).
- Needs a lot of supervision.
- Is frequently called out in class.
- Has difficulties awaiting turns in games or group situations.

Hyperactivity is used when the afflicted individual demonstrates two of the following:

- Runs about or climbs on things excessively.
- Has difficulty sitting still or fidgets excessively.
- Has difficulties staying seated.
- Moves about excessively during sleep.
- Is always "on the go" or acts as if "driven by a motor."

For reasons that are not understood, the disorder is 10 times more prevalent in boys than girls.

Attention Deficit Disorders among Children Exposed to Lead. In the early 1960s, David suggested that children who had been exposed to lead may develop an attention deficit disorder. There are several published studies in which elevated blood levels of lead have been found among children with such a deficit. However, in humans, it has been difficult to prove lead causation of ADD on the basis of either clinical observations or cross-sectional epidemiological studies. Many confounders have to be ruled out. It can be argued, for example, that hyperactive children are more prone than normal children to ingest contaminated soil. Therefore, hyperactivity may be the cause of increased levels of lead and not the other way around.

The association between lead and ADD remains an intriguing hypothesis only. Those advocating the lead-induced ADD hypothesis in humans have done little to rule out possible confounders by means of appropriate epidemiological study designs. Animal studies in the rat performed by Dr. Ellen Silbergeld at the Environmental Defense Fund in Washington, DC, however, seem to support the hypothesis that chronic exposure to lead is associated with hyperactivity. But in humans, this hypothesis still remains to be demonstrated in follow-up study designs, which are very difficult to plan and carry out.

TESTING CONCENTRATION

As a rule, clinical studies are limited to the demonstration that the sometimes subtle changes in the level of consciousness occur as a result of low levels of exposure to neurotoxic agents. Neuropsychologists are relying increasingly on the use of traditional and well-known tests originally developed for the assessment of brain damage to study these questions. The following is a brief description of some of the most widely known, widely used test instruments.

One of the oldest tests of concentration still in use is the Letter Cancellation test. The test can be constructed out of written material in any language. The examinee is presented with a written sentence and instructed to cancel out as many u's and a's as possible in 1 minute. The examiner then counts the number of letters correctly and incorrectly canceled, which becomes the raw score of the test. In the Bourdon–Wiersma Cancellation test the letters are replaced by groups of dots, substitutions that allow the use of the test among people who cannot read.

The letter cancellation test and the Bourdon–Wiersma cancellation test are easy to administer but cumbersome to score. In the former, for example, the examiner has to count all the letters that have been scanned as well as all the correct and incorrect responses. While using the unaided scoring procedure, the examiner literally has to administer the concentration test to himself or herself. The use of transparent plates that can be superimposed on the test sheets help somewhat in test scoring.

The Bourdon–Wiersma test is still popular in Europe and in Latin American countries but is rarely used in the United States. It has been extensively used by Dr. Helena Hänninen in Finland in her studies of the neurobehavioral effects of many toxic occupational agents (Hänninen and Lindström 1979). This author is unaware of any standardization of this test in the United States.

The ability to concentrate is basic and probably required or implied in the execution of all psychometric tests. (The tests described here are reviewed in detail in Chapter 4.) For example, in the execution of the Digit Symbol test, the subject needs to concentrate on the valid "menu" or digits/symbols throughout the test; in the Benton Visual Retention test, failure to retain the visual patterns represents a sure failure to reproduce them; the Embedded Figures test requires sharp scanning through competing interfering stimuli.

Short-term memory is also intimately related to concentration. Some of the psychometric tests that have been proposed for the measure of mental functions such as memory are also tests of concentration. For example, the Digit Forward test, a subtest of the Wechsler scale in which the subject repeats a series of numbers spoken to him or her, requires as much concentration as memory.

VIGILANCE AND VIGILANCE TESTS

Vigilance is the ability to detect meaningful signals during relatively long periods of time. The hunter in the woods who waits for visual and auditory cues of the presence of deer, the air traffic controller who watches the radar screen, and the mother who awakens from sleep to attend to her child are all examples of people performing vigilance tasks.

In contrast to tests of concentration, tests of vigilance often last several minutes. The relative time requirement of vigilance tests makes them unsuitable for medical field surveys, where time, as a rule, is at a premium.

Computer-based testing procedures that often combine vigilance with reaction-time tests now make it possible to test small groups of individuals. These procedures have greatly improved test-scoring as well. In a typical version of a computer-based test, the subject is asked to respond to a key letter—for example, "S"—by pressing a key. Errors and false alarms and the latency in which the response is executed are all measured and used in the evaluation.

One of the earliest studies in human behavioral toxicology involved the effect of an occupational toxic agent—carbon monoxide—on levels of consciousness, particularly vigilance. This is reviewed below.

Disturbances of Consciousness Produced by Carbon Monoxide Poisoning. Carbon monoxide is a colorless, odorless gas generated by the incomplete combustion of carbonaceous materials. It is found in the lower atmosphere as a ubiquitous air pollutant. Along with nicotine, it is present in cigarette smoke. Carbon monoxide is also generated naturally in the human body as a result of the normal degradation of the red blood cell. It combines with hemoglobin, a very important key to its toxic effects. The presence of carbon monoxide in the blood affects respiration by its direct effects on neural respiratory centers.

The toxic properties of carbon monoxide have been known since the work of Claude Bernard (1857) in France. Occupational carbon monoxide poisoning is relatively frequently encountered in industry and accounts for about 10% of all accidental exposures; it occurs in mines, garages, and, in general, where combustion products are released into enclosed areas. Carbon monoxide poisoning occurs frequently among garage workers who work in closed areas, particularly during wintertime; carbon monoxide in the cockpit, resulting in the pilot's loss of consciousness, has been implicated in plane accidents. Carbon monoxide is also frequently used for suicidal purposes (eg, leaving a car on in a closed garage).

The main clinical features of the acute phase of carbon monoxide poisoning are known from studies of suicide victims. But carbon monoxide poisoning may also occur as a complication of surgery and anesthesia, drug overdoses, the effects of naturally occurring toxins, or strangulation.

Disturbances of consciousness are the most common abnormalities observed in acute carbon monoxide poisoning. Psychophysiological experimentation reveals that perceptual deficits can occur when blood carboxyhemoglobin reaches a level of only 5% to 9% saturation (Steward 1976). (Carboxyhemoglobin is a measure of the combination of carbon monoxide and hemoglobin.) Confusion occurs when levels reach 40% to 50%. Coma and convulsions are observed at 50% to 60% levels. Cardiorespiratory failure and death occur at levels ranging between 70% and 80%.

The low-level, long-term effects of carbon monoxide exposure have been extensively studied in conjunction with cigarette smoking, which represents a very important source of individual exposure. Carbon monoxide is an important teratological agent. Injury to the fetus may result from maternal exposure during pregnancy (in smoking mothers or, to a lesser extent, mothers who are exposed to smoking as bystanders). But the cumulative effects of such exposures on neuropsychological functioning in adults have been difficult to study.

Carbon monoxide is also an environmental health problem. For example, toll collectors and tunnel operators are exposed to carbon monoxide from passing vehicles. Bus operators are subjected to the combined exposure to street vehicles in addition to their own.

Carbon monoxide produces many neuropathological alterations. One of the most striking is the appearance of delayed neurological deterioration days (and even weeks) after exposure in people who were deeply comatose as a result of carbon monoxide poisoning. The syndrome, which is often abrupt, exhibits a wide range of neurological and psychological abnormalities including sudden disorientation, confusion, excitement, restlessness, and apathy. Alterations of motor control are present in the form of severe rigidity or spasticity with Parkinson-like tremors.

For a review of the chemical, pharmacological, neurophysiological, and neuropsychological properties of carbon monoxide, see Ginsberg (1980). The technical publication by Vernon R. Putz and collaborators entitled *Effects of CO on Vigilance Performance,* published in 1976, is a good example of the experimental work performed on normal subjects under laboratory conditions.

Effects of Occupational Exposure to Neurotoxic Agents

The concern that occupational exposures to neurotoxic agents might lead to changes in attention and concentration, which in turn might cause accidents, has been raised since the 1960s. This concern has been voiced for workers who are exposed to neurotoxic agents that might cloud consciousness during the performance of life-threatening tasks. The following are examples.

Halothane. Anesthesiologists and personnel who work in the surgical theater have long been suspected of being especially vulnerable to anesthetic gases during the course of surgical interventions. For example, studies performed by Whitcher and collaborators, of the Department of Anesthesia at Stanford Medical School, were aimed at measuring levels of halothane in the environment and in the breath of people who participated in surgery. Both were shown to be elevated at the end of the working day. Importantly, residual concentrations in the breath were present in many individuals 16 hours after exposure.

But does the presence of anesthetic or other gases in the environment affect the concentration of people in a manner to disrupt performance? In addition to maintaining the patient's state of sleep, anesthesiologists have to monitor pulse rate, blood pressure, skin color and temperature, depth and frequency of respiration, electrocardiographic display, type and rate of intravenous infusion, degree of muscle relaxation, and color of blood of the patient. Thus, the anesthesiologist's task is a multidimensional vigilance task.

Whether halothane—or any other of the widely used anesthetic gases—affects vigilance is difficult to answer because there are very few studies reported that meet difficult study design problems. The usual study design is one in which repeated measures for a single individual are performed early in the morning before the exposure and again at the end of the day—ideally at the end of the work week—when maximal effects could be expected.

As a rule, studies in situ, close to the surgical theater where the anesthesiologists and technical personnel work, have failed to show a significant decrement in performance except for an increased prevalence of anesthetic-related symptoms. But experimental studies under laboratory conditions, such as those published in 1974 by Mary J. Bach and collaborators at the Department of Anesthesiology and Psychiatry of Northwestern University Medical School in Chicago, have shown that halothane does adversely affect behavior. Compared to controls, it was possible to demonstrate a significant decrement in performance following anesthetic exposure in tests involving recognition of changes in auditory and visual signals, among others.

Dichloromethane. Dichloromethane is used in industry as a solvent for several plastics as well as for metal degreasing and extraction processes. Dichloromethane is a central nervous system depressant that can cause narcosis when present at high concentrations. In 1976, Winneke and Fodor of the University of Düsseldorf in the Federal Republic of Germany published the results of a study to determine whether exposures to dichloromethane at levels comparable to those found at the workplace would produce significant changes in mental tasks requiring attention and concentration. Experiments were conducted in a special testing chamber where dichloromethane could be released at desired levels. The studies of Winneke and Fodor are important in that they show that while attention and concentration tasks might not be affected by exposure to dichloromethane, vigilance under similar testing conditions might be impaired.

Twenty-two female volunteers between the ages of 22 and 31 participated in experiments in which tests of attention and concentration were administered. The mental tasks consisted of the adding of numbers and letter cancellation. There were no performance differences that could be attributed to exposure to the solvent.

Eight female volunteers between the ages of 24 and 51 participated in the vigilance task. The subjects listened to a train of pulses of a hissing noise 0.35 seconds in duration. Normally these pulses were at 50 decibels of intensity. At random intervals, the intensity

was slightly decreased. These reductions in intensity had to be reported by the experimental subject by pressing a key. Errors of omission (misses) and errors of commission (false alarms) were recorded. False alarms were rare and did not merit further analysis.

Winneke and Fodor found that whereas performance under control conditions remained stable with dichloromethane, vigilance deteriorated as a function of the passage of time. The increased errors in performance were interpreted as having been caused by attention lapses associated with dichloromethane exposure.

SLEEP AND WAKEFULNESS

In spite of much research on sleep, we still do not know why we need to sleep and exactly how the activities of sleeping and dreaming occur. Most investigators agree, however, that sleep and the cyclic pattern of sleep and wakefulness can be viewed from at least four interrelated perspectives.

Perspectives of Sleep

Sleep is a psychological need. Many clinical and experimental studies in humans have shown that sleep deprivation, even for short periods, can cause profound psychological alterations, including psychosis. That one needs sleep can be proved experimentally by converting sleep into a motivation for a modification of behavior. For example, there are many reports around the world on the use of the unfulfilled need for sleep to break down the defenses of political prisoners, leading to "confessions."

Since the writings of Sigmund Freud, dreams have been interpreted as a psychological function. Freud's well-known theories (Freud 1967 translation) are fascinating and cannot be reviewed briefly without doing them an injustice. In short, external stimuli that reach the sleeper are transformed into dreams to prevent the sleeper's awakening. In addition, dreams represent the individual's unfulfilled needs that, when one is awake, are normally suppressed by an ever-watchful alter ego. Thus, knowing what an individual dreams about provides important cues to what these needs are.

Nightmares are often an important sequel of exposure to neurotoxic agents such as carbon disulfide, mercury, and lead. Nightmares can also be an accompanying symptom of stress, resulting from active participation in emotionally charged situations such as wars, plane accidents, or chemical accidents that destroy life and property. It is often very difficult to disentangle when a nightmare is the primary effect of a neurotoxic agent or an effect of stress.

Biologically, sleep and wakefulness form one of the many natural biorhythms of the body. Sleep and wakefulness are linked in a *circadian*—or daily—*rhythm,* since the duration of this cycle is about a day. The evolutionary advantages of the sleep–wake cycle are not fully understood, but it is known that the sleep–wake cycle is primarily attuned to the sun's cycle. However, experimental studies in humans who lived voluntarily in deep caves show that the human body has a much longer natural rhythm, lasting about 33 hours. Other examples of physiological changes in the body that follow circadian rhythms are fluctuations in body temperature, body electrolytes, and the secretion of various hormones.

Biochronology, until recently an obscure discipline, has recently emerged as an important field of study. Along with circadian rhythms lasting 1 day, other longer and shorter rhythms are now recognized. The menstrual cycle and seasonal variations in physiological functions are examples of *infradian rhythms* that last for several weeks and even months. Feeding, breathing, the heart rate, and the spontaneous discharge of nerve impulses are seen as progressively shorter expressions of *ultradian rhythms.*

Much has been learned about the possible neural mechanisms of sleep and wakefulness by means of electrophysiological studies. These advances can only be briefly summarized here. (The reader is directed to a comprehensive and easy-to-read source, such as Parkes 1985.) It was only in 1953 that the rapid eye movement (or *REM*) sleep was discovered. From that time, the convergence of electroencephalographic and electrooculographic techniques (both described in Chapter 5) made it possible to characterize five states of wakefulness and sleep. In experimental studies in humans under laboratory conditions, it has been possible to show that combined electroencephalographic/electrooculographic criteria define the behavioral and psychological status of the individual very well. The few available neurotoxicological studies have been aimed at showing—in a descriptive, often qualitative manner—how people exposed to neurotoxic agents suffer from alterations of these key functions.

Animal studies have also provided much insight into the individual mechanisms of the complex neural behavioral phenomena involved in the sleep–wake cycle. Some of these studies have been aimed at ascertaining the place within the brain where the rhythmic pattern of electrical activity originates. Although thalamic nuclei seem to account for the rhythmic pattern of the waveform, the existence of a single source of electric waves (a wave generator) postulated in the early 1950s is no longer accepted by most investigators. Some scientists have aimed at the structural and pharmacological characterization of small medullary nuclei—such as the raphe nuclei and the nucleus of the solitary tract—destruction of which causes insomnia.

Pharmacologically, the sleep–wake cycle might be related to changes in neurotransmitter activity. Jouvet (1983) and others have shown that arousal is associated with activity of noradrenergic fibers and that deep sleep is associated with activity of serotonergic fibers. The possibility that environmental and occupational neurotoxic agents produce modification of these neurotransmitter pathways, thus explaining alterations in the wakefulness and sleep patterns, is appealing but has not been systematically explored.

An integrated view of how these mechanisms account for all psychological, behavioral, electrophysiological, and pharmacological events related to sleep and wakefulness is often described at the level of a theory. One of these comprehensive theories, proposed by Hobson and McCarley of Harvard University in 1977, is primarily concerned with explaining the dream process.

Sleep Disorders

The Association of Sleep Disorder Centers (ASDC) defines more than 65 separate diagnostic entities grouped into four major classes of sleep disorders:

- Disorders of initiation and maintenance of sleep (eg, insomnia).
- Disorders of excessive somnolence. *Hypersomnia* refers to inappropriate and undesirable sleepiness during waking hours rather than to excessive total sleep time within a day.
- Disorders of the sleep–wake schedule.
- Dysfunctions associated with sleep, sleep stages, or partial arousals (*parasomnias*).

Insomnia is the inability to get enough sleep at night, with the result that it may interfere with the person's ability to function efficiently the next day. It may occur as a difficulty in falling asleep or frequent awakening during the night or too early waking in the morning. Insomnia is generally regarded as a symptom of an underlying problem. It can be transient, short-term, or long-term. If insomnia continues for at least 3 weeks, it is considered long-term insomnia.

Insomnia is frequently associated with depression, but there are many other psychiatric conditions—such as anxiety, unresolved psychological conflicts, phobias, and schizophrenia—that interfere with sleep. Drug use or withdrawal from drugs can produce insomnia. It is fairly well established that alcohol as well as immoderate use of barbituates may produce long-lasting sleep disorders such as insomnia. Caffeine, diet pills, and amphetamines also interfere with sleep. Some disorders that impair breathing may interfere with sleep.

Two disorders, sleep apnea and myoclonus, are detected by electrophysiological techniques in all-night testing. *Sleep apnea* is a condition characterized by brief halts in breathing lasting from 20 to 100 seconds. Those suffering from sleep apnea wake up during the night gasping for air. *Myoclonus* is a syndrome involving involuntary leg twitching that interrupts sleep. Sometimes, as many as 300 leg twitchings may occur during the night. As with sleep apnea, the sufferer may not be aware of the problem.

In Parkes (1985), the reader can find descriptions of other, relatively rare, forms of sleep disorders.

The Epidemiology of Sleep Disorders

Under the organizational aegis of Project Sleep and the Association of Sleep Disorder Clinics (ASDC), nearly 5000 patient records from 11 sleep–wake disorder clinics have been analyzed in a cooperative study (Coleman et al. 1982). Eighty percent of the patients underwent a polysomnographic study consisting of electroencephalography, electrooculography, electromyography, and electrocardiography. The diagnostic categories found were hypersomnia (51%), insomnia (31%), parasomnias (15%), and sleep–wake schedule disturbances (3%). Within the most prevalent diagnosis, hypersomnia, sleep apnea was found in 43% of subjects and narcolepsy in 25%. Psychiatric disorders accounted for the most frequent group of insomnia diagnoses (25%).

Sleep Disorders Linked to Environmental or Occupational Exposure to Neurotoxic Agents

Sleeping problems have sometimes been linked to environmental exposures to neurotoxic agents. But to this author's knowledge, there is not a single sound epidemiological study focused on alterations in the cycle of sleep and wakefulness in people exposed to neurotoxic agents that can be said to be good enough to serve as a model. (The few existing clinical studies have serious problems in study design and subject selection.)

There are many studies in which sleeping problems are one of the many neurological symptoms and signs studied. Hypersomnia, for example, has been linked to the accidental environmental exposure to polybrominated biphenyls (PBBs) in Michigan that occurred in 1973 (Anderson et al. 1979; Valciukas et al. 1979). A mixture of such compounds used as fire retardents was accidentally released into the environment in animal feed, causing widespread contamination of livestock including dairy and beef cattle, poultry, and eggs. Before the cause and dimensions of the problem were appreciated, contamination of milk, beef, pork, eggs, and poultry occurred. Sleepiness was found to be a prominent symptom when, in a large epidemiological study, the prevalence of neurological symptoms exhibited by Michigan residents was compared with the prevalence of neurological symptoms in nonexposed residents of Wisconsin serving as controls. A syndrome described in the exposed group included the symptoms of tiredness, headaches, nervousness, depression, dizziness, paresthesia, blurred vision, muscle weakness, and other neurological symptoms and signs. Sleepiness was also prominent when the time course of the syndrome was reconstructed.

At the time of the publication of the first studies in the middle 1970s it was argued that sleepiness may have been caused by PBBs (PBBs contain bromine molecules known to cause sleepiness in humans; bromine had been used in the past as a hypnotic). In addition, PBBs were found to be neurotoxic in animal models. However, a dose–response relationship between blood levels of PBB and symptoms was never found. In addition, some speculated that sleepiness may have been the result of a stress-related reactive depression. The latter etiology seemed to have been the case in patients admitted to local hospitals.

For a review of these studies and opposing views, see Valciukas et al. (1979).

Sleeping problems, including both hypersomnia and insomnia, are a frequently reported symptom among workers occupationally exposed to lead and neurotoxic metals, including mercury. Ruth Lilis and collaborators at the Mount Sinai School of Medicine in New York, for example, have published several studies in which they were able to show a dose–response relationship between biological indicators of lead exposure (blood lead levels) and absorption (zinc protoporphyrin levels) and neurological symptoms such as sleep problems (Lilis et al. 1985). The neural and neuropharmacological basis for the sleep disorders caused by lead or mercury is unknown.

CONCLUSIONS

Consciousness is a basic psychological function without which other sensory functions—such as perception, learning, recall, and cognition—cannot normally occur. Consciousness is intimately related to wakefulness and the wake–sleep cycle. Although concentration problems and sleep problems are common complaints in the clinic, there have been few systematic studies of dose–response relationships between neurotoxic exposures and disorders of consciousness except for studies on carbon monoxide and anesthetic gases. Sleep problems are frequent and often are an expression of much larger nerurological or psychiatric problems. The link between environmental or occupational toxic agents and sleep problems should be made only when possible alternative explanations can be satisfactorily ruled out.

Since the mid-1950s, important advances have been made in our understanding of the neural, electrophysiological, and pharmacological basis of wakefulness and sleep. Yet, these advances have yet to be integrated into the body of knowledge now existing on environmental and occupational health matters. Thus far, epidemiological studies have been largely descriptive, offering few cues to the possible environmental (toxic) determination of disorders of consciousness and the sleep–wake cycle.

REFERENCES

American Psychiatric Association (1987) *Diagnostic and Statistical Manual of Mental Disorders*, rev ed (DSM-III-R). Washington, DC: American Psychiatric Association.

Anderson, HA, Wolff, MS, Lilis, R, et al. (1979) Symptoms and clinical abnormalities following ingestion of polybrominated-biphenyl-contaminated food products. In *The Scientific Basis for the Public Control of Environmental Health Hazards*, WJ Nicholson and John A Moore (eds) pp. 684–702. New York: The New York Academy of Sciences.

Bach, MJ, Arbit, J, and Bruce, DL (1974) Trace anesthetic effect on vigilance. In *Behavioral Toxicology, Early Detection of Occupational Hazards*, C Xintaras, BL Johnson, and I DeGroot (eds) pp. 41–50. Washington, DC: US Department of Health, Education and Welfare, Public Health Center for Disease Control, National Institute for Occupational Safety and Health.

Bernard, C (1857) *Leçons sur les Effets des Substances Toxiques et Médicamenteuses*. Paris: J Balliere et Fils.

Coleman, RM, Roffwarg, HP, Kennedy, SJ et al. (1982) Sleep–awake disorders based on a polysomnographic diagnosis. *JAMA* 247(7):997–1003.

Freud, S (1967) *The Interpretation of Dreams* (translation). New York: Avon.

Ginsberg, MD (1980) Carbon monoxide. In *Experimental and Clinical Neurotoxicology*, PS Spencer and HH Schaumburg (eds) pp. 374–393. Baltimore: Williams & Wilkins.

Hänninen, H and Lindström, K (1979) *A Battery for Toxipsychological Evaluation*. Helsinki: Institute of Occupational Health.

Hobson, JA and McCarley, RW (1977) The brain as a dream state generator: An activation–synthesis hypothesis of the dream process. *Am J Psychiatry* 134:1335–1348.

Jouvet, M (1983) Neurobiology of dream. In *Functions of the Nervous System, Vol 4, Psycho-Neurobiology*, M Monnier and M Meulders (eds) pp. 227–248. Amsterdam: Elsevier.

Lilis, R, Valciukas, JA, Malkin, J, et al. (1985) Effects of low-level lead and arsenic exposure on copper smelter workers. *Arch Environ Health* 40(1):38–47.

Parkes, JD (1985) *Sleep and Its Disorders*. London: WB Saunders.

Putz, VR, Johnson, BL, and Setzer, JV (1976) *Effects of CO on Vigilance Performance. Publication DHEW (NIOSH) 77-124*. Cincinnati, OH: US Department of Health, Education and Welfare, US Public Health Service, Center for Disease Control, National Institute for Occupational Safety and Health.

Steward, RT (1976) The effects of carbon monoxide on humans. *J Occup Med* 18:304.

Valciukas, JA, Lilis, R, Wolff, M, et al. (1979) The neurotoxicity of polybrominated biphenyls: Results of a clinical field study. In *The Scientific Basis for the Public Control of Environmental Health Hazards*, WJ Nicholson and John A Moore (eds) pp. 684–702. New York: The New York Academy of Sciences.

Whitcher, CE, Cohen, EN, and Trundell, JR (1971) Chronic exposure to anesthetic gases in the operating room. *Anesthesiology* 35:348.

Winneke, G and Fodor, GG (1976) Dichloromethane produces narcotic effect. *Occup Health Saf* 45(2):34–35.

SUGGESTED READINGS

Allen, MD, Greenbraltt, DJ, and Noel, BJ (1979) Self-poisoning with over-the-counter hypnotics. *Clin Toxicol* 15(2):151–158.

Aschoff, J, Pöppel, E, and Wever, R (1969) Circadiene Periodik des Menschen unter dem Einfluß von Licht-Dunkel-Wechseln unterschiedlicher Periode. *Pflugers Arch Ges Physiol* 306:58–70.

Association of Sleep Disorders Centers (1979) Diagnostic classification of sleep and arousal disorders. *Sleep* 2:1–137.

Braddeley, AD (1966) Influence of depth on the manual dexterity of free divers. *J Appl Psychol* 50:81–85.

Beard, RR and Grandstaff, NW (1974) Carbon monoxide and human functions. In *Behavioral Toxicology*, B Weiss and VG Laties (eds) pp. 1–27. New York: Plenum Press.

Beningus, VA, Muller, KE, Barton, C et al. (1987) Effect of low level carbon monoxide on compensatory tracking and event monitoring. *Neurotoxicol Teratol* 9(3):227–234.

Bernstein, S and Leff, R (1967) Toxic psychosis from sleep medicines containing scopolamine. *N Engl J Med* 277:638.

Bixler, E, Kales, A, Soldatos, C, et al. (1979) Prevalence of sleep disorders: A survey of the Los Angeles metropolitan area. *Am J Psychiatry* 136:1257–1262.

Christensen, CL, Gliner, JA, Horvath, SM, et al. (1977) Effects of three kinds of hypoxias on vigilance performance. *Aviat Space Environ Med* 48:491–496.

Coleman, RM (1986) *Wide awake at 3:00AM: By Choice or by Chance?* New York: WH Freeman.

Colquhoun, WP, Paine, MWPH, and Fort, A (1979) Changes in the temperature rhythm of submariners following a rapidly rotating watchkeeping system for a prolonged period of time. *Int Arch Occup Environ Health* 42:185–190.

Crowell, DH, Kapuniai, LE, Boychuk, RB et al. (1982) Daytime sleep state organization in three-month old infants. *Electroencephalogr Clin Neurophysiol* 53:36–47.

Czeisler, CA, Moore-Ede, M, and Coleman, RM (1983) Resetting circadian clocks: Application to sleep disorders in medicine and occupational health. In *Sleep/Wake Disorders: Natural History, Epidemiology, and Long-Term Evolution,* V Guilleminault and E Lugaresi (eds) pp. 243–260. New York: Pergamon Press.

Czeisler, CA, Kronauer, RE, Allan, JS, et al. (1989) Bright light induction of strong (type O) resetting of the human circadian pacemaker. *Science* 244:1328–1333.

David, OJ (1974) Association between lower level lead concentration and hyperactivity in children. *Environ Health Perspect* 7:17.

David, OJ, Clark, J, and Voeller, K (1972) Lead and hyperactivity. *Lancet* 1:900–903.

Davis, DM, Jolly, EJ, Pethybridge, RJ, et al. (1981) The effects of continuous exposure to carbon monoxide on auditory vigilance in man. *Int. Arch Occup Environ Health* 48:25–34.

Dement, WC (1978) *Some Must Watch While Some Must Sleep.* New York: WW Norton.

Dement, W and Kleitman, N (1957) The relation of eye movements during sleep to dream activity: An objective method for the study of dreaming. *J Exp Psychol* 53:89–97.

Dinges, DF, Davis, MM, and Glass, P (1980) Fetal exposure to narcotics: Neonatal sleep as a measure of nervous system disturbances. *Science* 209:629–621.

Dreyfus-Brisad, C (1964) The electroencephalogram of the premature infant and full-term newborn: Normal and abnormal sleeping patterns. In *Neurological and Electroencephalographic Correlative Studies in Infancy,* P Kellaway and I Peterson (eds) pp. 186–207. New York: Grune & Stratton.

Dreyfus-Brisad, C (1968) Sleep ontogenesis in early human prematurity from 24 to 27 weeks of conceptual age. *Dev Psychobiol* 1:162–169.

Dreyfus-Brisad, C (1979) Neonatal electroencephalography. *Rev Perinat Med* 3:397–472.

Durham, WF, Wolfe, HR, and Quinby, GE (1965) Organophosphate insecticide and mental alertness. *Arch Environ Health* 10:55.

Ellington, RJ and Peters, JF (1980) Development of EEG and daytime sleep patterns in normal full-time infants during the first three months of life: Longitudinal study. *Electroencephalogr Clini Neurophysiol* 49:112–124.

Evarts, EV (1967) Activity of individual cerebral neurons during sleep and arousal. *Res Publ Assoc Res Nerv Ment Dis* 45:319–337.

Fodor, GG and Winneke, G (1972) Effect of low CO concentrations on resistence to monotony and on psychomotor capacity. *Staub Reinhalt Luft* 32:46–54.

Foret, J and Benoit, O (1980) Predictable effects on individual sleep patterns during a rapidly rotating shift system. *Int Arch Occup Environ Health* 45:49–56.

Gopinathan, PM, Pichan, G, and Sharma, VM (1988) Role of dehydration in heat stress-induced variations in mental performance. *Arch Environ Health* 43(1):15–17.

Halberg, F (1969) Chronobiology. *Annu Rev Physiol* 31:675–725.

Haldane, J (1895) The action of carbon monoxide on man. *J Physiol* 18:430.

Hallen, B, Ehner-Samuel, H, and Thomason, M (1970) Measurements of halothane in the atmosphere of an operating theatre and in expired air and blood of the personnel during routine anesthetic work. *Acta Anaesth Scand* 14:17–26.

Hanlon, JF (1974) Preliminary studies of the effects of carbon monoxide on vigilance in man. In *Behavioral Toxicology,* B Weiss and VG Laties (eds) pp. 61–75. New York: Plenum Press.

Hildebrandt, G and Stratmann, I (1979) Circadian system response to night work in relation to the individual circadian phase position. *Int Arch Occup Environ Health* 43:73–83.

Horne, J (1988) *Why We Sleep: The Functions of Sleep in Humans and Other Mammals.* New York: Oxford University Press.

Horvath, SM, Dahms, TE, and O'Hanlon, JF (1972) Carbon monoxide and human vigilance. *Arch Environ Health* 23:343–347.

Hunt, HT (1989) *The Multiplicity of Dreams: Memory, Imagination and Consciousness.* New Haven, CT: Yale University Press.

Inoué, S (1989) *Biology of Sleep Substance.* Boca Raton, FL: CRC Press.

Johnson, LC, Tepas, DI, Colduhoun, WP, et al. (eds) (1981) *The Twenty-Four Hour Workday: Proceedings of a Symposium on Variations in Work–Sleep Schedules.* Cincinnati: US Department of Health and Human Services, Public Health Service, Centers for Disease Control, National Institute for Occupational Safety and Health, Division of Biomedical and Behavioral Sciences.

Kales, JD (1987) Evaluation and treatment of insomnia. *Psychiatr Ann* 17:459–483.

Karacan, I, Thornby, J, Anch, M, et al. (1976) Prevalence of sleep disturbances in a primarily urban Florida county. *Soc Sci Med* 10:239–244.

Kellerman, H (1981) *Sleep Disorders: Insomnia and Narcolepsy.* New York: Brunner/Mazel.

Kelly, DD (1985) Sleep and dreaming. In *Principles of Neural Science,* 2nd ed, ER Kandel and JH Schwartz (eds) pp. 648–658. New York: Elsevier.

Kelly, DD (1985) Disorders of sleep and consciousness. In *Principles of Neural Science,* 2nd ed, ER Kandel and JH Schwartz (eds) pp. 659–672. New York: Elsevier.

Kleitman, N (1963) *Sleep and Wakefulness.* Chicago: University of Chicago Press.

Knauth, P and Rutenfranz, J (1976) Experimental shift work studies of permanent night, and rapidly rotating, shift systems: I. Circadian rhythm of body temperature and reentrainment at shift change. *Int Arch Occup Environ Health* 37:125–137.

Knauth, P, Rutenfranz, J, Schultz, H et al (1980) Experimental shift work studies of permanent night and rapidly rotating shift systems: II. Behavior of various characteristics of sleep. *Int Arch Occup Environ Health* 46:111–125.

Knauth, P, Landau, K, Schwitteck, M, et al. (1980) Duration of sleep depending on the type of shift work. *Int Arch Occup Environ Health* 46:167–177.

Kotok, D, Kotok, R, and Heriot, T (1977) Cognitive evaluation of children with elevated blood lead levels. *Am J Dis Child* 131:791–793.

Kubicki, S and Herrmann, W (eds) (1986) *Methods of Sleep Research.* New York: VCH Publishers.

Lindsley, DB (1960) Attention consciousness, sleep and wakefulness. In *Handbook of Physiology, Sec 1, Neurophysiology, Vol 3,* p. 1553. Washington, DC: American Physiological Society.

Lorry, M, Forer, J, and Laville, A (1979) Circadian rhythms and behavior of permanent nightworkers. *Int Arch Occup Environ Health* 44:1–11.

Luby, ED, Frohman, C, Grissel, JL et al. (1960) Sleep deprivation: Effect on behavior, thinking, motor performance and biological transfer system. *Psychosom Med* 22:182–192.

Ludy, ED, Grissel, JL, Frohman, CE et al. (1962) Biochemical, psychological and behavioral responses to sleep deprivation. *Ann NY Acad Sci* 96:71–79.

Moody, JA and Duggar, BC (1966) Alertness management in industry. *Am Ind Hyg Assoc J* 27:17–24.

Palca, J (1989) Sleep researchers awake to possibilities. *Science* 245:351–352.

Parrot, J and Petiot, J-C (1978) Less than 24 hour pseudoperiodicity in work schedules of train drivers, in relation to their sleep. *Int Arch Occup Environ Health* 41:179–188.

Peretz Lavie (1983) Sleep apnea in industrial workers. In *Sleep/Wake Disorders: Natural History, Epidemiology, and Long-Term Evolution,* V Guilleminault and E Lugaresi (eds) pp. 127–135. New York: Pergamon Press.

Peter, JH, Fuchs, F, Langanke, P, et al. (1983) The SIFA train function safety circuit: I. Vigilance and operational practice in psychophysiological analysis. *Int Arch Occup Environ Health* 52:329–339.

Peter, JH, Fuchs, F, Langanke, P, et al. (1983) The SIFA train function safety circuit: II. Inefficiency of a paced secondary task as a vigilance monitor. *Int Arch Occup Environ Health* 52:341–352.

Pompeiano, O (1967) The neurophysiological mechanisms of the postural and motor events during desynchronized sleep. *Res Publ Assoc Res Nerv Ment Dis* 45:351–423.

Rechschaffen, A and Kales, A (eds) *A Manual of Standardized Terminology Techniques and Scoring System for Sleep Stages of Human Subjects, National Institutes of Health Publication No. 204.* Washington, DC: US Government Printing Office.

Riley, TL (1985) *Clinical Aspects of Sleep and Sleep Disturbance.* Boston: Butterworth Publishers.

Rummo, N and Sarlans, K (1974) The effect of carbon monoxide on several measures of vigilance in a simulated driving task. *J Saf Res* 6:126–130.

Sagvolden, T and Archer, T (1988) *Attention Deficit Disorders.* Hillsdale, NJ: Lawrence Earlbaum Associates.

Silbergeld, EK and Goldberg, AM (1974) Hyperactivity: A lead induced behavioral disorder. *Environ Health Perspect* 7:227–232.

Silbergeld, EK and Goldberg, AM (1974) Lead-induced behavioral dysfunction: An animal model of hyperactivity. *Exp Neurol* 42:146–157.

Smith, P (1979) A study of weekly and rapidly rotating shiftworkers. *Int Arch Occup Environ Health* 43:211–220.

Steward, RD, Newton, PE, Hosko, MJ, et al. (1974) The effect of carbon monoxide on time perception, manual coordination, and arithmetic. In *Behavioral Toxicology,* B Weiss and VG Laties (eds) pp. 29–60. New York: Plenum Press.

Stoffer, DS, Scher, MS, Richardson, GA, (1988) A Walsh–Fourier analysis of the effect of moderate maternal alcohol consumption on neonatal sleep-state cycling. *J Am Stat Assoc* 83:954–963.

Tune, GS (1969) Sleep and wakefulness in a group of shift workers. *Br J Ind Med* 26:54–58.

Vokac, Z, Magnus, P, Jebens, E et al. (1981) Apparent phase shifts or circadian rhythms (masking effects) during rapid shift rotation. *Int Arch Occup Environ Health* 49:53–65.

Weitzman, ED (1981) Sleep and its disorders. *Annu Rev Neurosci* 4:381–417.

Woods, W, Gavica, J, Brown, W, et al. (1971) Implication of organophosphate pesticide poisoning in the plane crash of a duster pilot. *Aerospace Med* 42:1111–1113.

Xintaras, C, Sobecki, MF, and Ulrich, CE (1967) Sleep: Changes in rapid-eye-movement phase in chronic lead absorption. *Toxicol Appl Pharmacol* 10:384.

Zerubavel, E (1985) *The Seven Day Circle: The History and Meaning of the Week.* Chicago: University of Chicago Press.

22

Chemical Senses

Chemical senses are used by living organisms to gather chemical information from the external and internal environment. From the evolutionary point of view, chemical senses, particularly taste and olfaction, are the oldest channels of information. In spite of the efforts of several generations of scientists, many fundamental processes underlying the sensations of olfaction and taste are poorly understood.

Chemical reception can be demonstrated in the simplest of organisms, such as microbes. One such organism is the ciliated protozoan *Paramecium tetraurelia.* Tetraurelia exhibits *chemotaxis,* that is, modulation of behavior that results from sensing the chemical composition of its immediate environment. Chemotaxis can also be demonstrated in bacteria and in many invertebrates such as nematodes. Leukocytes (white blood cells) present in the human bloodstream act as scavengers clearing the debris resulting from damaged tissue and microorganisms—chemotaxis is also involved in this process.

Chemical senses are responsible for mediating numerous biological processes and species behavior. Ethology has helped to uncover many of these chemical cues. There is much evidence that organisms throughout the phylogenetic spectrum from simple to complex living things use chemical signals in species and individual recognition. An intriguing hypothesis proposed by Lewis Thomas in 1974 is that the process of odor recognition of self and nonself is akin to that of immunologic recognition, where the recognition of "foreign" cells or substances is crucial to the body's defense system.

Many organisms use chemical signals called *pheromones* to attract a member of the opposite sex within the same species. Pheromones are hormones secreted by an organism into its external environment, where they are sensed by members of the same or opposite sex. Hormones secreted by endocrine glands have long been known to be related to the chemical senses. Some women exhibit marked changes in olfactory thresholds during the menstrual cycle.

On the molecular level, all senses are chemical. However, the concept of "chemical senses" has traditionally been reserved for those processes observed in chemical reception in lower organisms, sensory organs such as taste and olfaction, and certain interoreceptors—sensors that intervene in the regulation of the internal environment—such as those that maintain the optimum degree of oxygenation of the human blood.

The effects of toxic agents on taste and

olfaction have not been as extensively studied as have effects on other sensory systems such as vision. However, techniques and methods for the evaluation of these two chemical senses do exist to gather information on an epidemiological scale. It is difficult to speculate on the reasons for this selective ignorance. Since vision and hearing dominate our lives, one possibility is that we attach a relatively low value to our chemical senses. Cultural mores may also play a role.

TASTE

In organisms such as fish, taste and olfaction are one and the same. In fish—as well as in the earliest stages of the development of the human embryo—chemoreceptors are located both inside and outside the body. In the fish, taste buds found externally are involved in food selection, whereas taste buds closest to the alimentary canal are related to ingestive and protective reflexes.

It has been postulated (Finger and Morita 1985), that there are two gustatory (relating to taste) systems in humans, one supported by the facial and the other by the vagal nerve. Support for this theory can be found in the functional organization of neural pathways mediating taste in lower organisms. In the fish, for example, there appear to be two separate neural pathways in the brainstem for facial and vagal gustation. The facial gustatory system is connected to the reticular formation and trigeminal nuclei. The primary sensory nucleus of the vagal gustatory system is connected to neurons involved in swallowing. It is thought that these two separate but overlapping systems may also be found in higher vertebrates, including humans.

Taste Qualities and Receptors

Psychophysical and electrophysiological studies have shown that all tastes can be classified into four qualities: bitter, salty, sour, and sweet. There is a regional distribution of

gustatory receptors for the optimal perception of each of these tastes:

- The tip of the tongue is sensitive to all four taste qualities but is optimally sensitive to sweet.
- The lateral portion of the tongue (tip to back) senses the sour quality.
- The lateral portion of the tongue (anterior third only) detects salty qualities.
- The back of the tongue senses the bitter quality.

Taste is modified by the chemical composition of saliva. For example, it is thought that saliva is responsible for the taste alterations found in many metal intoxications such as lead and mercury.

Gustatory receptors are located in the tongue as large anatomic structures, the *papillae*, that can be recognized with the naked eye. There are also gustatory receptors in the epiglottis, the upper third of the esophagus, and the palate of the mouth. There are three types of papillae: fungiform, foliate, and circumvallate. How their different shapes contribute to the sensory codings is unknown. The taste receptor cells, concentrated in groups with sometimes as many as 50 to a group, are contained in the taste buds. Between the receptor cell and the afferent (sensory) fiber there is a synapse.

Neural Pathways

Taste sensations are conveyed by two different cranial nerves, VII and IX. The neural pathways of the gustatory system are uncrossed, an exception to the pattern exhibited by all other sensory pathways (Fig. 22.1). The anterior two-thirds of the tongue is innervated by the corda tympani, a branch of the facial nerve (cranial nerve VII); the cell bodies of these bipolar cells are located in the geniculate nucleus. The posterior third of the tongue is innervated by the lingual branch of the glossopharyngeal nerve (cranial nerve IX);

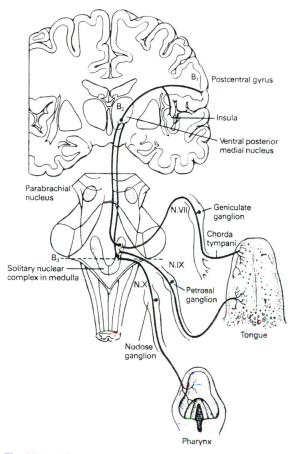

Fig. 22.1. The neural pathways of the gustatory system.
(From Kandel and Schwartz 1985.)

the cell bodies of these bipolar cells are located in the petrosal ganglion. All these first-order neurons conveying gustatory messages from the tongue converge into the solitary nuclear complex located in the medulla, the lowest portion of the brainstem.

In the medulla, neurons carrying taste messages synapse with the cell bodies of second-order neurons. The fibers of the second-order neurons synapse in the thalamus in the ventral posterior medial nucleus. The third-order neuron projects into the cortex of the brain in the area where the somesthesic representation of the tongue is found. Another group of fibers project into the insular cortex. There are also projections into the limbic system and the hypothalamus that may account for

the affective and emotional quality of gustatory sensations.

Stimulus Transduction and Coding of Gustatory Stimuli

A plausible explanation of how the stimulus of gustation might be transduced into a neural stimulus is the assumption that the oral cavity contains receptors that are sensitive to the chemical configuration of certain molecules. This is called the *stereochemical theory of chemical transduction* (proposed for both taste and olfaction). Molecules of a given shape will fit receptor sites the way a key fits a keyhole; the successful match between the molecular shapes and receptor sites will initiate the action potential. Although many molecules of known shapes are associated with predictable tastes, there are a large number of substances that do not fit the taste predicted by theory. Those interested in the history and context of some other theories may consult Beidler (1971) and Cain (1978).

Many facts about the neural coding of taste are known. Carl Pfaffmann and his students (Pfaff 1985) have proposed a theory of taste in which taste sensation is coded in labeled lines and the analysis of gustatory sensation is achieved by comparison of the patterns of neural activity across labeled lines.

A taste fiber can code all tastes. A fiber that is primarily sensitive to sweet is also sensitive to acids, a fiber that is primarily sensitive to acids is also sensitive to bitter, and so forth. Thus, the taste fiber "labels" all tastes with a maximum sensitivity to one of the four primary taste qualities. (The reader may recognize the similarity of this theory with that of the primary colors that explains color vision, to be reviewed in Chapter 26.) Taste is not identified by a single neuron. In order to accomplish taste identification, a comparison between the patterns of several labeled lines must be made.

Taste as a Psychological Experience

Palatability of foods depends on gustatory, somatosensory, and olfactory mechanisms. Some of us appreciate the "crunchiness" of nuts added to salads; some others do not like the "chewiness" of game meat. These sensory and motor cues are provided by the trigeminal nerve and its neural connections to the brain. There are many experimental studies in humans and animals supporting the view that the trigeminal nerve interacts with gustatory pathways to explain the palatability of food (Cain 1974).

The pleasure we get from savoring a meal before we eat it also depends on olfaction. Part of the reason why food is distasteful when we have a cold is that the olfactory cues with which we usually associate our favorite meals are lost. Enjoyment of food is also heavily influenced by the culture in which we live as well as by education.

Linda Bartoshuk of the John B. Pierce Laboratory in New Haven, Connecticut is one the world's leaders in the field of taste psychophysics. Many of the complex sensory cues that account for "taste" are now understood because of her extensive work on this subject.

Experimental and Clinical Procedures to Assess Taste

There are no universally accepted experimental procedures for the scientific examination of taste. Some authors apply drops of liquids of known concentrations onto several areas of the tongue. Most of the experimental conditions in the laboratory are rather artificial because in everyday situations the active movement of the tongue is involved in the full appreciation of flavors. The technical difficulties encountered in the design of good equipment for stimulus delivery are minor compared to those found in olfaction. Recording of subjective responses in humans is achieved by means of psychophysical procedures, particularly those derived from the new psychophysics (explained in Chapter 25, on the auditory system, where these methods have been extensively applied). Multidimensional scaling of taste (rating of multiple attributes at the same time) is also used.

Factors That Modify the Sense of Taste

There are many physiological and medical conditions that affect the sense of taste. Among them are the action of natural taste modifiers. For example, the taste of pure water is sweet after one has savored artichokes. The red berries of the the miracle fruit *Synsepalum dulcificum* cause sour substances to taste sweet. Bartoshuk and collaborators (1972, 1974) have described many naturally occurring substances that act as taste modifiers.

Taste changes can also serve as preclinical or concomitant manifestations of many acute and chronic diseases—eg, liver failure, hypothyroidism, and cancer. Taste changes have also been noted under certain nutritional conditions such as lack of vitamin A (Bernard and Halpern 1968).

Occupational Neurotoxic Agents That Modify the Sense of Taste. A number of metals, including lead, selenium, zinc, silver, and manganese, and solvents such as tetrachloroethane, butanol, and xylene, modify the sense of taste. There are numerous case reports where a bitter metallic taste in the mouth and garlicky breath contribute to the positive diagnosis of selenium poisoning. Alderman and Bergin (1986) reported a 21-year-old female college student working in a university electrical engineering research laboratory who was exposed to hydrogen selenide at least once a week for approximately a year. (Hydrogen selenide is a nonmetallic compound used in the manufacture of solar panels and in semiconductor industries; selenium is an essential trace element required by the body.) Garlicky breath was again an important cue to establish such a diagnosis.

The experimental work by Taniewski (1975) in Poland using gustatometric and psychophysical procedures is the only report on an epidemiological scale (of which this author is aware) on abnormalities in the sense of taste resulting from occupational exposure to toxic agents. Taniewski studied threshold levels of the taste sensation to grape sugar, citric acid, domestic salt, and quinine hydrochloride in several different occupational groups. The groups included clinical cases of occupational poisoning (eg, lead poisoning), workers in a chocolate factory, those handling paints and varnishes and styrene, and workers in ship engine rooms. (The occupational exposures of the latter group are difficult to ascertain from this report.) Concentrations were increased logarithmically. The battery of tests consisted of the determination of the threshold for taste sensitivity,

the ability to differentiate between taste stimuli, and temporary threshold shifts in taste sensation before and after work.

Although his work has merit nonetheless, Taniewski's experimental study does not match standards of quality we are used to in the West. As a result, some questions may be raised in understanding his findings. For example, it is not clear whether he controlled for temperature, since temperature is an important taste modifier. The level of consciousness in patients admitted to a clinic for acute cases of poisoning is also not discussed. Consciousness is known to affect results of psychophysical experiments. In spite of these shortcomings, several interesting observations are worth noting:

1. For clinical patients with diagnosed saturnism (lead poisoning), higher thresholds for taste were demonstrated for all flavors, most distinctly sweet and bitter tastes. The changes were chronic in character. In nine cases of zinc poisoning, higher values for all thresholds were also observed, particularly for the acid and bitter tastes. As a group, the 14 patients performed significantly worse than normal controls.

2. A comparative study of several occupational groups has revealed that the greatest handicap of taste is found in the workers of paint and varnish factories. Others include those with occupational exposures to styrene.

3. Alterations in acid and bitter tastes were most commonly found; disturbances in sweet tastes were rare.

4. In cases of acute poisoning, taste alterations disappear in the normal course of recuperation from the illness.

OLFACTION

Olfactory Quality and Receptors

As a result of the success of the notion that taste and vision result from primary sensations—ie, mixtures of primary taste qualities and primary colors, respectively—scientists have long speculated that similar principles must exist for olfaction. Seven or more primary odors have been proposed. These include camphoraceous, musky, floral, pepperminty, ethereal, pungent, and putrid.

John Amoore (1974) put forward a theory that links the initiation of the receptor potential to the successful entrapment of molecules of specific shapes by olfactory receptors. In his view, the odoriferous molecules are absorbed by the mucous layer of the olfactory epithelium. The successful locking of molecules with their receptor sites causes the opening of sodium ion (Na$^+$) and potassium ion (K$^+$) channels, thus initiating the receptor potential. There are about 600 substances whose odors can be predicted using this theory, but the odor of a much larger number of molecules cannot be predicted on the basis of their shape.

The olfactory receptors are confined to the olfactory epithelium, an area of about 5 cm^2 lining the nasal cavity. The receptor cell is a modified neuron that can divide (as a rule, neurons in the human nervous system cannot). The olfactory receptors turn over rapidly, and new receptors are generated approximately every 60 days. The olfactory receptor cell has a short peripheral process where cilia are found. The cilia are embedded in the olfactory mucosa. The short peripheral process and the cilia are thought to contain the mechanism(s) by which the transduction of a specific molecule to a neural signal is accomplished. The unmyelinated fibers of the long central processes form the olfactory nerve (cranial nerve I). The olfactory nerve is very short, extending from the olfactory epithelium to the olfactory bulb, penetrating the cribiform plate. The cribiform plate, containing perforations, is present in the ethmoid bone and receives its name from its similarity to a colander.

Neural Pathways

The olfactory nerve synapses in spherical synaptic areas of the olfactory bulb called glomeruli; the olfactory messages travel through

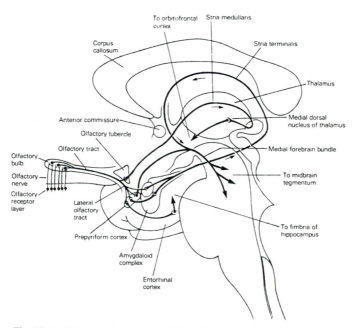

Fig. 22.2.   The neural pathways of the olfactory system. (From Kandel and Schwartz 1985.)

the glomeruli and then reach the neurons in the olfactory bulb. The bulb contains four types of cells: mitral cells, tufted cells, periglomerular cells, and granule cells. The afferent axons of the mitral and tufted cells are distributed to the olfactory cortex. There is also an extensive network of lateral innervations.

There are at least five areas of the olfactory cortex where olfactory information is relayed (Fig. 22.2): the anterior olfactory nucleus, the olfactory tubercle, the prepyriform cortex, the cortical nucleus of the amygdala, and the entorhinal area.

Whether the olfactory sensation is primarily discriminative (ie, the information can be used to tell differences between different olfactory sensations) or affective (ie, the olfactory sensation can produce a feeling or emotion) is thought to depend on the ultimate fate of the neural pathways. The neural pathways that are directly or indirectly connected with the medial dorsal nucleus of the thalamus and the olfactory neocortex are thought to be mainly responsible for the conscious perception of smell leading to discriminative sensations. Those relayed to the amygdala, the hippocampus, and the hypothalamus seem to account for the affective or emotional component of the olfactory sensations.

Coding of Olfactory Stimuli

Olfactory coding seems to rely on two basic processes: labeled lines and spatial coding. The codes used by a single fiber are a frequency code and labeling. The greater the magnitude of the olfactory stimulus, the more frequent is the rate of response. As shown in other receptor processes, olfactory fibers are capable of responding to one or more qualities. Thus, the fiber "labels" the relative magnitude to which it is sensitive. The olfactory centers of the cortex do not seem to have a one-to-one representation of the world as the visual system does. In the visual system, for example, different points of the visual field are coded in a specific area of the

brain cortex. This is called the *receptotopic* organization of the cerebral cortex. No such organization exists for olfaction. In the olfactory system, physical space seems to be used for the representation of different basic odors.

Experimental and Clinical Procedures for the Study of Smell

These can be characterized by the equipment used to deliver the olfactory stimulus and the procedures used to record the response. The delivery of olfactory stimuli under controlled conditions is one of the most difficult tasks in experimental psychophysiology. There are so many factors to consider that early attempts to create the perfect olfactometer have been abandoned.

The nature of the stimulus is important. The stimulus must act on the olfactory epithelium while having a minimal effect on the somatosensory functions served by branches of the trigeminal nerve. Odoriferous substances dissolved in alcohol, for example, are likely to stimulate sensory endings of the trigeminal nerve. People who have both of their olfactory nerves sectioned as a result of accidents can still "smell" some irritant substances because of the nasal cavity's somatosensory innervation. Other stimulus factors to be controlled are temperature, mode of delivery (ie, whether the person must actively inhale the substance or the substance is passively injected by means of a stream of air of known gaseous properties), and humidity.

An important subjective characteristic is the individual's state of *olfactory adaptation*. One can adapt to odors very quickly; therefore, under laboratory conditions it is sometimes necessary to increase the concentration of the stimulus several logarithmic units in order to elicit the same response. This is one of the primary reasons why olfaction cannot be trusted for the occupational monitoring of odoriferous chemical substances. (Another, even more important, reason is that many lethal chemical substances have no odor.)

Most of the current research on humans is conducted by using one of the following methods: (1) small sealed envelopes similar to those used to sample perfumes or scratch-and-smell kits and (2) small bottles containing the odoriferous substance embedded in cotton balls (the bottle sometimes has two narines—tubes that attach to the nostrils—from which the subject actively inhales.

There are many well-established procedures to record response. In laboratory animals (fish, rabbits, dogs) and in humans, it is possible to record an electrical response associated with the olfactory stimulation: the *electroolfactogram*. As a result of the work by Ottoson (1954) in Sweden, it has been possible to establish that the electroolfactogram is the record of the olfactory epithelium's generator potential. Because of the many technical difficulties in obtaining an electroolfactogram, plus the factors associated with the delivery of the stimulus, it is unlikely that this experimental and clinical electrophysiological procedure could be used for large-scale experimental studies of olfaction in the near future.

Toxic Agents That Modify Olfaction

There are at least three fundamental mechanisms by which toxic agents in the environment and the workplace may affect the sensation of olfaction.

Particle deposition can occur in the nasal cavity, trachea, and lungs. Metals such as cadmium, manganese, mercury, nickel, and zinc may produce olfactory alterations through this process. These metal layers deposited on the surface areas are invariably associated with a decrease or marked reduction of olfactory function. Wood dust may produce similar effects. Interestingly, zinc can also affect olfaction through a still poorly understood metabolic mechanism. Anomalies in zinc metabolism can produce smell and taste al-

terations that can be partially corrected by supplemental zinc ingestion.

There may be a **direct effect** on sensory receptors. Olfactory receptors are directly exposed to the external environment. Neurotoxic agents such as many industrial solvents actually dissolve these receptors through the solvents' lipophilic action. The rarely used term "olfactory toxicity" should be reserved only for neurotoxic agents that act in this manner. The scant literature available points to both changes in the quality of odors and elevation of the threshold for odor detection as being results of solvent exposure.

Some agents can have a **metabolic effect**. Garlic remains on the breath for many hours because it is quickly absorbed in the bloodstream and is exhaled through the lungs. There are neurotoxic agents that may act through this process, causing qualitative alterations in olfactory perception. Occupational exposure to selenium is reported to be associated with "garlic taste." Many of the metabolic conditions that affect taste (discussed above) also affect smell (Schiffman and Dackis 1975).

Smell Identification and Age

Doty and collaborators (1984) conducted an extensive cross-sectional study on the effect of age on odor identification. The sample consisted of 1955 presumably normal individuals employed at the University of Pennsylvania, residents at homes for the elderly, persons attending regional health fairs and other public events, university students, and youngsters enrolled at summer camps. Ages ranged from 5 to 99. The task, the University of Pennsylvania Smell Identification Test, consisted of four envelope-sized 10-odorant booklets with associated multiple-choice questions. The major findings were the following:

- Average ability to identify odors reaches a peak between 20 and 40 years of life, declining very drastically thereafter.

- A large proportion of the elderly are *anosmic* (unable to smell): 80% of those over the age of 80 exhibited major olfactory impairment, and nearly 50% were anosmic. These findings do not seem to be an expression of memory or other cognitive problems.
- Women of all ages outperform men in odor identification tasks.

The authors conclude that their findings explain why the elderly seem to complain about lack of food flavor and the disproportionate number of home accidents involving gas poisoning. A major flaw of this and similar studies conducted to examine the status of sensory function with age is that the study design is cross-sectional. Cross-sectional study designs tend to maximize age effects; there can be many other reasons apart from age why individuals at one point in time fail a sensory detection test. Prospective (follow-up) studies are more likely to show realistic aging trends but obviously are more difficult and costly to perform.

Representative Research

There are two distinctive lines of research: (1) odor pollution and control and (2) the influence of occupational exposure to neurotoxic agents on olfaction. These are intimately related. Odors, too, sometimes trigger mass psychogenic illnesses (see Chapter 34). There are totally innocuous water vapor fumes that can cause community concerns; however, there are also deadly neurotoxic agents such as carbon monoxide and nerve gas that are odorless and colorless.

William S. Cain and collaborators from the John B. Pierce Foundation Laboratories in New Haven, Connecticut, have performed numerous psychophysical studies on the chemical senses, particularly olfaction. Their early research work, concentrated primarily on psychophysical studies of odoriferous substances, has helped in our understanding of stimulus factors intervening in olfactory perception.

More recently, they have carried out important studies that almost overlap with the experimental questions social psychologists ask—eg, how perceived conditions of crowding affect judgments of odors in the environment. Their findings suggest that odor pollution is far from being solely a "nose" problem.

One intriguing piece of research (Cain et al. 1983) dealt with the requirement for ventilation of occupied spaces. This included estimates of ventilation requirements for tobacco smoke derived from subjective measures of acceptability and objective measures of contaminants. Psychophysical experiments on occupancy odor involved 47 different combinations of occupancy density, temperature, humidity, and ventilation rate. Experimenters collected judgments both from visitors, who smelled air from the chamber only once every few minutes, and from occupants, who remained in the chamber for an hour at a time. Visitors sampled the air from a sniffing box attached to the chamber.

The most significant factors affecting the judgment of visitors and occupants alike were a combination of temperature and humidity. There seemed to be no need for greater ventilation per person when there were, say, 12 persons in a chamber than under lower occupancy density (four or eight occupants). These results imply that there is little rationale for increased ventilation where odor is the principal offender.

CONCLUSIONS

Chemical senses are sometimes indicators of both acute and chronic neurotoxicity. In rare cases, taste and olfactory alterations have been demonstrated as signs of neurotoxic absorption. A good arsenal of techniques has now been accumulated allowing the assessment of taste and olfactory functions in a rapid manner, as is required for medical field surveys. However, because of practical considerations of time and resources—and the general perception that chemical senses rank low in the relative value we attach to our sense organs—chemical senses have not been extensively studied from a toxicological point of view. Most of the existing information comes from clinical observations and experimental studies under laboratory conditions; epidemiological studies are scant.

REFERENCES

Alderman, LC and Bergin, JJ (1986) Hydrogen selenide poisoning: An illustrative case with review of the literature. *Arch Environ Health* 41(6):354–358.

Amoore, JE (1974) Evidence for the chemical olfactory code in man. *Ann NY Acad Sci* 237:137–143.

Bartoshuk, LM, Gentile, RL, Moskowitz, HR, et al. (1974) Sweet taste induced by miracle fruit (*Synsepalum dulcificum*) *Physiol Behav* 12:449–456.

Bartoshuk, LM, Lee, C-H, and Scarpellino, R (1972) Sweet taste of water induced by artichoke (*Cynara scolymus*) *Science* 178:988–990.

Beidler, LM (ed) (1971) *Handbook of Sensory Physiology, Vol. IV: Chemical Senses Part 2: Taste.* New York: Springer-Verlag.

Bernard, RA and Halpern, BP (1968) Taste changes in vitamin A deficiency. *J Gen Physiol* 52:444–464.

Cain, WS (1974) Contributions of the trigeminal nerve to perceived odor magnitude. *Ann NY Acad Sci* 237:28–34.

Cain, WS (1978) History of research on smell. In *Handbook of Perception, Vol. 6A, Tasting and Smelling,* EC Carterette and P Friedman (eds) pp. 197–229. New York: Academic Press.

Cain, WS, Leaderer, BP, Isseroff, R, et al. (1983) Ventilation requirements in buildings: Control of occupancy odor and tobacco smoke. *Atmos Environ* 17:1183–1197.

Doty, RL, Shaman, P, and Dann, M (1984) Development of the University of Pennsylvania Smell Identification Test: A standardized microencapsulated test of olfactory function. *Physiol Behav* 32:489–502.

Finger, TE and Morita, Y (1985) Two gustatory systems: Facial and vagal nuclei have different brainstem connections. *Science* 227:776–778.

Kandel, ER and Schwartz, JH (1985) *Principles of Neural Science.* New York: Elsevier.

Ottoson, D (1954) Sustained potentials evoked by olfactory stimulation. *Acta Physiol Scand* 32:384–386.

Pfaff, DW (ed) (1985) *Taste, Olfaction, and the Central Nervous System: A Festschrift in Honor of Carl Pfaffman.* New York: Rockefeller University Press.

Schiffman, SS and Dackis, C (1975) Taste of nutrients: aminoacids, vitamins and fatty acids. *Percept and Psychoph* 17:140–146.

Taniewski, M (1975) The sense of taste in some occupational exposures. *Bull Inst Marit Trop Med (Gdynia)* 26:329–336.

SUGGESTED READINGS

Adams, RG and Crabtree, N (1961) Anosmia in alkaline battery workers. *Br J Ind Med* 18:216–221.

Ahlaström, R, Berglund, B, Berglund, U, et al. (1986) Impaired odor perception in tank cleaners. *Scand J Work Environ Health* 12(6):574–581.

Alarie, Y (1973) Sensory irritation by airborne chemicals. *Crit Rev Toxicol* 2(1):299–363.

Amoore, JE and Hautela, E (1983) Odor as an aid to chemical safety: Odor thresholds compared with threshold limit values and volatilities for 214 industrial chemicals in air and water dilution. *J Appl Toxicol* 3:272–290.

Amoore, JE and Ollman, BG (1983) Practical test kits for quantitatively evaluating the sense of smell. *Rhinology* 21:49–54.

Barrow, CS (1986) *Toxicology of the Nasal Passages, Chemical Industry Institute of Toxicology Series.* Washington, DC: Hemisphere.

Bartoshuk, LM (1975) Taste mixtures: Is mixture suppression related to compression? *Physiol Behav* 14:643–649.

Bartoshuk, LM (1978) The psychophysics of taste. *Am J Clin Nutr* 31(6):1068–1077.

Bate-Smith, EC (1968) Odor qualities: A glossary of usage. *Br J Psychol* 59:231–252.

Beetsm, MGJ (1978) *Structure–Activity Relationship in Human Chemoreception.* London: Applied Science Publishers.

Berglund, B (1974) Quantitative and qualitative analysis of industrial odors with human observers. *Ann NY Acad Sci* 237:35–51.

Berglund, LG and Dunn, JD (1981) *Ventilation Requirements for Control of Occupancy and Tobacco Smoke Odor: Laboratory Studies Final Report.* Berkeley: Lawrence Berkeley Laboratory, University of California, LBL-12589 UC-41.

Berglund, U, Berglund, B, Ekman, G et al. (1971) Individual psychophysical functions for 28 odorants. *Percept and Psychoph* 9:379–384.

Berglund, B, Berglund, U, and Lindvall, T (1976) Psychological processing of odor mixtures. *Psychol Rev* 83:432–441.

Berning, C, Griffith, J, and Wild, J (1982) Research on

the effectiveness of denatonium benzoate as a deterrent to liquid detergent ingestion by children. *Fund Appl Toxicol* 2:44.

Black, A, Evans, JC, Hadfield, EH, et al. (1974) Impairment of nasal mucociliary clearance in woodworkers in the furniture industry. *Br J Ind Med* 31:10–17.

Blackadder, ES and Manderson, WG (1975) Occupational absorption of tellurium: A report of two cases. *Br J Ind Med* 32:59–61.

Breipohl, W (ed) (1986) *Ontogeny of Olfaction: Principles of Olfactory Maturation in Vertebrates.* New York: Springer-Verlag.

Bridge, KC and Fentress, JC (1985) Trigeminal–taste interaction in palatability processing. *Science* 228:747–750.

Buchan, RT (1974) Garlic breath odor. *JAMA* 227:559–560.

Cain, WS (ed) (1974) Odors: Evaluation, utilization and control. *Ann NY Acad Sci* 237:1–439.

Cain, WS (1974) Scope and evaluation of odor counteraction and masking. *Ann NY Acad Sci* 237:427–439.

Cain, WS (1975) Odor intensity: Mixtures and masking. *Chem Sens Flavor* 1:339–352.

Cain, WS (1976) Olfaction and the common chemical sense: Some psychophysical contrasts. *Sens Process* 1:57–67.

Cain, WS (1977) Differential sensitivity for smell: "Noise" at the nose. *Science* 195:796–798.

Cain, WS (1979) To know with the nose: Keys to odor identification. *Science* 203:467–470.

Cain, WS (1982) Odor identification by males and females: Predictions vs performance. *Chem Senses* 7:129–142.

Cain, WS and Gent, J (1986) Use of odor identification in clinical testing of olfaction. In *Clinical Measurement of Taste and Smell,* HL Meiselman and RS Rivlin (eds) pp. 170–186. New York: Macmillan.

Cain, WS and Krause, RJ (1979) Olfactory testing: Rules for odor identification. *Neuro Res* 1:1–9.

Cain, WS, Gent, J, Catalonotto, FA, et al. (1983) Clinical evaluation of olfaction. *Am J Otolaryngol* 4:253–256.

Cain, WS, Goodspeed, RB, Gent, JF, et al. (1988) Evaluation of olfactory dysfunction in the Connecticut chemosensory clinical research center. *Laryngoscope* 98(1):1–5.

Cain, WS, Isseroff, R, Leaderer, BP, et al. (1980) Interaction between chemoreceptive modalities of odor and irritation. *Nature* 284:255–257.

Chapman, RF, Bernays, EA, and Stoffolano, JG (1987) *Perspectives in Chemoreception.* New York: Springer-Verlag.

Cowart, BJ (1981) Development of taste perception in humans: Sensitivity and preference throughout the lifespan. *Psychol Bull* 90:43–73.

Crocker, EC (1935) Seeking a working language for odors and flavors. *Ind Eng Chem* 25:1225.

Deane, M, and Sanders, G (1978) Annoyance and health reactions to odor from refineries and other industries in Carson, California. *Environ Res* 15:119–132.

Deane, M., Sanders, G, and Jonsson, E (1977) Trends and community annoyance reactions to odors from pulp mills in Eureka, California. *Environ Res* 14:232–244.

Desor, J, Maller, O, and Andrews, K (1975) Ingestive responses of human newborns to salty, sour, and bitter stimuli. *J Comp Physiol Psychol* 89:966.

Doty, RL (1979) A review of olfactory dysfunction in man. *Am J Otolaryngol* 1:57–79.

Doty, RL (1983) *The Smell Identification Test,*™ Philadelphia, Sensonics, Inc.

Doty, RL, Applebaum, SL, Zusho, H, et al. (1985) A cross-cultural study of sex differences in odor identification ability. *Neuropsychologia* 23:667–672.

Doty, RL, Gregor, T, and Monroe, C (1986) Quantitative assessment of olfactory function in an industrial setting. *J Occup Med* 28:457–460.

Doty, RL, Newhourse, MG, and Azzalina, JD (1985) Internal consistency and short-term test–retest reliability of the University of Pennsylvania Smell Identification Test. *Chem Senses* 10:297–300.

Doty, RL, Shaman, P, Appebaum, SL, et al. (1984) Smell identification ability: Changes with age. *Science* 226:1441–1443.

Doving, KB (1974) Odorant properties correlated with physiological data. *Ann NY Acad Sci* 237:184–192.

Emmet, EA (1976) Parosmia and hyposmia induced by solvent exposure. *Br J Ind Med* 33:196–198.

Engen, T (1972) The effect of expectation on judgment of odor. *Acta Psychol Austr* 36:450–458.

Finger, TE and Silver, W (eds) (1987) *Neurobiology of Taste and Smell.* New York: Wiley-Interscience.

Firestein, S and Werblin, F (1989) Odor-induced membrane currents in vertebrate olfactory receptor neurons. *Science* 244:79–82.

Flesh, RD (1974) Social and economic criteria for odor control effectiveness. *Ann NY Acad Sci* 237:320–327.

Gent, JF, Goodspeed, RB, Zagraniski, RT, et al. (1987) Taste and smell problems: Validation of questions for the clinical history. *Yale J Biol Med* 60:27–35.

Gilbert, AN and Wysocki, CJ (1987) The smell survey: Results. *Natl Geogr* Sept:514–525.

Glover, JR (1970) Selenium and its industrial toxicology. *Ind Med Surg* 39(1):50–54.

Goodspeed, RB, Gent, JF, and Catalonott, FA (1987) Chemosensory dysfunction: Clinical evaluation results from a taste and smell clinic. *Postgrad Med* 81:251–260.

Halpern, BP (1985) Environmental factors affecting chemoreceptors: An overview. In *Toxicology of the*

Eye, Ear and Other Special Senses, AW Hayes (ed) pp. 195–211. New York: Raven Press.

Hellman, TM (1974) Characterization of the odor properties of 101 petrochemicals using sensory methods. *J Air Pollut Control Assoc* 24:979–982.

Henkin, RI (1967) Abnormalities of olfaction and taste in various disease states. In *Chemical Senses and Nutrition,* MR Kare and O Maller (eds), pp. 95–113. Baltimore: The Johns Hopkins Press.

Henkin, RI (1984) Zinc in taste function: A critical review. *Biol Trace Elem Res* 6:263–280.

Henkin, RI (1987) Taste and smell disorders. In *Encyclopedia of Neuroscience,* Vol 2, G Adelman (ed) pp. 1185–1186. Boston: Birkhäuser.

Holness, DL, Tarashuk, IG, and Nethercott, JR (1989) Health status of copper refinery workers with specific reference to selenium exposure. *Arch Environ Health* 44(5):291–297.

Jones, DT and Reed, RR (1989) G_{olf}: An olfactory neurone specific G protein involved in odorant signal transduction. *Science* 244:790–795.

Judd, SC (1971) Ancient stench and present-day effluent. *Calif Med* 114:44–48.

Lancet, D (1986) Vertebrate olfactory system. *Annu Rev Neurosci* 9:329–355.

Lawless, HT, Hammer, LD, and Corina, MD (1982) Aversion to bitterness and accidental poisonings among preschool children. *J Toxicol* 19(9):951–964.

Leonardos, G, Kendall, D, and Barnard, N (1969) Odor threshold determinations of 53 odorant chemicals. *J Air Poll Control Assoc* 19:91–95.

Leonardos, G (1974) A critical review of regulations for the control of odors. *J Air Poll Control Assoc* 24:456–468.

Liddel, K (1976) Smell as a diagnostic marker. *Postgrad Med J* 52:136–138.

Liddel, K and White, J (1975) The smell of cancer. *Br J Dermatol* 92:215–217.

Lindvall, T (1970) *On Sensory Evaluation of Odorous Air Pollutant Intensities: Measurements of Odor Intensity in the Laboratory and in the Field with Special Reference to Effluents of Sulfate Pulp Factories.* Stockholm: Department of Environmental Hygiene, Karolinska Institutet, and the Department of Environmental Hygiene, National Institute of Public Health.

Lindvall, T (1974) Monitoring odorous air pollution in the field with human observers. *Ann NY Acad Sci* 237:247–260.

Lindvall, T and Stevenson, LT (1974) Equal unpleasantness matching of malodorous substances in the community. *J Appl Psychol* 59(3):264–269.

Lockman, DS (1981) Olfactory diagnosis. *Cutis* 27:645–647.

Marks, LE (1974) *Sensory Processes: The New Psychophysics.* New York: Academic Press.

Mateson, JF (1955) Olfactometry: Its techniques and apparatus. *J Air Poll Control Assoc* 5:167.

Mattes-Kuling, DA and Henkin, RI (1985) Energy and nutrient consumption of patients with dysgeusia. *J Am Diet Assoc* 85:822–826.

Mitchell, MJ and Gregson, RAM (1971) Between-subject variation and within-subject consistency of olfactory intensity scaling. *J Exp Psychol* 89:314–318.

Moskowitz, HR (1977) Profiling of odor compounds and their mixtures. *Sensory Processes* 1:212–226.

Moulton, DG (1976) Spatial patterning of response to odors in the peripheral olfactory system. *Physiol Rev* 56:578–593.

Nader, JS (1958) An odor evaluation apparatus for field and laboratory use. *Am Ind Hyg Assoc J* 19:1–7.

Naus, A (1975) *Olphactoric Properties of Industrial Matters.* Prague: Charles University.

Opdyne, DL (1973) Monographs on fragrance of raw materials. *Food Cosmet Toxicol* 11:855–876.

Pihl, RO, Shea, D and Costa, L (1978) Odor and marijuana intoxication. *J Clin Psychol* 34:775–779.

Pinching, AJ (1977) Clinical testing of olfaction reassessed. *Brain* 100:377–388.

Rabin, MD and Cain, WS (1979) Determinants of measured olfactory sensitivity. *Percept Psychophys* 39:281–286.

Riddle, L (1988) Uproar over odor persists despite plans to close fish plant. *New York Times,* May 15.

Rothe, M (1988) *Introduction to Aroma Research* [translated from the German edition]. Norwell, MA: Kluwer.

Ryan, CM, Morrow, LA, and Hodgson, M (1988) Cacosmia and neurobehavioral dysfunction associated with occupational exposure to mixtures of organic solvents. *Am J Psychiatry* 145(11):1442–1445.

Sandmark, B, Broms, I, Löfgren, L, et al. (1989) Olfactory function in painters exposed to organic solvents. *Scand J Work Environ Health* 15(1):60–63.

Schemper, T, et al. (1981) Odor identification in young and elderly persons: Sensory and cognitive limitations. *J Gerontol* 36:446–452.

Schechter, PJ and Henkin, RI (1974) Abnormalities of taste and smell following head trauma. *J Neurol Neurosurg Psychiatry* 37:802–810.

Schiffman, SS (1974) Contributions to the physicochemical dimensions of odor: A psychophysical approach. *Ann NY Acad Sci* 237:164–183.

Schiffman, SS, et al. (1976) Thresholds of food odors in the elderly. *Exp Aging Res* 2:389–398.

Schwartz, BS, Doty, L, Monroe, C, et al. (1989) Olfactory function in chemical workers exposed to acrylate and methacrylate vapors. *Am J Pub Health* 79(5):613–618.

Sherman, AH, Amoore, JE, and Weigel, V (1979) The pyridine scale for clinical measurement of olfactory threshold: A quantitative reevaluation. *Otolaryngol Head Neck Surg* 87:717–733.

Stevens, SS (1969) Sensory scales of taste intensity. *Percept Psychophys* 6:302–308.

Tapia, C (1978) Environment and odours. *Int Rev Appl Psychol* 27(1):39–51.

Temple, AR and Stremming, K (1975) Taste as a deterrent in pediatric poisoning. *Clin Toxicol* 8(5):541–546.

Theimer, ET (ed) (1982) *Fragrance Chemistry: The Science of Sense and Smell*. New York: Academic Press.

Turk, A, Johnston, JW, and Moulton, DG (eds) (1974) *Human Responses to Environmental Odors*. New York: Academic Press.

Venstrom, D and Amoore, JE (1968) Olfactory threshold in relation to age, sex, or smoking. *J Food Sci* 33:264–265.

Vickers, ZM, Nielsen, S, and Theologides, A (1981) Odor aversion in cancer patients. *Minn Med* 64:277–279.

Westerman, ST (1981) An objective approach to subjective testing for sensation of taste and smell. *Laryingoscope* 91:301–303.

Wohlers, HC (1963) Odor intensity and odor travel from industrial sources. *Int J Air Water Poll* 7:71–78.

Wood, RW (1978) Stimulus properties of inhaled substances. *Environ Health Perspect* 26:69–76.

Wright, RH (1982) *The Sense of Smell*. Boca Raton, FL: CRC Press.

23

Somatic Sensory Systems

The *somatic sensory*—or *somatosensory*—*system* is a group of sensory submodalities that convey and interpret sensory information originating in the skin and muscles. There are numerous neurotoxic agents and drugs that can affect the somatic sensory system. These include agents such as metals and metallic compounds (eg, lead, mercury, arsenic), solvents (eg, trichloroethylene, styrene, methyl *n*-butyl ketone, carbon disulfide), alcohol, "sniffers" such as toluene, and household products such as acetone. How (and, whenever possible, why) the somatic sensory system is particularly vulnerable to these neurotoxic agents is reviewed in this chapter. These neurotoxin-induced conditions must be distinguished from hereditary, metabolic, traumatic, and viral or other causes that may produce similar effects on the peripheral nervous system.

SOMATIC SENSIBILITY

Four types of somatic sensations are recognized: pain, temperature, discriminative touch, and proprioception.

Proprioception is the sense of balance, position, and movement of the limbs. Limb position sense is the sense of the stationary positions of the limbs. *Kinesthesia* is the sense of limb movement. The sense of balance is largely mediated by the specialized receptors of the vestibular apparatus—the otolithic organs and the semicircular canals (described in Chapter 24).

The Skin Senses

The skin is not at all a homogeneous structure. Structurally and functionally, the skin varies very much from region to region, and these variations profoundly affect our cutaneous perceptions. For example, the two-point discrimination threshold, which measures the minimal distance we can detect between two sharp points applied to the skin, is about 2 mm for the fingertips, about 2 cm for the arms, and even larger for the back. The two-point discrimination threshold varies in proportion to the population of cutaneous receptors present in the skin. The skin is an accessory structure for cutaneous perception. Its thickness, natural temperature and humidity, whether hairs are present, and calluses developed as a result of occupational mechanical friction, all are factors to be taken into consideration for the evaluation of skin sensitivity.

The skin accomplishes many sensory functions—thus the term "cutaneous sensation." Touch, temperature, pressure, vibration sensations, and superficial pain are carried out by sensory processes located in the skin.

In the 19th century, it was thought that the four sensory qualities were associated with specific receptors. In support of this view, a complex taxonomy of skin receptors was described in histology textbooks. Presently, however, a much simpler classification of sensory receptors prevails: free neural endings and encapsulated organs. The receptors for pain and temperature are simply free neural endings, with unmyelinated afferent fibers of slow conduction velocity. The receptors for touch and proprioception are contained in encapsulated organs. The hand's glabrous skin contains four different types of encapsulated organs: the Pacinian corpuscle, the Meissner corpuscle, the Ruffini corpuscle, and the Merkel receptor. Joint receptors and muscle spindles, which are responsible for limb position sense and kinesthesia, are also encapsulated receptors. The base of the hair also houses an encapsulated receptor.

The Stimuli for Skin Senses

Controlled stimuli for the study of skin senses can be created under laboratory conditions. In the middle of the 19th century, hairs of horses' tails were used to study touch and pressure. Wooden compasses were utilized to study two-point discrimination thresholds. More sophisticated equipment was developed when psychophysics experienced a renaissance in the 1940s and 1950s. For example, Hardy et al. (1940) developed an infrared stimulator for the study of the sensation of pain. Stevens and Mack (1959) used rods of known contacting area and weight to study sensations of passive force. Vibration sensations, which—as will be seen later—are

conducted by well-defined receptors and neural pathways, are studied by means of vibrators originally created to calibrate accelerometers (devices for the measure of mechanical vibration such as those produced by air flow in the wings of airplanes).

Nociceptors are the receptors for pain. The stimulus for pain is tissue destruction, chemical irritation, or heat. On the basis of extensive clinical, electrophysiological, and psychophysical research three types of nociceptors have been identified. *Mechanical nociceptors* are activated by strong mechanical stimulators or by sharp objects. During the course of a clinical examination, a pinprick may be sufficient to assess the functional status of pain sensations. *Heat nociceptors* respond when the skin temperature is raised above 45°C, the heat pain threshold for humans. Psychophysical experiments for the determination of input–output relationships in heat nociception have been carried out by means of heat generated by infrared sources. *Polymodal nociceptors* respond equally well to mechanical, heat, or chemical stimulation. Chemical stimulation is sometimes accomplished by the use of cantharidine, an irritant substance secreted by certain insects. This substance produces blisters, which are removed in order to apply chemical substances (the nociceptive stimulus) to the exposed area. Stringent institutional ethical codes have now restricted this type of research in humans as well as in animals.

The stimulus for temperature sensation is radiant heat. As in the case of pain, simple tests in clinical use can easily be made available (eg, ice cubes, a mildly warmed iron). However, because of the presence of homeostatic mechanisms—processes by which the organism maintains a state of physiological equilibrium, such as normal levels of temperature, water, salt, etc, in the face of changes in the external environment—the study of temperature sensations under laboratory conditions is difficult. Sweating is one aspect of these homeostatic mechanisms. In addition, regional variation in the physical properties of the skin contributes to the difficulty of studying temperature sensations.

There are specialized receptors for hot and cold. Joseph Arezzo, of the Albert Einstein College of Medicine in New York City, has developed an ingenious device for the study of hand and foot temperature sensations using cryogenic plates. A cryogenic plate—commonly used in the laboratory to cool biological specimens rapidly for study under the microscope—is a metal plate the temperature of which can be markedly reduced by passing an electric current through it. This technique has been applied for the study of the effect of neurotoxic agents on neural pathways conveying temperature sensations.

The stimulus for discriminative touch is mechanical stimulation of the skin. A great deal of research on somatic sensations has been carried out with vibratory stimuli because this type of stimulation is easy to define quantitatively. Many of the basic concepts used in the definition of acoustic stimuli have also been applied for the characterization of vibratory stimuli.

The stimuli for vibration threshold studies are described in terms of three interrelated measures of the stimulus: displacement, velocity, and acceleration. Displacement is the wave amplitude (ie, the distance between the peaks and valleys of the vibration wave). Although the skin receptors can detect displacement of a few micrometers, this unit is not used because displacement per se is not an adequate stimulus. Single skin receptors such as Pacinian corpuscles are sensitive to the acceleration of the vibrating stimulus.

The stimulus for proprioception is the mechanical stretch of muscle spindles and joint receptors (described in Chapter 27).

Stimulus Transduction and Neural Coding

The details of how the stimuli for the various receptors of the somatic sensory system produce a depolarization that ultimately triggers the action potential are poorly understood in most individual somatic sensory receptors

except for the Pacinian corpuscle. The onion-shaped capsule that is characteristic of this receptor seems to be essential for the stimulus transduction of touch and vibration.

Each somatic sensory receptor is linked to a neural fiber that transmits only one specific type of sensory information. For example, the neural fibers linked to a touch receptor result in the sensation of touch; those linked to pain receptors result in pain sensations. The fact that each receptor line transmits only one kind of sensation is known as *Müller's law of specific energy*. Modern neurophysiologists think of these receptors and their fibers as "committed" lines ("committed" to touch; "committed" to pain) or "labeled" lines ("labeled" for touch; "labeled" for pain).

The neural codes that the somatic sensory receptors use are similar to other sensory systems: the frequency code and the population code. The intensity of the stimulus is coded by a *frequency code:* the neural fiber attached to the individual receptors fires more quickly in proportion to the intensity of the stimulus. It has been shown in humans (Vallbo et al. 1979) that the activity of the individual neural fibers parallels that of the subjective impression of touch and exhibits similar thresholds for sensation. In addition, the input–output relationship at both neural and subjective levels is a power function (see Chapter 25). The intensity of the stimulus is also encoded in a *population code*. As the stimulus increases in intensity, more and more receptors are recruited to convey the information.

Receptor adaptation is also a form of coding, called "feature extraction." The sensation of touch rapidly adapts. For example, we do not feel the constant contact of our clothing on our skin. The sensation of pain, however, does not adapt: we feel pain as long as the nociceptive stimulus lasts. These characteristics of different sensations are explained by the speed of adaptation of single receptors.

Those interested in a more detailed description of the functioning of the somatic sensory system at the receptor level may refer to Martin (1985).

Neural Pathways

The chain of central neurons carries sub-modality-specific somatic sensory information for the arms, legs, and trunk. The projections from the face are mediated by the trigeminal nerve, described below.

Somatic sensory information for pain, temperature, discriminative touch, and proprioception is mediated via peripheral nerves. Some of the nerves used in the evaluation of neurotoxic effects in humans include the ulnar, the peroneal, the median, and the sural nerves. The evaluation of the conduction velocity of the peripheral nerves is a measure of the status of their functioning. (The details of how this is accomplished are described in Chapter 5.)

As the peripheral nerves enter the spinal cord, they become organized into easily recognizable and fairly symmetrical anatomic structures called the spinal nerves. As shown in Chapter 1, four regions of the spinal cord where spinal nerves enter or exit are identified: cervical, thoracic, lumbar, and sacral. A *dermatome* is the area of the skin innervated by a single spinal nerve. An expert clinical neurologist knows which nerves innervate specific regions of the skin. This knowledge has clinical value for localizing neural lesions.

Figure 23.1 contains a schematic representation of a cross section of the spinal cord. Even with the naked eye it is possible to recognize a butterfly-shaped, relatively darker area in the center of the spinal cord, called the gray matter, surrounded by white matter. The gray matter contains the nerve cell bodies and unmyelinated fibers. The white matter is formed entirely of myelinated fibers.

The appearance of the cross section of the spinal cord varies from level to level. At the lumbar level of the spinal cord, only the fibers from the lower limbs are present. As a result, the spinal cord, and the white matter (the fibers) in particular, are smaller than in other sections of the spinal cord. As higher and higher levels are examined—for example, the thoracic—the white matter becomes much larger compared to the gray matter. At higher levels, the myelinated fibers of the upper limbs are added outside the existing fibers from the lower limbs, like the rings of a tree. We can think of the spinal cord as a core of neural bodies and unmyelinated fibers to which layers of fibers are added as we go toward the brain.

Experienced investigators and clinical neurologists can recognize several zones in the gray and white matter that are only a few square millimeters in size. In numerous clinical observations and animal experiments carried out over the past two centuries, it has been firmly established that lesions of specific areas of the spinal cord are related to motor, autonomic, and sensory loss.

Bell (1774–1842) and Magendie (1783–1855) discovered that the anterior portion of the spinal cord mediates predominantly motor function, whereas the posterior portion of the spinal cord mediates somatic sensory functions. In old textbooks, this predictable relationship between structure localization and function was referred to as the Bell–Magendie law (Boring 1950). Lateral portions of the spinal cord contain autonomic preganglionic neurons.

The two major ascending systems that convey somatic sensory information are the dorsal column (touch and proprioception) and the anterolateral column (pain and temperature). Selected lesions on each of these columns (or both) are accompanied by fairly localized loss of sensory information in the body.

The basic neural circuitry of the somatic sensory system is formed by a circuit of three neurons. The sensory fibers have their cell bodies in the dorsal root ganglion located outside the vertebral column. Thus, the ganglion cells are the first-order neurons of the somatic sensory system. These cells cross to the opposite side of the brainstem at the level of the medulla and meet their second-order neurons in the gracile and cuneatus nuclei, where the second-order neurons are located. The fibers originating in these two nuclei end in the thalamus. The thalamic nucleus that relays somatic sensory information is pri-

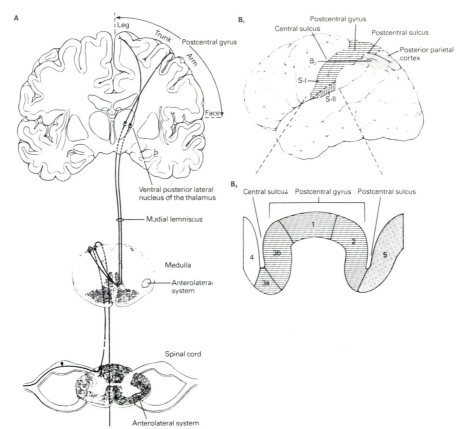

Fig. 23.1. Cortical representation of the somatosensory system. (From Kandel 1985.)

marily the ventral posterior lateral nucleus. The primary somatic sensory areas of the cortex are shown in Figure 23.1. These cortical areas receive the inputs from the major ascending somatic sensory systems.

There are numerous lesion, stimulation, and recording studies showing how touch is represented in the somatic sensory cortex. One important feature derived from animal experimentation—particularly in the monkey—is that the cerebral cortex contains a topographic representation of somatic sensory function, particularly touch. In an experimental animal in which recording electrodes have been implanted in the somatic sensory area, touching specific areas of the body surface is followed by a sensory evoked potential in a specific area of the cortex.

Pain and temperature sensations have a cortical representation also, but this representation is not as sharp as that for touch. In addition, about two decades ago, it was discovered that the brain contains a neural system to suppress pain. This is accomplished by a pharmacological process in which peptides of the opioid families are involved.

Three branches of the trigeminal nerve—the ophthalmic, the maxillary, and the mandibular—mediate somatic sensory information of the face. These converge in the semilunar ganglion from which they are distributed to numerous other relay sensory, motor, and autonomic nuclei of the medulla, pons, and midbrain. Most of the somatic sensory information from the head is conveyed by fibers that, after crossing to the opposite side of the brainstem, end up in the ventral posterior nucleus of the thalamus. A small contingent of neural fibers reach the thalamus by means of an ipsilateral projection. In the cerebral cortex, there is a well-defined area where sensations of the face are represented.

SENSORY MANIFESTATIONS OF PERIPHERAL NEUROPATHIES

A *peripheral neuropathy* is a disease involving the peripheral nervous system (described in Chapter 1). There are many conditions—genetic, vascular, traumatic, metabolic, etc—that affect somatosensory functions. The most frequent in occupational settings are carpal tunnel syndrome and peripheral neuropathies associated with diabetes and chronic alcoholism.

Carpal tunnel syndrome is the most commonly reported nerve entrapment syndrome (Taylor and Wasserman 1988). It presents as tingling sensations and pain in the thumb, index, middle finger, and portion of the ring finger. In chronic conditions, it may result in muscle weakness and wasting. It results from the compression of the median nerve—a mixed nerve containing motor as well as sensory fibers—as it passes through the wrist.

REPRESENTATIVE RESEARCH

Peripheral Neuropathy Induced by Methyl *n*-Butyl Ketone

Some neuropathological studies conducted by Peter S. Spencer and H. H. Schaumburg and their collaborators at Albert Einstein College of Medicine in New York City have aimed at establishing how and where in the nervous system certain neurotoxic agents, such as industrial solvents, produce their deleterious effects. Some of these studies have been precipitated by outbreaks of neurotoxic illness at the workplace.

In the summer of 1973, 79 workers engaged in the printing of polyvinyl fabrics at a plant in Columbus, Ohio developed clinical symptoms of peripheral neuropathy. Neurological examination revealed a mixed sensorimotor neuropathy with a distal symmetrical distribution.

The most severely affected individuals were those employed in printing rooms, where they applied colored inks dissolved in volatile solvent mixtures to surfaces of polyvinyl fabrics. For years, the solvent mixtures in use consisted of 90% methyl ethyl ketone (MEK) and 10% methyl isobutyl ketone (MIBK). Methyl *n*-butyl ketone (MBK) was suspected to be the harmful agent because MBK had been introduced into the printing process less than a year prior to the neurotoxic outbreak. The workers were exposed via inhalation and dermal absorption.

Spencer and Schaumburg (1976) performed a clinical and neuropathological study in cats chronically exposed to MBK and MIBK inhalation to determine the relative neurotoxicity of these two agents. Fifteen young adult cats were exposed for up to 4 months to MBK or to MIBK, and three were normal controls. Pronounced symmetrical foot drop and proximal limb and forelimb weakness developed between the third and fourth months of exposure to MBK. Neuropathological studies revealed massive local axonal enlargements containing abnormally large numbers of neurofilaments and dying-back axonal degeneration. ("Dying back" is a neuropathological process in which the more distal structures of the peripheral nervous system are destroyed first.) Cats exposed to MIBK showed minimal distal axonal change but remained neurologically intact. This study firmly established MBK as a powerful neurotoxic agent.

Lead Exposure and Nerve Conduction Velocity: The Differential Time Course of Sensory and Motor Nerve Effects

Automobile assembly plant workers are exposed to lead during finishing of automobile body panels. Solder, which contains lead, is applied to gaps and then smoothed by grinding to produce an even surface. This manufacturing process is common in automobile assembly plants around the world. Singer et al. (1983) measured the nerve conduction velocity (NCV) of the median motor, median sensory, peroneal motor, and sural nerves in 40 lead-exposed automobile production workers as part of a comprehensive health survey carried out in an automobile assembly plant in New Jersey. Blood lead (Pb-B) and blood zinc protoporphyrin (ZPP) were also measured. The control group consisted of workers without lead exposure. All subjects were screened for the possible presence of confounding medical conditions such as limb, neck, or back injury, diabetes, neurological diseases, and excessive alcohol consumption.

The investigators found that NCVs were slowed in the lead-exposed group for two sensory nerves: the median sensory and the sural nerves. A subsample of workers exposed for less than 10 years showed slowing of the median sensory and the sural nerves; Pb-B and ZPP levels correlated inversely with NCVs of the sural nerve. In a subsample of workers exposed for more than 10 years, slowing of the median motor as well as the median sensory and sural nerves was observed; ZPP levels were inversely correlated with median and peroneal motor nerve velocity. A time course of effects was noted in which slowing of sensory NCV was seen to occur earlier than motor NCV slowing.

Historically, particular attention has been given to the motor manifestation of lead-induced neurological illness, as motor effects are more obvious to the observer. As environmental and occupational levels of lead have been effectively reduced over recent decades, however, the extreme picture of lead poisoning characterized by motor paralysis is now rarely seen. As subclinical effects of lead began to be investigated, it was seen that the motor nerves were likely candidates to exhibit early subclinical toxic changes. Consistent with this view, electrophysiological studies of lead neurotoxicity

had shown that motor NCV changes preceded the onset of neurological findings; NCV changes may be present without neurological signs of illness. However, investigators around the world arrived at this conclusion before taking a close look at the sensory nerves.

The determination of sensory NCV has often been plagued with technical difficulties that prevented such measurements during medical health surveys and even in the clinic. The demonstration that sensory peripheral nerves may be involved even earlier than motor nerves after lead absorption gave impetus to the search for alternative techniques for the monitoring of lead-induced health effects. Current developments of psychophysical procedures for that specific purpose are reviewed below.

Psychophysical Procedures for the Determination of Neurotoxin-Induced Peripheral Nerve Changes. In 1980 Arezzo and Schaumburg described a technique to assess vibratory thresholds using the Optacon™, a device composed of vibrating rods which is used to help blind people read Braille. The vibrating pattern consisted of an array of 144 rods vibrating at 230 Hz. The amplitude of the vibration could be varied by means of a digital voltmeter. [The equipment and the procedure for testing have been extensively modified since the original publication (see Fig. 23.2). The basic psychophysical procedure—forced choice—has also been changed in favor of the traditional methods of limits, which is more likely to be understood by the subject.]

It is only recently that investigators in the field of environmental and occupational neurotoxicology have begun testing vibratory sensations along the lines of what is known in psychophysics. Before, there were many reports that described the stimulus being measured in terms of the voltage applied, when in fact the stimulus for the sensation of vibration is thought to be either displacement,

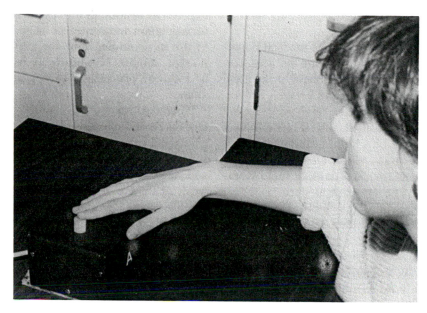

Fig. 23.2. Psychophysical determination of vibratory thresholds. (Courtesy of Dr. Richard Letz, Division of Environmental and Occupational Medicine, Mount Sinai Medical School, New York City; reproduced by permission.)

velocity, or acceleration of the vibratory stimulus. Also, by using a single frequency—230 Hz in the original description of the equipment—it was impossible to detect changes that might have occurred in the higher-frequency range. Finally, in none of the reports was the control of temperature—an important confounding variable—mentioned.

Maurissen and Weiss (1980) described a procedure for testing vibratory thresholds in monkeys and humans. Two features of this report are noteworthy: vibration sensations were assessed within a wide range of frequencies (the skin has a range extending between 25 and 500 Hz), and an attempt was made to control pressure. Vibration sensitivity was measured at 10 frequencies ranging from 25 to 400 Hz. The vibrator, fixed to precision equipment that allows control of the pressure applied to the skin, causes indenting of the skin by 0.5 mm. At the time of this writing, this system has not been used for the study of the effects of neurotoxic agents on somatic sensations in humans.

ISSUES

Confounding Factors

Environmental and occupational neurotoxicologists have concentrated on the study of both toxin-induced changes in somatosensory perception in humans and its morphological and neurochemical mechanism in animal models. This is primarily because in the past 20 years numerous chemical compounds such as solvents have surfaced as occupational health problems with the peripheral nervous system as a target. A classification of neurotoxic agents proposed by Spencer and Schaumburg (1980), for example, is based on extensive research on toxin-induced neuropathies. Thus, there are numerous studies on discriminative touch and temperature among people affected by neurotoxic agents.

However, somatic sensations can be affected by a large variety of medical conditions, physical agents, and chemical intoxications. The ones named below only serve as illustrations.

Most common among the medical conditions of blue-collar workers are diabetes, carpal tunnel syndrome (numbness of the hand caused by pinching of hand nerves), and excessive use of alcohol.

The frequent use of vibrating tools may induce a condition similar to Raynaud's syndrome, known as vibration syndrome. Although pneumatic tools causing rapid vibration were in general use as early as 1883, vibration syndrome was reported for the first time in 1911 (McCallum 1971). The vibration syndrome consists of stiffness or numbness of hands, loss of muscle control, inability to hold, grab, or manipulate objects, finger swelling, reduced sensibility, paresthesia (tingling sensations in the hand), cyanosis, and a characteristic blanching of fingers when exposed to cold. Pyykkö and collaborators (1982) pointed out that mechanical vibration might be the common etiology of hand–arm somatic sensation alterations and hearing loss among Finnish lumberjacks.

Tight boots might affect somatic sensations in the feet.

Excessive cigarette smoking can affect hand blood flow and indirectly affect somatic sensations.

Mild injury by heat can induce hyperalgesia (painful reaction to the slightest touch).

The clinical and epidemiological conclusion that somatic sensory changes are caused by industrial toxic agents can therefore be made only after these possible causes of peripheral neuropathy have first been ruled out.

The Narrow View of the Somatic Sensory Systems

One of the major problems inhibiting the study of the effects of neurotoxic agents on somatosensory mechanisms is the narrow view that somatic sensations should be considered in terms of neurophysiology only. This shortcoming makes it very difficult to translate experimental findings into useful information for regulation and control of neurotoxic agents in the environment and the workplace. At present, somatic sensations are seen in terms of receptor processes and neural pathways alone.

However, somatic sensations are important for communication, affection, feeling, and emotional behavior. In perception of musical sound and communication, for example, skin and deep tendon receptors complement the work of the ear in the reception of low-frequency tones. These sensations are also involved in feelings and affection, such as kissing, hugging, and erotic play.

Sharing of Knowledge Necessary

A body of knowledge was accumulated in clinical neurology during the time when the concept of "minimal brain damage" was very much in vogue. The concept of "minimal brain damage" was subsequently rejected after it was found that the term was used as a catchall label to designate neuropsychological dysfunction of, sometimes, multiple etiology. The variety of techniques that were developed for exploring evidence of minimal or subclinical brain damage was also (unjustifiably) rejected. Some techniques for the examination of the somatic sensory system in individuals suspected to be neurologically impaired might aptly be incorporated into the arsenal of techniques now available in human neurotoxicology.

Let's consider, for example, a test of intrasensory loading such as "double simultaneous stimulation." The examiner taps the patient with the index and middle fingers simultaneously in two different regions of the body—say, the left side of the face and the upper part of the lower limbs. A child and an elderly individual are likely to report the face as being tapped. (The stimulation of the face inhibits the perception of the upper limb.) Young individuals affected by organic mental syndrome exhibit similar effects. It would be important to know if young people affected by neurotoxic agents show similar effects. The double simultaneous stimulation test is now rarely described except by the first and second generations of Dr. Morris Bender's students.

In conclusion, a much greater collaboration is needed between neurotoxicologists, clinical neurologists, and neuropsychologists for a fresh look at designing effective procedures for monitoring possible early effects of neurotoxic agents. It is very likely that as a result of this integration, special tests for the exclusive evaluation of neurotoxin-induced peripheral nervous system dysfunction might be developed in the future. These tests must be firmly rooted in the existing knowledge of the neurosciences, psychophysics, and clinical neuropsychology.

REFERENCES

Arezzo, JC and Schaumburg, HH (1980) The use of the Optacon™ as a screening device: A new technique for detecting sensory loss in individuals exposed to neurotoxins. *J Occup Med* 22:461–464.

Boring, EG (1950) *A History of Experimental Psychology.* New York: Appleton-Century-Crofts.

Hardy, JD, Wolff, HG, and Goodell, H (1940) Studies on pain: A new method for measuring pain thresholds observations on spatial summation of pain. *J Clin Invest* 19:649–657.

Kandel, ER (1985) Central representation of touch. In *Principles of Neural Science,* 2nd ed, ER Kandel and JH Schwartz (eds) pp. 316–330. New York: Elsevier.

Martin, JH (1985) Anatomical substrates for somatic sensation. In *Principles of Neural Science,* 2nd ed, ER Kandel and JH Schwartz (eds) pp. 301–315. New York: Elsevier.

Maurissen, JPJ and Weiss, B (1980) Vibration sensitivity as an index of somatosensory function. In *Experimental and Clinical Neurotoxicology,* PS Spencer and HH Schaumburg (eds) pp. 767–774. Baltimore: Williams and Wilkins.

McCallum, RI (1971) Vibration syndrome. *Br J Ind Med* 28:90–99.

Pyykkö, I, Hyvärinen, H, and Färkkilä, M (1982) Studies in the etiological mechanisms of the vasopressive component of the vibration syndrome. In *Vibration Effects on the Hand and Arm in Industry,* AJ Bram-

mer and W Taylor (eds) pp. 31–25. New York: John Wiley & Sons.

Singer, RM, Valciukas, JA, and Lilis, R (1983) Lead exposure and nerve conduction velocity: The differential time course of sensory and motor nerve effects. *Neurotoxicology* 4:183–202.

Spencer, PS and Schaumburg, HH (1976) Feline nervous system response to chronic intoxication with commercial grades of methyl *n*-butyl ketone, methyl isobutyl ketone, and methyl ethyl ketone. *Toxicol App Pharm* 37:301–311.

Spencer, PS and Schaumburg, HH (1980) Classification of neurotoxic disease: A morphological approach. In *Experimental and Clinical Neurotoxicology,* PS Spencer and HH Schaumburg (eds) pp. 92–99. Baltimore: Williams & Wilkins.

Stevens, JC and Mack, JD (1959) Scales of apparent force. *J Exp Psychol* 58:405–413.

Taylor, W and Wasserman, DE (1988) Occupational vibration. In *Occupational Medicine: Principles and Practical Applications,* Zenz (ed) pp. 324–333. Chicago: Year Book Medical Publications.

Vallbo, ÅB, Harbarth, KE, Torebjord, HE, et al. (1979) Somatosensory, proprioceptive, and sympathetic activity in human peripheral nerves. *Physiol Rev* 59:919–957.

SUGGESTED READINGS

Agate, NJ (1949) An outbreak of cases of Raynaud's phenomenon of occupational origin. *Br J Ind Med* 4:144–163.

Araki, S, Murata, K, and Aono, H (1986) Subclinical cervico-spino-bulbar effects of lead: A study of short-latency somatosensory evoked potentials in workers exposed to lead, zinc, and copper. *Am J Ind Med* 10:163–175.

Araki, S, Murata, K, and Aono, H (1987) Central and peripheral nervous system dysfunction in workers exposed to lead, zinc and copper: A follow-up study of visual and somatosensory evoked potential. *Int Arch Occup Environ Health* 59:177–187.

Arezzo, JC, Schaumburg, HH, and Spencer, PS (1982) Structure and function of the somatosensory system: A neurotoxicological perspective. *Environ Health Perspect* 44:23–30.

Arezzo, JC, Schaumburg, HH, and Peterson, CA (1983) Rapid screening for peripheral neuropathy: A field study with the Optacon™. *Neurology (NY)* 83:626–629.

Bender, MB (1952) *Disorders in Perception.* Springfield, IL: Charles C Thomas.

Carlson, WS, Samueloff, S, Taylor, W, et al. (1979) Instrumentation for measurement for sensory loss in the fingertips. *J Occup Med* 21:260–264.

Fullerton, GS and Cattel, JMcK (1892) *On the Perception of Small Differences*. Philadelphia: University Press.

Halonen, P, Halonen, J-P, Lang, HA, et al. (1986) Vibratory perception thresholds in shipyard workers exposed to solvents. *Acta Neurol Scand* 73(6):561–565.

Hardy, JD and Oppel, TW (1938) Studies in temperature sensation: IV. The stimulation of cold by radiation. *J Clin Invest* 17:771–778.

Hardy, JD, Stolwijk, JA, and Hoffman, D (1968) Pain following step increase in skin temperature. In *The Skin Senses*, DR Kenshalo (ed) pp. 444–457. Springfield, IL: Charles C Thomas.

Heinonen, E, Färkkilä, M, Forsström, J et al. (1987) Autonomic neuropathy and vibration exposure in forestry workers. *Br J Ind Med* 44:412–416.

Hellstrom, B and Myhre, K (1971) A comparison of some methods of diagnosing Raynaud phenomena of occupational origin. *Br J Ind Med* 28:272–279.

Hirata, M, Miyajima, K, Kosaka, H, et al. (1980) Somatosensory evoked response of lead-exposed workers. In *Proceedings of the Osaka Prefectural Institute of Public Health, Osaka, Japan*, pp. 23–28 [in Japanese].

Hirosawa, I (1983) Original construction of thermoesthesiometer and its application to vibration disease. *Int Arch Occup Environ Health* 52:209–214.

Hirosawa, I, Watanabe, S, Fukuchi, Y, et al. (1983) Availability of temperature sense indices for diagnosis of vibration disease. *Int Arch Occup Environ Health* 52:215–222.

Hubbard, JI (1974) *The Peripheral Nervous System*. New York: Plenum Press.

Iggo, A and Andres, KH (1982) Morphology of cutaneous receptors. *Annu Rev Neurosci* 5:1–31.

Jewett, DL, Heard, GS, and Chimento, TC (1985) Peripheral neurotoxicity testing by pairs of stimuli. *Neurobehav Toxicol Teratol* 7(4):525–528.

Jones, SJ (1982) Somatosensory evoked potentials: The normal waveform. In *Evoked Potentials in Clinical Testing*, AM Halliday (ed) pp. 393–427. Edinburgh: Churchill Livingstone.

Katims, JJ, Naviasky, EH, Lorenz, KY, et al. (1986) New screening device for assessment of peripheral neuropathy. *J Occup Med* 28:1219–1221.

Katz, D (1925) *Der Aufbau der Tastwelt*, Leipzig: JA Barth.

LeQuesne, PM (1978) Neurophysiological investigation of subclinical and minimal toxic neuropathies. *Muscle Nerve* 1:392.

Marks, RM, Barton, SP, and Edwards, C (eds) (1987) *The Physical Nature of the Skin*. Boston, MTP Press.

Mathers, LH (1985) *The Peripheral Nervous System:*

Structure, Function and Clinical Correlations. Menlo Park, CA: Addison-Wesley.

Maurissen, JOJ (1979) Effects of toxicants on the somatosensory system. *Neurobehav Toxicol* 1 (Suppl 1):23–31.

Muijser, H, Hooisma, J, Hoogendsijl, EMG, et al. (1986) Vibration sensitivity as a parameter for detecting peripheral neuropathy. I. Results in healthy workers. *Int Arch Occup Environ Health* 58:297–299.

Murata, K and Araki, S (1985) The effects of age, height, and skin temperature on short-latency somatosensory evoked potentials. *Jpn J EEG EMG* 13:152–158 (in Japanese).

Okada, A, Yamashita, T, Nagano, C, et al. (1981) Studies on the diagnosis and pathogenesis of Raynaud's phenomenon of occupational origin. *Br J Ind Med* 28:353–357.

Sallé, HJA and Verberk, MM (1984) Comparison of five methods for measurement of vibratory perception. *Int Arch Occup Environ Health* 53:303–309.

Schaumburg, HH and Spencer, PS (1979) Clinical and experimental studies of distal axonopathy—a frequent form of brain and nerve damage produced by environmental chemical hazards. *Ann NY Acad Sci* 329:14–29.

Schaumburg, HH, Spencer, PS, and Thomas, PK (1983) *Disorders of Peripheral Nerves*. Philadelphia: FA Davis.

Schaumburg, HH, Wisniewski, HM, and Spencer, PS (1974) Ultrastructural studies of the dying-back process: I. Peripheral nerve terminal and axon degeneration in systemic acrylamide intoxication. *J Neuropathol Exp Neurol* 33:260–284.

Seppäläinen, AM (1970) Nerve conduction in the vibration syndrome. *Work Environ Health* 7:82–84.

Snook, SH, Hinds, WC, and Burgess, WMA (1966) Respirator comfort: Subjective response to force applied to the face. *Am Ind Hyg J* 26:93–97.

Spencer, PS and Schaumburg, HH (1974) A review of acrylamide neurotoxicity. I. Properties, uses and human exposure. *Can J Neurol Sci* 1:143–150.

Summer, AJ and Asbury, AK (1975) Physiologic studies of the dying-back phenomenon: Muscle stretch afferents in acrylamide neuropathy. *Brain* 98:91–100.

Taylor, W (1974) *The Vibration Syndrome*. London: Academic Press.

Thomas, PK (1980) The peripheral nervous system as a target for toxic agents. In *Experimental and Clinical Neurotoxicology*, PS Spencer and HH Schaumburg (eds) pp. 35–47. Baltimore: Williams & Wilkins.

WHO Study Group (1980) *Peripheral Neuropathies, Technical Reports Series 654*. Geneva: World Health Organization.

24

The Vestibular System

The vestibular and auditory systems are both mechanoreceptors and have a common evolutionary origin; thus, their functions are intimately related. The vestibular system detects the position and motion of the head and mechanical vibrations imparted to the whole body; the auditory system—discussed in Chapter 25—is specifically designed to detect air vibrations in the acoustic range. Figure 24.1 shows the range of frequencies at which both sensory systems are sensitive.

The *membranous labyrinth* contains the receptors of both the vestibular apparatus and the cochlea, the main sensory organ of hearing. In addition, neural messages originating from these receptors are conveyed by a single nerve, cranial nerve VIII. As a result of this intimate anatomic relationship, neurological conditions that affect vestibular functions are also likely to affect auditory functions. An example is Ménière syndrome, in which both auditory and vestibular functions are affected. The condition is characterized by sudden and transient attacks of dizziness and vertigo, tinnitus (ringing in the ears), and inability to stand or walk. Because of these intimately related functions, the toxicology of the vestibular system is often discussed along with that of the auditory system under the name *ototoxicology*. There is growing literature showing selective effects of some occupational neurotoxic agents—particularly industrial solvents—on the vestibular system.

FUNCTIONAL ORGANIZATION

The receptors for the vestibular apparatus and for hearing are contained in the membranous labyrinth, which is comprised of the *cochlea,* the *otolithic organs,* and the *semicircular ducts.* The membranous labyrinth floats inside the *bony labyrinth,* carved deep in the temporal bone, and is separated from the bony labyrinth by the *perilymph.* The membranous labyrinth is filled with a liquid called the *endolymph.* The endolymph has a high concentration of potassium compared to the perilymph. This differential potassium concentration is thought to be involved in the initiation of the neural impulses by receptor cells.

The otolithic organs and the semicircular ducts are "accelerometers"—they are designed to detect the vectors of acceleration due to gravity and accelerations experienced by the head (Fig. 24.2).

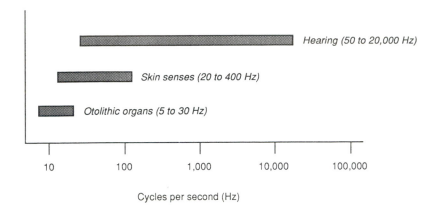

Cycles per second (Hz)

Fig. 24.1. The range of mechanical vibrations detected by the three sensory systems: the otolithic receptors of the vestibular system, the skin (somatosensory) senses, and hearing.

Otolithic Organs

The otolithic organs are primitive sensory organs present in all living organisms, including plants. (The fact that plants and trees grow away from earth is called negative geotaxis, and is possible as a result of mechanisms that help the plant to sense the direction of the acceleration of gravity.) In humans, the otolithic organs are involved in the initiation of balance and corrective postural movements as well as movements of the eyes.

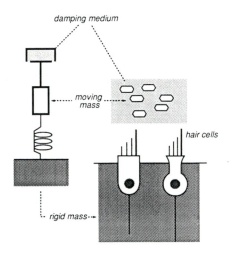

Fig. 24.2. The receptor organs of the vestibular apparatus are accelerometers. (See text.)

The major divisions of the otolithic organs are the *utricle*, in anatomic proximity to the semicircular ducts, and the *saccule*, in anatomic proximity to the cochlea (Fig. 24.3). The utricle and the saccule contained the *otoliths*, small stones of calcium carbonate embedded in a gelatinous substance. The otoliths rest on a roughly horizontal receptor called the *macula* (Latin for "spot"). When the head is moved, let's say, from side to side, the otoliths, embedded in the gelatinous substance, move passively. The gelatinous substance provides mechanical damping. The otolithic organs, particulary the saccule, are also thought to be involved in the detection of low-frequency sounds and mechanical vibrations.

The receptor cells of the otolithic organs, the semicircular ducts, and the cochlea are similar, revealing their common evolutionary and embryologic origin. These are *hair cells* containing a single *kinocilium* and 40 to 70 *stereocilia*. The hair cells exhibit a morphological polarization; ie, they are built so that they sense the direction in which movement occurs. A movement toward the kinocilium is associated with depolarization of the hair cells and an increase of impulse frequency typical of excitation. A movement away from the kinocilium is associated with hyperpolarization of the hair cells and a decrement in the impulse frequency typical of inhibition.

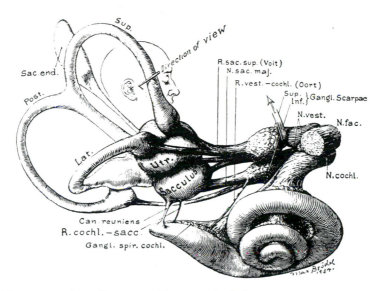

Fig. 24.3.   A classic illustration of the anatomic relation between vestibular organs and cochlea.

Within the macula, the hair cells are found to be morphologically polarized into clearly defined fields. The *striola,* located in the utricle macula, for example, separates two fields in which the hair cells are polarized in exactly opposite directions. The significance of these fields of morphological polarization of hair cells is still poorly understood.

Semicircular Ducts

At constant velocity, the endolymph contained inside the ducts does not move. As we sit inside a plane, for example, accelerations will be felt when the plane increases or decreases speed. At a constant motion of the plane, however, we can walk inside the plane without difficulty or even sensing motion. Similarly, the endolymph responds to changes of velocity (accelerations) experienced by the head. The inertia of the fluid explains this process. If the acceleration is exerted in one direction, the endolymph will push the ampulla in the opposite direction.

The ampulla is formed by a gelatinous substance that tightly fills the space between the ampullary crest and the roof of the cupula. The angle of displacement of the cupula is proportional to the acceleration of the head.

The hair cells are located at the base of the cupula on top of the ampullary crest, their cilia embedded in its gelatinous medium. The hair cells are activated by the movements of the ampulla.

The utricle is generally taken as a reference point to describe the movements of the ampulla. Thus, the ampulla is described as moving either toward or away from the utricle.

There are three pairs of semicircular ducts oriented orthogonally: the lateral, posterior, and anterior pairs. The semicircular ducts work in pairs. The lateral semicircular ducts act synergistically to detect accelerations occurring around the anterior–posterior axis of the body. The right anterior semicircular duct works synergistically with the left posterior duct. The left anterior semicircular duct works synergistically with the right posterior duct.

Neural Pathways

By the interrelated function of the otolithic organs and the semicircular ducts, the vestibular system accomplishes two functions: static functions (mediated primarily by the otolithic organs, enabling the control of the position of the head and posture) and dynamic functions (mediated primarily by the semicircular ducts, allowing the detection of head accelerations). These functions are possible through the relay of information to multiple sensory and motor nuclei in the brainstem and the cerebellum.

Fibers originating from the hair cells of the otolithic organs and the semicircular ducts have their cell bodies in the vestibular ganglion, also called *Scarpa's ganglion.* Like many first-order neurons in most sensory systems, this is a bipolar neuron. The central portion of the axon, the one that enters the nervous system, forms the vestibular division of the VIII cranial nerve, which carries acoustic as well as vestibular sensory information.

The VIII nerve enters the brain at the level of the pons, where second-order neurons are found in the vestibular nuclear complex formed by four distinctive nuclei:

- The *lateral vestibular nucleus,* also called Deiters' nucleus. The cells of this nucleus are functionally connected with motor neurons of the spinal cord that control antigravity muscles—muscles that pull the body against gravity—involved in postural reflexes. They also receive input from the cerebellum.
- The *medial vestibular nucleus* and the *superior vestibular nucleus.* These two groups of neurons mediate the reflex control of neck muscles and eye movements.
- The *inferior* or *descending vestibular nucleus.* This nucleus is the major link between the vestibular system and the cerebellum. These connections mediate the coordination of fine motor movement and the programming of motor acts.

Sensory input of the vestibular system also interacts with proprioceptive and visual information. (Proprioception is information originating in the muscles; it is proprioception that allows us to elevate the right arm to the same height as the left with our eyes closed.) Patients with vestibular disorders, for example, are unable to suppress the influence of visual and proprioceptive inputs (Nashner et al. 1982).

Unlike vision and audition, the stimulation of the vestibular system is not normally accompanied by conscious experience except under very sophisticated laboratory conditions. It is only under certain stimulus conditions—such as those accelerations that elicit motion sickness—that we notice the unpleasant consequences of the normal work of the vestibular system. Much of the literature on the normal function of the vestibular system in humans originated during World War II in the training of Navy personnel and in the late 1950s in the training of test pilots and astronauts.

EXAMINATION OF THE VESTIBULAR SYSTEM

Currently proposed batteries of tests for the examination of possible targets of neurotoxic action do not include the vestibular system. The literature on humans is scant and does not seem to justify their inclusion. (Some investigators have performed important studies using animal models, but this research has yet to find a human counterpart.) However, clinical tests of vestibular function are indispensable for the differential diagnosis of many neurological diseases.

There are numerous vestibulooculomotor reflexes that are mediated by inputs from the semicircular ducts. One such reflex is the *postrotatory nystagmus.* (Nystagmus is the involuntary, repetitive movement of the eyes.) This test can be performed with a five-wheeled office chair (for maximal stability) and the help of an assistant. The subject, sitting in the chair, is rotated either clockwise or counterclockwise in a normally lighted room; after the subject has spun gently several turns, he or she is stopped suddenly. As the subject rotates to the left with eyes open, the eyes undergo a slow conjugate deviation to the right while attempting to fixate on objects of the visual space. This is the slow phase of the nystagmus. Because visual objects are kept in the central region of the retina (called the fovea), the eyes experience a quick movement to the left when the limit of the eye excursion is reached. This is called the fast phase of the nystagmus.

As the chair is stopped suddenly, the endolymph of the horizontal ducts is suddenly moved in the opposite direction. This is accompanied by a total reversal of the phases of the nystagmus. The slow phase now occurs to the left with fast phases to the right. This test provides a gross evaluation of the functional status of the vestibular system.

In the clinic, vestibular nystagmus can also be produced by the use of hot or cold water injected into the external ear by means of a specially designed syringe. Cold and hot air can also be used. As a result of this stimulation, a convection current is created in the endolymph, a current that is strong enough to stimulate the cupula and produce nystagmus. This form of nystagmus is called caloric nystagmus; it is not the normal manner in which the semicircular ducts are stimulated.

Vestibular and caloric nystagmus, as used in the clinic without special instruments, are not sensitive enough to reveal neurotoxin-induced changes in the vestibular system. Many neurology and ear–nose–throat clinics around the world have sophisticated equipment with which subclinical alterations of oculomotor behavior can be studied in detail. (The principles of oculography have been reviewed in Chapter 5.)

There have been clinical and epidemiological studies and studies on experimental animal models of the effects of neurotoxic agents on the vestibular system. These studies take advantage of the fact that oculomotor behavior is controlled to a great extent by the vestibular system. Other sensory and motor inputs and confounding factors need to be taken into account, however. For example:

- It is estimated that a quarter of the human population exhibits nystagmus on lateral fixation. This epidemiological information is important to bear in mind so as not to attach undue significance to spontaneous nystagmus.

- Acute ingestion of alcohol and chronic alcoholism may be associated with abnormal eye movements and changes that could be interpreted as "vestibular." (Conversely, some solvent-induced motor changes, such as slurring of speech, could be interpreted as drunkenness.)

- Aging and dementia of the Alzheimer's type can produce changes in oculomotor reaction time as a result of the diffuse involvement of cortical regions controlling eye movements (Pirozzolo and Hansch 1981).

- Chronic absence of light can precipitate spontaneous nystagmus (eg, miners' nystagmus).

REPRESENTATIVE RESEARCH

There have been numerous studies on motion sickness and the effect of drugs designed for its effective control. This line of research is an example of the early interest in the effect of neurotoxic agents and drugs on the vestibular system. Motion sickness was a major health problem in World Wars I and II when large numbers of soldiers were exposed to accelerations that caused chronic vomiting and malaise. Dimenhydrinate (Dramamine) was discovered as a result of this research.

The literature on the effect of drugs on the vestibular system is extensive. Dichgans and Brandt (1973) and Brandt and collaborators (1974), working at the University of Freiburg, Federal Republic of Germany, have reviewed the comparative effectiveness of drugs—including belladonna, an alkaloid—in motion sickness.

Interest in the study of changes in the vestibular system produced by industrial solvents is relatively new in the United States. In Europe, however, there has been an uninterrupted line of work extending over 20 years.

Effect of Inhaled Solvents on the CNS as Measured by Nystagmus in Humans

One of the earliest reports on the use of oculographic methods for the assessment of neurotoxic agents is that of Kylen and collaborators in Sweden in 1967. They studied 12 subjects exposed to 1000 ppm of trichloroethylene for 2 hours and then tested for optokinetic nystagmus. (*Optokinetic nystagmus* is a repetitive pattern of eye movements, in response to stimulation such as that produced by looking out the window of a moving vehicle.) Optokinetic nystagmus was recorded by means of electrophysiological procedures similar to those described in Chapter 5. Kylen et al. were interested in determining whether trichloroethylene affected the optokinetic fusion limit, the highest speed of a striped stimulus that can produce optokinetic nystagmus. They found that "a number of subjects" showed a clear reduction in the optokinetic fusion limit; ie, they could not follow the stripes as fast as when nonexposed. Alcohol produced an even more marked effect.

Effects of Solvent Exposure on Vestibular Function Using Clinical Criteria

Because of the difficulties in interpreting clinical and epidemiological findings, some investigators propose that strict adherence to clinical criteria be observed in the evaluation of neurotoxin-induced effects. The following is an example.

Binaschi and Cantù (1983) speculate that the vestibular syndrome associated with solvent exposure is similar to that of toxic nucleoreticular vestibular syndrome. This syndrome consists of slight, usually short-lasting vertigo influenced by head movements, alterations in eye movements, and reduced reflex activity of the vestibular system. The

syndrome presumably results from the impairment of the vestibular apparatus at the level of the central vestibular nuclei and reticular pathways to the brainstem. The authors argue that because of its complexity, the syndrome is missed if only a superficial testing of the status of the vestibular system is attempted. They rightly point out that examinations of this type sometimes measure caloric nystagmus, which is unlikely to be disturbed during the subclinical manifestation of solvent-induced illness.

To make a clinical diagnosis of toxin-induced effects of neurotoxic agents on the vestibular system, the clinical examination therefore needs to be comprehensive, with a clear understanding of which levels of nervous system function are measured by the different tests. Thus, a judgment needs to be made on the meaning of the clinical findings. The clinical protocol includes the observation of spontaneous and provoked vestibular symptoms, evaluation of the stapedial acoustic reflex, electroencephalography, and a psychiatric examination.

Studies On Effects of Lead Exposure on Oculomotor Function Using Epidemiological Criteria

The study by Glickman et al. (1984) is one of the very few in which the status of the oculomotor system has been studied in individuals occupationally exposed to neurotoxic agents in the context of a medical field survey.

Glickman et al. conducted quantitative measures on saccadic eye movements in 52 lead-exposed workers and 52 age-matched controls with no history of occupational lead exposure. (Saccadic eye movements are rapid movements of the eye in following a moving target.) Three characteristics of saccadic eye movements were studied: saccade accuracy, number of overshoots, and maximal velocity.

The results indicated that workers exposed to inorganic lead showed a decrease in saccadic accuracy and an increase in overshoots compared to controls. In addition, saccade accuracy was negatively correlated with both blood lead levels and zinc protoporphyrin levels. It was concluded that these findings were consistent with a relatively rapid buildup of metabolically active lead burden observed in the study group. Neuropathological studies have shown that lead has a primary affinity for cerebellar structures.

REFERENCES

Binaschi, S and Cantù, L (1983) Vestibular function in solvent exposure; clinical criteria. In *Neurobehavioral Methods in Occupational Health*, R Gilioli, MG Cassitto, and V Foà (eds) pp. 205–210. New York: Pergamon Press.

Brandt, T, Dichgans, J, and Wagner, W (1974) Drug effectiveness on experimental and vestibular motion sickness. *Aerospace Med* 45:1291–1297.

Dichgans, J and Brandt, T (1973) Optokinetic motion sickness and pseudo-coriolis effects induced by moving visual stimuli. *Acta Otolaryngol* 76:339–348.

Glickman, L, Valciukas, JA, Lilis, R, et al. (1984) Occupational lead exposure: Effects on saccadic eye movements. *Int Arch Occup Environ Health* 54:115–125.

Kylen, B, Axell, K, Samuel, HE, et al. (1967) Effect of inhaled tricholoethylene on the CNS: As measured by optokinetic nystagmus. *Arch Environ Health* 15:48–52.

Nashner, LM, Black, FO, and Wall, C (1982) Adaptation to altered support and visual conditions during stance: Patients with vestibular deficits. *J Neurosci* (5):536–544.

Pirozzolo, FJ and Hansch, EC (1981) Oculomotor reaction time in dementia reflects degree of cerebral dysfunction. *Science* 214:349–351.

SUGGESTED READINGS

Arlien-Søborg, P. Zilstroff, K, Grandjean, B, et al. (1981) Vestibular dysfunction in occupational chronic solvent intoxication. *Clin Otolaryngol* 6:285–290.

Aschan, G, Bergstedt, M, Goldberg, L, et al. (1956) Positional nystagmus in man during and after alcohol intoxication. *Q J Stud Alcohol* 17:381–405.

Aschan, G and Berglund, M (1975) Positional alcohol nystagmus (PAN) in man following repeated alcohol doses. *Acta Otolaryngol Suppl* 330:15–29.

Aschan, G, Bunnfors, I, Hydén, D, et al. (1977) Xylene exposure: Electronystagmographic and gaschromatographic studies in rabbits. *Acta Otololaryngol* 84:370–376.

Aschoff, JC (1968) Veränderum raschen Blickbewegungen (Saccaden) beim Menschen unter Diazepam (Valium). *Arch Psychiatr Nervenkr* 211:325–332.

Baloh, RW and Honrubia, V (1990) *Clinical Neurophysiology of the Vestibular System*, 2nd ed. Philadelphia: FA Davis.

Barber, HO and Sharpe, A (1988) *Vestibular Disorders*. Boca Raton, FL: CRC Press.

Barnes, GB (1975) The role of the vestibular system in head–eye coordination. *J Physiol (Lond)* 246:351–369.

Biscaldi, GP, Mingardi, M, Pollini, G, et al. (1981) Acute toluene poisoning: Electrophysiological and vestibular investigations. *Toxicol Eur Res* 3:271–273.

Brown, RD and Wood, CC (1980) Vestibular pharmacology. *Trends Pharmacol Sci* 1:150–153.

Carpenter, RHS (1977) *Movements of the Eyes*. London: Pion.

Cohen, B (1974) The vestibulo-ocular reflex. In *Handbook of Sensory Physiology, Vol VI, Part 1, Vestibular Mechanisms: Basic Mechanisms*, HH Kornhuber (ed) pp. 477–540. New York: Springer-Verlag.

Cohen, B (1977) Use of Frenzel glasses in diagnosis of lesions of the vestibular system. *J Vertigo* 2:1–27.

Cramptom, GH (1989) *Motion and Space Sickness*. Boca Raton, FL: CRC Press.

De Oliveira, JAA (1989) *Audiovestibular Toxicity of Drugs*. Boca Raton, FL: CRC Press.

Franck, MC and Kuhlo, W (1970) Die Wirkung des Alcohols auf dir raschen Blickzielbewebefungen (Saccaden) beim Menschen. *Arch Psychiatr Nervenkr* 213:238–245.

Fukuda, T (1984) *Statokinetic Reflexes in Equilibrium and Movement*. Tokyo: University of Tokyo Press.

Goździk-Żolnierkiewicz, T, and Mosyyński, B (1969) VIIth nerve in experimental lead poisoning. *Acta Otolaryngol* 68:85–89.

Graham, MD and Kemink, JL (eds) (1987) *The Vestibular System: Neurophysiologic and Clinical Research*. New York: Raven Press.

Koch, C and Serra M (1962) Effetti dell'intossicazaione da piombo tetraetile sugli apparati accustico e vestibolare. *Acta Med Ital Med Trop Subtrop Gastroenterol* 17:77–80.

Larsby B, Tham, R, Ödkvist, LM, et al. (1978) Exposure of rabbits to styrene: Electronystagmographic findings correlated to the styrene level in blood and cerebrospinal fluid. *Scand J Work Environ Health* 4:60–65.

Larsby, B, Tham, R, Ödkvist, LM, et al. (1978) Exposure of rabbits to methylchloroform: Vestibular disturbances correlated to blood and cerebrospinal fluid levels. *Int Arch Occup Environ Health* 41:7–15.

Nauton, RF (ed) (1975) *The Vestibular System*. New York: Academic Press.

Ödkvist, LM, Larsby, B, Fredrickson, JMF, et al. (1980)

Vestibular and oculomotor disturbances caused by industrial solvents. *J Otolaryngol* 9(1):53–59.

Ödkvist, LM, Larsby, B, Tham, R, et al. (1978) Positional nystagmus elicited by industrial solvents. In *Vestibular Mechanisms in Health and Disease,* JD Hood (ed) pp. 188–194. London: Academic Press.

Precht, W (1979) Vestibular mechanisms. *Annu Rev Neurosci* 2:265–289.

Savolainen, K and Linnavuo, M (1979) Effects of *m*-xylene on human equilibrium measured with a quantitative method. *Acta Pharmacol Toxicol* 44:315–318.

Wilpizeski, C (1974) Effects of lead on the vestibular system: Preliminary findings. *Laryingoscope* 84:821–832.

Wilson, AT (1968) Acute vertigo and the lead content of food and drink. *Practitioner* 200:282–285.

25

The Auditory System

Because of its interdisciplinary nature, the literature on hearing is extensive. In the early 1950s S. S. Stevens (1906–1973), director of the Laboratory of Psychophysics at Harvard University, compiled the available worldwide literature on hearing, its psychophysical and neurophysiological basis, the study of auditory perception throughout the phylogenetic scale, noise assessment in the environment, and hearing loss prevention at the workplace. Even then, the literature amounted to tens of thousands of titles.

The literature on drug-induced hearing loss is also somewhat extensive. The properties of certain chemical agents—such as quinine (used in the treatment of malaria) and salicylates (eg, aspirin for the treatment of pain)—that cause alterations in hearing were recognized in the late 19th century. But drug-induced hearing damage became a major medical problem when antibiotics for the treatment of tuberculosis were introduced in the middle 1940s. Arsenical compounds used in the treatment of trypanosomiasis and syphilis also caused hearing problems. Since then, there have been numerous clinical observations and experimental studies on laboratory animals documenting the effect of drugs on hearing

(Stebbins and Rudy 1978; Hybels 1979; Prosen and Stebbins 1980).

Unlike the body of information on noise-induced or drug-induced damage to the auditory system, however, the body of knowledge concerning the effects of environmental and occupational neurotoxic agents in humans is scant and controversial. A corpus can barely be reconstructed at this time. The major single difficulty in evaluating the effects of E & O neurotoxic agents on the human auditory system is the need to rule out normal hearing loss caused by age and alterations in hearing induced by other conditions. These include occupational exposure to noise (eg, in people who use jackhammers or many other noisy power tools such as drills, borers, saws, etc or those who drive noisy vehicles such as tractors, subway trains, etc), recreational noise (eg, in professional rock musicians, disco dancers, people who listen to personal tape-playing systems, etc), neurotoxic drugs, and preexisting medical conditions suspected of causing hearing impairment (eg, diabetes).

The basic methodology for studying neurotoxin-induced hearing loss is similar to that available for the evaluation of noise-induced hearing loss. In this chapter we will review this knowledge and methodology, the stimulus for the auditory system, and the functional organization of the auditory system. This is followed by a discussion of noise as an environmental "pollutant."

The term "ototoxicity" (meaning "toxicity of the ear") which is often found in neurotoxicological literature, particularly that of therapeutic drugs, is a misnomer: neurotoxic agents act not only on the ear (the cochlea, to be more precise) but also on peripheral and central neural pathways. The phrase "toxicology of the auditory system" is preferred.

PSYCHOPHYSICS

Psychophysics is a discipline dealing with the quantitative relationships between the physical properties of environmental stimuli and the subjective attributes of sensation. Psychophysical methods are a collection of techniques and procedures for the study of these quantitative relationships.

Psychophysical procedures are applied to the study of the attributes of sensation in all the sensory systems—eg, taste, olfaction, somatosensory, vision, vestibular reflexes. In these other sensory systems the methods are largely used by trained observers under laboratory conditions. (A trained observer is a subject who, as a result of extensive training or experience, is able to participate in complex experiments requiring keen observational skills and attention to detail. For example, a psychophysical study in color perception might require the observation of changes in hues as a result of the simultaneous change of the brightness and wavelength of the light, changes that most of us would not detect.) Since this book deals with clinical observations and epidemiological observations of the "average" person, I have chosen not to include these important methods of experimental psychology. Results obtained from trained observers may not be representative of "normal" people.

Psychophysics is one of the oldest branches of experimental psychology. Weber (1795–1878) and Fechner (1801–1887) are recognized as the founders of psychophysics (Boring 1950). Stevens (1906–1973) was responsible for the modern revival of psychophysics in the middle 1950s. Weber is said to be the first to use the concept of "threshold," ie, the minimal energy necessary to produce a sensation. Since the middle of the last century, this concept of threshold has been borrowed and used by many other scientists in many other disciplines.

Psychophysicists ask questions such as: What is the relationship governing the growth of sensation of brightness of a light vis-à-vis the intensity of the light source?; How much energy strikes the ear drums when one hears the faintest noise?; and What is the minimum difference necessary between two wavelengths in order to perceive the difference as two separate colors? These are basic questions that characterize "classical psychophysics."

Psychophysics also provides the experimental foundation for the validity and reliability of subjective estimations, such as those made by interviewees during surveys: What is the relationship between the dollar and the subjective value of goods? What is the relative prestige of various occupations? How do we define well-being? How do we define environmental risk, and how can we rank the relative risk of different hazardous conditions? Psychophysics provides a theory of measurement and quantitative tools, such as scales of measurement, to study these problems.

Scaling is a systematic method of assigning numbers to objects and events according to preestablished rules. Scaling procedures have been used for the study of important problems such as the subjective estimate of environmental and occupational problems. In the social and behavioral sciences, the terms "scaling" and "measuring" mean the same thing when used in the context of the measurement of subjective phenomena.

As the significance of other factors in the interpretation of psychophysical experiments became known—eg, the role of the consequences of one's choices—the field of psychophysics expanded even further. Presently, many of the well-known problems in psychophysics are being reexamined in terms of a new discipline: signal detection.

The Measurable Properties of the Auditory Stimulus

The term "stimulus" has specific meanings for different scientific disciplines. In sensory physiology, stimulus is defined as a form of energy change that can produce a sensation. The following is a description of sound as a sensory stimulus.

Auditory stimuli have two fundamental attributes: intensity (the loudness of a sound) and quality (the beauty of a melody, the roughness of a sound). First, measurements of intensity are reviewed.

Sound is produced by the periodic compression and expansion of any acoustically conducting medium such as air, water, ground, metals, artificial materials, etc. The present discussion is restricted to the propagation of sound in air. If the successive compression and expansion of air that occurs in the production of a "pure" sound is plotted on graph paper, we see a sinusoidal pattern. However, pure sounds are rarely heard in real life. Pure sounds are generated by mechanical devices (such as a tuning fork or a flute) or electronic oscillators (such as an electronic synthesizer). A whistle is also close to a pure tone.

The pitch of a sound is primarily determined by the frequency of its sound waves, measured in Hertz (Hz), and secondarily by its intensity. An increase in the intensity of a sound of 1000 Hz, for example, is perceived as an increase in pitch, whereas an increase in the intensity of a sound of frequency less than 1000 Hz is perceived as a lower pitch. Interestingly, the pitch of a pure tone of 1000 Hz does not change as its intensity is increased or decreased. That is why fundamental calibrations in acoustic research depend on a pure tone of 1000 Hz as a reference sound.

The loudness of a tone is primarily determined by the intensity of the sound.

Psychoacoustic research has revealed that sounds have the dimensions of both volume and density. Volume and density of sound result from different permutations of their frequencies and amplitudes of the sinusoidal sound waves. Thus, low-frequency tones are perceived in general as occupying more "space" than high-frequency tones. Sounds of high frequency and high amplitude—for example, a "piercing sound"—are perceived as being "denser" than sounds of low frequency and low amplitude. There are several other sound attributes not thoroughly studied. A whistle, for example, is described as being "clean."

The detection of sound is primarily accomplished by the auditory sensory system, but sound is also detected by the skin, receptors located in the joints, and the otolithic organs, a component of the vestibular system. The present discussion is confined to the acoustic reception that occurs via the auditory system. Auditory stimuli have properties of intensity that can be measured in terms of our reaction to them. These reactions can be measured by their lower thresholds, upper thresholds (not measurable in all sensory systems), and range and resolution.

The *lower (absolute) threshold* is the minimal energy that can be detected by a specific sensory system. In environmental health, knowledge of the lower threshold for hearing is important in the design of instruments that simulate human hearing organs.

Upper thresholds are more difficult to define than lower thresholds. The *upper threshold* for hearing is that level of sound (subjectively arrived at) that is so loud that the sound is either irritating or painful. However, under normal living conditions, people are exposed to explosive sounds (eg, rock music) that would be intolerable to a research volunteer. The context in which the sound occurs makes a difference. The context where sound is produced, to be discussed below, determines the relative annoyance of the sound.

The range of sound is the range of intensities (or frequencies) that can be detected. The range of intensities detectable by humans extends from 0 to 140 dB; the range of frequencies from 60 Hz to 20 kHz. The upper limit of the ranges varies for every person, as we lose approximately 50 Hz per year of life.

The Decibel as a Measure of Intensity. The *decibel* is a unit for expressing the intensity of sound. To understand this commonly used unit of measurement, it is best to reconstruct the historical context within which the measurement of sound developed: electrical engineering and acoustics.

Once the absolute threshold for audition was known for a tone of 1000 Hz, scientists began to ask the following question: "When we measure the level of energy that produces a sound, how far are we from the absolute energy that is needed to produce the absolute threshold for sound?" Using symbols, this question can be translated as: I/I_0, where I is the level of energy that is being measured, and I_0 the absolute threshold for hearing.

Let's consider the following example. If the level of energy I is 2000 ergs/cm^2 and the estimated level I_0 is 0.0002 erg/cm^2, then we have the ratio I/I_0 = 2000/0.0002 = 10,000,000. For people moving about in busy laboratories, these long numbers represent an inconvenience. Expressing the number as its logarithm is much more concise. (The logarithms for common numbers are: log 1 = 0; log 10 = 1; log 100 = 2; log 1000 = 3; and so on.)

The logarithm of the ratio I/I_0 (the measured intensity of the sound vis-à-vis its reference point) became known as the *Bel* (originally "Bell") after the famous Scottish-American physicist (1847–1922). Thus

$$Bel = \log I/I_0$$

In our example, there are seven logarithmic units between the reference level and the level of the sound that one is measuring.

Soon after beginning to work with Bels, scientists needed finer units of measurements, so they multiplied the Bel by 10, thus creating the "decibel."

$$decibel = \log I/I_0 \times 10$$

The definition of decibel is expressed verbally as the logarithm of the ratio between the measured intensity of sound and a reference intensity of sound, multiplied by 10. A sound that is 10,000,000 times the level of the reference standard I_0 has 70 decibels (70 dB).

Decibels are flexible units because they are *relative units* of measurement. The reference standard, for example, does not have to be a measurable quantity; the level of I_0 is a conventional unit of measurement set at 0.0002 erg/cm^2. As does any other measure of human performance, the absolute threshold for hearing a tone of 1000 Hz varies from individual to individual; 0.0002 erg/cm^2 is the threshold of the ideal observer.

An "ideal observer" should not be confused with a "trained observer." An ideal observer is an imaginary entity whose performance or sensory organs have quantitative features specified by convention among scientists. For example, the ideal observer has an ideal eye, an essential concept for the design of optical instruments in which many of the structures of the eye, such as the lens and the cornea, have been geometrically defined. In acoustics, the sound level meter (to be described below) is the ideal ear, that is, the "ear" that nobody has but that researchers agree to use as a reference. The quantitative values of an ideal observer do not have a statistical distribution (eg, mean and standard deviations).

A "subject"—often abbreviated S—is any individual participating in a study. A subject may or may not be a trained observer, and is never an ideal observer.

The reference level need not always be specified when one needs to measure two different levels of intensity in the clearly audible acoustic range. For example, the difference between 70 dB and 30 dB is 40 dB.

The decibel scale does not predict the manner in which sounds of different intensities and frequencies will be heard. Psychophysics flourished in the 1950s when methods were introduced for the study of how real people—not ideal observers—judge sounds in relation to the physical properties of the auditory stimulus.

Foundations of Psychophysical Methods

As the intensity of the stimulus increases, in what proportion is the sensation increased? Classical psychophysicists, notably Fechner, had a philosophical interest in the subject (Boring 1950). Fechner tried to understand the laws governing the relationships between the physical world and the human mind. [Present-day scientists and engineers have more practical purposes in mind, such as the need to construct sound and noise meters (personal noise level meters are already available) or the need to control glare or manufacture glare-free crystals for reading panels.] Only the most basic principles of these psychophysical laws can be reviewed here.

Fechner argued that sensations increase with the logarithm of the intensity of the stimulus causing the sensation. If we designate the sensation as S and the intensity of the stimulus as E (for energy), Fechner proposed that $S = \log E$ (Fig. 25.1, left). He arrived at this conclusion on the basis of a large variety of simple laboratory experiments that he and other scientists had performed, most notably his fellow countryman Weber. That is why the logarithmic law linking sensations to stimuli is also known as the *Weber–Fechner law*.

To perform his experiments, Fechner developed numerous ingenious methods for stimulus presentation. Some of his psychophysical methods, such as the method of limits, are increasingly used in neurotoxicology and thus are reviewed here.

The Weber–Fechner law was accepted for almost a century until it was superseded by *Stevens' power law* (Stevens 1975). Again, on the basis of numerous experiments—first on the sensation of hearing but then extended to other sensory dimensions and even social phenomena—Stevens proposed a more general, and probably more elegant, model to describe how sensations are related to their stimuli.

Stevens argued that sensations can be rated. One can say "Stimulus A is 100 times more intense than stimulus B." If one obtains the logarithmic value of these quantitative sub-

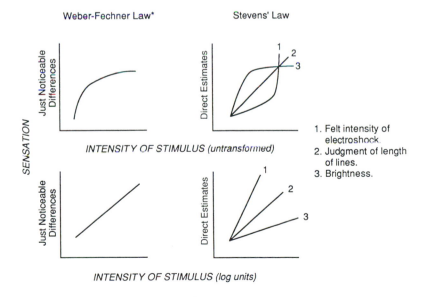

Fig. 25.1. The Weber–Fechner law compared to Stevens' law (see text). (*Note that Fechner never published a visual representation of how his law worked for different sensory modalities.)

jective ratings and plots these values against the logarithmic value of the level of energy of the stimulus, one observes a straight line:

$$\log S = \log E$$

The line linking the sensation to its stimulus can be calculated mathematically:

$$Y = a + bX$$

where Y, the vertical axis—the dependent variable—is a measure of sensation, and X, the horizontal axis, is the independent variable. The constant a is the point where the line intersects the vertical axis. The constant b is the slope of the line, calculated as the ratio of the increment of Y over the increment of X. Because the vertical and horizontal axes have been logarithmically transformed, the mathematical equation describing the relationship can to be written as follows:

$$\log Y = a + b \log X$$

The equation can also be expressed as:

$$Y = aX^b$$

Stevens' now widely known law is generally expressed in Greek letters:

$$\psi = \kappa \Phi^\beta$$

where ψ is the magnitude of the sensation, Φ is the magnitude of the physical stimulus, β is the exponent of the power function, and κ is usually referred to in the literature as "the constant of proportionality," which depends on the unit of measurement. (In fact, it is simply the Y-intercept; Fig. 25.1, right.)

Stevens' law is considered a more accurate way of describing raw laboratory data than that which led Fechner to propose his logarithmic law. (Some of Stevens' followers would argue that the difference is fundamental.) For audition, it is widely accepted that the power law matches more closely how people hear sounds than the decibel scale does. However, the power law has even wider applications. It appears to be valid at the elementary neural level (eg, the description of the relationship between light intensity and the firing of neural fibers), the psychological level describing the behavior of a single individual (the context in which it was first developed and described), and the description of the behavior of social groups and quantitative human factors (eg, the worth attached to goods). Those measures are important in creating models in econometry.

Following Fechner's steps, Stevens had to develop or adapt experimental methods to study his insights. Three of these scientific procedures became widely known and are still used in psychological research: the methods of subjective estimation, magnitude production, and matching are described below, under the heading "Methods for Assessment of Dose–Response Relationships in Audition."

Stevens provided many fundamental contributions in his long and productive career. Like Fechner, he proved once more that subjective estimates follow definite laws vis-à-vis what an individual perceives. Thus, Stevens is credited with providing the most comprehensive scientific foundation for subjective rating scales.

Stevens was less successful than Fechner in describing laboratory procedures, however. Fechner, on the one hand, kept methods simple and wrote in a language that is still understood by an educated person. Stevens, on the other hand, wrote for his peers and thus employed technical language. Only in his posthumous publications (eg, Stevens 1975) was an effort made to express his views in a more understandable fashion for the benefit of the public at large.

Methods for (Intensity) Threshold Determinations

Two methods are widely used in psychophysiological research. The method of limits, well known to psychologists, is used in laboratory-based studies on the effects of neurotoxic agents. The method of adjustment is also well known to experimental psychologists: it has a potential role in neurotoxicological research, particularly in research performed under laboratory conditions. However, this is not familiar to most neurotoxicologists. Sometimes these methods are built into special testing equipment (eg, the Békésy audiometer).

Method of Limits. This method can be used for determinations of both the threshold of intensity and the quality of the stimulus. Here, we discuss the former. The intensity of the stimulus of a given quality (eg, a tone of 1000 Hz) is either reduced until the subject no longer perceives it (in a *descending series*) or increased until it is perceived (in an *ascending series*). Figure 25.2 illustrates the method used in sound pitch discrimination.

Most modern audiometers have these protocols built into the circuitry, and the device has a printer producing a hard copy of the threshold contours. Protocols like these are difficult to follow. They are time consuming, and subjects are not likely to cooperate, particularly when the research is performed under field conditions.

It should be emphasized that the method of limits requires minimal use of language on the part of the person being examined. A simple hand gesture or a turn of a switch is enough for the subject to tell the status of the stimulus: above threshold, just about threshold, or below threshold. The method is easily understood by most subjects.

Tracking Methods. The method of tracking can be used for a variety of purposes, as can the method of limits. The intensity of the stimulus is under the subject's control. The subject is instructed to keep a switch on until the intensity of the stimulus decreases to an imperceptible level. When the stimulus is below threshold, the subject releases the switch, and the intensity of the stimulus increases automatically.

Békésy (1899–1972) designed a new method of audiometry that is based on this procedure. In it, the frequency of the sound increases automatically from lower to higher frequencies, and the subject hears the slowly increasing sound pitch. The subject controls the increment of the intensity of the stimulus by pressing the switch when he/she can hear the sound, and the switch is to be released when the sound becomes imperceptible. Figure 25.3 is a plot of a typical audiogram using the tracking method. Although developed for hearing studies, it can be adapted for other sensory modalities.

As stated earlier, there are many variations of psychophysical procedures for threshold determinations. The reader who is interested in pursuing this topic further should consult some of the many excellent sources available (Marks 1974).

A threshold value is inversely proportional to the sensitivity of a sensory system: the greater the sensitivity, the lower the threshold.

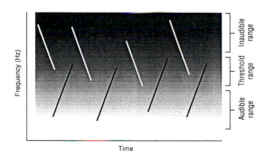

Fig. 25.2. Schematic representation of the psychophysical method of limits as used in sound pitch discrimination.

When using commercially available testing equipment, a serious investigator carefully reads the claims of the inventors and manufacturers of such equipment. For example, at exactly what levels should a hearing threshold value be declared "abnormal"?

In many instances, the role of confounding variables, such as age, is assumed to be known by the experimenter or the technician who determines

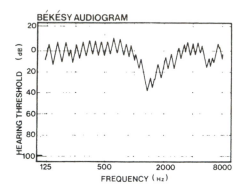

Fig. 25.3. Békésy method of tracking. (See text.)

auditory thresholds. However, confounding variables are not corrected automatically in the "reading" made by equipment designed to measure sound levels.

Obvious as this may seem, many manufacturers' claims are not supported by standardization procedures. One should be particularly cautious about studies in which a judgment of neurotoxicity is made on the basis of built-in normal values "memorized" in the testing equipment.

Methods for Assessment of Dose–Response Relationships in Audition

As stated earlier, Stevens developed several psychophysical procedures to study the "laws" governing the relationship between the physical (or chemical) stimulus and its corresponding sensation. Three methods are described: subjective estimation, magnitude production, and cross-modality matching.

The method of **subjective estimation** is called a direct method. The subject attaches numbers to his or her perceptions which are proportional to an agreed-upon standard. The experimenter presents the subject with a luminous circle of known intensity and asks him/her to pay attention to its brightness. The experimenter may ask the research subject to attach an arbitrary number to the brightness. Alternatively, the experimenter himself/herself may set such a standard (eg, 100). In successive trials, the intensity of the circle is

reduced below or increased above the set standard in easy-to-recognize steps. The experimenter asks the subject to attach numbers to the various luminosity steps in proportion to how far above or below the standard the subject perceives them. Given a standard of 100, the subject would assign the number 200 to a stimulus perceived as being "double" the amount of the standard; conversely, if the subject were to perceive the stimulus as only a quarter of the value of the standard, then the number 25 would be assigned.

The method of **magnitude production** is the opposite of the method of subjective estimation. Here, the experimenter calls up numbers, and the subject in turn increases or decreases the value of the stimulus in proportion to his/her subjective judgment. For example, the subject has to adjust the sound of a fixed frequency (ie, 1000 Hz) to correspond to the numbers called up by the experimenter. The data are analyzed and plotted in essentially the same way as those obtained in studies employing the method of subjective estimation. The dose–response relationships—or psychophysical functions as they are called in psychophysics—are found to be similar to those obtained by the method of subjective estimation.

The method of **cross-modality matching** does not require the use of numbers. The subject is presented with stimuli of, let's say, varying light brightness, and he/she has to adjust another stimulus, say a tone of 1000 Hz, in proportion to the levels of the luminous target. Typically, the graphic representation consists of two axes, one that represents levels of brightness and the other representing the intensity levels of the sound. Logarithmic coordinates are used. The slope of this log–log plot is the exponent of the power function.

Some of these scaling procedures have been successfully applied to study the annoyance of environmental pollutants such as odors and noise. Although they have a potential use in human neurotoxicology, current representative examples are lacking.

ASSESSMENT OF ENVIRONMENTAL NOISE

Acoustically, noise is a complex sound waveform having no esthetic or judgmental value; psychologically, noise is any unwanted sound. The bass sounds of rock music escaping from someone's personal tape-playing system, for example, a sound that may measure no more than 40 dB, can be mental torture for a bus rider who is trying to read a novel. Thus, both the acoustic characteristics of sounds and the context within which sound occurs intervene in the definition of "noise."

Noise is often listed as one of the top 10 industrial health problems. In spite of the fact that the technology for noise abatement and hearing impairment assessment has existed for several decades, noise has yet to be eradicated. There is no single explanation why noise is so difficult to control.

It is unlikely that a neurotoxicologist may be called upon to assess environmental or occupational levels of noise. But in many cases, a clinical neurotoxicologist must make evaluations of environmental and occupational conditions—to rule out confounding effects of noise, for example—without having access to objective data. The following is only a brief coverage of this topic. Interested readers can consult many of the excellent sources available (Kryter 1985).

The Sound Level Meter

The *sound level meter* is the basic instrument to measure noise. It contains three weighting networks (electronic circuitry that reproduces different acoustic characteristics of the human ear): A, B, and C. The A network is an ideal ear reacting to the characteristics of the sound very much as the human ear does. To imitate human hearing, the A network, for example, "hears" high-frequency tones louder than lower-frequency tones of the same decibel level. The A network is used in environmental monitoring because it is sensitive to high-frequency tones, which are the most damaging to the ear.

The noise level meter functions as the ear of an ideal observer placed in the environment to measure sounds as humans would perceive them, and is used by pretending a human being is there. For example, noise measurements are made at the ear level of the worker, so that the sound level meter registers the same amount of noise the worker does. The significance of the level meter can be appreciated most in the case of measuring sounds too intense to be assessed by humans.

Environmental noise is measured in octaves. An octave is a concept borrowed from music. In piano playing, the distance from the note A_3 to A_4 is an octave. A_4 has double the frequency of vibration of A_3. For example, if A_3 vibrates at 440 Hz, A_4 vibrates at 880 Hz. Thus, an octave is always double the frequency of a sound taken as a reference.

We saw earlier that a sound of 1000 Hz is, by convention, a reference sound. Octaves are measured up and down vis-à-vis 1000 Hz. For example, in environmental monitoring the octave scales are sounds of 125, 250, 500, 1000, 2000, 4000, and 8000 Hz. The sound level meter measures the concentration of acoustic energy in each of these bands of frequencies (eg, 125–250, 250–500, and so on). For precision measurements, sometime a third of an octave is measured.

Personal noise dosimeters have been designed that allow the measuring of daily doses of sound. The dosimeter's microphone is placed on the workers' shoulder or collar. Personal monitors are based on the principle of piezoelectricity, in which sound energy is transformed into electrical signals. After the duration of exposure is calculated, the cumulative sound energy for the day is transformed into a "sound dose." If on any given day the dosimeter measures, for example, over 100%, that day the worker has been exposed to excessive noise. The advantage of personal monitoring devices over the sound level meters is that workers' exposures are measured directly as they actually occur under working conditions.

The Noise Survey

A *noise survey* is the characterization of the sounds in a given environment in terms of frequency and intensity in relation to people who live or work in the area where noise is a problem—the engine room of a ship, the room where metal automobile parts are molded by riveting, a neighborhood close to an airport, etc. Thus, the report of a noise survey usually contains a simplified layout of where the noise survey was conducted, with recognizable components of such an environment, the registered values in decibels, and, most importantly, the probability of incurring hearing damage at the levels of noise that have been measured. The report usually contains a conclusion as to whether measured levels are hazardous to hearing and, if they are, recommendations as to the elimination of the problem.

In walk-throughs aimed at planning a noise survey, experts get a "sense" of the trouble spots. As a rule of thumb, a sound is damaging in the long term:

- If the sound interferes with human speech between two people talking at arm's length, so that they are forced to raise their voices in order to be heard. A sound of 50 dB, for example, will interfere with speech; at 60 dB one is forced to speak loudly; at 65 dB, communication is possible by shouting. (There is also a "frequency factor" that contributes to the interference of voice communication: low-frequency tones mask high-frequency tones.)
- If tinnitus—ringing of the ear—is present after brief exposure to the source of noise.
- If temporary loss of hearing that muffles speech occurs at the completion of a work shift.

Some very experienced experts can judge the prevailing level of sound within an error margin of a few decibels.

Current Standards of Maximal Exposure to Noise

The Occupational Safety and Health Agency (OSHA) recommends permissible exposure to sound, but individual states have the power to enforce less or more stringent levels. The current recommended standard is 90 dB A (ie, 90 dB measured in the A network) for an 8-hour period. However, it is generally agreed that 85 dB would be a safer level. Higher intensity levels are permitted for briefer periods of time.

A "dose" of noise is defined as:

$$\text{Dose} = \frac{C_1}{T_1} + \frac{C_2}{T_2} + \frac{C_3}{T_3} \cdots \frac{C_n}{T_n}$$

where C stands for "concentration," ie, the intensity of the sound, and T is the maximal allowable level for that frequency. This equation—sometimes called "the hygienic effect" in European sources—leads to a number that varies in proportion to its individual components. In an environment where the average level of noise is less than the maximum allowable level, the dose will be less than 1; where the average level of noise exceeds the maximum allowable level, the dose will be greater than 1.

The Annoyance of Sounds

Noise is sometimes unwanted or unpleasant even at levels known not to impair hearing. Thus, the difference between acoustic and contextual characteristics that make sounds annoying needs to be clearly recognized. Among the acoustic, loudness is an important factor; in general, the louder the more annoying. However, the spectral composition of the sound is important as well. For example, the roaring sound of waterfalls—a "white noise" because it contains most of the audible sound frequencies—in a tropical mountain setting is generally considered pleasant; intermittent hammering of metal sheet (acoustically, an intermittent noise concentrated in the high frequencies) at a construction site across the street where one lives is not.

In general, higher frequencies are more annoying than lower frequencies. For example, to an adult, the noise that a small child makes when moving a squeaky door back and forth in the kitchen can be maddening. The low-frequency sounds of distant thunder heard during a particularly warm summer day may be considered pleasant. In certain contexts, however, low-frequency sounds can be very annoying. House walls filter the high-frequency sounds of music; if the upstairs neighbor has a party with rock music, the tune is effectively eliminated by the walls, and what is left to hear is the pounding sound of bass sounds that makes the rhythm.

Most important are the contextual characteristics within which sound occurs. An important factor is whether the subject is a passive receiver of the sound or the active generator of the noise. The noise that a mosquito makes during a summer night is an example. The noise—which is rather unpredictable—can be annoying to the point of interfering with sleep.

In general, a sound that interferes with speech is annoying. To the aged individual, even the voices of other people interfering with the speech of the interlocutor may be annoying.

The vast research that has been performed on the annoyance of sounds should be inspirational for environmental neurotoxicology. However, a cross-fertilization of these disciplines has yet to materialize.

THE FUNCTIONAL ORGANIZATION OF THE AUDITORY SYSTEM

The details of how the ear processes sounds and creates a neural code that ultimately results in the subjective impression of sounds,

speech, and music have attracted the brightest minds in each generation of experimental scientists. Investigators have been attracted by the ingenious ways the ear senses sounds and transforms them into a neural code. It is difficult to avoid a deep feeling of awe when considering the simplest facts about what the cochlea is capable of doing.

The ear by itself performs several forms of energy transformation: the sound pressure is first transformed into movement by means of mechanical processes involving several stages (to be described below); mechanical movement then produces a unique biophysical process, the traveling wave; the traveling wave moves the basilar membrane, where receptors are located, and the receptors rub against a flexible membrane, thus initiating the neural code.

The need for a process of energy transformation is best understood if some features of the evolution of the auditory apparatus are reviewed. In the fish, the receptor cells for the detection of acoustic signals in water are located outside the body, in an organ called the lateral line. The receptors of the lateral line are activated by acoustic vibrations of the surrounding water. When living organisms that had lived in the sea began to move about on the surface of the earth, the acoustic communication formerly mediated by water was now mediated by air. Bones were added to transform air vibrations into mechanical movements that in turn activate hydraulic processes in the cochlea. These bones—the ossicles—were originally involved in mastication (chewing).

This is just one of the many examples of how we still carry functions that were originally evolved from our sea-living ancestors. Mechanisms to maintain optimum sodium levels in the blood and the existence of water inside the semicircular duct, water whose movement allows the detection of the body's own acceleration, are other examples.

The following is a review of the major events that occur in a space whose total volume approximates that of a small cherry.

Transformation of Sound Pressure into Mechanical Movement

The ear has three major components: The external ear, represented primarily by the concha; the middle ear, where the ossicles are found; and the inner ear, where the organ of Corti is located.

The two *conchas* attached to the head are suited for the localization of the sources of sounds in space. The orienting reflex—the turning of the head toward the source of an unexpected sound—is mediated by neural pathways linking the auditory pathways with neck and other body muscles that move the head. The convoluted structure that is the concha mechanically filters and enhances frequencies that are vital for speech communication.

Figure 25.4 shows the elements of the middle and inner ear. Sound waves are propagated through the *external auditory meatus* (Latin for "opening") to reach the *tympanic membrane*, causing its vibration. The *malleus* (Latin for "hammer") is attached to the tympanic membrane, so when the tympanic membrane vibrates the malleus vibrates. The malleus transmits this mechanical vibration to two ossicles linked in succession, the *incus* (Latin for "anvil") and the *stapes* (Latin for "stirrup"). The *oval window* is normally closed tightly by the oval-shaped base of the stapes. The movement imparted by the stapes to the oval window is similar to that of a piston.

The ossicles create very little mechanical damping and in fact amplify sounds. Sound amplification is achieved because the base of the stapes receives approximately the same mechanical energy as the tympanic membrane on an area that is smaller than that of the tympanic membrane.

The ossicles are controlled by the tiniest muscles in the human body. These muscles modify the mechanical transmission characteristics of the ossicle.

Until the 1920s very little was known about what happens next. In that year George Békésy initiated a series of brilliant experiments with mechanical models, experiments that helped to destroy several different theories of how sound waves are transformed into a neural code. (The author was privileged to work with such models left by Békésy during a series of lectures in Argentina. Békésy won the Nobel prize for his work.)

How Mechanical Movement Creates the Traveling Wave

The oval window is a key interface between the ossicles and the *cochlea*, a liquid-filled structure where the transduction of sounds

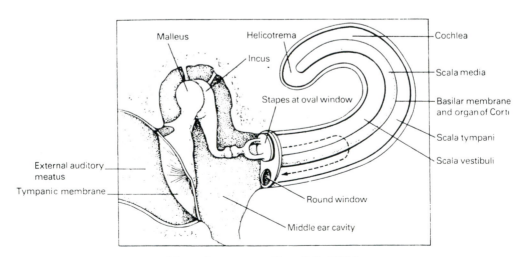

Fig. 25.4. The peripheral organs of the auditory system. (From Kelly 1985.)

to neural signals is accomplished. The cochlea is shaped like a shell spiraling two-and-a-half turns around a central pillar, the modiolus. The spiral architecture of the cochlea seems to have a space-saving function. Mechanical models of the cochlea constructed to understand its mechanohydraulic properties are usually uncoiled versions of the cochlea. The visualization of the cochlea as a tube having three inner compartments facilitates the understanding of the function of its different elements.

The cochlea has three compartments (see Fig. 25.4): the *scala tympani,* which follows the outer contours of the cochlea; the *scala vestibuli,* which follows the inner contours of the spiral; and the *scala media,* wedged between the scala tympani and scala vestibuli.

The cochlea is filled with liquid: the *endolymph.* Liquids are incompressible, and when the stapes pushes the endolymph inside the scala vestibuli the liquid is forced to flow into the scala tympani through an opening called the *helicotrema.* The helicotrema connects the scala vestibuli with the scala tympani. Each of the piston-like compressions of the stapes is followed by a bulge of the membrane covering an opening—the *round window*—in the scala tympani. When the ossicles are surgically removed, as in cases of hardening of the little bones, the membrane of the round window can function as a resonant membrane, a function of the tympanic membrane.

The *basilar membrane,* which separates the scala tympani from the scala media, plays a major role in the transduction of the auditory stimulus. Békésy was the first to understand its function. Until Békésy began his experimental work it was thought—after Herman L. F. von Helmholtz (1821–1894), an influential German scientist—that the striations of the basilar membrane acted as resonators (Boring 1950). Individual resonators positioned along the basilar membrane would vibrate in unison with the frequency of the sound. Short striations at the base of the basilar membrane were thought to be respon-

sible for the detection of high-pitched sounds, while the relatively longer striations of the apex of the basilar membrane were thought to be responsible for the detection of low-frequency sounds.

Békésy used mechanical models to discern how the basilar membrane functions. He was an engineer by training, so he understood the workings of biophysical structures when the essential features of these structures were reproduced in physical models. Very early in his career, he manufactured a rubber model of the basilar membrane. He noted that the base of the basilar membrane was narrow and thick, whereas the apex, near the helicotrema, was wide and thin. How would a membrane having such features behave when vibrations of various frequencies and intensities were applied to it?

Békésy performed such experiments and noted that when mechanical oscillations were applied, a wave was generated. The peak of this wave would be located close to the base for low-frequency sound and close to the apex for high-frequency sounds. Békésy discovered that the receptors of the cochlea are activated by a traveling wave. In his lectures, Békésy would carry such a model and invite members of the audience to place an arm on top of his model to feel the movement of the wave "licking" various areas of the skin as a function of the varying frequency of the sound wave.

The *organ of Corti* sits in the basilar membrane. It is now believed that the peak of the traveling wave pushes the organ of Corti upward forcing the cilia of the hair cells to rub against the tectorial membrane. As a result of the rubbing movement of the hair cells against the tectorial membrane, the cilia are bent. Hair cells have kinocilia and several stereocilia. The cilia have directional sensitivity—a feature shared by the cells of the lateral line organs of fish, where hair cells are believed to have originated. Thus, movement in one direction is excitatory, and movement in the opposite direction is inhibitory. The mechanical stimulation of the hair cells depolarizes or hyperpolarizes the cells, creating the receptor potential.

Hair cells also have mechanical resonance. Hair cells positioned at the apex are long and flexible, whereas the hair cells of the base are shorter and relatively inflexible.

Auditory Neural Pathways

The auditory pathways consist of at least four neurons, with extensive branching to other neural cells of the brainstem and cerebellum involved in acoustic reflexes (Fig. 25.5). The *spiral ganglion*—so shaped because it follows the turns of the cochlea—contains the ganglion cell; the cells of the spiral ganglion thus receive the fibers from the hair cells. The

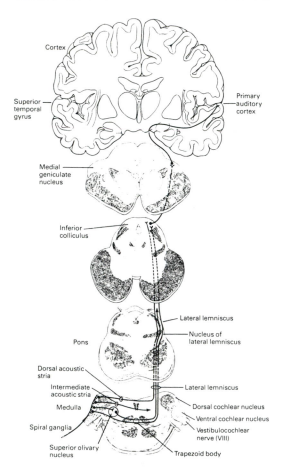

Fig. 25.5. The neural pathways of the auditory system. (From Kelly 1985.)

acoustic nerve is formed from the fibers leaving the spiral ganglion. The acoustic nerve ends in the cochlear nucleus, whose neurons are the second-order neurons in the transmission of sound information to the cerebral cortex. The cochlear nucleus has a ventral and a dorsal division. Some ascend to higher neural centers ipsilaterally (on the same side), and other fibers cross to the opposite site, synapsing with the nucleus of the superior olive. Ipsilateral and contralateral fibers synapse with neurons of the *inferior colliculus* and then with neurons of the *medial geniculate bodies,* from which they reach the auditory cortex.

The auditory neural pathways exhibit a "tonotopic" representation—ie, the spatial organization of the neural elements is such that similar sound frequencies are represented in adjacent neural areas. The neural fibers are organized in such a manner that even at cortical levels, it is always possible to tell from which region of the cochlea the sound information comes. Thus, the neural code is provided by the spatial distribution of the neural elements.

Unilateral cortical lesions do not cause deafness because of the extensive bilateral representation of the auditory pathways.

Those interested in a review of the functional organization of the neural pathways and additional references should consult Kelly (1985).

ASSESSMENT OF HEARING IMPAIRMENT

The transient and the chronic effects of noise on the human auditory system are fairly well established by now. Deficits have been characterized at the psychophysical, electrophysiological, and anatomic levels.

The Audiogram

Audiometry is performed in a sound-insulated room or portable booth by means of earphones. Hearing thresholds are determined for each ear at frequencies of 125, 250, 500, 1000, 2000, 4000, and 8000 Hz. To this octave scale, some audiologists add other sound frequencies such as 750, 1500, 3000, and 6000 Hz. Amplitude is varied, usually in 5-dB steps, and hearing thresholds are recorded as decibels above the zero level (the reference level) of the audiometer. For example, a typical threshold measurement would be 30 dB above this standard. The audiogram is the plot of the thresholds for each ear at all chosen frequencies.

During threshold determination the contralateral ear is masked with a white noise—a hissing noise having all acoustic frequencies. This is necessary because of the possibility that while the "bad" ear is being tested, the subject could still hear with the "good" ear.

Air Conduction and Bone Conduction

In the clinic, the differential diagnosis between the sensory (ie, cochlear) and neural (ie, acoustic nerve) etiology of hearing impairment is essential. Sound can be heard as a result of bone conduction. All bones—in particular the temporal bone where the cochlea is contained—conduct sounds, which ultimately reach the acoustic nerve. Should the cochlea be impaired—eg, as a result of occupational exposure to noise—sounds can still be heard as a result of bone conduction and the direct influence of sound on the acoustic nerve. When the nerve is damaged—eg, as a result of the effect of an ototoxic drug—bone conduction is lost, and hearing is profoundly deteriorated or lost. Thus, bone-conduction audiometry is sometimes required along with sound audiometry.

Conditions Affecting Auditory Thresholds

There are numerous conditions affecting the sensibility to sound. Only age and some medical conditions will be discussed. The child can hear tones as high as 20,000 Hz or more.

Our pitch sensitivity is reduced at a rate of between 50 and 100 Hz per year. There are wide individual variations in this rate of age-related decrease.

The normal rate of decrease in hearing with age makes the evaluation of the effect of neurotoxic agents and drugs on hearing difficult. From the epidemiological point of view, in the clinic, hearing thresholds are measured at a single point in time. Individual trends of hearing loss as a function of age are detected in follow-up studies performed over a number of decades, information that is rarely available. Thus, whether thresholds are reduced as a result of normal aging or as a result of noise or toxic exposure is always difficult to ascertain because these follow-up trends are not available for comparison.

There are numerous medical conditions that affect hearing. For example, hearing loss can occur as a result of diabetes. The peripheral neuropathy associated with diabetes mellitus is responsible for a number of autonomic and somatic syndromes. Progressive somatic neuritis affects sensory fibers, leading to neural and bone and articulatory changes. The typical hearing loss is described as a progressive bilateral sensory-neural deafness (ie, involving the cochlea as well as the acoustic nerve) of gradual onset that affects predominantly high frequencies and older patients.

Clinical reports seem to show that diabetes causes hearing impairment. Friedman et al. (1975), for example, studied 20 diabetic patients with peripheral neuropathy, and the results were compared with 32 age-matched controls. Although the patients had no history of hearing loss or ear disease, 11 (55%) had symmetrical hearing loss involving at least one acoustic frequency.

Diabetes causes a thickening of the capillary wall of the stria vascularis—a blood vessel in the cochlea—leading to a thickening of the vessels to 10 to 20 times normal (Taylor and Irwin 1978). However, neural changes caused by diabetes have also been suggested.

Epidemiological studies aimed at studying the interactions between diabetes and noise are inconclusive, however.

Evaluation of the Auditory System of the Child

Deafness at birth can cause mental retardation, as language cannot be acquired. Thus, assessment of suspected hearing impairment in the young child is essential.

In the child, hearing impairment is assessed by clinical and electrophysiological procedures. The blinking reflex is an unconditioned reflex—a reflex one is born with—of closing the eyes as a result of a sudden and loud noise. The suspicion that young babies do not hear is indicated by the absence of the blinking reflex. The blinking reflex can be elicited in the unborn at as early as 24 weeks of gestation and detected by the use of acoustic imaging.

Hearing impairment in the child can also be assessed by means of evoked sensory potentials as described in Chapter 5. In the normal child, ear stimulation with sounds is associated with an evoked electrical potential in the brain cortex. Failure to record auditory evoked potentials is an indication of a severe hearing impairment.

The Effect of Lead on Hearing

Blood Lead and Hearing Thresholds. Lead can cause hearing impairment in the child. Clinical studies in children performed by means of electrophysiological studies of event-related potentials—slow electrical waves in the brain cortex—seem to indicate that lead produces a change in these potentials at levels of 25 μg/dL of lead in blood.

Schwartz and Otto (1987) published a study linking an elevation of hearing threshold with elevated blood lead level in children and youth. The study was carried out during the Second National Health and Nutrition Survey (NHANES II) on samples taken to be representative of the civilian noninstitutionalized U.S. population aged from 6 months to 74 years of age. A total of 20,322 people were examined. Blood lead levels were obtained

for a subsample of 9932 also chosen to be representative of the U.S. population. Audiometric testing was conducted on a nationally representative subsample of 5717 children and youths aged 4 to 19 years. Of those, blood lead levels were available for 4519. Medical examinations included medical history, physical examination, anthropometric measurements, dietary information, laboratory tests, electrocardiograms, and radiographs.

Audiometric testing procedures were carried out in a sound-treated chamber, and tests were conducted at 500, 1000, 2000, and 4000 Hz on each ear. To prevent systematic bias, the order of testing the left and right ears was alternated between subjects. Pure-tone thresholds were determined using a modified method of limits commencing with 20 dB at 1000 Hz. Intensity was decreased in 10-dB steps until no response occurred and then was increased in 5-dB steps until response resumed. Subjects were grouped at hearing thresholds of 0 dB, 5 dB, and 10 dB, greater decibel values indicating worse hearing than lower decibel values.

The relationships between blood lead levels and hearing thresholds, age at which the child first sat up, walked, and spoke, as well as diagnosed speech impairment and hyperactivity were examined using multiple-regression analysis. Possible confounding factors included demographic characteristics of the child and parents, medical conditions, etc. Logistic multiregression procedures—described in Chapter 19—were employed because the variable "threshold impairment" is a categorical variable (0 dB, 5 dB, or 10 dB). All conclusions were drawn after possible confounding variables had been accounted for.

Blood lead levels were found to be associated with increased right and left hearing threshold at 500, 1000, 2000, and 4000 Hz. Effects persisted down to the lowest measured lead levels; an individual with a blood lead level of 20 μg/dL was 10% to 20% more likely to have an elevated hearing threshold than an individual with a blood lead level of 4 µg/dL. The most important covariates (other than lead) were family income (poorer children were more likely to have higher hearing thresholds) and race (blacks had better hearing thresholds than whites). Lead was not associated with a diagnosis of speech difficulty but was associated with a diagnosis of hyperactivity.

The Acoustic Basis of Speech Intelligibility

In psychoacoustics, speech intelligibility describes the ability to detect spoken words as a result of the acoustic characteristics of the verbal message. For example, one is able to understand a message even if all the frequencies above 3 kHz (1 kHz is 1000 Hz) are eliminated from a taped spoken message by means of acoustic filters. However, the intelligibility of the message is impossible if the lower frequencies are eliminated. Often, the difficulty an aging individual has comprehending instructions results from deficits in cognition, but the possibility of severe hearing impairment can never be ruled out.

Auditory Perception Underlies Many Psychometric Tests

Many psychometric tests assume that the subject, patient, or defendant (or plaintiff) has normal hearing. It is essential that the examiner make a quick evaluation of whether there is any suspicion of hearing loss before the administration of a test.

Simple examinations of the status of the auditory system can be performed, such as with the ticking of a mechanical watch. The watch is progressively removed from the subject's ear until its ticking ceases to be perceived. Unilateral traumatic rupture of the tympanic membrane is not unusual among industrial workers. Other simple tests may involve the utilization of the hissing sound produced by rubbing the index finger against

the thumb. When there is doubt, a thorough evaluation by a professional hearing specialist is required.

Auditory Perception and Cognition Are Intimately Related

Most of us are constantly attuned to our auditory environment. Quick or unexpected noise elicits the orienting reflex, which is the tendency to turn the head in the direction of the sound. However, a hobbyist, a scientist, or a musician deeply involved in his/her thoughts may not hear trivial auditory changes in the surroundings. Some severely disturbed individuals—such as autistic children or schizophrenics—show total apathy even to the loudest noises. Finally, people who are non-English speakers or who do not have a total command of the language may not react to an auditory message born English speakers do. These factors are important and must be taken into account in the psychometric evaluation of the foreign-born.

Some auditory-based perceptual characteristics are affected by age. For example, the "cocktail party phenomenon" is severely affected in people of advanced age. The cocktail party phenomenon is our ability to follow the conversation of a friend while hearing other voices simultaneously. It is not clear how the nervous system accomplishes this feat. Historically, there have been alternative explanations, some favoring the primary sensory functions of the cochlea and some invoking cognitive mechanisms. The cocktail party phenomenon is the auditory counterpart of the phenomenon of figure–ground relationships known to exist in vision, touch, and in the chemical senses.

CONCLUSIONS

The possibility that occupational neurotoxic agents may impair hearing has been raised several times during the past decade, particularly in connection with occupational solvent exposure, but incontrovertible evidence is rare. The main body of relevant literature originates from reports of isolated clinical cases.

There are numerous suggestions that possible synergistic effects exist compounding the effects of industrial solvents and of noise on hearing loss. As a working hypothesis, this suggestion is interesting. But at present, the solid clinical, epidemiological, and statistical foundations that are needed to support such speculations are lacking (Mills 1985).

REFERENCES

Boring, EG (1950) A History of Experimental Psychology. New York: Appleton–Century-Crofts.

Friedman, SA, Shulman, RH, and Weiss, S (1975) Hearing and diabetic neuropathy. Arch Intern Med 135:573–576.

Hybels, RL (1979) Drug toxicity of the inner ear. Med Clin North Am 63(2):309–319.

Kelly, JP (1985) Auditory system. In Principles of Neural Science, ER Kandel and JH Schwartz (eds) pp. 396–408. New York: Elsevier.

Kryter, KD (1985) The Effects of Noise on Man, 2nd ed. New York: Academic Press.

Marks, LE (1974) Sensory Processes. New York: Academic Press.

Mills, JH (1985) A review of environmental factors affecting hearing. In Toxicology of the Eye, Ear, and Other Special Senses, AW Hayes (ed) pp 231–247. New York: Raven Press.

Prosen, CA and Stebbins, WC (1980) Ototoxicity. In Experimental and Clinical Neurotoxicology, PS Spencer and HH Schaumburg (eds) pp. 62–76. Baltimore: Williams & Wilkins.

Schwartz, J and Otto, D (1987) Blood lead, hearing thresholds, and neurobehavioral development in children and youth. Arch Environ Res 42(2):153–160.

Stebbins, WC and Rudy, MC (1978) Behavioral ototoxicology. Environ Health Perspect 26:43–51.

Stevens, SS (1975) Psychophysics: Introduction to its Perceptual, Neural and Social Prospects. New York: John Wiley & Sons.

Taylor, IG and Irwin, J (1978) Some audiological aspects of diabetes mellitus. J Laryngol 92:99–113.

SUGGESTED READINGS

Baker, SR and Lilly, DJ (1977) Hearing loss from acute carbon monoxide poisoning. Ann Otolaryngol 86:232–328.

Békésy, G von (1960) Experiments in Hearing. New York: McGraw-Hill.

Békésy, G von (1967) Sensory Inhibition. Princeton, NJ: Princeton University Press.

Bergholtz, LM and Odkvist, LM (1984) Audiological findings in solvent exposed workers. Acta Otolaryngol 412:109–110.

Berlin, CI (ed)(1984) Hearing Science. San Diego, CA: College-Hill Press.

Birnholtz, JC and Benacerraf, BR (1983) The development of human fetal hearing. Science 222:516–518.

Department of Labor, Occupational Health Administration (1981) Occupational noise exposure: Hearing conservation amendment. Federal Register Jan 16, pp. 4078–4179.

Department of Labor, Occupational Health Administration (1983) Occupational noise exposure: Hearing conservation amendment. Federal Register, March 8, pp. 9738–9785.

Fawcett, HH (1961) Speech transmission through respiratory protective devices. Am Ind Hyg Assoc J 21:170–174.

Hodgson, MJ, Talbott, E, Helmkamp, JC, et al. (1987) Diabetes, noise exposure and hearing loss. J Occup Med 29(7):576–579.

Hudspeth, AJ (1985) The cellular basis of hearing: The biophysics of hair cells. Science 230:745–752.

Hulse, SH and Dooling, RJ (1989) Complex Acoustic Perception: The Comparative Psychology of Audition. Hillsdale, NJ: Lawrence Erlbaum Associates.

Miller, JJ (1985) Handbook of Ototoxicity. Boca Raton, FL: CRC Press.

Møller, AR (1975) Noise as a health hazard. Ambio 4:6–13.

Møller, AR and Jannetta, PJ (1981) Compound action potential recorded intracranially from the auditory nerve in man. Exp Neurol 74:862–874.

Moody, DB and Stebbins, WC (1985) Detection of the effects of toxic substances on the auditory system by behavioral methods. In Nervous System Toxicology, CL Mitchell (ed). New York: Raven Press.

Nauton, RF and Fernandez, C (eds)(1978) Evoked Electrical Activity in the Auditory Nervous System. New York: Academic Press.

Peterson, EA, Augenstein, JS, Tanis, DC, et al. (1981) Noise raises blood pressure without impairing auditory sensitivity. Science 211:1450–1452.

Romand, R (ed)(1983) Development of Auditory and Vestibular Systems. New York: Academic Press.

Rosellini, L (1981) Noise control loses its priority, and

expert sees his job vanish. *The New York Times,* May 27.

Sullivan, MJ (1986) *Ototoxicity of Toluene in Rats.* Doctoral Thesis, University of Michigan Microfilms, Ann Arbor.

Schwartz, J and Otto, D (1987) Blood lead, hearing thresholds and neurobehavioural development in children and youth. *Arch Environ Health* 42:153–160.

US Department of Health, Education and Welfare, National Institute of Occupational Safety and Health (1972) *Occupational Exposure to Noise.* Washington, DC: DHEW.

Welch, BL and Welch, AS (1970) *Physiological Effects of Noise.* New York: Plenum Press.

Worthington, EL, Lunin, LF, Heath, M, et al. (1973) *Index-Handbook of Ototoxic Agents.* Baltimore, MD: The Johns Hopkins Press.

26

The Visual System

The toxic properties of chemical agents that might affect the eye and visual perception have long been recognized. This is in part because of the value we ascribe to vision—the loss of vision is what we fear most. *Ophthalmic toxicology* is a catch-all term that refers to the study of the effects of toxic agents and drugs on the eyes, their receptors, and their associated neural pathways.

Knowledge and characterization of the effects of industrial chemical agents and drugs on the eye and visual perception have been compiled in comprehensive sources since the 19th century. An early book on the subject was published by Galezowski in 1878. Several other classical treatises followed: Uhthoff (1911), Lewin and Guillery (1913), Grant (1974), and Frauenfelder (1982).

A review of the functional organization of the visual pathways follows. Those interested in an up-to-date treatment of the subject are encouraged to consult the chapters by Bayley and Gouras (The Retina and Phototransduction), Kelly (Anatomy of the Central Visual Pathway), Kandel (Processing of Form and Movement in the Visual System), and Gouras (Color Vision) in Kandel and Schwartz's *Principles of Neural Science* (1985).

FUNCTIONAL ORGANIZATION

Figure 26.1 shows the gross functional organization of the visual neural pathways. The following anatomic structures can be identified: the *retina,* containing the photoreceptors; the *visual pathways,* including the optic nerve, the optic chiasma, the optic tract, the lateral geniculate bodies, the superior culliculus and pretectum, and the visual cortex; and the anatomic structures responsible for the control of eye movements, without which vision would be impossible.

Visual Receptor Processes

There are five kinds of neurons that are present in the retina: receptor cells, bipolar cells, horizontal cells, amacrine cells, and ganglion cells. There are two types of receptor cells, *rods* and *cones.* These are called photoreceptors or phototransductors because of their property of translating light into a neural code. The rods, the more numerous photoreceptors, are located in the periphery of the retina and are more sensitive to light than the cones; the latter are concentrated in the center of

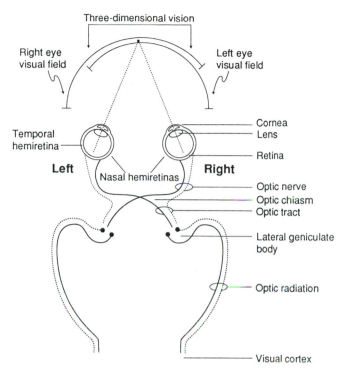

Fig. 26.1. Neural pathways of the visual system.

the retina, the fovea. Color vision is possible because of the cones.

The basic biochemical process underlying the transformation of light into a neural code is now fairly well characterized. These processes differ somewhat in rods and cones.

Rods contain rhodopsin, a photosensitive chemical capable of absorbing photons, arranged in the outer segment of the photoreceptor in one single layer. Rhodopsin is bleached by light to form retinal and opsin. Retinal is an aldehyde of vitamin A and is responsible for absorbing light. Opsin is a protein.

When hit by photons, retinal undergoes a reversible transformation—often referred to as a cycle—from the 11-cis (an isomer) to the all-trans form. Exposure to an intense light breaks down most of the rhodopsin to the all-trans form. For example, after one has been outside for a number of hours on a particularly bright summer day, most of the rhodopsin is transformed into its all-trans form. Immediately after one moves into the

dark, the all-trans retinal is reisomerized and transformed back into the 11-cis form, which is photosensitive.

There are two forms of visual adaptation. Photochemical adaptation is explained by changes in the chemical composition of the rhodopsin as the level of light increases or decreases. There is also a neural adaptation of the photoreceptor, in which the rate of response of the receptors drops when exposed to light of constant brightness. Neural adaptation occurs in a shorter period of time than photochemical adaptation.

Cones also contain the protein opsin (called cone opsin) and the light-absorbing molecule 11-cis retinal. It is now fairly well established that the retinas of primates contain three types of the colorless protein opsin. The sensitivity of the retinal molecule to light depends on the type of opsin to which retinal is bound. As will be seen below, color vision is possible in part because of these three types of molecular configurations.

The mechanisms by which light is transformed into a neural code is now beginning to be understood. Briefly, the structural changes taking place *in rhodopsin in the rods and cones when exposed to light cause closure of sodium ion (Na$^+$) channels. The Na$^+$ channels are normally open when the eye is in the dark. The photoreceptors are known to produce an inward continuous flow of Na$^+$, that is, from the outer segment to the synaptic terminal. Light is inhibitory. A single molecule of rhodopsin when stimulated can close several hundred Na$^+$ channels. This is thought to be accomplished by means of a mechanism of amplification involving the enzyme phosphodiesterase. Light produces inhibitory effects in the receptor: it produces a hyperpolarization of the receptor. Dark does the opposite. Dark is excitatory: it depolarizes the receptor.*

Receptor cells synapse with bipolar cells, which in turn synapse with ganglion cells. The ganglion cells relay visual information from the retina to the lateral geniculate body, the superior colliculus, and other brainstem nuclei.

Two types of *interneurons* modulate information originating from the photoreceptor and transmitted to the bipolar and ganglion cells: the *horizontal cells* are located between the receptor and the bipolar cells; the *amacrine* cells are located between the bipolar cells and the ganglion cells.

The photoreceptors and these four types of cells give rise to three clearly identifiable layers of the retina: the outer layer, formed exclusively by photoreceptors (rods and cones); the inner layer, formed by bipolar, horizontal, and amacrine cells; and the ganglion cell layer, formed exclusively by ganglion cells.

Two facts on the relationship between photoreceptors and neurons are noteworthy. First, rods and cones do not generate action potentials, but, because of their physical proximity to the bipolar cells, photoreceptors can nonetheless influence the bipolar cells' rate of depolarization. Second, the synapses between photoreceptors and bipolar cells do not have a threshold for transmitter release. Rather, neurotransmitters are constantly present in the synapses existing between the photoreceptor and the bipolar cells. The neurotransmitter substance is thought to be the amino acid glutamate.

The cones synapse with two types of bipolar cells: *on-center* and *off-center cells*. The on-center cells are inhibited by the neurotransmitters, whereas the off-center cells are excited by the neurotransmitters. In addition, the two types of neurons are morphologically distinct.

Although the vast majority of the synapses in the retina are chemical—that is, function via a neurotransmitter—some of them are electrical synapses. These are called gap junctions. In a gap junction, the electrical messages pass from a cell directly into another cell without the aid of a chemical messenger.

The horizontal cells are responsible for sharpening visual edges. For example, when a white vertical bar is placed against a gray bar, in the place where the white meets the gray, white is seen whiter and gray darker. This visual phenomenon is called *Mach bands* and for many years was thought to be a visual illusion. Now it is understood that these bands are produced by the horizontal cells (Ratliff 1965).

Horizontal cells change the polarization of the bipolar cells by modifying the receptor fields of a neuron. The receptor field is the area of the retina that, when stimulated, produces a change in the electrical activity of the neuron. The amacrine cells enhance the response at the center of the receptor field and decrease the response at the periphery of the receptor field. Luminance gradients, such as those that form the contours of objects, are then enhanced by this neural network.

Ganglion cells are of three types. The W cells have small bodies and large dendrites; these cells project into the superior colliculus and are involved in head and eye movements. The X cells have medium-sized cell bodies; these cells participate in high-acuity vision, the ability to see detail. The Y cells have the largest bodies; the cells project to a greater extent to the lateral geniculate body and to a lesser extent into the superior colliculus.

The Visual Pathway from the Retina to the Thalamus and the Visual Cortex

The axons of the W, X, and Y cells exit the retina converging first at the optic disk. In the *optic nerve,* they become myelinated, and in the optic chiasma the nerves of the left and right eyes meet (see Fig. 26.1). Fibers from the nasal portion of the retina (that close to the nose) cross to the other side of the midline. Fibers from the temporal portion of the retina (that close to the temples) do not cross. The temporal fibers of the right eye and the nasal fibers of the left eye form the right *optic tract.* The temporal fibers of the left eye and the nasal fibers of the right eye form the left optic tract.

The fibers of the optic tract have a relay station in the *lateral geniculate body.* In primates, the lateral geniculate body has six layers numbered 1 to 6. Fibers from the contralateral nasal retina relay in layers 6, 4, and 1; fibers from the ipsilateral side end in layers 5, 3, and 2. From the lateral geniculate body, fibers project to the *primary visual cortex,* also called the striate cortex, located in the occipital lobe. The axons that form this projection, called the *optic radiation,* make up an easily recognized anatomic bundle of fibers. Fibers from the inferior parts of the retina make a loop inside the temporal lobe called the *Meyer's loop.* The striate cortex has layers of fibers and cells, each one receiving specific projections.

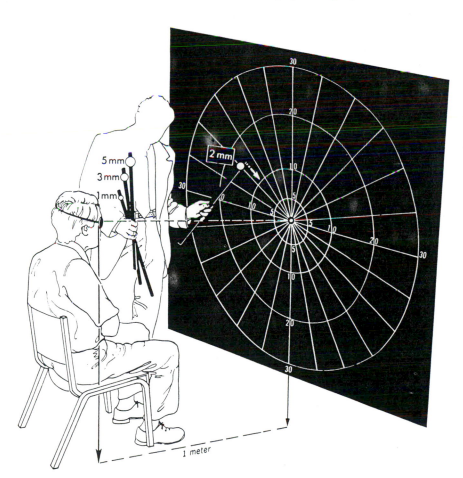

Fig. 26.2. Assessment of the visual field. (From Anderson 1982.)

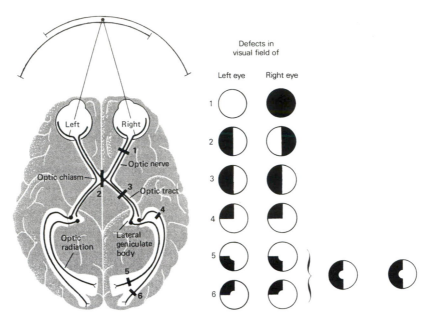

Fig. 26.3. Patterns of alteration of the visual field caused by lesions at various levels of the visual pathway.

Black areas in the visual field diagrams (right) indicate loss of vision. (From Kandel and Schwartz 1985.)

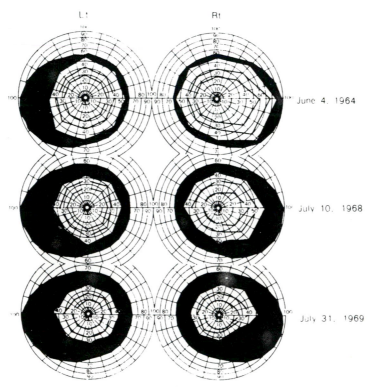

Fig. 26.4. Progressive constriction of the visual field in a patient affected by Minamata disease. Black areas

indicate loss of vision. (Courtesy of Professor K. Iwata, reproduced by permission.)

The *visual field* is the field of view seen by the two eyes without moving the head. Figure 26.2 shows one method of assessing visual field in a subject. Figure 26.3 is a simplified view of the alterations in the visual fields produced by lesions in the optic pathway. It is important to understand this pattern of visual alterations for the differential diagnosis of neurological diseases. Neurotoxic agents rarely produce *homonymous hemianopsia*—half visual fields of identical configuration in both eyes (3 in Fig. 26.3)—or incomplete (or quadratic) field defects. *Tunnel vision,* in which the peripheral area of the visual field is lost and foveal vision is spared, may be seen in people poisoned by either methanol or methylmercury (Fig. 26.4).

The Ocular Effects of Methyl Alcohol Poisoning

Case reports and epidemics of methyl alcohol (methanol) poisoning are often reported in the literature. For example, an epidemic of methyl alcohol poisoning involving 320 persons occurred in Atlanta in October 20, 1951. A large quantity of bootleg whiskey containing 35% methyl alcohol and 15% ethyl alcohol had been distributed in that city, and people sought medical care attributable to this mixture. Twenty-four persons died before or shortly after reaching the hospital and 13 died in the medical wards, making a total of 37 deaths. The article by Cooper and collaborators published in 1952 contained a detailed account of the methyl alcohol epidemic as well as a reference to a Christmas Eve cocktail party in 1946 responsible for 12 deaths from similar causes.

The symptoms of acute methyl alcohol poisoning developed within 18 to 48 hours after ingestion, but in a few instances transitory symptoms were observed within an hour. The patients complained of visual disturbances, weakness, abdominal pains, nausea and vomiting, headache, dizziness, and shortness of breath. Here, only the ocular manifestations of methyl alcohol poisoning are de-

scribed in detail, as described by Benton and Calhoun in 1953.

The most striking symptom was visual disturbance. The initial visual symptoms ranged from photophobia and spots before the eyes to complete blindness. There was no close correlation between the severity of the symptoms and the quantity of methyl alcohol consumed. Many patients complained of whitish or grayish misty vision. Some experienced full recovery of vision during the first hour of treatment with intravenous alkaline fluids.

The typical alteration of the visual field was a scotoma of considerably density. Frequently, this type of scotoma was incomplete, arched above or around the fixation point, and did not impair central visual acuity. After 2 or 3 months, profound alterations of the visual field occurred with severe peripheral constriction of most of the visual field.

The Visual Reflex Center of the Superior Colliculus and the Pretectum

The superior colliculus receives the input from the retina and from the visual cortex. The *tectospinal tract* is formed by axons that have their cells in the superior colliculus. These axons cross the midline and descend to an area adjacent to the third ventricle. This tract is involved in the reflex control of the head, neck, and eye movements. Turning the head and eyes toward the source of a visual stimulus is a reflex mediated by this tract. The tectopontine axons link the superior colliculus with nuclei of the pons. The tract relays visual information to the cerebellum.

The pretectal area mediates pupillary light reflexes. When light is shone in one eye, the pupil of that eye constricts, and the pupil of the other eye also constricts. The pupillary constriction of the two eyes as the result of shining light into one eye is called *consensual response.*

Axons originating in the pretectal area project to preganglionic parasympathetic neurons that innervate the ciliary ganglion. The postsynaptic neurons that control the smooth muscles of the pupil's sphincter originate in the ciliary ganglion.

The pupil can be chronically dilated or constricted as a result of neurotoxic agents and drugs. Both eyes are equally affected, and the most common disturbance is *mydriasis*— pupil dilation. Mydriasis is observed as a side effect of numerous drugs (eg, antispasmodics, antiparkinsons, antidepressants, tranquilizers, central nervous system stimulants), botulism, plant poisoning (eg, belladonna, horse chestnut, arum, nightshade, snakeweed), mushroom poisoning, chemical substances (eg, carbon monoxide, DDT, tetramethyl butanediamide), snakebite, etc. *Mioisis*—pupil constriction—is also observed as a side effect of drugs (eg, analgesics, narcotics, antihypertensives), plant poisoning (marijuana smoke), mushroom poisoning, agricultural pesticides (eg, Parathion, Meta-Systox), chemical weapons (Sarin, Tabun), scorpion venom, etc. A good source for a detailed review of pupillary changes caused by poisoning is Alexandridis (1985).

The absence of pupillary light reflexes is seen during massive damage to the brain and in toxin-induced coma, for example.

Visual Perception Cannot Occur without Eye Movements

Vision is an active phenomenon. We see after scanning the world around us, locating objects in our environment, focusing on targets of particular interest, and tracking moving objects. Experiments performed by Pritchard in the 1950s (Pritchard 1961) showed that if a miniature slide projector is attached to the cornea and patterns are projected onto the retina, the images disappear very quickly. That is why we do not see the blood vessels of our own retinas.

Vision cannot occur without eye movements. At rest, the eyes exhibit *physiological nystagmus,* quick and small-amplitude movements of the eye. Retinal images do not fade because of the presence of these almost imperceptible eye movements.

The eyes can be moved horizontally from side to side and vertically up and down. The eyeballs can also rotate around an anterior–posterior axis. Eye movements are controlled by three pairs of muscles: the lateral and medial recti, the superior and inferior oblique and the superior and inferior recti.

Eye movements are controlled by a system that contracts some ocular muscles at the time others are relaxed. The small muscles that move the eyes are controlled by the oculomotor nuclei of the midbrain, nuclei that in turn are controlled by input from the superior colliculus, the cerebellum, the vestibular system, and the cerebral cortex. This system is particularly vulnerable to the effects of neurotoxic agents and psychotropic drugs. Some forms of dizziness and, in severe cases, vertigo might be a manifestation of the effects of toxic agents on the oculomotor system. In these cases, the visual fields apparently move as the result of the retina's passive movement. Double vision, which occurs after moderate or advanced stages of alcohol consumption, for example, results from the disrupting effects of ethanol on the neural pathways that control the mechanisms of eye convergence. (Vergent eye movements are those that allow the focusing of the two eyes on a single object.)

It has been recognized that five separate types of control systems keep the fovea on visual targets:

1. Saccadic eye movements
2. Smooth pursuit movements
3. Vestibulooculomotor reflexes
4. Optokinetic nystagmus
5. Vergence eye movements

All five share the same effector pathways.

Saccadic Eye Movements.   A saccade is an extremely fast movement of the eye responsible for bringing the target to the fovea. Human saccades can occur at speeds as high as 700° of visual angle per second. The system controlling saccadic eye movements computes both the retinal position of the visual target and the position of the eye.

How saccadic eye movements are accomplished is still not completely understood. The nervous system is constantly fed information about the position of the eye. This information, called corollary discharge, allows us to see the world as stationary in spite of the movements of our eyes, head, and body. If one closes one eye with one hand and presses gently with a finger the side of the other eye, the visual scene moves as a result of the finger pressure. This happens as a result of the failure by the oculomotor system to collect the information that the system itself generates.

Saccadic eye movements can be recorded by means of special recording equipment. In Chapter 6 a technique for recording eye movement by means of an infrared system is described.

It has been shown that alcohol effectively reduces the speed of the saccades (Franck and Kuhlo 1970). Saccades are also altered by mercury (Tsutsui 1980). In Chapter 24 a reference is made to an epidemiological study in which eye movement was used as a subclinical indicator of lead neurotoxicity (Glickman et al. 1984). The results indicated that workers exposed to inorganic lead showed a decrease in saccadic accuracy and an increase in overshoots compared to controls. In addition, saccade accuracy was negatively correlated with both blood lead levels and zinc protoporphyrin levels.

Smooth Pursuit Movements. Smooth pursuit eye movements keep the fovea on the visual target once the target is located. In the clinic, this system is examined by asking the patient to follow the movement of the examiner's finger from side to side. Some laboratories of clinical neurology have special stimulation and recording equipment to examine the status of this system. The examiner's finger is replaced by a mechanically driven visual target that moves from side to side with controllable frequency and amplitude. In normal subjects, a recording of such movements is very close to a sinusoid. In patients suffering from neurological disorders of the oculomotor system a disrupted pattern of drifts and flicks is observed. Mercury poisoning produces such patterns.

Vestibulooculomotor Reflexes. The vestibular system, particularly that portion controlled by the otolithic organs, stabilizes the eye against changes in head position. In a normal subject, the passive tilting of the head from side to side is accompanied by rotations of the eyeball that compensate to a certain extent for the tilting of the head. The rotational movements of the eye can be easily observed by means of specially designed magnifying glasses such as the Fresnel glasses.

Other vestibulooculomotor reflexes are initiated by the semicircular ducts. The physiological stimulus for the activation of these reflexes is a change in the speed of the head movements. Head accelerations occurring in any spatial plane are accompanied by predictable movements of the eyes. Eye movements can also be elicited by changes of the temperature of the ear.

Optokinetic Nystagmus. Nystagmus is a repetitive movement of the eyes. Optokinetic nystagmus: is present when the eyes attempt to follow a moving visual target. Two types of movements complete a cycle of optokinetic nystagmus: the slow and the fast phase of eye movements. The speed of the slow phase is roughly proportional to that of the moving target. A quick saccade to the opposite side—the return or quick phase of the nystamus—terminates the cycle.

Optokinetic nystagmus is mediated by many neural structures, both visual and oculomotor. Thus, an examination of its intactness is always part of a comprehensive neurological examination. In the clinic, the examiner places the patient inside a rotating drum having vertical stripes. Eye movements are recorded by means of electrooculographic procedures.

Vergence Eye Movements. Depth perception is possible because of the presence of two eyes. (However, there are also powerful monocular cues of depth as, for example, visual texture.) As the target moves toward or away from the subject, the eyes converge or diverge to maintain the target in the fovea. This system works in close association with pupil and lens accommodation reflexes.

Color Vision

Color perception is achieved by a neural system, often described as a "computer," that analyzes the physical parameters of the light reflected by objects. The system is said to perform an "abstraction" of visual information. But "abstraction" has no cognitive connotations here.

The human retina is sensitive to light wavelengths in the range of 400 to 700 nanometers (nm). This range covers the perception of the blue, green, yellow, orange, and red portion of the spectrum. Studies performed early in the 19th century suggested the existence of three types of cones responsible for color perception. This view has been confirmed by the demonstration of three different pigments in the cones. The rods do not detect color.

The outer segments of the human cone photoreceptors absorb different spectra of light: short waves (S) strongly contribute to the perception of blue; middle-ranged waves (M) strongly contribute to the perception of green; long waves (L) strongly contribute to the perception of red. Single cones cannot "see" colors. Targets that are very small—and presumably perceived by single cones—are colorless. Rather, color perception depends on the integration of outputs of several cones.

In its simplest form, a minimum output of two cones is required for color perception to occur. If the output of cones tuned for optimal reception of short wavelengths is greater than the output tuned for the optimal reception of higher wavelengths, the object will be seen as blue. On the other hand, if an object reflects all wavelengths in equal amounts, the object will be seen as white.

Alteration or deficits in color perception can be genetic or acquired. Neurotoxic agents and drugs can produce alterations in color perception called acquired *achromatopsia*.

From the subjective point of view, color has three semi-independent dimensions: hue, saturation, and brightness. The *hue* of a color is what gives the color its quality: eg, blue, yellow, or red. Psychophysical experiments have demonstrated that about 200 different colors can easily be distinguished, although we do not have names for all of them. The *saturation* of a color is that amount of black or white a given hue contains. If white is added to red, the color will appear pink; if, on the other hand, black is added, the red changes to a deep red resembling burgundy wine. The *brightness* of a color is given by its intensity and is roughly proportional to the energy of the source. All color television sets, for example, have a knob for changing the brightness of the color. By manipulating this knob, the quality of the color can be changed; one notices that as the intensity changes, the quality of the colors also changes.

Hue, saturation, and brightness are interrelated. Permutations of the three dimensions of color permit the perception of about two million different colors (500 gradations of brightness times 200 gradations of hue times 20 gradations of saturation).

Color perception is achieved when *trichromacy*—the ability to detect all color by means of three primary colors—and a color opponent process are integrated. *Color opponency* is a concept derived from Hering's theory of vision, which proposes that green antagonizes red, blue antagonizes yellow, and white antagonizes black (Gouras 1985).

It is currently thought that color perception and form perception might be mediated by different pathways. There are both clinical observations and anatomic and electrophys-iological studies that seem to support this view.

VISUAL PERCEPTION

Our understanding of the neural basis of visual perception has changed substantially over the past 20 years. Many of the abstracting functions that occur in normal visual perception and were thought to be performed at higher levels of the brain—particularly the cerebral cortex—are now known to be performed at the retinal level. In consulting original sources, alert readers will notice that human neurotoxicological studies are often performed disregarding advances in the neurosciences and even standard practices of clinical neurology. This is regrettable because many areas of human visual perception that may be affected by neurotoxic agents still remain virtually unexplored. Many of the facets of human visual perception were already well characterized more than a century ago. It is possible that when the integration of human neurotoxicology and the neurosciences is finally achieved in the future, many obscure laboratory curiosities might turn out to have important assessment and even diagnostic value in neurotoxicology.

At this early stage in the development of neurotoxicology, it is essential to refer to key principles of human visual testing as well as the methods of clinical neurology of the visual system that are used for detecting brain damage. Two principles will be discussed: masking and loading. *Masking* is an increased threshold for perception or a decrease in the subjective intensity of a stimulus as a result of the simultaneous presence of another stimulus that inhibits it. *Loading* is a "weight" added to a visual or other sensory stimulus that makes its detection more difficult. These two principles share the common property of making visual tasks more challenging. "Challenge" is an important test attribute in the assessment of people who exhibit subclinical manifestations of neurotoxin-induced illness.

Visual Masking

Visual masking and visual loading are both expressions of the same fundamental perceptual process. In our daily life we do not see squares, triangles, or circles. We see people, houses, trees, or mountains. Simple geometric figures are laboratory simplifications of visual stimuli. These simplifications are necessary in order to study perceptual variables experimentally, one at a time. What we miss in this process is the fact that what we actually see in practice is markedly influenced by the surroundings, sometimes called field effects. These field effects can make perception either less effective—ie, create inhibitory influences—or more effective. By masking and loading, one can effectively challenge the subject's visual system. Thus, the importance of these principles: we can study how subjects acutely or chronically affected by neurotoxic agents respond to those challenges.

In 1921 Rubin proposed the distinction between "figure" and "ground" in perception, and since that time there has been a vast literature on the phenomenon of figure–ground relationships. The selection process involved is a basic perceptual mechanism occurring in all sensory channels: vision, audition, skin senses, etc. Gestalt psychologists (Wertheimer 1912; Köhler 1929; Koffka 1935) used a variety of perceptual tasks in humans and animals to demonstrate the generality of this perceptual mechanism.

During the same and later periods, neurologists such as Gottschaldt (1926), Goldstein (1942), and Morris B. Bender (1952) devised ingenious perceptual tests to challenge the visual system in order to unveil subtle brain dysfunction hithertofore hidden during neurological examinations. Many of these tests were designed to evaluate distortions in the perception of figure–ground relationships. One of these tests, the Gottschaldt test, consists of a test figure presented either alone or within different geometric patterns. The subject's task is to detect the test figure in each of the different background configurations.

Unfortunately, the wealth of knowledge accumulated in the study of brain damage during World War II (Teuber 1960; Teuber et al. 1951; Teuber and Weinstein 1956; Battersby et al. 1953; Newcombe 1969) has not yet been transferred to the testing of people exposed to neurotoxic agents at the workplace or in the environment at large. The development of the Embedded Figures test based on the figure–ground principles (discussed below) was an early attempt to create a bridge

Hidden Pictures
Squirrel House

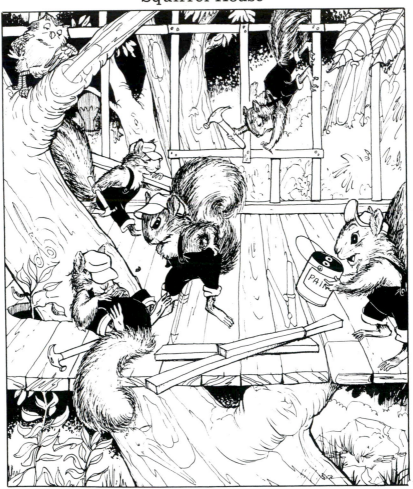

In this big picture find the umbrella, scissors, clothespin, hen, arrow, baseball bat, hot dog, pelican, mushroom, horse's head, shoe, book, vase, sheep dog, and trowel.

Fig. 26.5. An example of hidden pictures game from a children's magazine; this has potential as an Embedded Figures test. (Reproduced by permission of *Highlights for Children*.)

between classical neuropsychological research and clinical neurotoxicology.

The Embedded Figures Test.

The test of the embedded figures (Valciukas and Singer 1982) was developed for the evaluation of adults suspected of suffering from chronic or acute exposure to neurotoxic agents in the environment or the workplace. It was inspired by similar tests that have historically been developed for the evaluation of minimal brain damage. These classical tests—meant to be used for patients suffering traumatic brain injuries—were found by the author to be nonchallenging for workers whose brain functions might be affected but who were "normal" enough to be able to go to work and to fulfill their daily responsibilities.

For a review of the pathology of figure–ground relationships in the child see Teuber (1960); for an historical account of the test see Corkin (1979).

The construction of the test plates in the Embedded Figures test proceeded as follows. The outlines of familiar objects were traced from illustrations from children's books. Each plate, 8½ × 11 inches and containing the outlines of 10 different objects, was produced in the following manner. A photocopy of the first outline of the group of 10 was placed on top of the paper tray that fed paper to a photocopying machine, while the second outline rested on the photocopying area. Then the second outline was copied onto the first. As a result of this process, the collecting tray contained a new pattern consisting of two overlapping outlines, which in turn was placed on top of the paper tray. Then the third outline was placed on the photocopying area and copied onto the two overlapping outlines, thus forming three overlapping outlines. The process was continued until 10 overlapping outlines were obtained. Figure 4.5 (Chapter 4) illustrates the four plates currently in use. Administration instruction and scoring procedures are found in Valciukas and Singer (1982).

A children's version of the Embedded Figures test needs to be developed. The version developed by Ghent (1956) is meant for children with brain damage and as a result is too easy for the normal child. Many puzzles that appear in children's magazines have good potential; Figure 26.5 is one example.

The Tangled Lines test (Rey 1964) measures similar functions (Fig. 26.6). The subject is presented with 16 horizontal superimposed labyrinths, and has to follow each labyrinth visually—that is, without the aid of

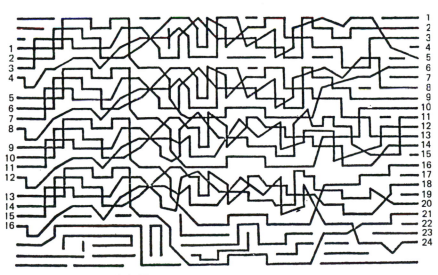

Fig. 26.6.   Rey's Tangled Lines test.

hands—starting from the left and indicate its ending on the right.

The Bender–Gestalt Test.

This test, created by Dr. Loretta Bender, consists of the presentation and reproduction of nine cards containing drawings inspired by the Gestalt theory of visual perception. In the correct reproduction of the figures, the relationship between the components of the designs (eg, a circle attached to a square), periodic groupings, overlapping of two figures, etc must be recognized. Although this test requires drawing, the results are not heavily dependent on motor abilities. Education is an important factor. The test has been widely used in neuropsychology and in clinical neurotoxicology. The major drawback of the test is the scoring, which requires interpretation by the test administrator. There have been attempts to quantify the test (Lacks 1984).

Intrasensory Visual Loading

There are two kinds of loading: intrasensory (eg, within the visual system) and intersensory (ie, joint effects of other sensory systems). Visual intrasensory loading can be achieved by:

- Decreasing the luminance of the stimulus
- Increasing the complexity of the stimulus
- Changing the target eccentricity (ie, placing the target away from the fovea)
- Reducing the exposure time
- Delaying the presentation of the visual stimulus
- Creating interference with other visual stimuli

The influence of the luminance of the stimulus on visual perception has been known for several generations. To put it simply, the lower the stimulus luminance the more difficult a visual task becomes. There are numerous neurophysiological mechanisms that explain this relationship. In part, it is because the cones are involved in the perception of detail at high luminance levels. At reduced luminance levels, such as when driving at night in the countryside, visual perception is mediated by rods. Rods are extremely sensitive to light but cannot detect detail.

Loading by **reduction of stimulus luminance** has been effectively used to explore the effects of lead on scotopic vision in the monkey (Bowman and Bushnell 1980). (Scotopic vision is that performed at low illumination, after the eyes have become dark-adapted.) In human as well as animal research, one needs to become familiar with the numerous genetic, metabolic, and acquired conditions that may lead to changes in scotopic vision, particularly lack of vitamin A. A claim that lead has an effect on scotopic vision, for example, can legitimately be made only when nutritional factors leading to avitaminosis can be ruled out.

An **increase in stimulus complexity** is an effective way to achieve visual loading. The literature generated by Morris Bender and his collaborators in the use of stimulus complexity for the detection of minimal brain damage is staggering. Stimulus complexity is difficult to define. A drawing of a square is a "simple" stimulus, whereas a tree is a "complex" stimulus. Psychometric tests used in environmental and occupational neurotoxicology are based on "simple," often geometric, visual stimuli. With the advent of desktop publishing by means of personal computers, the possibility of access to banks of "icons"—complex visual stimuli found in everyday life—are now possible.

The influence of **target eccentricity** on perception is not fully appreciated in neurotoxicological testing. The use of critical fusion frequency (CFF, the frequency of a flickering light at which the light appears to be continuous) for assessment of the neurotoxic effects of mercury is a case in point. An effective method for testing the subclinical manifestations of mercury toxicity is likely to be the determination of CFF with point targets in the periphery of the visual field. In advanced stages of mercury intoxication, "tunnel vision" (foveal vision) can be observed. **Foveal**

CFF has been dropped from the arsenal of potentially useful neurotoxicological techniques because it is claimed to be insensitive. Yet, there is an abundance of information on the value of **peripheral** CFF as a subclinical indicator of minimal brain damage.

Reduced exposure time and **delayed stimulus presentation** are two of the most important ways "time" can be manipulated to produce visual loading. As a rule, reduced exposure time is a powerful visual loading factor leading to a proportional decrease in the detection of a visual stimulus. But, because visual reaction time increases with age, the role of the examinee's reaction time needs to be taken into account. People in their eighties can perform the most difficult designs of the Block Design test if enough time is allowed. The fact that 120 seconds is allocated to reproduce the most difficult designs is an example of loading by limiting the time in which the task should be executed. Delayed presentation creates a type of loading that transforms visual tasks into recent memory tasks. One of the optional administration techniques for the Benton Visual Retention test includes a delayed reproduction of the drawing.

Visual interference is in most cases—such as in the readability of a message—considered an undesirable feature of the test situation. However, visual interference can be manipulated to increase the loading of visual tasks. In 1987, this author proposed a test of iconic pairs with interference stimuli that takes advantage of this powerful loading principle. The test follows the paradigm of the word "pair-associates" in which two words are initially memorized and one word is then presented as a recalling stimulus. Between the recalling stimulus and the response an interference is presented to make the recalling more difficult.

Intersensory Loading

Intersensory loading is the inhibition or alteration of visual perception by the simultaneous stimulation of other sensory systems. Intersensory loading can be achieved, for example, by the simultaneous presence of auditory and motor cues, hot bath tests, and visual fixation with passive head movements.

EXPERIMENTAL AND CLINICAL METHODS FOR STUDYING THE EFFECTS OF NEUROTOXIC AGENTS

There are numerous experimental and clinical methods for the study of peripheral and central visual system functions. Their full potential for the study of the effects of neurotoxic agents on humans remains unexplored. Grant (1980) has grouped these techniques as follows:

- Visual acuity measurements
- Ophthalmoscopic examinations
- Visual fields
- Color vision studies
- Electroretinography
- Visual evoked responses

Visual Acuity

Visual acuity is the ability to detect, resolve, and perceive fine details of a visual display; it can be assessed by simple means—for example, by presenting samples of reading material of different sizes similar to those used during a routine ophthalmoscopic examination.

The importance of assessing visual acuity before any psychometric testing is attempted cannot be overestimated, since visual acuity is essential for the performance of numerous psychometric tests.

Visual acuity plays different roles depending on the context of the research. In experimental studies of humans under laboratory conditions, the assessment of visual acuity is essential, and in reports in the scientific literature the status of the subject's visual acuity is often stated. As a rule, people with poor vision do not participate in such studies. In clinical or large-scale epidemiological investigations, subjects cannot be dismissed from testing because of reduced visual acuity. The investigator needs to account for this factor in the interpretation of the results.

In clinical field surveys it is relatively common to encounter subjects who forget to bring their reading glasses in spite of being instructed to do so. In such cases, test administrators need to write notes on the probable influence of lack of reading glasses in the performance of the task. It is as frequent to find subjects who insist on being tested in spite of the fact that they do not have reading glasses as to have subjects who refuse to perform the test because of the lack of them. Experience and common sense are necessary to resolve these situations.

The issue of whether people with extensive visual scotomas have normal acuity is still a matter of controversy. Grant (1980) states that "it is worth keeping in mind . . . that a patient can be blind over the entire visual field except for a tiny central island, yet have normal visual acuity." Normal acuity in ophthalmological tests is just a curiosity. Behavioral adaptations (eg, pointing the seeing "island" to the objects they need to see) reveal profound alterations in visual perception. In addition, perceptual disorders are often detected through the use of sensitive techniques such as critical fusion frequency or color perception.

Ophthalmoscopic Examination

This examination is performed with the aid of an ophthalmoscope. A physician, neurologist, or ophthalmologist can detect important qualitative features of the retina and the nervous system using this examination. This is possible because the retina is the only portion of neural tissue directly observable from outside. The optic disk—the site where the optic nerve originates—may be found to be abnormal, edematous, or hyperemic (with a bloody appearance). The optic disk can show pallor, discoloring, or whitening, indicative

of atrophy. The retina sometimes may show changes in pigmentation indicating alterations in the retinal pigment epithelium. To determine whether these changes are consistent with toxic poisoning needs experienced clinical judgment. One of the best compendia on the toxicology of the nervous system from a clinical point of view is that of Grant (1974).

Refractive Errors as Confounders in Tests of Visual Perception. Refractive errors are a family of visual problems associated with the optical properties of the eye [eg, deformities in the cornea (astigmatism), near- or farsightness]. There are epidemiological reports indicating that biological and environmental factors may be associated with refractive errors (Angle and Wissmann 1980; Gehring 1971). Many physical and chemical agents, such as radiation and chemical corrosive agents, cause eye damage by affecting the cornea (Coe and Douglas 1988).

Cataractogenic Properties of Drugs and Toxic Agents. A large variety of drugs and toxic agents affect vision through their ability to produce cataracts. *Cataract* is a condition of partial to complete opacification of the lens of the eye. There are numerous clinical and experimental reports dealing with the cataractogenic effects of drugs and other chemicals, including sugars (eg, D-glucose, D-galactose, D-xylose), antibiotics, corticosteroids, anticholinesterase agents, antipsychotic and anticonvulsive drugs, drugs aimed at reducing cholesterol levels, naphthalene, trinitrotoluene (TNT), many sympathomimetic drugs (drugs that act on the sympathetic division of the autonomic nervous system), fungicides, oral contraceptives, heptachlor, and many others. Although dated, Gehring (1971) is still a good review of the cataractogenic properties of chemical agents and drugs.

Cataracts can also be observed among workers excessively exposed to infrared radiation. It is important to consider these factors in the neuropsychological examination of workers exposed to multiple physical and toxic agents.

Visual Fields

The *visual field* is a quantitative estimation of the extent of our vision. It is obtained through a routine examination called the visual fields examination. The subject fixates his or her eyes at the center of an apparatus while visual colored targets are moved away and toward the center. The blind spot, the place where the optic nerve leaves the retina and which contains no visual receptors, is readily apparent in the assessment of a person's visual field. Visual fields are important sources of information, for example, to make the clinical diagnosis between intracranial and peripheral lesions. This is possible through knowledge of the functional organization of the visual system's neural pathways. Students of neuroanatomy learn early to relate alterations in the visual field to different lesions of the visual pathway.

Gross alterations of the visual field can be detected by means of simple testing methods. The examiner needs to position himself/herself in front of the subject and ask the subject to fixate his or her eyes on the examiner's nose. With extended arms, the examiner moves a colored pencil vertically and horizontally about the subject's visual field until the subject can no longer see it. Experienced test administrators recognize hemilateral scotoma as a result of left–right differences in the drawing of symmetrical figures. In general, people with hemilateral scotoma tend to ignore the blind area of their immediate environment; they may or may not be conscious of this.

Marked changes in visual fields occur as a result of methylmercury poisoning. Visual fields become progressively constricted from the periphery to the center, creating tunnel vision. Central vision may or may not be spared in visual acuity testing.

Alterations of the visual fields may be produced by migraine headaches. During a migraine attack many people experience visual phenomena ranging from phosphenes—bright moving lights—to elaborate flickering "fortification" illusions.

Color Vision in Neurotoxicological Studies

Chronic exposure to neurotoxic agents may lead to acquired *dyschromatopsia,* a dysfunction in color perception. A dose–response approach is necessary in order to establish the link between chronic exposure and visual effects. Prevalence studies of dyschromatopsia in control and exposed groups—particularly if the study groups are small—need to be interpreted with caution because "color blindness" and many varieties of alterations in color perception are common in the general population.

There are many valid and reliable techniques for the quick assessment of color vision—to be described in conjunction with some representative studies below. The classical tests for color perception based on the Ishihara plates, which are commercially available, should be avoided. The task is based on figure–ground discrimination, which in itself can be altered by acute or chronic exposure to neurotoxic agents. In fact, the Ishihara plates can be used as embedded figures plates for a much less challenging task, required for people seriously affected by brain lesions.

Effects of Pharmacological Agents on Color Perception.   Color perception can be altered by the use of medications. Alterations in color perception as a result of drug and pharmacological agents are well documented in the scientific literature (Grant 1974, 1980). Aronson and Ford (1980) have used such tests to demonstrate changes in color perception resulting from ingestion of toxic levels of digoxin, a therapeutic cardiovascular drug.

Impairment in Color Perception among Workers Exposed to Carbon Disulfide. Raitta and collaborators (1981) performed a study to determine whether occupational exposure to carbon disulfide is associated with alterations in color perception. The groups tested were 62 workers in a viscose rayon factory and 40 nonexposed men. Color discrimination was assessed with the Farnsworth–Mussel 100-Hue test (Farnsworth 1957). The exposure history of the exposed group was 6 to 26 years. Test scores of the exposed and control populations were plotted in histograms. The test scores of workers exposed to carbon disulfide showed a significant shift toward impaired color discrimination when compared with controls. The findings seemed consistent with an impaired receptiveness of the ganglion cells for polarizing and depolarizing signals generated by the cones. This phenomenon is similar to that found in workers exposed to n-hexane (Seppäläinen et al. 1979).

Blain and Mengler (1986) evaluated color discrimination among 89 workers occupationally exposed to organic solvents with the aid of the Lanthony D-15 desaturated panel. Quantitative and qualitative analysis revealed that among nonexposed workers, the prevalence of tritanomalies (a rare form of dichromatism characterized by a deficiency in seeing blue and yellow) and color confusion expressed in a "confusion index" increased with age. However, among the exposed workers, the prevalence of dyschromatopsia (alterations in color perception) and the mean color confusion index increase with age and exposure level.

The authors concluded that chromatic discrimination impairment may be an important indicator of neuroophthalmologic changes associated with occupational exposure to organic solvents. Chromatic discrimination impairment associated with solvent exposure reflects neural rather than ocular damage. From this report, however, it is not clear how the authors ruled out cognitive factors in the aged as an alternative explanation for color confusion.

Electroretinography and Visual Evoked Potentials

As mentioned in Chapter 5, the electroretinogram and the measurement of visual evoked potentials are experimental techniques that have been proposed for evaluating the effects of neurotoxic agents on the visual system. For now, their potential use is more valuable in humans under clinical conditions and in experimental animals under laboratory conditions. In the United States acute exposure in humans under experimental conditions have not been encouraged for ethical reasons. However, ethical standards vary from country to country. Koopowitz (1974) has reviewed the history, recording techniques, equipment needed to deliver the visual stimuli, animal and human preparations, and measurements and interpretations in electroretinographic studies.

Because of the technical difficulties in the preparation of subjects and the expert clinical judgment that needs to be made in the interpretation of the recorded waveforms, electroretinography (ERG) and visual evoked potentials (VER) at the present time are reserved for the study of mechanisms of action of neurotoxic agents and for the differential diagnosis of neurological diseases. Even if some of these technical difficulties could be overcome, ERG has not been proposed as a screening procedure or as a routine test in medical field surveys.

The electroretinogram measures the action potential that is generated in quick response to a flash of light. The powerful effects of solvents on retinal functions have been known since Granit (1955) used solvents to produce structural changes in the retina of experimental animals (the frog) and observed subsequent alterations in the ERG. Gerritsen (1971) also has studied the effects of anesthesics on the the ERG of the rabbit.

SOURCES OF INFORMATION ON DRUGS AND SUBSTANCES THAT MAY AFFECT THE VISUAL SYSTEM

Grant (1980) has listed at least 90 different substances known or suspected of affecting the peripheral visual system. We are fortunate to have his useful encyclopedic book, *Toxicology of the Eye,* published in 1974, as a source. Grant sees neurotoxicology from the viewpoint of a clinical ophthalmologist, so one cannot rely on this source for information on perceptual (ie, psychological) dysfunctions produced by neurotoxic agents. As a consequence, studies that originated within the framework of behavioral toxicology are not reviewed there.

As stated in other sections of this volume, one should consult compilations of neurotoxic substances affecting the visual system with a critical mind. The sources for judging a substance as having the visual system as a target can be as varied as biochemical studies in vitro, electrophysiological preparations of isolated nerves, behavioral studies in laboratory animals, medical field surveys, and case reports.

The vast literature on the effects of naturally occurring toxins, drugs, and neurotoxic agents on the visual system of laboratory animals such as the rat, mouse, cat, or monkey have not been adequately reviewed. However, multiauthored books containing chapters describing contemporary research are available. In most cases, important classical sources are not mentioned.

ILLUMINATION

"Lighting" is an engineering discipline that deals with the optimal visibility of objects and awareness of space needed for people to perform their daily activities. Performance, safety, and comfort are intimately related to lighting. "Glare" is a serious environmental problem leading to accidents. Light can also be a pollutant. A discussion of lighting terminology, the purposes of lighting, recommended illumination of industrial environments, industrial lighting equipment, lighting design, a special review of laser sources, and lighting surveys is beyond the scope of this chapter.

A good introduction to lighting is the chapter by Kaufman on illumination in *The Industrial Environment: Its Evaluation and Control,* published by the National Institute for Occupational Safety and Health in 1973.

Sliney and Wolbarsht's book *Safety with Lasers and Other Optical Sources,* published in 1980, is also a valuable handbook. Visual perception and industrial labeling are intimately related topics. Those interested in labeling design may consult *Handbook of Chemical Industry Labelling,* edited by O'Connor and Lirtzman in 1984.

REFERENCES

Alexandridis, E (1985) *The Pupil.* New York: Springer-Verlag.

Anderson, DR (1982) *Testing the Field of Vision.* St. Louis: CV Mosby.

Angle, J and Wissmann, DA (1980) The epidemiology of myopia. *Am J Epidemiol* 111(2):220–228.

Aronson, JK and Ford, AR (1980) The use of colour vision measurements in the diagnosis of digoxin toxicity. *Q J Med* 193:273–282.

Battersby, WS, Krieger, EP, Pollack, M, et al. (1953) Figure–ground discrimination and the "abstract" attitude in patients with cerebral neoplasms. *AMA Arch Neurol Psychiatry* 70:703–712.

Bender, MB (1952) *Disorders in Perception.* Springfield, IL: Charles C Thomas.

Benton, CD and Calhoun, FP (1953) The ocular effects of methyl alcohol poisoning: Report of a catastrophe involving 320 persons. *Am J Ophthalmol* 36:1677–1685.

Blain, L and Mengler, D (1986) La dyschromatopsie chez des personnes exposées professionnellement aux solvants organiques. *J Fr Ophthalmol* 9(2):127–133.

Bowman, RE and Bushnell, PJ (1980) Scotopic visual deficits in young monkeys given chronic daily low levels of lead. In *Neurotoxicology of the Visual System,* WH Merigan and B Weiss (eds) pp. 219–231. New York: Raven Press.

Coe, JE and Douglas, RB (1988) Ocular responses to chemnical and physical injury. In *Occupational Medicine: Principles and Practical Applications,* 2nd ed, C Zenz (ed) pp. 166–173. Chicago: Year Book Medical Publishers.

Cooper, MN, Mitchell, GL, Bennett, IL, et al. (1952) Methyl alcohol poisoning: An account of the 1951 Atlanta epidemic. *J Med Assoc Georgia* 11:48–51.

Corkin, S (1979) Hidden-figures-test performance: Lasting effects of unilateral penetrating head injury and transient effects of bilateral cingulotomy. *Neuropsychologia* 17:585–604.

Farnsworth, D (1957) *The Farnsworth–Munsell 100-Hue Test for the Examination of Color Discrimination, Revised Manual.* Baltimore: Munsell Color Co.

Franck, C and Kuhlo, W (1970) Die Wirkung des Alkohols auf die raschen Blickziebewegungen (Saccaden) beim Menschen. *Arch Psychiatr Nervenkr* 213:238–245.

Frauenfelder, FT (1982) *Drug-Induced Ocular Side Effects and Drug Interaction,* 2nd ed. Philadelphia: Lea & Febiger.

Galezowski, X (1878) *Des Amblyopies et des Amauroses Toxiques.* Paris: P Assaebin.

Gehring, PJ (1971) The cataractogenic activity of chemical agents. *CRC Crit Rev Toxicol* 1(1):93–118.

Gerritsen, BG (1971) The effect of anesthetics on the electroretinogram and the visually evoked response in the rabbit. *Doc Ophthalmol* 29:289–330.

Ghent, L (1956) Perception of overlapping and embedded figures by children of different ages. *Am J Psychol* 69:576–587.

Glickman, L, Valciukas, JA, Lilis, R, et al. (1984) Occupational lead exposure: Effects on saccadic eye movements. *Int Arch Occup Environ Health* 54:115–125.

Goldstein, K (1942) *Aftereffect of Brain Injuries in War.* New York: Grune & Stratton.

Gottschaldt, K (1926) Über den Einfluss gehaufter Einprägnung von Figure auf ihre Sichbarkeit in umafassended Konfigurationen. *Psychol Forsch* 8:261–317.

Gouras, P (1985) Color vision. In *Principles of Neural Science,* 2nd ed. ER Kandel and JH Schwartz (eds) pp. 384–395. New York: Elsevier.

Granit, R (1955) *Receptors and Sensory Perception.* New Haven: Yale University Press.

Grant, WM (1974) *Toxicology of the Eye,* 2nd ed. Springfield, IL: Charles C Thomas.

Grant, WM (1980) The peripheral visual system as a target. In *Experimental and Clinical Neurotoxicology,* P Spencer and HH Schaumberg (eds) pp. 77–91. Baltimore: Williams & Wilkins.

Kandel, ER and Schwartz, JH (ed) (1985) *Principles of Neural Science,* 2nd ed. New York: Elsevier.

Kaufman, JE (1973) Illumination. In *The Industrial Environment: Its Evaluation and Control,* pp. 349–356. Washington, DC: US Department of Health, Education, and Welfare, Public Health Service, Center for Disease Control, National Institute for Occupational Safety and Health.

Koffka, K (1935) *Principles of Gestalt Psychology.* New York: Harcourt, Brace.

Köhler, W (1929) *Gestalt Psychology.* New York: Liveright.

Koopowitz, H (1974) The electroretinogram. In *Bioelectric and Recording Techniques, Part C,* RF Thompson and MM Patterson (eds). New York: Academic Press.

Lacks, P (1984) *Bender Gestalt Screening for Brain Dysfunction.* New York: John Wiley & Sons.

Lewin, L and Guillery, H (1913) *Die Wirkung von Arzneimittelm und Giften auf das Auge, Vols 1 and 2.* Berlin: A Hirschwald.

Newcombe, F (1969) *Missile Wounds of the Brain: A Study of Psychological Deficits.* New York: Oxford University Press.

O'Connor, CJ and Lirtzman, SI (1984) *Handbook of Chemical Industry Labeling.* Park Ridge, NJ: Noyes Publications.

Pritchard, RM (1961) Stabilized images on the retina. *Sci Am* 204:72–78.

Raitta, C, Teir, H, Tolone, M, et al. (1981) Impaired color discrimination among viscose rayon workers exposed to carbon disulfide. *J Occup Med* 23:189–192.

Ratliff, F (1965) *Mach Bands: Quantitative Studies on Neural Networks in the Retina.* San Francisco: Holden-Day.

Rey, A (1964) *L'Examen Clinique in Psychologie.* Paris: Presses Universitaires de France.

Rubin, E (1921) *Visuelle wahrgenommene Figuren.* Copenhangen: Glyldendolske Goghandel.

Seppäläinen, AM, Raitta, C, and Huuskonen, M (1979) *n*-Hexane-induced changes in visual evoked potentials and electro-retinograms of industrial workers. *Electroencephalogr Clin Neurophysiol* 47:492–498.

Sliney, D and Wolbarsht, M (1980) *Safety Lasers and Other Optical Sources: A Comprehensive Handbook.* New York: Plenum Press.

Taylor, HR (1981) Racial variation in vision. *Am J Epidemiol* 113(1):62–80.

Teuber, H-L (1960) Perception. In *Handbook of Physiology, Section I, Vol III, Neurophysiology,* J Field, HW Magound, and VE Hall (eds) pp. 1595–1668. Washington, DC: American Physiological Society.

Teuber, H-L, Battersby, WS, and Bender, MB (1951) Performance of complex visual tasks after cerebral lesions. *J Nerv Ment Dis* 114:413–419.

Teuber, H-L and Weinstein, S (1956) Ability to discover hidden figures after cerebral lesions. *Arch Neurol Psychiatry* 76:369–379.

Tsutsui, J (1980) Clinical and pathological studies of eye movement disorders in Minamata disease. In *Neurotoxicity of the Visual System,* WH Merigan and B Weiss (eds) pp. 187–202. New York: Raven Press.

Uhthoff, W (1911) Die Augenstörungen bei Vergiftungen. In *Graefe-Saemisch Handbuch der Gesamten Augenheilkunde, II,* pp. 1–180. Leipzig: Engelman.

Valciukas, JA and Singer, RM (1982) An embedded figures test in environmental and occupational neurotoxicology. *Environ Res* 28:183–198.

Wertheimer, M (1912) Experimentelle Studies über das Sehen von Bewegung. *Z Psychol* 61:161–265.

SUGGESTED READINGS

Åkesson, B, Bergtsson, M, and Florén, I (1986) Visual disturbances after industrial triethylamine exposure. *Int Arch Occup Environ Health* 57:297–302.

Åkesson, B, Florén, I, and Skerfving, S (1985) Visual disturbances at experimental human exposure to triethylamine. *Br J Ind Med* 42:848–850.

Araki, S, Murata, K, and Aono, H (1987) Central and peripheral nervous system dysfunction in workers exposed to lead, zinc and copper: A follow-up study of visual and somatosensory evoked potential. *Int Arch Occup Environ Health* 59:177–187.

Armington, JC (1974) *The Electroretinogram.* New York: Academic Press.

Baumach, GL, Cancilla, PA, Martin-Amat, G, et al. (1977) Methyl alcohol poisoning: IV. Alterations of the morphological findings of the retina and optic nerve. *Arch Ophthalmol* 95:1859.

Bender, L (1938) *A Visual Motor Gestalt Test and Its Clinical Use, Research Monographs, No. 3.* New York: American Orthopsychiatric Association.

Bender, MB (1964) *The Oculomotor System.* New York: Harper & Row.

Bender, MB (1970) Perceptual interactions. In *Modern Trends in Neurology,* F Williams (ed) pp. 1–28. London: Butterworths.

Bizzi, E (1974) The coordination of eye–head movements. *Sci Am* 231:100–106.

Blain, L, Lagace, JP, and Mengler, D (1985) Sensitivity and specificity of the Lanthony D-15 desaturated panel to assess chromatic discrimination loss among solvent-exposed workers. *Environ Health* 3:105–109.

Blain, PG, Nightingale, S, and Stoddart, JC (1982) Strychnine poisoning: Abnormal eye movements. *J Toxicol* 19(2):215–217.

Bowman, KJ (1982) A method for quantitative scoring of the Farnsworth panel D-15. *Acta Ophthalmol* 60:907–915.

Bowman, KJ and Cameron, KD (1984) A quantitative assessment of colour discrimination in normal vision and senile macular degeneration using some colour confusion tests. *Doc Ophthalmol Proc Ser* 39:363–370.

Bowman, KJ, Collins, MJ, and Henry, J (1984) The effect of age on the Panel D-15 and desaturated D-15: A quantitative evaluation. *Doc Ophthalmol Proc Ser* 38:227–231.

Brandt, T, Wist, E, and Dichgans, J (1975) Foreground and background in dynamic spatial orientation. *Percep Psychophys* 17(5):497–503.

Braun, CM, Daignealth, S, and Gilbert, B (1989) Color discrimination testing reveals early printshop solvent neurotoxicity better than a neuropsychological test battery. *Arch Clin Neuropsychol* 4(1):1–13.

Brown, JW (1989) *Neuropsychology of Visual Perception.* Hillsdale, NJ: Lawrence Erlbaum Associates.

Bushnell, PJ, Bowman, RE, Allen, JR, et al. (1977) Scotopic vision deficits in young monkeys exposed to lead. *Science* 196:333–335.

Cohn, NB, Dustman, RE, and Bradford, DC (1984) Age-related decrements in Stroop Color Test performance. *J Clin Psychol* 40:1244–1250.

Cornsweet, TM (1980) *Visual Perception.* New York: Academic Press.

Davson, H (1980) *Physiology of the Eye,* 4th ed. New York: Academic Press.

Dempsey, LC, O'Donnel, JJ, and Hoff, JT (1976) Carbon monoxide retinopathy. *Am J Ophthalmol* 82:692–693.

Derakhshan, I and Forough, M (1978) Progressive visual loss after eight years on clioquinol. *Lancet* 1:715.

Duke-Elder, S (1972) *System of Ophthalmology, Vol XIV, Part 2, Non-Mechanical Injuries,* S Duke-Elder and PA MacFaul (eds). St. Louis: CV Mosby.

Evans, HL (1978) Behavioral assessment of visual toxicity. *Environ Health Perspect* 26:53–57.

Fox, SL (1973) *Industrial and Occupational Ophthalmology.* Springfield, IL: Charles C Thomas.

François, J and Verriest, G (1961) On acquired deficiency of color vision, with special reference to its detection and classification by means of the tests of Farnsworth. *Vis Res* 1:201–219.

Goldstein, K (1942) *Aftereffects of Brain Injuries in War.* New York: Grune & Stratton.

Graham, CD (ed) (1965) *Vision and Visual Perception.* New York: John Wiley & Sons.

Grant, WM (1986) *Toxicology of the Eye: Effects on the Eyes and Visual System from Chemicals, Drugs, Metals & Minerals, Plants, Toxins & Venoms,* 3rd ed. Springfield, IL: Charles C Thomas.

Häkkinen, L (1984) Vision in the elderly and its use in the social environment. *Scand J Soc Med Suppl* 35:23–24.

Harrower, MR (1939) Changes in figure–ground perception in patients with cortical lesions. *Br J Psychol* 30:47–51.

Havener, WH (1978) *Ocular Pharmacology.* St. Louis: CV Mosby.

Helve, J and Krause, U (1972) The influence of age in the Panel D-15 colour test. *Acta Ophthalmol* 50:896–900.

Hiller, R, Giacometti, L, and Yuen, K (1977) Sunlight and cataract: An epidemiologic investigation. *Am J Epidemiol* 105:450–459.

Hollows, F and Moran, D (1981) Cataract—the ultraviolet risk factor. *Lancet* 2:1249–1250.

Humphreys, GW and Riddoch, MJ (1987) *To See But Not To See: A Case Study of Visual Agnosia.* Hillsdale, NJ: Lawrence Erlbaum Associates.

Humphreys, GW and Riddoch, MJ (1988) *Visual Object Processing: A Cognitive Neuropsychological Account.* Hillsdale, NJ: Lawrence Erlbaum Associates.

Jacobiec, FA (1982) *Ocular Anatomy, Embryology and Teratology.* Philadelphia: Harper & Row.

Jaensch, PA (1958) *Augenschädigungen in Industrie und Gewerbe.* Stuttgart: Wissenschaftliche Verlagsgesellschaft.

Johnston, CW and Pirozzolo, FJ (1988) *Neuropsychol-*

ogy of Eye Movements. Hillsdale, NJ: Lawrence Erlbaum Associates.

Judd, DB and Wyszecki, G (1975) *Color in Business, Science, and Industry,* 3rd ed. New York: John Wiley & Sons.

Karai, I, Horiguchi, S, and Nishikawa, N (1982) Optic atrophy with visual field defect in a worker occupationally exposed to lead for 30 years. *J Toxicol* 19(4):409–418.

Karai, I, Sugimoto, K, and Goto, S (1983) A fluorescein angiography study on carbon disulfide retinopathy among workers in viscose rayon factories. *Int Arch Occup Environ Health* 53:91–99.

Keane, JR (1978) Toluene optic neuropathy. *Ann Neurol* 4:390.

Kolata, G (1988) Zinc shows promise in slowing disease that causes blindness. *New York Times,* March 10.

Krill, AE and Fishman, GA (1971) Acquired color vision defects. *Trans Am Acad Ophthalmol Otolaryngol* 75:1095.

Lakowski, R (1969) Theory and practice of colour vision testing: A review, Part 1. *Br J Ind Med* 26:173–189.

Lakowski, R (1969) Theory and practice of colour vision testing: A review, Part 2. *Br J Ind Med* 26:265–288.

Lerman, S and Tripathi, RC (1988) *Ocular Toxicology.* New York: Marcel Dekker.

Lewin, L and Guillery, H (1913) *Die Wirkung von Arzneimitteln und Giften auf das Auge,* Vols 1 and 2. Berlin: A Hirschwald.

Livingstone, M and Hubel, D (1988) Segregation of form, color, movement, and depth: Anatomy, physiology and perception. *Science* 240:740–749.

Mäntyjärvi, M, Karppa, T, Karvonen, P, et al. (1986) Comparison of six colour vision tests for occupational screening. *Int Arch Occup Environ Health* 58:53–59.

Martin-Amat, G, Tephly, TR, McMartin, KE, et al. (1977) Methyl alcohol poisoning: II. Development of a model for ocular toxicity in methyl alcohol poisoning using the rhesus monkey. *Arch Ophthalmol* 95:1847–1850.

Meir-Ruge, W (1972) Drug induced retinopathy. *Crit Rev Toxicol* 1(3):325–360.

Merigan, WH (1979) Effects of toxicans on visual system. *Neurobehav Toxicol* 1:15–22.

Merigan, WH (1980) Visual fields and flicker thresholds in methylmercury-poisoned monkeys. In *Neurotoxicity of the Visual System,* WH Merigan and B Weiss (eds) pp. 149–162. New York: Raven Press.

Merigan, WH, Barkdoll, E, and Maurissen, JPJ (1982) Acrylamide-induced visual impairment in primates. *Toxicol Appl Pharmacol* 62:342–345.

Merigan, WH, Maurissen, JPJ, Weiss, B, et al. (1983) Neurotoxic actions of methylmercury on the primate visual system. *Neurobehav Toxicol Teratol* 5:649–658.

Merigan, WH and Weiss, B (eds) (1980) *Neurotoxicity of the Visual System.* New York: Raven Press.

Miranda, MN (1980) Environmental temperature and senile cataract. *Trans Am Ophthalmol Soc* 173:255–264.

Mista, UK, Nag, D, Mista, NK, et al. (1985) Some observations on the macula of pesticide workers. *Hum Toxicol* 4:135–145.

Nathans, J (1989) The genes for color vision. *Sci Am* 261(1):42–49.

Nathans, J, Thomas, D, and Hogness, DS (1986) Molecular genetics of human color vision: The genes encoding blue, green and red pigments. *Science* 232:193–202.

Newcombe, F (1969) *Missile Wounds of the Brain: A Study of Psychological Deficits.* New York: Oxford University Press.

Plestina, R and Piukovic-Plestina, M (1978) Effects of anticholinesterase pesticides on the eye and on vision. *CRC Crit Rev Toxicol* 6(1):1–23.

Potts, AM, Praglin, J, Farkas, I, et al. (1955) Studies on the visual toxicity of methanol, VIII. Additional observations of methanol poisoning in the primate test object. *Am J Ophthalmol* 40:76–82.

Raitta, C, Sepäläinen, AM, and Huuskonen, MS (1978) *n*-Hexane maculopathy in industrial workers. *Albrecht Graef von Arch Klin Exp Ophthalmol* 209:99–110.

Raitta, C and Tolonen, M (1975) Ocular pulse wave in workers exposed to carbon disulfide. *Albrecht von Graefes Arch Klin Ophthalmol* 195:149–154.

Raitta, C and Tolonen, M (1980) Microcirculation of the eye in workers exposed to carbon disulfide. In *Neurotoxicology of the Visual System,* WH Merigan and B Weiss (eds) pp. 73–96. New York: Raven Press.

Reed, ES (1989) *James J Gibson and the Psychology of Perception.* New Haven, CT: Yale University Press.

Rice, DC and Gilbert, SG (1982) Early chronic low-level methylmercury poisoning in monkeys impairs spatial vision. *Science* 216:759–761.

Richard, W (1971) The fortification illusions of migraines. *Sci Am* 224:88–96.

Schaumburg, HH and Spencer, PS (1978) Environmental hydrocarbons produce degeneration in cat hypothalamus and optic nerve. *Science* 199:199.

Schneider, B, Hood, DC, Cohen, H, et al. (1977) Behavioral threshold as a function of Vitamin A deprivation in the rat. *Vis Res* 17:799–806.

Smith, MB (1976) *Handbook of Ocular Toxicity.* Acton, MA: Publishing Sciences Group.

Specchio, LM, Bellomo, R, Pozio, G, et al. (1981) Smooth pursuit eye movements among storage battery workers. *Clin Toxicol* 18(11):1269–1276.

Spector, A (1970) Aging of the lens and cataract formation. In *Aging and the Human Visual Functions,* R Sekuler, D Kline, and R Dismukers (eds) pp. 27–43. New York: Alan R Liss.,

Spillmann, L and Werner, JS (eds) (1990) *Visual Perception: The Neurophysiological Foundations.* San Diego: Academic Press.

Sugimoto, K, Goto, S, and Hotta, R (1976) An epidemiological study on retinopathy due to carbon disulfide: CS$_2$ exposure level and development of retinopathy. *Int Arch Occup Environ Health* 37:1–8.

Sugimoto, K, Goto, S, and Hotta, R (1976) Studies on chronic carbon disulfide poisoning: A 5-year follow-up study on retinopathy due to carbon disulfide. *Int Arch Occup Environ Health* 37:233–248.

Sugimoto, K, Goto, S, Taniguchi, H, et al. (1977) Ocular fundus photography of workers exposed to carbon disulfide: A comparative epidemiological study between Japan and Finland. *Int Arch Occup Environ Health* 39:97–101.

Tateishi, J, Kuroda, S, Saito, A, et al. (1972) Experimental myeolo-optico neuropathy induced by clioquinol. *Acta Neuropathol* 24:304.

Taylor, H (1980) The environment and the lens. *Br J Opthalmol* 64:303–310.

Teuber, H-L, Battersby, WS, and Bender, MB (1960) *Visual Defects after Penetrating Missile Wound of the Brain.* Cambridge, MA: Cambridge University Press.

Toates, FM (1972) Accommodation function of the human eye. *Physiol Rev* 52:828–863.

Tolor, A and Schulberg, HC (1963) *An Evaluation of the Bender Gestalt Test.* Springfield, IL: Charles C Thomas.

van Heyningen, R (1976) What happens to the human lens in cataract. *Sci Am* 233:70–81.

Vernon, RJ and Ferguson, RK (1969) Effects of trichloroethylene on visual–motor performance. *Arch Environ Health* 18:894–900.

Verries, G (1963) Further studies on acquired deficiency of colour discrimination. *J Opt Soc Am* 53(1):185–195.

Vigliani, EC (1950) Clinical observations on carbon disulfide intoxication in Italy. *Ind Med Surg* 19:240–242.

Walsh, FB and Hoyt, WF (1969) *Clinical Neuro-Ophthalmology,* 3rd ed. Baltimore: Williams & Wilkins.

Weale, RA (1983) Senile cataract: The case against light. *Ophthalmology* 90:420–423.

Werner, H and Strauss, AA (1941) Pathology of figure–ground relation in the child. *J Abnorm Soc Psychol* 36:236–248.

Wilmer, WH (1921) Effects of carbon monoxide upon the eye. *Am J Ophthalmol* 4:73.

Wolter, JR and Clark, RL (1972) Ocular involvement in acute intermittent porphyria. *Am J Ophthalmol* 74:666–674.

Zigman, S, Datiles, M, and Torczynski, E (1979) Sunlight and human cataracts. *Invest Ophthalmol Vis Sci* 18:462–467.

27

Motor Behavior

INTRODUCTION TO MOTOR FUNCTION

"Motor" is a term designating movement, but movement can be viewed from at least four broad points of view: our abilities to walk, grab an object, lift a paper clip, move our eyes to follow a target, run, or communicate through body language or speech are all examples of motor functions that are voluntary and mediated predominantly, but not exclusively, by skeletal muscles; the work of the heart, the need to breathe, the urge to urinate or defecate, thirst, hunger, sex, the emotions of fear, anger, etc are only partially controlled by will and are mediated predominantly, but not exclusively, by the autonomic nervous system; the nervous system also is intimately related to endocrine functions through the neuroendocrine system controlling the secretion of hormones; finally, it is now beginning to be understood that the nervous system also controls immunologic functions through the neuroimmunologic system.

This chapter reviews some basic facts on the effects of neurotoxic agents on motor functions that are mediated by the musculoskeletal system. Chapter 28 reviews effects of neurotoxic agents on motor functions mediated by the autonomic system. Although neuroendocrinology and, more recently, neuroimmunology are part of the corpus of neurosciences, human and animal information on the effects of toxic agents on those systems is scant.

Chapters 22 to 26 reviewed the effects of toxic agents on sensory systems and dealt with afferent systems—ie, neural organizations that are primarily designed to bring information from the external or internal environment to the nervous system. Motor and autonomic functions described in this chapter and in Chapter 28 are examples of efferent systems—ie, neural organizations that exert control over the external environment via the musculoskeletal system or the internal environment via the autonomic system. (Afferent and efferent systems cannot be conceived as separate entities because there are many "motor" mechanisms involved in sensory processes and almost all motor controls can be achieved only as a result of "sensory" processes.)

The *effector* is the unit of analysis of any motor system. The effector can be skeletal muscle (eg, that controlling the movement of the tongue), smooth muscle (eg, that controlling the dilation or opening of blood vessels), or glands (eg, hypophysis, pituitary, or testes).

PERSPECTIVES ON MOTOR BEHAVIOR

Motor behavior can be viewed from a biological, neural, or psychometric point of view. These views complement each other.

From a **biological point of view**, motor behavior is studied in order to ascertain its genetic and environmental determining factors, the role of motor behavior in evolutionary adaptation (eg, bipedalism, the advantages of an opposing thumb), and the relationship of the motor behavior of animals to their living environment. The biological point of view provides a common frame of reference for describing the basic mechanisms of motor behavior, integrating neural mechanisms and performance. Discussion of the biological view, essential as it is, is omitted here because it has been grossly underrepresented in neurotoxicological literature in contrast to the other two views. (Those interested in this topic are referred to Section IV of *Neurobiology* by G. M. Shepherd, published in 1983.)

The **neural point of view** is that represented by the neurosciences, clinical neurology, and experimental neuropathology; it studies movement and motor behavior at the gross morphological, cellular, and molecular levels. This view is essential for the understanding of why neurotoxic agents produce their effects and for the adequate diagnosis and treatment of neurotoxic illness. Some probes that neurologists and clinical neuropsychologists use—such the Romberg test for the assessment of whole-body balance—are based on our understanding of essential facts of the gross anatomy and physiology of the nervous system. Some electrophysiological techniques for the assessment of motor behavior in the clinic originated within this context. An example is the measurement of tremor by means of tremography.

The **psychometric point of view** of motor behavior sees motor functions as part of the abilities and skills of the individual; it looks for the basic motor skills on which complex abilities are based and contributes the supporting (statistical) theory and equipment for measuring what the individual can do. Many techniques for the assessment of motor functions that are currently used in human neurotoxicological research are based on the psychometric approach. Examples are reaction time, dexterity, and motor coordination testing.

_____

By the early 1960s the need for objective and quantitative methods for evaluating motor functions in environmental and occupational neurotoxicology had been firmly established. By the mid-1970s reports on quantitative methods for the evaluation of steadiness, resting tremor, sustained tremor, and static–intention tremor for use in clinical trials began to appear (Potvin et al. 1975a,b). However, American "behavioral toxicologists" did not find their inspiration in those; rather, they began from scratch, based on concepts of human factor engineering. For example, when Chaffin (1975), Miller et al. (1975), and Langolf et al. (1978) at the University of Michigan began working on the neurotoxicity of mercury in the early 1970s, they did the work within the framework of human factor engineering.

There has been a cross-fertilization among professionals who see behavior from either the biological, neural, or psychometric points of view. For example, many tests psychologists use for the assessment of individual differences in skills were born in the neurological clinic. The neurologist in the clinic may ask the patient to unbutton and then button his shirt, a test that only the profoundly impaired fail. The neuropsychologist may design a test that captures the essential skills involved in buttoning the shirt such as lifting, rotating, and inserting wooden pegs in special holes. Once a pegboard test is developed, the test developer might make the tests more difficult in order to assess the limits of motor skill.

Other tests were originally born in the clinic, but when they became adapted for use in other research contexts they lost their clinical meaning. In certain industries depending on manual labor-

ers, for example, occupational psychologists may administer to prospective workers simple motor tests to assess current levels of skills. Tests of motor performance that are currently used in human neurotoxicology have been adapted from those available in the examination of individual differences in skills.

No biological theories successfully explain individual differences. However, such biological theories were proposed in the past, some of them in support of "scientific racism." In 1981, Dr. Stephen Jay Gould from Harvard University published The Mismeasure of Man, *containing an excellent historical review of this pseudoscience.*

In this chapter the effects of E & O neurotoxic agents on selected motor functions are reviewed. We will discuss neural and behavioral characterization of motor functions; the importance of reaction-time measurement in neuropsychological assessment; and the effect of neurotoxic agents on speech. As will be seen, knowledge of how (or whether) exposure to neurotoxic agents induces speech pathology has yet to be adequately summarized and integrated into the larger body of E & O neurotoxicology.

THE NEURAL BASIS OF MOTOR ACTS

Knowledge of the neural basis of motor functions has progressed based on clinical studies in humans and neuropathological observations of experimental animals, many originating in the 18th century and even earlier. Since the 1960s the genetics and neuropharmacology of some movement disorders have begun to be understood.

Motor functions are accomplished by the coordinated action of several structures. The most obvious is the muscle itself, including its receptors, and the mechanical relationships among muscles, joints, and bones. The *final common pathway* is the neuron where all the motor impulses, regardless of their origin, finally converge. The muscles that ultimately produce movement are called effectors. Other tissues that contribute to motor functions include neural fibers and the unique neural network they form to optimize muscle tone; motor and sensory nerves that carry information to and from the central nervous system; and neural centers in sensory ganglia and in the spinal cord, brainstem, motor cortex, and precentral cortex.

Structural Basis for Muscle Contraction

Skeletal muscles are those that move bones and joints. Skeletal muscles are also called striated muscles because of the striated (striped) appearance of the muscle fiber under light microscopy. Light microscopy also reveals the presence of bands on the muscle fiber. The bands reflect the division of each muscle fiber into *sarcomeres,* the contractile units of the muscle fiber. Each sarcomere contains a set of *myofilaments,* and each myofilament contains the proteins *actin* and *myosin* organized in a highly regular fashion (Fig. 27.1).

Until 1954 the mechanism of muscle contraction was poorly understood. That year, two groups of British scientists—Hugh Huxley and Jean Hanson in London and Andrew Huxley and Robert Niedergerke in Cambridge—proposed independently the *sliding-filament model* of muscle fiber contraction. It was previously thought that muscle contraction was brought about by shortening or crumpling of individual filaments. Now it is recognized that the actin filaments and the myosin molecule slide past each other bringing about changes in the widths of the bands in the sarcomere without changing the length of the individual filaments (see "Introduction: The Nature of Motor Function," in Shepherd 1983).

In order to understand how a myofilament can create longer or shorter structures without altering its own length, the reader first needs to imagine tightly packed toothpicks firmly held by one's hand and individual toothpicks moving out from the pack and then coming back into the pack. One then has to modify this view slightly and imagine

SKELETAL MUSCLE

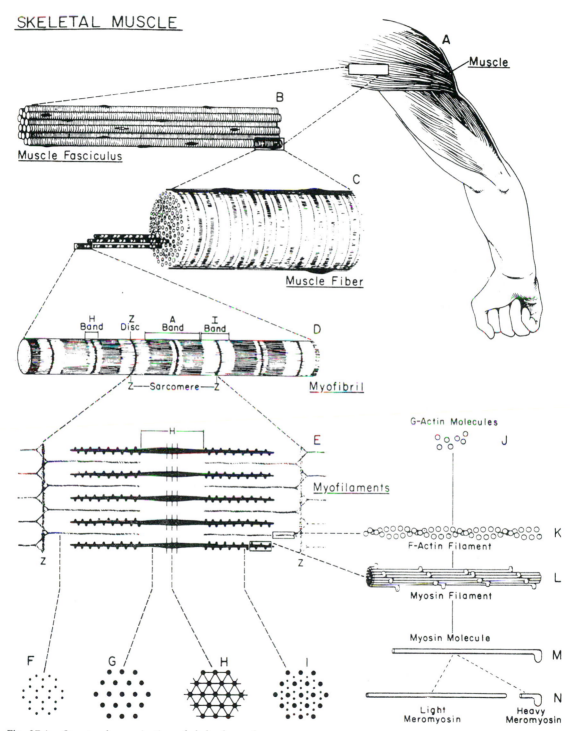

Fig. 27.1. Structural organization of skeletal muscle, from the whole muscle to the molecular level. (From Bloom and Fawcett 1975.)

that each toothpick (representing a myofilament), when looked at closely, looks like golf irons (the individual head of an iron is the myosin head) oriented in opposite directions. Actin is displaced by a series of molecular events occurring between the myosin head and the actin filaments.

Striated muscle fibers are of two types: extrafusal and intrafusal. The *extrafusal fibers* are the ones that contract as a result of the electrochemical events that occur in the synapses linking nerve and muscle fibers. The *intrafusal fibers* contain receptors that sense the muscle fiber contraction (to be described below).

Motor fibers are contracted by motoneurons as a result of electrochemical events occurring at the neuromuscular junctions.

Motor Neurons

A *motoneuron* (or *motor neuron*) is a neuron characterized by both its location in the nervous system and where its axons end. Motoneurons are located either in the spinal cord or the brainstem of the central nervous system. They have axons that leave the central nervous system via the ventral spinal roots of the spinal cord or cranial nerves.

Motoneurons are the largest neurons in the nervous system. They are unique in that they are the only central nervous system neurons that innervate nonneural tissue: the muscle fiber.

The Motor Unit

The *motor unit* is the combination of a motoneuron and all the muscle fibers innervated by the motoneuron. The central nervous system controls muscles through this functional link between neural fibers and muscles.

The Neuromuscular Junction

The *neuromuscular junction* is the synapsis existing between a single fiber of a motoneuron and a single muscle fiber. The simplicity and the accessibility of this neuromuscular junction resulted in a great deal of experimentation on structural, electrophysiological, and neurochemical events that occur at this meeting place between neuron and muscle fiber. Thus, in spite of the fact that the neuromuscular junction is not a typical synapse, it is often considered a model for the structure and function of all other synapses in the nervous system.

As in other synapses, the neuromuscular junction is the site where the electrical signal carried by the neural fiber releases the neurotransmitter (in this case, acetylcholine) generated at the presynaptic membrane into the synaptic cleft; acetylcholine reaches its receptor at the postsynaptic membrane, leading to the contraction of the muscle fiber; and acetylcholine is then either hydrolyzed by the enzyme acetylcholinesterase or is stored in synaptic vesicles.

Many naturally occurring neurotoxins contain substances that block the receptor for acetylcholine, causing a flaccid paralysis of the respiratory muscles and eventual death. For example, the arrow poison curare—originally developed by South American Indians for animal hunting—and the poisons of many snakes are receptor-blocking agents.

Some other neurotoxins prevent the release of acetylcholine, causing similar effects. For example, the neurotoxin responsible for botulism and the venom of the black widow spider act on this principle.

In myasthenia gravis, a progressive neurological disease characterized by generalized weakness and fatigability of skeletal muscles, the affected individual generates his or her own antibodies, which are directed against the acetylcholine receptor.

Mammalian Muscle Receptors

Muscle tissue contains a variety of receptors involved in the reception of mechanical vibration, temperature, and pain. But the control of muscle force and length is largely mediated by two receptors: the tendon organs and muscle spindles.

The *tendon organ,* located in the tendon between the bone and the muscle, operates like a strain gauge. The tendon organ fires when the tendon is stretched either as a result of a neural command from the motoneuron or by the passive mechanical stretch of the muscle.

The *muscle spindle,* located in the intrafusal muscle filament, provides information about the length of the muscle. The intrafusal muscle fibers do not contribute to the overall tension of the muscle but regulate the tone by means of mechanically deforming receptors.

Muscle Tone

Tone is the normal degree of vigor or tension of the muscle, the resistance to passive elongation and stretch. However, in spite of the fact that dead muscle has a certain physical measure of malleability, the tone of the muscle is largely determined by a neural mechanism. Thus, muscle tone is an active process of negative feedback in which the muscle fibers stimulate the tendon receptors and muscle spindles and the contraction of muscle fibers is regulated by the activity of muscle receptors.

Neural regulation of muscle tone is accomplished by a neural "wiring," a detailed description of which is beyond the scope of this chapter. Those interested in this topic are referred to Chapters 34 ("Muscle and Muscle Receptors" by Carew and Ghez) and 35 ("The Control of Reflex Action" by Carew) in *Principles of Neural Science* (2nd ed) edited by Kandel and Schwartz (1985).

There are several terms that refer to alterations in tone. *Hypertonus* is a muscle contraction that persists in spite of an effort by the patient to relax. The hypertonus of Parkinsonism—a neurological syndrome caused by faulty neurotransmission in the basal ganglia—is an example. *Spasticity* is an exaggerated reaction to applied stretch, resulting in exaggerated movement. Sudden releases in reflex muscle contraction is called the clasp-knife reaction and can usually be observed in alterations of the "upper" motoneurons (discussed below). *Rigidity* is a state originally described in experimental animals where extensor muscle contraction of all limbs results from a lack of cortical modulating influences. However, the simplistic view that these animal experiments provide an explanation for human spasticity is no longer held.

Muscle Sense

Muscle sense, or *kinesthesia,* is the awareness of movement of body and limbs, whether muscles are exerting effort or not. The concept of muscle sense is closely related to proprioception, a term usually reserved to indicate the awareness of the position of body and limbs in space. Although the existence of a muscle sense is obvious to all of us—we are aware of where our limbs are and what they do—the neural mechanisms by which this information is obtained and processed are still not completely understood. There are two important questions to be solved: What are the receptors for muscle sense, and is there an alternative mechanism for explaining muscle sensations?

It is still a matter of speculation what the receptors might be that are involved in muscle sense. Receptors located in the joints, muscles, tendons, and skin, singly or in combination, have all been proposed to be the receptors for coding muscle sense. For a review of the relative merits of each of these theories, see Matthews (1982).

A provocative hypothesis is that motor centers would supply sensory centers with copies (called corollary discharges) of the outgoing messages. The hypothesis of the corollary discharge sounds logical but is difficult to prove experimentally. Intuitively, it can be recognized that the motor system controlling limb movements, for example, is more efficient having an instantaneous copy of the force and extent of the commands sent by motor centers to limb muscles rather than waiting for the sensory information on the effector's degree of muscle contraction.

Corollary discharges are known to exist in the visuooculomotor system. We always know when we move and when the physical world around us moves. But if one pushes the eyeball gently with a finger from the side while closing the opposite eye, for example, the visual scene moves in unison with the pressure of the finger. This visual movement when neither we nor the world moves is explained by the absence of the corollary discharge from brain centers indicating that eyes have been ordered to move. The relative absence of receptors in the muscles controlling eye movements seems to support the notion that corollary discharge is the predominant mechanism by which the instantaneous positions of the eyes are always known.

The Organization of the Motor System

The motor system exhibits both a hierarchical and a parallel organization. (Figure 27.2 shows the organization of the motor pathways and some illnesses associated with each.) In a *hierarchical organization*, higher levels control the lower levels of functional organization. Thus, the brainstem controls the function of the spinal cord, the motor cortex controls the function of the brainstem and the spinal cord, and the premotor cortex controls all of them. In addition, the cerebellum and the basal ganglia are neural structures functionally related to this hierarchy.

These centers of motor control are linked to one another by neural pathways or tracts, which often take their names from their origin and termination. Thus, the corticospinal tract is responsible for sending motor com-

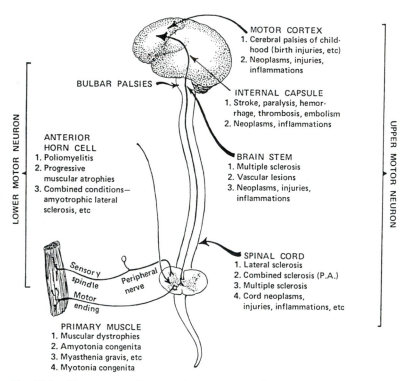

Fig. 27.2. The motor pathways and some associated illnesses. (Modified and reproduced from Chor 1936.)

mands from the cortex to the spinal cord, the corticobulbar tract is responsible for sending motor commands from the cortex to the brainstem, and so on.

The spinal cord is the lowest component of the motor hierarchy. It is capable of organizing automatic and stereotyped movements. The cat whose brainstem connections have been removed surgically, for example, still withdraws the limbs from painful stimuli. Even the coordinated movements of swimming are possible through the reflex responses of the spinal cord. Some of the neural circuits that control these behaviors are relatively simple, involving almost direct contact of sensory information with motor centers of the spinal cord.

The brainstem integrates motor commands descending from higher levels of the motor organization such as the motor cortex and from specialized sense organs such as the visual and vestibular systems. The vestibulospinal tract originating in the brainstem, for example, is essential for muscle adjustments necessary to stabilize posture.

The motor cortex exerts its control over the lower components of the motor hierarchy through the corticospinal and the corticobulbar tracts. The corticospinal tract mediates the cortical motor centers with spinal cord centers; the corticobulbar tract controls neural centers of the brainstem.

The premotor cortex is often depicted as the site where the planning and programming of motor acts occur. This is possible through corticocortical tracts that link sensory and motor areas of the cortex with the motor cortex.

The meaning of two terms can now be clarified: lower and upper neurons and higher brain function. Clinical neurotoxicological literature refers to diseases of the lower and upper neurons. "Lower" neuron usually means a neuron located in the spinal cord that mediates the final common pathway. "Upper" neuron usually means a neuron in the brainstem, motor cortex, or premotor cortex.

Neuroscientists see the classification of diseases of the lower and upper neurons as an oversimplified view of the neural mechanisms of motor function. For example, for a long time the neurological picture of spasticity—chronic contraction of muscles—was viewed as an "upper" neuron syndrome resulting from the lack of control of upper neural centers that were supposed to regulate spinal centers. (Flaccid paralysis, on the other hand, was generally viewed as the result of an impairment of the "lower" neuron.)

Experimental studies in animals do not support this view of spasticity as a condition resulting from an "upper" neuron condition. For example, sectioning of the corticospinal tract—which one would predict to cause spasticity—produces a decrease in muscle tone rather than spasticity. Spasticity is now believed to be caused by damage to the corticobulbar tracts or descending tracts originating in the brainstem.

In the neurological and neuropsychological literature, particularly that inspired by the Pavlovian tradition, the expression "higher brain function" is used when most would use the term "cognitive." "Higher brain function" means the psychological functions that are most likely mediated by neural centers higher up in the hierarchy. The reason for the use of the term "higher brain function" is that neuropsychologists inspired by the Russian tradition wanted to avoid the implication that a "thought"—a mental act—could initiate a motor act. No one knows how thoughts are produced, but most neuroscientists adhere to the view that thoughts themselves are ultimately the expression of neural activity. The view that thoughts reflect neural processes is rejected by those who interpret it as a negation of human freedom. (If everything that I "think" is caused by the activity of my brain, why should I be accountable for my individual behavior, such as committing a crime?)

The cerebellum acts as a comparator of sensory inputs and motor commands; it compares the signals of intended motor actions with the actual trajectory (as seen by the eyes, for example). The cerebellum is thus essential for the execution of coordinated movements.

The relationship of the basal ganglia to the

other components of the motor hierarchy is still poorly understood. The basal ganglia receive inputs from all cortical areas and are involved in pathological neurological conditions such as the presence of involuntary movements—as in Parkinson's disease—and normal posture.

The motor system also exhibits a *parallel organization*. This means that the spinal cord, the brainstem, and the motor cortices can act independently on the motoneurons of the final common pathway. Parallel organization allows the modification or suppression of commands initiated by other levels of the hierarchical organization.

Neurogenic and Myopathic Diseases

The distinction between neurogenic and myopathic diseases is essential to establish the differential diagnosis in clinical neurotoxicology. A *neurogenic disease* is one caused by pathological alterations of some components of the nervous system. Thus, a neurogenic disease can be a motoneuron disease or a peripheral neuropathy. A *myopathic disease* is caused by pathological alterations of the muscle with little change in the motoneurons. The differential diagnosis between neurogenic and myopathic diseases is established, in part, as a result of clinical and laboratory criteria. L. P. Rowland's "Diseases of the Motor Unit, the Motor Neuron, Peripheral Nerve, and Muscle" in *Principles of Neural Science* (2nd ed), edited by Kandel and Schwartz (1985), provides a good introduction to this topic.

PERIPHERAL NEUROPATHIES

A *neuropathy* is any disease of the nervous system. A *toxic polyneuropathy* is a neurological disease in which many components of the nervous system—such as the autonomic system, the brain, the cerebellum, the basal ganglia, the peripheral nervous system—are affected by a neurotoxic agent or drug. Many occupational neurotoxic agents (eg, lead, mercury, solvents, pesticides) cause polyneuropathies.

A *peripheral neuropathy* is a disease involving the peripheral nervous system (described in Chapter 1). [There are a hundred or so causes of human peripheral neuropathy, with considerable variability in symptoms and neurological deficits. This variability depends on which nerves and class of fibers are affected, how severely and where in their proximal to distal length they are affected, and the rate and kind of structural alteration (Dyck 1987).]

The causes of peripheral neuropathy are many. Inflammation (eg, Guillain–Barré syndrome), metabolic disorders (eg, diabetes, uremia, porphyria, endocrine dysfunction), alcoholism, hereditary conditions, vascular conditions, malnourishment, and virus infections, among others, can cause the syndrome of peripheral neuropathy.

Of particular interest to us are the peripheral neuropathies caused by working conditions and environmental and occupational neurotoxic agents, of which only a brief mention can be made within the scope of this chapter. (Those wishing to consult additional sources may consult *Disorders of Peripheral Nerves* by Schaumburg, Spencer, and Thomas, published in 1983; an early source, *Experimental and Clinical Neurotoxicology* by Spencer and Schaumburg, published in 1980, contains many references to the clinical manifestations and mechanisms of action of environmental and occupational neurotoxic agents.)

Following are one example of a commonly encountered peripheral neuropathy in the workplace (the carpal tunnel syndrome) and a review of the motor effects of four well-established neurotoxic agents: mercury, lead, pesticides, and solvents.

Carpal Tunnel Syndrome

Carpal tunnel syndrome is the most commonly reported nerve entrapment syndrome.

It presents itself as tingling sensations and pain in the thumb, index, middle finger, and a portion of the ring finger. In chronic conditions, it may result in muscle weakness and wasting. It results from the compression of the median nerve—a mixed nerve containing motor as well as sensory fibers—as it passes through the wrist.

There are nonoccupational as well as occupational factors associated with the carpal tunnel syndrome. Nonoccupational factors include several chronic diseases (eg, rheumatoid arthritis, gout, diabetes mellitus, hypothyroidism), congenital deficits (eg, anomalous muscles, acute trauma to the wrist, age, use of birth control pills), etc. Occupational factors include forceful or excessive use of the hand including repetitive hand motions, awkward postures, mechanical stresses at the base of the palm, repetitive jobs (and in particular, high-force repetitive jobs), unaccustomed use of the hand (eg, carrying boxes, pulling weeds, chopping wood), etc. For a review of occupational factors leading to carpal tunnel syndrome, see Taylor and Wasserman (1988).

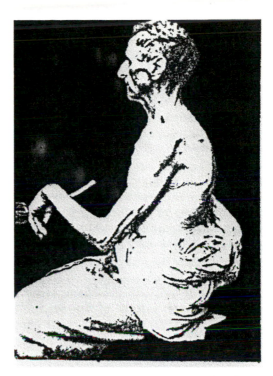

Fig. 27.3.   A victim of chronic lead poisoning, showing wrist drop. (From Hunter 1978.)

Lead-Induced Peripheral Neuropathy

The neuropathy caused by lead is a motor neuropathy affecting upper limbs before lower limbs in adults and lower limbs before upper limbs in children (Krigman et al. 1980). (However, sensory effects can be demonstrated by using either vibratory threshold determinations or nerve conduction velocity determination or both.) In lead poisoning, adults exhibit wrist drop from paralysis of the distal portion of the upper extensor muscles innervated by the radial nerve (Fig. 27.3). Leg weakness results in foot drop.

The neuropathology of human lead neuropathy is still not clear (it is not certain that animal models mimic neuropathological changes observed in humans). Most investigators agree that lead damages peripheral nerves, and that pathological changes are similar to those observed during axonal Wallerian degeneration (see Chapter 2). The degree and extent to which anterior nerve roots and the spinal cord are involved is controversial (Krigman et al. 1980).

Neuropathy Induced by Organophosphorus Compounds

Organophosphorus compounds—known in the literature as OP compounds—have three applications: as insecticides, as petroleum additives, and as modifiers of plastics. With such a variety of uses, OP compounds are pervasive in the human environment. Organophosphorus compounds include "nerve gas" used as a chemical weapon in World War I (to be reviewed in Chapter 35). In humans, acute poisoning by OP compounds results in involuntary defecation and urination, excessive lacrimation, muscular twitching, and convulsions. Death occurs as a result of respiratory arrest.

One class of OP compounds are the cholinesterase inhibitors. Cholinesterase is an enzyme that hydrolyzes the neurotransmitter acetylcholine once it is released into the synaptic cleft. Thus, acetylcholine cannot be effectively removed and builds up in the synaptic cleft, exciting skeletal as well as smooth muscles. The neurological picture of OP poisoning is then explained by the effect of this cholinesterase inhibitor on the autonomic and skeletal motor systems.

There have been numerous episodes of OP poisoning. One of the most tragic occurred in the United States in the 1930s. A massive outbreak of paralysis occurred as a result of the consumption of an alcohol substitute called "ginger jake" (Smith et al. 1930). This ginger extract was diluted with an oil named Lindol, which consisted mainly of tri-*ortho*-tolyl phosphate (TOTP) or tri-*ortho*-cresyl phosphate (TOCP). As many as 20,000 persons were paralyzed during the outbreak.

Delayed Neurotoxicity of Organophosphorus Pesticides. The term "pesticide" designates various chemical compounds manufactured for the purpose of destroying some forms of life that society deems undesirable. This includes fungicides, herbicides, insecticides, rodenticides, and fumigants. Organophosphorus compounds have replaced the chlorinated pesticides such as DDT. Although they have a relatively short persistence in the environment, OPs are more toxic to humans.

Tri-*ortho*-cresyl phosphate causes a delayed peripheral neuropathy. Neurological (motor) signs and symptoms and observable pathological findings occur days, sometimes weeks, after a single acute or chronic exposure. Many neurotoxic agents—such as alcohol, acrylamide, carbon monoxide, carbon disulfide, and hexanedione—are now known to produce peripheral axonopathies. But the phenomenon of delayed neurotoxicity was first observed in 1930 as a result of the "ginger jake" paralysis discussed above. Several episodes of food poisoning with TOCP have since been reported.

In experimental animals no other neuropathological findings are observed before the signs and symptoms of paralysis occur. Curiously, the chicken appears to respond more consistently in reproducing the dose- and time-dependent signs of human poisoning. In rats, rabbits, and other rodent species, delayed neurotoxicity is not readily induced. Guinea pigs develop the syndrome only after extensive administration of this class of neurotoxic compounds. The dog shows signs of flaccid paralysis only after extended delay periods. Testing for delayed neurotoxicity has only recently been incorporated into the protocols for the assessment of toxicity of chemical compounds.

For a review of the delayed neuropathy produced by some organophosphorus esters, see Johnson (1975), Baron (1976), and Davis and Richardson (1980).

Solvent-Induced Neuropathy

Chronic occupational exposure to organic solvents may produce a polyneuropathy. The most common symptoms associated with long-term occupational exposure to solvents are increased fatigue, concentration difficulties, memory disturbances, decreased libido and sexual potency, and sometimes personality changes.

However, in advanced stages of chronic exposure to solvents, a variety of motor disturbances can be observed. Some of them are the expression of pathological changes in the peripheral nervous system (eg, paresthesias). Other signs and symptoms have their origin in the central nervous system and include tremor, disturbances in gait, cerebellar signs, and vestibular signs (such as loss of balance and incoordination).

In 1985 the Regional Office for Europe of the World Health Organization published the important document *Chronic Effects of Organic Solvents on Central Nervous System and Diagnostic Criteria*. In it, the neurological changes associated with acute and chronic exposure to solvents, acute and chronic symptoms, and neurological and psychological evaluation are summarized. The sensory manifestations of solvent exposure have been reviewed in Chapter 23.

MOVEMENT DISORDERS AND TREMOR

Parkinsonism

Parkinsonism is a neurological syndrome—a set of signs and symptoms—characterized by "tremor, muscular rigidity, difficulty in initiating motor activity, and loss of postural reflexes. It is one of the most frequently encountered of the basal ganglia disorders and is a prominent cause of neurological disability in adults" (Yahr 1987). The prevalence of the disease is close to one million cases in the United States, with 50,000 new cases a year. A deficiency of dopamine—a neurotransmitter—in the striatal nucleus is common to all types of parkinsonism.

The disease in all of its forms is characterized by:

- Progressive tremor, most prominent at rest, usually in the upper limbs and involving hands and digits.
- Stiffness of the limbs associated with slowing of movement and inability to carry out daily activities.
- Change in facial expression, appearing mask-like with loss of eye blinking and lack of emotional expression ("poker player face").
- Slow speech, diminished in tone and monotonous in quality.
- Stooped body posture.
- Shuffling gait with loss of arm swing.
- Overall picture of impaired motor activity associated with lack of spontaneity.

Two types of parkinsonism have been described (Yahr 1987). *Primary parkinsonism* (Parkinson's disease or paralysis agitans) is of unknown etiology and characterizes the largest number of cases. The disease usually has an onset between the ages of 50 and 65 years. *Secondary* or *symptomatic parkinsonism* is brought about by a heterogeneous group of conditions such as infections (postviral encephalitis), atherosclerosis, metabolic disorders (parathyroid dysfunction or hypoparathyroidism), tumors of the basal ganglia, acute or chronic head trauma (such as those occurring among professional boxers), and many degenerative diseases causing multisystem atrophy.

Of particular interest is the symptomatic parkinsonism caused by neurotoxic agents in the environment and the workplace. Carbon monoxide, carbon disulfide, manganese, and temporary anoxic states such as those occurring as a result of drowning are known to cause symptomatic parkinsonism.

Myoclonus

Myoclonus refers to to the sharp, sudden involuntary muscle jerking observed in many diseases of the brain or spinal cord as well in normal physiological functioning. Elementary myoclonus involves part or all of one muscle; complex myoclonus, of several muscles. The muscle jerking can be unilateral or bilateral, rhythmic or disrhythmic, synchronous or asynchronous (Przumtek 1987).

Myoclonus of the oculomotor system is called opsomyoclonus. Myoclonus can also be present in the palate, pharynx, larynx, tongue, etc. *Essential myoclonus,* or myoclonus of unknown origin, is a normal motor phenomenon that occurs at the onset of sleep in many individuals.

Symptomatic myoclonus indicates myoclonus associated with other known diseases. These include infectious or immunologic disorders such as Creutzfeldt–Jakob disease, encephalitis lethargica, herpes zoster encephalitis, and malaria. Of particular interest here is symptomatic myoclonus observed in intoxications, such as with hydantoins and dichloroethane.

Tremulousness Associated with Alcohol Withdrawal.

Sufferers from chronic alcoholism who suddenly stop drinking often develop tremulousness associated with irritability, gastrointestinal symptoms such as constipation, or autonomic symptoms such as tachycardia (a fast heartbeat). Incoordination sometimes may be present, such as in the inability to lift a glass of water without spilling. (The affected individual may hide the handicap by lifting the glass with two hands.) Tremulousness may also be present after a drinking spree lasting several hours or days.

Alcohol-induced tremulousness is recognized because the individual can prevent its onset or halt its ocurrence by further drinking. Thus, tremulousness may not be seen in a mildly intoxicated individual. Alcohol-related tremulousness may last for 2 or 3 days—or even longer—after complete alcoholic withdrawal.

Involuntary Movements Associated with Chronic Mercury Poisoning.

Clonus caused by neurotoxic exposure at the workplace has been documented for a long time. In 1943, Alice Hamilton, one of the founders of occupational medicine in the United States, wrote in her autobiographical book:

> I have seen hatters, who could do their work satisfactorily at the accustomed bench when nobody was noticing them, go to pieces and shake like a leaf if I asked them to stop and show me something. . . . I heard of a hatter whose muscles jerked so violently that he could walk to work only if he pushed a baby carriage in front of him; but once his mates had guided him to his sizing bench, he could carry on (Hamilton 1943, p. 281).

It has been known since antiquity that tremor is an important sequel to mercury poisoning. Wood and Weiss (1973) studied hand tremor induced by industrial exposure to inorganic mercury in two female patients during their recovery. Subjects were instructed to maintain a force with the forefinger between two limits (10 and 40 g). Performance progressively improved after cessation of exposure, reaching base-line levels at about 3 months. These changes were associated with a reduction in plasma levels of mercury.

Miller and collaborators (1975) and Langolf and collaborators (1978) from the Department of Operations Engineering, The University of Michigan, performed an evaluation of workers in the chloralkali and electrical equipment industries exposed to vapors of elemental mercury, using quantitative tests of tremor, neuromuscular functions, and psychomotor testing. Tests were those of human factor engineering with a heavy emphasis on performance. (The report by Miller and collaborators contains detailed photographs of the techniques utilized.) Historical indices of mercury exposure included: average urine mercury concentrations for the previous 3, 6, and 12 months; the number of peak concentrations over 0.15, 0.25, and 0.50 mg/L in the previous 3, 6, and 12 months; the highest peak urine mercury concentration ever recorded for the individual; and the individual's duration of mercury exposure.

Forearm tremor was recorded from a transducer attached to a weight, converted into an electrical signal, and recorded for further spectral analysis. Electromyography (EMG) was recorded from the biceps brachii muscle using a monopolar electrode. In the second study, tremor and biceps EMGs were recorded under two load conditions—"high" (6.8 kg weight) and "low" (285 g)—suspended on the subject's wrist.

Myotatic (stretch) reflexes were measured by means of a pointing task. The subject's forearm was placed on a platform that was firmly supported by an electromagnet. When a quiet EMG signal was observed on the oscilloscope, the electromagnet was unexpectedly released, causing the subject's forearm to fall. This elicited the myotatic reflex in the biceps muscle; reflex latency and arm drop amplitude were determined through analysis of the EMG and pointer displacement signals.

Psychomotor tests included choice reaction time, rapid pointing, finger tapping, Michigan maze, and critical target tests.

The spectral analysis of the EMG indicates a shift in the peak of the power spectrum. In the second study, these effects were detectable only with light muscular loading. Subjects with the highest urinary mercury tended to show a relative increase in neuromuscular tremor amplitude. In exploring the various indices of urine mercury, the number of peak levels exceeding 0.5 mg/L was the most significant predictor of increased neuromuscular tremor.

Miller and collaborators subjected the data to multiregression analysis. (This technique is explained in Chapter 19; at the time of publication few investigators in the world performed such analyses.) In the regression analysis record of hypertension, reports of insomnia and "factors associated with plant 1" were included as predictors. Reflex testing revealed some minor but statistically significant changes in the myotatic reflex related to urine mercury. Three psychomotor test measures showed statistically significant changes related to urinary mercury.

proach provides information on human motor behavior that complements the information provided by the neuroscientist and the clinical neurologist. In the clinic, the results of psychometric testing of motor behavior in either the child or the adult is essential for assessing what the individual can or cannot do—eg, getting up from a chair, dressing oneself, washing or bathing, combing the hair, lifting common objects in the household, walking, shopping, playing some sports. This information is important for detecting the extent to which an exposure to a neurotoxic agent can affect the life of the individual, to assess his or her rehabilitation potential, to design rehabilitation strategies, and, if neurotoxicologic impairment is a matter of litigation, to estimate the extent of the liability.

Psychometric tests are objective procedures, usually (though not always) designed to yield quantitative information about certain aspects of the motor behavior of an individual. Thus, in epidemiological studies, when an association between the level of neurotoxic exposure and level of motor performance is suspected, psychometric tests are usually found to be a more sensitive technique than the standard neurological evaluation for the assessment of specific motor functions.

THE PSYCHOMETRIC VIEW OF MOTOR BEHAVIOR

A *psychometric test* is a formalized procedure for the observation of human behavior that compares the results (the test scores) of a single individual to that of a group sharing similar demographic characteristics. In Chapter 4, the general purposes of psychometric testing have been reviewed, the rationale behind the evaluation of the single individual explained, and representative examples illustrated. Those psychometric tests used exclusively for the assessment of motor behavior are reviewed here.

In neurotoxicology, the psychometric ap-

Varieties of Motor Behavior

Many psychometric studies for assessing motor abilities in personnel selection were developed in response to practical considerations, the Army Tests developed to select recruits during World War I being a prime example. In peacetime, army-based laboratories have continued to provide essential information for the understanding of motor behaviors leading to successful human performance.

The series of studies by Edwin A. Fleishman and collaborators at the Advanced Research Resources Organization in Washington published in the 1960s is one of the best examples of the psychometric approach to the study of motor performance. Fleishman attempted to ascertain the basic dimensions of motor abilities; he performed a factor-analytical study (a statistical technique described in Chapter 19) of the results of 27 apparatus-based and 11 paper-and-pencil-based tests of abilities. The research was conducted at the Skill Component Research Laboratory of the Air Force Personnel and Training Research Center.

The complete battery of 38 tests was administered to 400 basic trainee airmen. No demographic information on the group is given—they are presumed to be white men in their 20s. Two hundred of the subjects received the tests in one order of administration, while the remaining 200 received exactly the reverse administration order to minimize any possible influence of the administration sequence.

Fleishman's work was important in that his factor-analytical study provided a psychometric explanation of what motor tests of ability actually measure. Only a sample of the tests employed by Fleishman, still in use in their original or modified form, are described here.

Precision–steadiness. The subject is seated before a rectangular box-like apparatus containing two openings. Each opening is the entrance to a straight passageway, which the subject must negotiate with a long stylus. The stylus is moved forward at slightly below shoulder height and at arm's length. The subject must move the stylus slowly and steadily away from his body trying not to hit the sides of the cylindrical passage. As the subject reaches the end of the passage, he strikes a contact point and withdraws the stylus, again trying to avoid hitting part of the passageway. Then he negotiates the second passageway. Electrical counters record the number of contacts, and clocks record the amount of time in contact, the two independent scores of the test. Six trials with no time limit are allowed.

Steadiness–aiming. The subject must keep a delicately balanced stylus centered in a small hole. Any contact with the sides of the hole is recorded on a clock. The scores record the number of seconds in contact. Six 40-second trials are allowed.

Track tracking. The subject is required to negotiate an irregular slot pattern with a T-shaped stylus. He sits at arm's length from the apparatus box and moves slowly and steadily through the pattern from right to left, depresses a plunger at the end of the pattern with the stylus, and then returns through the pattern. Errors are recorded each time any part of the stylus touches the top, bottom, or back of the slot. Also recorded is the time in contact. Thus, errors and time are the two independent scores. Six trials with no time limit are allowed.

Two-plate tapping. The subject is required to strike two adjacent metal plates with a stylus as rapidly as possible. He strikes the plates successively, that is, first one and then the other, making as many taps as possible on the plates in the time allowed. The number of taps is recorded on counters. Six 30-second trials are allowed.

Key tapping. The subject stands by a standard telegraph key and must tape the key as rapidly as possible with the index finger. The number of taps is recorded on counters. Six 30-second trials are allowed.

Visual reaction time. The subject is seated before an upright panel containing a single amber light. He is required to respond as rapidly as possible when the light appears. The subject responds by striking a button with his hand, which turns off the light. Before the light appears, the subject must keep his hand on a small cross located 6 inches in front of the button. A click provides the subject with a ready signal before each light stimulus is present. The foreperiod—between clicks and light—varies in a random order from 0.5 to 1.5 seconds. The score is the cumulative reaction time between the appearance of the stimulus and completion of the response for each setting. The subject receives two trials consisting of two reactions each.

Auditory reaction time. This test utilizes the same apparatus and scoring as the visual reaction time test except that the light does not appear. The subject now responds to a buzzer when it sounds. The subject receives two trials of 20 reactions each.

Minnesota rate of manipulation—placing. The subject is required to place 60 cylindrical blocks in the proper holes as rapidly as possible. The score is the number of blocks placed. Two 40-second trials are allowed.

Minnesota rate of manipulation—turning. This test uses the same apparatus as above. The subject is required to remove the blocks from the holes with one hand, turn them over with the hand, and replace them in the same holes, moving from block to block as rapidly as possible. The score is the number of blocks turned. Two 35-second trials are allowed.

Purdue pegboard—right hand, left hand, and both hands. The subject is required to place a number of small pegs individually in a series of small holes as rapidly as possible with the right hand. The score is the number of pegs placed. One 30-second trial is allowed. In the Purdue pegboard—left hand, the subject is required to perform the same as above but with the left hand. The use of the nondominant hand is implied. In the Purdue pegboard—both hands, the subject is required to pick up two pins at a time, one with each hand from different trays, and to place them simultaneously in two different holes. The score is the number of pegs placed. One 30-second trial is allowed for any of the three variations of this test.

The Santa Ana Dexterity test. The subject is required to rotate a number of square pegs with circular tops 180° in their holes, moving from peg to peg as rapidly as possible. The score is the number of pegs rotated. Two 35-second trials are allowed.

Rotary pursuit. The subject attempts to keep a stylus in contact with a small metallic target set in a rapidly revolving disk. The score is the total time in the target. Fifteen 20-second trials are allowed.

Complex coordination. The subject is re-quired to make complex motor adjustments of stick-and-pedal controls in response to successively presented patterns of visual signs. The score is the number of completed matchings. The test period lasts 8 minutes.

Dynamic balance. The subject stands on a teeter-totter platform. Next to the platform is a panel of two parallel rows of five lights each. A red stimulus light appears in one of the rows, and the subject is required to shift his weight on the platform in order to match up a green light in the other row with the stimulus light. The position of the green light is controlled by the position of the platform. When the platform is tilted appropriately and a correct matching is achieved and held for a short time delay, the stimulus light shifts to another position. The subject must accomplish as many of these matchings as possible. The score is the number of matchings accomplished and the amount of time spent in the correct position.

Postural vertical discrimination. The subject sits in a tilting chair arrangement that can be displaced to various positions by the test administrator. The subject is blindfolded and strapped into the chair. The subject's task is to return that chair as closely as possible to the perceived upright position. The subject readjusts the chair by means of buttons on the arm rests. The score is the average deviation (number of degrees) of the subject's readjustments from the "true" upright position. Twelve trials are allowed without any time limit.

Postural angular discrimination. This test utilizes the same apparatus as above. However, this time the subject is displaced to a given angular position, held in that position briefly, and told to remember it. He is then displaced and is told to reproduce that position as closely as possible. The score is the average deviation (in degrees) from the correct position. Twelve trials (displacements) are allowed without time limit.

Rudder control. The subject sits in a mock cockpit which his own weight throws off balance unless the subject applies proper correction by means of foot pedals. The task is to keep the cockpit lined up with one of three target lights. The score is total time on target. There are three 30-second center target trials and three 112-second triple target trials.

The paper-and-pencil tests from Fleishman's battery include:

Medium tapping. The subject is required to make three dots in each of a series of circles 3/8 inch in diameter, working as rapidly as possible. Two 15-second trials are allowed.

Pursuit aiming I. The subject is required to follow a pattern of small circles 3/16 inch in diameter, working as fast and as accurately as possible. The score is the number of dots correctly placed. There are two 15-second trials.

Pursuit aiming II. This test is the same as above except that the patterns are more difficult and the circles are smaller—1/8 inch in diameter. Two 60-second trials are allowed.

Steadiness. The subject must trace between a pair of narrowly separated lines (1/16 inch) that form a pattern. The score is the number of segments negotiated without touching the lines. Two trials are allowed with no time limit.

Marking accuracy. The subject is given an answer sheet in which one of the alternatives to each item has been overprinted with a small circle. The alternatives that are circled are randomly determined from item to item. The subject's task is merely to mark the answer sheet as rapidly as possible under the indicated circles. The score is the number of items completed minus errors. Two 40-second trials are allowed.

The Basic Dimensions of Motor Abilities

For a long time, psychologists have attempted to determine what the basic dimensions are in which behavior can be described. Since the beginning of this century, investigators such as Galton, Spearman, and Thurstone have devoted significant portions of their professional careers to developing strategies to answer these questions. The concept of intellectual quotient (IQ) was born as a result of these investigations.

It was soon realized that cognitive functions—such as our ability to think of opposites in meaning—are not correlated with motor functions—such as our ability to lift and rotate a wooden peg. Thus, on the one hand, to research-oriented psychologists who use the technique of factor analysis (described in Chapter 19), motor behavior and cognition are usually considered to be independent factors, or *primary dimensions,* of human behavior. Psychologists who perform disability assessments, on the other hand, consider these "independent dimensions" as inborn motor capacities and skills that are developed and changed during one's lifetime.

As a result of a factor-analytical study, Fleishman concluded that psychomotor skills can be described in nine primary dimensions:

1. **Wrist–finger speed.** This dimension represents the speed with which rapid wrist–finger movements can be made. The best test to assess this function is finger tapping. No visual control seems to be necessary for the execution of these tests.

2. **Finger dexterity,** or fine dexterity. Tests that measure this skill are those requiring grasping and releasing and manipulation of small objects (eg, pegs or pins). The Purdue Pegboard test measures this basic skill.

3. **Rate of arm movement.** This skill appears to be confined to apparatus-based tests, all of which emphasize the speed with which gross rapid arm movements can be made.

4. **Manual dexterity.** These tests require the skill involved in the manipulation of larger blocks or objects in which the whole hand is used to grasp, release, turn, or position the objects. An example of a test that assesses this skill is the Santa Ana Dexterity test and the Minnesota Rate of Manipulation.

5. **Arm–hand steadiness.** This is best measured by tests that emphasize precise, accurate arm–hand movements of the type that minimize strength or speed.

6. **Reaction time.** This is a separate skill that depends on both perceptual (visual, auditory) and motor components.

7. **Aiming (eye–hand) coordination.** This is characterized by the ability to perform quickly and precisely a series of accurately directed movements requiring eye–hand coordination. Pursuit and aiming tests assess this ability.

8. **Psychomotor coordination.** This factor reflects either coordination of the large muscles of the body in movements of moderate scope or coordination of such movements with the perception of a visual stimulus. The Rotary Pursuit test, the Rudder Control test, the Complex Coordination, and the Dynamic Balance test assess these skills.

9. **Postural discrimination.** This is characterized by the ability to make use of postural cues in making precise body adjustments in the absence of visual cues. The Postural Discrimination—Angular and Postural Discrimination—Vertical assess these skills.

SUBCLINICAL INDICATORS OF MOTOR DYSFUNCTION: REACTION TIME

Reaction time is the time (in milliseconds) elapsed between the detection of a stimulus and the reaction to it. Reaction time testing has a fascinating history.

Early, simplistic efforts at localizing the neural pathways responsible for reaction time have been largely abandoned. But it is generally recognized that sensory pathways, neural processing centers, and motor pathways must be intact for the proper execution of this basic form of behavior. In the middle of the last century, many experimental psychologists thought that if the conduction time of sensory and motor nerves were subtracted from reaction time, one would have a good quantitative estimation of the time it takes for psychological functions to be processed. Thus, the measurement of reaction time made such estimations possible.

For the past two decades, in experimental studies designed against the background of information theory, measures of reaction time have been valuable for providing an estimate of the human channel capacity. In neurotoxicology research, reaction time has become an empirical measure. In the most recent literature there is little discussion of neural loci or the mechanism by which a given neurotoxic agent may lengthen reaction time. Born first as strictly physical and then changed to a physiological tool, reaction time is now part of the arsenal of psychometric techniques. An operational approach underlies its measures. Boring (1950) provides a scholarly account of the importance of reaction time studies in the early development of experimental psychology.

The Essential Components of a Reaction Timer

Reaction timers are among the oldest pieces of equipment in experimental psychology (Boring 1950). Early investigators had subjects position their hands around a fixed graduated cane, without touching it. The cane was then released with the simultaneous presentation of a signal. Subjects were instructed to react to the signal as quickly as possible by closing a hand on the cane. Readings of the graduations provided a measure of the reaction time. A light (or a sound), a lever, and a timing mechanism are all that is needed to build a mechanical reaction timer. The reaction timers should be able to measure the milliseconds it takes from the presentation of the visual or auditory stimulus to the moment the the subject reacts to it. There are hundreds of types of reaction timers around the world, each reflecting the level of local technology. Computer-based procedures are now used to measure reaction time in the United States and other developed countries.

Factors Accounting for Reaction Time

Contrary to common-sense expectations, simple reaction time is a much more sensitive indicator of neurotoxicity than "complex reaction time." Complex reaction time is measured under certain rules ("if the red light appears, press the right switch; if the green light appears, press the left switch; if both red and green lights appears, then press the middle switch).

After Gamberale, a leading Italian neurotoxicologist residing in Sweden who has made extensive use of this test (Gamberale and Hultengren 1974), most experimenters in the field choose high-density signals in their studies. The rate at which the signals are presented is about 16 per minute for the reaction time test, with intertrial intervals varying between 2.5 and 5.0 seconds in steps of 0.25 seconds. A random series of 32 intertrial intervals that is repeated five times is common. The testing is often preceded by a 1-minute training period.

Complex reaction time does not deteriorate over time as much as simple reaction time does. Gamberale speculates that during the execution of complex reaction time tasks, the level of alertness is very high, minimizing the decline of the response. On the other hand, because of the intrinsically noninteresting nature of the task, attention may wane in the execution of the simple reaction time test. As a test tool, simple reaction time is thus more "loaded" than complex reaction time.

Psychological literature contains innumerable laboratory studies of factors that account for reaction time. Another Italian scientist, Maria Grazia Cassitto (1983), thinks that there are three groups of factors influencing measures of reaction time:

1. **Physical factors** originating in the equipment design. These include stimulus intensity, intertrial interval, timing characteristics between warning and test signal—known as foreperiod—occurring during stimulus presentation, and physical characteristics of the warning signal.

2. **Environmental factors** occurring at the moment of testing. Room temperature and illumination and distractors are among the most important environmental factors.

3. **Physiological** and **psychological factors** originating in the subject being tested. These include response characteristics associated with any signal detection task—namely, the "false alarms" (reaction to a nonexisting stimulus) and "missings" (no reaction when the stimulus is present). Among the psychophysiological factors considered to be important is the time of day: reaction time is affected by the individual's own circadian rhythm.

The Use of Reaction Time in Psychometric Tests

In a large number of psychometric tests presently used in the assessment of nervous system function, execution time or performance in a fixed time is the basis for scoring. An example of time-of-execution scoring is that for the Block Design test. Let us say that if the third pattern of the Block Design test is executed in less than 15 seconds, the score is 4; if it is completed between 16 and 30 seconds, the score is 3; if between 31 to 45, 2; and finally, if the task is finished between 46 to 60 seconds, the score is 1. No score is provided for the successful completion of the task in more than 60 seconds. Digit Symbol is an example of a test whose scores reflect performance in a fixed time. The score is the number of correct symbols completed in 90 seconds. Thus, complex reaction time is directly or indirectly measured in most psychometric tests.

Environmental Monitoring by Means of Reaction Time Measurement

It has been known by many generations of students that neurotoxic agents (notably alcohol) can lengthen reaction time. It is not surprising then that many efforts to control drunken driving have been directed at the measurement of reaction time and motor dexterity of suspected individuals. Indeed, alcohol has often been given to experimental subjects (in most cases, college students) in order to calibrate the sensitivity of the equipment. The important contribution of Gamberale's group in the use of reaction time testing for environmental control of neurotoxic substances has been recognized.

Reaction Time in Epidemiological Studies Of Chronic Exposure To Organic Solvents. Reaction time measurements have been favored in the study of the neurotoxicity of solvents. The work of Francesco Gamberale and collaborators in Sweden and Nicola Cherry and collaborators (1983) in Great Britain are representative.

In a multiauthored work published in 1980 (Elofsson et al. 1980), Gamberale and coworkers investigated whether changes in psychological functions occurred as a result of chronic low-level exposure to solvents. Simple reaction time measurements were one of the 18 psychometric tests employed in this important work. It was found that the solvent-exposed group performed significantly worse than controls in measures of simple reaction time, manual dexterity, perceptual speed, and memory.

In an analysis of group differences by means of variance analysis, the mean reaction time of the solvent-exposed group was found to be significantly higher (impaired) than controls. The significant differences were found at a probability level of less than one in 1000, a level rarely observed in epidemiology research involving psychometric procedures.

The lengthening of reaction time was found to be an important component of solvent-induced changes. In a comparison between solvent-exposed and control groups, a simple reaction test had nearly half of the discriminative power of the entire test battery. This means that in discriminant analysis (a statistical analytical procedure discussed in Chapter 19), reaction time measurements alone were better able to predict group membership than the entire test battery.

Finally, reaction time measurements were analyzed in 1-minute time blocks over the 10 minutes it takes to administer the test. Changes in reaction time over time were approximately linear for both the control and the solvent-exposed group, the latter exhibiting a statistically significant difference in the slope of the time change compared to controls.

Cherry and collaborators conducted studies on two groups of men exposed to styrene-based resin. Concentration levels of early morning urinary mandelic acid (a metabolite resulting from styrene absorption) after 2 days without exposure were correlated with reaction time measurements on arrival at work. The men were found to differ considerably in their rate of clearance of mandelic acid, those with slow clearance having slower reaction times. Although this effect is long-lasting, it appears to be reversible when exposure is discontinued or drastically reduced (Cherry et al. 1983). This conclusion is important to bear in mind for study designs aimed at the detection of chronic neuropsychological changes as a result of long-term, low-level occupational exposure to solvents.

THE MOTOR COMPONENT OF SPEECH

The effect of neurotoxic agents and drugs on speech and language is easily recognized. For example, an individual consuming even moderate amounts of alcohol may become loquacious and experience exhilaration; at increased levels of alcohol, however, speech becomes slurred to the point of becoming unintelligible. At this advanced stage of intoxication, a sad or aggressive mood may prevail. For another example, amphetamine ingestion is associated with increased levels of consciousness and accelerated thought processes; speech becomes quicker. Importantly, the speaker may lose the capacity to be "in tune" with the audience, giving the impression of selfishness.

Speech and language are areas of research that lag considerably behind other areas of the neurosciences. This is primarily because of the complexity of speech and language as objects of scientific research and difficulty in quantifying them. There are many functions that intervene in speech production, speech recognition, and human communication; there are many factors that need to be disentangled. Even if one chooses to restrict communication to sound communication (humans also communicate by body language, signs, and writing), the task is formidable. As Shepherd (1983) has stated: "Apart from the identification of the speech area of the human cortex, the subject of mammalian vocal mechanisms does not even exist as far as most textbooks are concerned."

It is not surprising then that study of the effects of E & O neurotoxic agents on speech and language has had a similar fate. Apart from fragmented clinical observations and isolated studies on children, this essential area of knowledge remains virtually untapped.

The topic of sound characteristics of speech is dealt with in Chapter 25. In this chapter, the motor components of human speech are reviewed. The cognitive aspects of language are reviewed in Chapter 22.

The Origins of Human Speech

Humans developed speech by adapting a system originally evolved for breathing and mastication. The main components involved in the mechanics of sound production in humans are a source of air pressure, a set of vibrating elements, and a system of resonators and articulators.

Air pressure is created by taking air into the lungs (inspiration) and expelling it (expiration). This is accomplished by the respiratory muscles, particularly the diaphragm, the intercostal muscles, and the abdominal muscles.

The **vibrating elements** are the vocal folds within the larynx. Both are controlled by the laryngeal muscles. As air rushes through the widely open vocal cords, a white noise is generated. (A white noise is a sound composed of many sound frequencies.) This is the sound we hear while panting after vigorous exercise.

The **resonators** and **articulators** are structures of the upper respiratory tract such as the pharynx, mouth, tongue, lips, sinuses, and related structures.

The sounds required in normal speech are produced primarily by the vocal cords. When the vocal folds are closed, air accumulates under them; when they are open, a sound is emitted. The sounds required for human speech have a spectral composition varying between 100 and 7000 Hz. The quality of the sound depends on how the vocal cords are opened (the vocal cords have several degrees of freedom) and the intensity of the air flow. The mouth is critical in the production of vowel sounds. The tongue, lips, teeth, hard palate, and soft palate are primarily involved in the production of consonants. A discipline called *psychoacoustics* studies the physical composition of the sounds as they are produced by the human phonation system.

In patients whose vocal cords have been surgically removed, speech can be reconstructed. An artificial larynx—a battery-powered source of sound—is placed in the neck area under the jaw, and the afflicted individual can still use the articulators to produce monotonic but intelligible speech. Sounds can also be produced without the vocal folds, as in whispering or whistling.

Neural Control of Speech

Speech is produced by the orchestrated activity of muscles of the abdomen, chest, larynx, head, and neck. The motoneurons that control these muscles are distributed from the upper part of the spinal cord to the cerebral cortex.

The muscles that control air pressure are innervated by motoneurons located in the upper levels of the spinal cord. The motoneurons that control the movements of the diaphragm are cervical segments 3 to 5; those motoneurons controlling the intercostal muscles are thoracic segments 2 to 5; and those controlling the abdominal muscles are thoracic segments 6 to 12.

The muscles that control the larynx are innervated by the vagus (cranial nerve X) and accessory (cranial nerve XI) nerves. The laryngeal nerve supplies all the intrinsic muscles of the larynx except the cricothyroid. The laryngeal nerve is so essential to speech that functional loss from infection or injury leaves the afflicted individual able to speak only in whispers.

The muscles that control the resonators and articulators are innervated by motoneurons of cranial nerves V, VI, VII, X, XI, and XII.

The human phonation system is also innervated by sensory nerves. Proprioceptive information on the positions of the diverse elements of the speech production system is essential. An example of this is the difficulty we experience in speaking after returning from the dentist after local anesthesia has been applied to the mouth, spilling to the tongue and inner walls of the mouth. Another example of the importance of the proprioceptive input is recognized by linguists who learn the correct pronunciation of vowel and consonant sounds in many languages.

REFERENCES

Baron, RL (1976) *Pesticide Induced Delayed Neurotoxicity, Proceedings of a Conference Feb 19–20.* Washington, DC: US Environmental Protection Agency, WEPA-600/1-76.

Bloom, W and Fawcett, DW (1975) *A Textbook of Histology,* 2nd ed. Philadelphia: WB Saunders.

Boring, EG (1950) *A History of Experimental Psychology.* New York: Appleton-Century-Crofts.

Carew, TJ (1985) The control of reflex action. In *Principles of Neural Science,* ER Kandel and JH Schwartz (eds) pp. 457–468. New York: Elsevier.

Carew, TJ and Ghez, C (1985) Muscle and muscle receptors. In *Principles of Neural Science,* ER Kandel and JH Schwartz (eds) pp. 443–456. New York: Elsevier.

Cassitto, MG (1983) Reaction times. In *Neurobehavioral Methods in Occupational Health,* R Gilioli, MG Cassitto, and V Foà (eds) pp. 131–136. New York: Pergamon Press.

Chaffin, DB (1975) Ergonomic guide for the assessment of human static strength. *Am Ind Hyg Assoc J* 36:505–511.

Cherry, N, Venables, H, and Waldron, HA (1983) The use of reaction time in solvent exposure. In *Neurobehavioral Methods in Occupational Health,* R Gilioli, MG Cassitto, and V Foà (eds) pp. 191–195. New York: Pergamon Press.

Chor (1936) Some problems in muscle disorders. *Physiother Rev* 16:2.

Davis, CS and Richardson, RJ (1980) Organophosphorus compounds. In *Experimental and Clinical Neurotoxicology,* PS Spencer and HH Schaumberg (eds) pp. 527–544. Baltimore: Williams & Wilkins.

Dyck, PJ (1987) Neuropathy, peripheral. In *Encyclopedia of Neuroscience,* G Adelman (ed) pp. 832–834. Boston: Birkhäuser.

Elofsson, SA, Gamberale, F, Hindmarsh, T, et al. (1980) Exposure to organic solvents: A cross-sectional epidemiologic investigation on occupational exposed can and industrial spray painters with special reference to the nervous system. *Scand J Work Environ Health* 6:239–273.

Gamberale, F and Hultengren, M (1974) Exposure to styrene. II. Psychological functions. *Work Environ Health* 11(2):86–93.

Gould, SJ (1981) *The Mismeasure of Man.* New York: WW Norton.

Hamilton, A (1943) *Exploring the Dangerous Trades.* Boston: Little, Brown.

Hunter, D (1978) *Diseases of Occupation,* 6th ed. Boston: Little, Brown.

Johnson, MK (1975) The delayed neuropathy caused by some organophosphorus esters: Mechanisms and challenge. *Crit Rev Toxicol* 3:289–316.

Kandel, ER and Schwartz, JH (1985) *Principles of Neural Science,* 2nd ed. New York: Elsevier.

Krigman, MR, Bouldin, TW, and Mushak, P (1980) Lead. In *Experimental and Clinical Neurotoxicology,* PS Spencer and HH Schaumberg (eds) pp. 490–507. Baltimore: Williams & Wilkins.

Langolf, GD, Chaffin, DB, Henderson, R, ct al. (1978) Evaluation of workers exposed to elemental mercury using quantitative tests of tremor and neuromuscular functions. *Am Ind Hyg Assoc J* 39:976–984.

Matthews, PBC (1982) Where does Sherrington's "muscle sense" originate? Muscles, joints, corollary discharge. *Annu Rev Neurosci* 5:189–218.

Miller, JM, Chaffin, DB, and Smith, RG (1975) Subclinical psychomotor and neuromuscular changes in workers exposed to inorganic mercury. *Am Ind Hyg Assoc J* 36:725–733.

Potvin, AR, Stribbly, PF, Pew, RW, et al. (1975a) A battery of tests for evaluating steadiness in clinical trials. *Med Biol* 13(6):914–922.

Potvin, AR, Tourtellotte, WW, Snyder, DN, et al. (1975b)

Validity of quantitative tests for measuring tremor. *Am J Phys Med* 54(5):243–252.

Przumtek, H (1987) Choreoathetosis. In *Encyclopedia of Neuroscience,* G Adelman (ed) p. 236. Boston: Birkhäuser.

Rowland, LP (1985) Diseases of the motor unit: The motor neuron, peripheral nerve, and muscle. In *Principles of Neural Science,* ER Kandel and JH Schwartz (eds) pp. 196–208. New York: Elsevier.

Schaumberg, HH, Spencer, PS, and Thomas, PK (1983) *Disorders of Peripheral Nerves.* Philadelphia: FA Davis.

Shepherd, GM (1983) *Neurobiology.* New York: Oxford University Press.

Smith, MI, Elvove, E, Valaer, PJ, et al. (1930) Pharmacological and chemical studies of the cause of so-called ginger paralysis. *US Public Health Rep* 45:1703.

Spencer, PS and Schaumburg, HH (eds) (1980) *Experimental and Clinical Neurotoxicology.* Baltimore: Williams & Wilkins.

Taylor, W and Wasserman, DE (1988) Occupational vibration. In *Occupational Medicine: Principles and Practical Applications,* C. Zenz (ed) pp. 324–333. Chicago: Year Book Medical Publications.

Wood, RW, Weiss, AB, and Weiss, B (1973) Hand tremor induced by industrial exposure to inorganic mercury. *Arch Environ Health* 26:249–252.

World Health Organization (1985) *Chronic Effects of Organic Solvents on the Central Nervous System and Diagnostic Criteria.* Copenhagen: WHO.

Yahr, MD (1987) Parkinsonism. In *Encyclopedia of Neuroscience,* G Adelman (ed) pp. 926–929. Boston: Birkhäuser.

SUGGESTED READINGS

Audo-Gianotti, GB (1932) Le parkinsonisme sulfo-carbone professionel. *Presse Med* 2:1289–1291.

Banister, PA and Smith, FV (1972) Vibration-induced white fingers and manipulative dexterity. *Br J Ind Med* 29:264–267.

Barbeau, A (1984) Manganese and extrapyramidal disorders. *Neurotoxicology* 5(1):13–36.

Beard, RR and Grandstaff, W (1974) Carbon monoxide and human functions. In *Behavioral Toxicology,* B Weiss and VG Laties (eds) pp. 1–27. New York: Plenum Press.

Buxton, PH and Hayward, M (1967) Polyneuritis cranialis associated with industrial trichloroethylene poisoning. *J Neurol Neurosurg Psychiatry* 30:511–518.

Cain, WS (1973) Nature of perceived effort and fatigue: Roles of strength and blood flow in muscle contractions. *J Motor Behav* 5:33–47.

Cain, WS and Stevens, JC (1971) Effort in sustained and phasic handgrip contractions. *Am J Psychol* 84:52–65.

Cain, WS and Stevens, JC (1972) Constant-effort contractions related to the electromyogram. *Med Sci Sports* 5:121–127.

Campbell, A, Williams, E, and Baltrop, D (1970) Motor neurone disease and exposure to lead. *J Neurol Neurosurg* 33:877–885.

Cavanagh, JB (1973) Peripheral neuropathy caused by chemical agents. *CRC Crit Rev Toxicol* 2:365–417.

Damasio, AR and Gerschwind, N (1985) The neural basis of language. *Annu Rev Neurosci* 7:127–147.

David, OJ (1974) Association between lower lead concentrations and hyperactivity in children. *Environ Health Perspect* 7:17–25.

DeJesus, PV and Pleasure, DE (1973) Hexachlorophene neuropathy. *Arch Neurol* 29:180–182.

Desmedt, JE (ed) (1983) *Advances in Neurology, Vol 39, Motor Control Mechanisms in Health and Disease.* New York: Raven Press.

Dichgans, J and Jung, R (1985) Oculomotor abnormalities due to cerebellar lesions. In *Basic Mechanisms of Ocular Motility and Their Clinical Implications,* G Lennerstrand and P. Bach-y-Rita (eds) pp. 281–298. New York: Pergamon Press.

Domino, EF, Albers, JW, Potvin, AR, et al. (1972) Effects of *d*-amphetamine on quantitative measures of motor performance. *Clin Pharm Ther* 13:251–275.

Fahn, S, Marsden, CD, and Calne, DB (1988) *Dystonia 2.* New York: Raven Press.

Fawer, RF, DeRibaupieree, Y, Guillemin, MP, et al. (1983) Measurement of hand tremor induced by industrial exposure to metallic mercury. *Br J Ind Med* 4:204–208.

Feldman, RG, Haddow, J, Kopito, L, et al. (1973) Altered peripheral nerve conduction velocity: Chronic lead intoxication in children. *Am J Dis Child* 125:39.

Findley, LJ and Capildeo, R (eds) (1984) *Movements Disorders: Tremor.* New York: Oxford University Press.

Fleishman, EA and Quaintance, MK (1984) *Taxonomies of Human Performance: The Description of Human Tasks.* Orlando, FL: Academic Press.

Gerhart, JM, Hong, JS, Uphouse, LL, et al. (1982) Chlordecone-induced tremor: Quantification and pharmacological analysis. *Toxicol Appl Pharmacol* 66:234–243.

Geschwind, N and Levitsky, W (1968) Human brain: Left–right asymmetries in temporal speech region. *Science* 161:186–187.

Gonzalez, EG and Downew, JA (1972) Polyneuropathy in a glue sniffer. *Arch Phys Med Rehab* 53:333–337.

Grabsky, DA (1961) Toluene sniffing producing cerebellar degeneration. *Am J Psychiatry* 118:461.

Granit, R (1970) *The Basis of Motor Control.* London: Academic Press.

Graybiel, A and Fregly, AR (1966) A new quantitative ataxia test battery. *Acta Otolaryingol (Stock)* 61:292–312.

Gregersen, P and Stigby, B (1981) Reaction time of industrial workers exposed to organic solvents: Relationship to degree of exposure and psychological performance. *Am J Ind Med* 2:313–321.

Gregory, RJ and Mohan, PJ (1977) Effects of asymptomatic lead exposure on childhood intelligence: A critical review. *Intelligence* 1:381–400.

Halliday, AM and Redfearn, JWT (1956) An analysis of the frequencies of finger tremor in healthy subjects. *J Physiol* (Lond) 134(3):600–611.

Herskowitz, A, Ishii, N, and Schaumburg, HH (1971) *n*-Hexane neuropathy: A syndrome occurring as a result of industrial exposure. *N Engl J Med* 285:82–85.

Hopkins, AP and Gilliatt, RW (1971) Motor and sensory nerve conduction velocity in the baboon: Normal values and changes during acrylamide neuropathy. *J Neurol Neurosurg Psychiatry* 34:415–426.

Jager, KW, Roberts, DV, and Wilson, A (1970) Neuromuscular function in pesticide workers. *Br J Ind Med* 27:273–278.

Jakobson, R, Fant, G, and Halle, M (1969) *Preliminaries to Speech Analysis.* Cambridge, MA: MIT Press.

Kelly, TW (1975) Prolonged cerebellar dysfuncions associated with paint sniffing. *Pediatrics* 56:605–606.

Kilburn, KH, Warshaw, R, Thornton, JC, et al. (1989) An examination of factors that could affect choice reaction time in histology technicians. *Am J Ind Med* 15:679–686.

Kirk, L and Baastrup, PC (1972) Propranolol and lithium-induced tremor. *Lancet* 1:839.

Kornhuber, HH (1971) Motor functions of the cerebellum and basal ganglia: The cerebellocortical saccadic (ballistic) clock, the cerebellonuclear hold regulator, and the basal ganglia ramp (voluntary speed smooth movement) generator. *Kybernetic* 8:157–162.

Mallow, JS (1976) MBK neuropathy among spray painters. *JAMA* 235:1455–1457.

Manu, P, Lilis, R, Lancrajan, J, et al. (1970) The value of electrophysiological changes in the early diagnosis of carbon disulfide peripheral neuropathy. *Med Lavoro* 61:102–108.

Mathers, LH (1985) *The Peripheral Nervous System: Structure, Function and Clinical Correlations.* Boston: Butterworths.

Mayfield, SA (1983) Language and speech behaviors of children with undue lead absorption: A review of the literature. *J Speech Hearing Dis* 26:362–368.

Metcalf, RL (1982) Historical perspective of organo-phosphorus ester-induced delayed neurotoxicity. *Neurotoxicology* 3(4):269–284.

Perino, J and Ernhart, C (1974) The relation of subclinical lead level to cognitive and sensorimotor impairment in black preschoolers. *J Learning Dis* 7:616–620.

Randall, JE and Stiles, RN (1964) Power spectral analysis of finger acceleration tremor. *J Appl Psychol* 19:357–360.

Roels, H, Abdeladim, S, Braun, M, et al. (1989) Detection of hand tremor in workers exposed to mercury vapor: A comparative study of three methods. *Environ Res* 49:152–165.

Sanes, JN, Colburn, TR, and Morgan, NT (1985) Behavioral motor evaluation for neurotoxicity screening. *Neurobehav Toxicol Teratol* 7(4):329–337.

Singh, S (ed) (1975) *Measurement Procedures in Speech, Hearing, and Language.* Baltimore: University Park Press.

Snyder, RD (1972) The involuntary movements of chronic mercury poisoning. *Arch Neurol* 26:379–381.

Somjen, GC, Herman, SP, and Klein, R (1973) Electrophysiology of methyl mercury poisoning. *J Pharmacol Exp Ther* 186:579–592.

Spencer, PS and Schaumburg, HH (1982) The pathogenesis of motor neuron disease: Perspectives from neurotoxicology. *Adv Neurol* 36:249–266.

Spencer, PS, Schaumberg, HH, Raleigh, RL, et al. (1975) Nervous system degeneration produced by the industrial solvent methyl *n*-butyl ketone. *Arch Neurol* 32:219–222.

Spyker, JM, Spoarber, SB, and Goldberg, AM (1972) Subtle consequences of methylmercury exposure: Behavioral deviations in offspring from treated mothers. *Science* 177:621–623.

Taylor, JR (1985) Neurological manifestations in humans exposed to chlordecone: Follow-up results. *Neurotoxicology* 6(1):231–236.

Teichner, WH and Krebs, MJ (1971) Laws of visual choice reaction time. *Psychol Rev* 81:75–98.

Vocate DR (1987) *The Theory of AR Luria: Functions of Spoken Language in the Development of Higher Mental Processes.* Hilldale, NJ: Lawrence Erlbaum.

Vogel, SA (1975) *Syntatic Abilities in Normal and Dyslexic Children.* Baltimore: University Park Press.

Yamins, JG (1977) *The Relationship of Subclinical Lead Intoxication to Cognitive and Language Functioning in Preschool Children.* Doctoral Dissertation (Hofstra University), Dissertation Abstracts International, 37:4176B (University Microfilms No. 77-2802).

Zemlin, WR (1968) *Speech and Hearing Science: Anatomy and Physiology.* Englewood Cliffs, NJ: Prentice-Hall.

28

Motivation, Emotions, and Moods

Whole areas dealing with the effects of neurotoxic agents on drives, motivation, emotion, moods, affects, and feelings do not receive specific attention in clinical and epidemiological neurotoxicology. These basic dimensions of behavior, often buried in reports on "neurobehavioral" or "neuropsychological" function, will be reviewed here. Since the autonomic nervous system provides the main neural basis for drives and emotions, the functional organization of this system is reviewed below.

THE AUTONOMIC NERVOUS SYSTEM

The animal (including human) body is recognized as having two major neural components: the visceral portion, innervating the internal organs, and the somatic portion, innervating the skeletal muscles and skin. The autonomic nervous system is that part of the nervous system controlling the activity of the visceral components of the animal and human body. It is called "autonomic" because it performs its functions automatically, meaning that its functioning cannot be controlled at will.

Smooth Muscles

The muscles of the viscera—except for the heart—are called smooth muscles. Like skeletal muscles, smooth muscles also contain the two proteins actin and, in smaller proportions, myosin. Unlike skeletal muscles, they do not present the regular organization of sarcomeres, the contractile units of the muscle fiber. Heart muscle has characteristics of both skeletal and smooth muscle. In addition, the heart exhibits *myogenic activity*—it contracts and relaxes on its own for several hours after its neural innervation has been severed.

The neuromuscular coupling in smooth muscles differs from that in skeletal muscles. In skeletal muscles, the neuromuscular junction is the link between the nerve and the muscle fibers. In smooth muscle, there is no neuromuscular junction; the nerve endings enter the muscle, spreading in all directions. The depolarization inside the smooth muscle therefore is much slower than that in skeletal muscles.

Finally, smooth muscle has the unique characteristic of exhibiting spontaneous contractions, such as that shown by the gut. To a large extent, the autonomic nervous system regulates the smooth muscles' spontaneous activity.

Different Views on the Organization and Function of the Autonomic Nervous System

The autonomic nervous system has been experimentally investigated over the past 300 years, and the vocabulary that has accumulated to describe its function and significance is sometimes confusing. (The functional organization of the autonomic nervous system is shown in Chapter 1.) The autonomic nervous system is complex, and the terminology often reflects the different points of view from which it is studied.

The autonomic nervous system can be described, for example, from an anatomic point of view. The system has two main components: the sympathetic and the parasympathetic nervous system. The sympathetic nerves, controlling visceral activity, arise from the thoracic and lumbar portions of the spinal cord; parasympathetic nerves arise from the brainstem and the sacral portion of the spinal cord. Both the sympathetic and the parasympathetic nerves have ganglia (groups of nerve cell bodies) between the neural fibers leaving the spinal cord and effectors (smooth muscles, the heart, and glands). The positions of these ganglia differ for the sympathetic and the parasympathetic system. In the sympathetic system, the ganglia are located near the spinal cord; in the parasympathetic system, they are located close to the organs they control.

From a physiological point of view, no single generalization can be made about the manner in which the sympathetic and the parasympathetic nervous systems control different body organs. In most cases, visceral organs are innervated by both systems. The heart, for example, is innervated both by sympathetic nerves, whose excitation produces an acceleration of the heartbeat, and by parasympathetic nerves, whose excitation produces a slowing of the heartbeat. Either system can stimulate or inhibit the organs it innervates. Some organs are predominantly or exclusively controlled by one system or the other.

From the pharmacological point of view, there is no single neurotransmitter associated with either sympathetic or parasympathetic functions, as was once believed. The old view that acetylcholine was the predominant transmitter of the autonomic system had to be abandoned when new classes of neurotransmitters and neuromodulators were found—eg, dopamine, serotonin, purines, and various neuropeptides.

The main function of the autonomic nervous system can be viewed (in what may be called the adaptive point of view) as maintenance of homeostasis and adaptation of the animal body to its external environment. *Homeostasis* is the state of equilibrium of body functions which the body actively and continuously tries to maintain; the control of body temperature, water, and electrolytes are all examples of homeostatic processes. The French physiologist Claude Bernard (1813–1878), the American Walter B. Cannon (1871–1945), and the Canadian Hans Selye are the originators of this view (Bernard 1987–1879; Cannon 1929, 1939).

Cannon and Selye, in particular, have stressed the important links between the autonomic nervous system and the endocrine organs. Interactions between the nervous system and immunologic functions are possible through the autonomic nervous system. Emotions that originate from the autonomic nervous system can be expressed via the skeletal muscles.

Neuroscientists have recently revived the behavioral point of view of the autonomic nervous system. Galen (AD 131–201), who was the first to identify the nerves innervating the viscera, suggested that the autonomic nerves carried the "sympathies," ie, the visceral–emotional reactions of the body (thus, the origin of the term "sympathetic" nervous system). This is the view adopted in this chapter. After a review of motivational states—which makes learning, the topic of the next chapter, possible—an examination of emotions and moods is undertaken.

To recapitulate, it needs to be emphasized that the autonomic nervous system can be considered from a number of different points of view, the anatomic (including neuropathological), physiological, pharmacological, adaptive, and behavioral points of view. The pharmacology of many therapeutic agents and those involved in drug abuse have been extensively studied (eg, Goodman Gilman et al. 1980). But except for organophosphates used in the manufacture of pesticides, information on the effects of environmental and occupational neurotoxic agents on the autonomic nervous system has yet to be systematically compiled.

GENETIC DETERMINANTS OF BEHAVIOR: INSTINCTS AND DRIVES

The notion that behavior might have a genetic component has been embraced and repelled by scientists many times during the past decades. Whether certain forms of human behavior are instinctive—that is, unlearned and therefore genetically determined—has been the subject of heated debate in biology, psychology, theology, and education. The debate continues to this date.

There are extreme positions taken on both sides; sometimes, representatives of one or the other view seem to take untenable positions as a result of these debates. Charles Darwin, late in the 19th century, and William McDougall and Sigmund Freud at the beginning of this century contended that many aspects of human behavior are instinctive. Behaviorism as a school of psychology was created as a result of an intellectual manifesto written by John B. Watson (1878–1958) in which it was argued that human behavior is to a great extent learned.

The study of instinctive behavior again gained respectability when in Europe, Konrad Lorenz

(1903–1989) and Nikolaas Tinbergen (1907–1988) created the discipline of ethology. Ethology deals with the observation of the behavior of organisms in their natural habitat. Lorenz and Tinbergen had remained relatively isolated from genetic versus environmental debates taking place in the United States and thus were able to take an impartial look at the role of instincts in (animal) behavior.

No clinical, experimental, or even theoretical work of significance has addressed the issue of the possible influence of neurotoxic agents on instincts, and therefore the subject will not be reviewed further. However, there are isolated references to effects of toxic agents on drives.

Motivational states are internal conditions that energize and direct voluntary behavior. They are called "motivational states" because behavior can be modified through their manipulation. Examples of how motivational states lead to behavior modification are the use of food for animal training and verbal praise for human learning.

Specific motivational states are called *drives*. In humans, inhalation and exhalation of air, urination, defecation, thermoregulation, thirst, hunger, and sex are examples of primary drives. Curiosity, need for prevention of excessive sensory stimulus, need for movement, and need for social companionship are examples of acquired, or secondary, drives. The hypothalamus is the main neural center for the integration of primary drives.

Thermoregulation

When the body temperature is above or below a set point—the normal temperature of the body—complex behavioral responses are initiated. Importantly, hot and cold environments induce motivational states leading to reduction or increases in body temperature.

The neural basis of thermoregulation is fairly well understood. The hypothalamus controls the body's set point through a number of autonomic, skeletomuscular, and endocrine responses. Vasoconstriction, shivering, and "goose bumps"—primitive responses of piloerection (raising of the body hair) in response to cold—are examples of autonomic responses.

Skeletomuscular responses to cold include semiconscious acts of rubbing the fingers, cuddling to avoid excessive escape of heat, getting up during sleep to pick up a blanket, etc. The autonomic and motor responses to hot temperatures include vasodilation (expansion of the diameter of the blood vessels) and prostration (utter exhaustion), respectively.

It has been postulated that prostaglandins—hormone-like substances normally generated by the brain—are involved in short-term thermoregulation. It has been known for some time that long-term exposure to cold increases body metabolism by increasing the release of the hormone thyroxin.

The hypothalamus is the integration center for peripheral and central temperature information. Temperature receptors are located throughout the body and within the hypothalamus itself, where neurons are differentially sensitive to cold and hot temperatures of the blood. The hypothalamus also contains fairly well-defined centers for the control of heat dissipation and conservation. The anterior portion of the hypothalamus (the preoptic area) contains a heat-dissipation area. When stimulated electrically it evokes dilation of the blood vessels and suppression of shivering. Experimental lesions lead to chronic hyperthermia (overheating). Electrical stimulation of the posterior portion of the hypothalamus produces shivering and many other behavioral responses associated with heat conservation. Its destruction, on the other hand, appears to have little effect on experimental animals if they are kept at room temperature. If such animals are exposed to cold, they become hypothermic (having low temperature) as a result of failure to initiate mechanisms for heat conservation.

The evidence for the acute effects of environmental and occupational neurotoxic agents on thermoregulation is incidental. Fever, for example, is possibly associated with normal (but indirect) responses to tissue damage or antiinflammatory responses. Little research has been performed on the effect of neurotoxic agents on thermoregulation. The discovery of the antipyretic properties of aspirin, however, has a long and fascinating history (Flower et al. 1980).

Thirst

Thirst is a complex sensation the magnitude of which is roughly proportional to the degree of water depletion. The sensation of thirst, the act of drinking, and the feeling of water satiation are all controlled by multiple cues. The subjective sensation of thirst ranges from a pleasant need to have something to drink (knowing that a source is available), to an unpleasant dryness of the mouth, hyperthermia, and restlessness when an immediate source is uncertain, to an obsession with water, delirium, and desperate attempts to obtain water or substitutes of it when sources of water are not available.

There is no specific time course for the onset of sensations of thirst, since water depletion can occur very quickly (such as after excessive bleeding or while walking through a desert), or it can occur over a period of several days, such as in reported cases of shipwreck victims. A book by Wolff (1958) contains a vivid description of the normal and pathological sensation of thirst; it is one of the most impressive sources ever assembled on the subject.

Much is now known about the behavioral and neurophysiological aspects of drinking. Drinking is controlled by tissue osmolarity and vascular fluid volume. The hypothalamus seems to contain receptors that detect blood sodium levels (osmic receptors), but the local action of sodium on the tongue can also regulate drinking. Vascular volume is detected by pressure receptors (baroreceptors) located inside the large veins of the circulatory systems.

Low blood volume is a stimulus that produces an increase in the secretion of *renin,* a kidney enzyme. Renin produces blood plasma changes leading to the production of angiotensin II, which elicits drinking and appropriate mechanisms for compensation of water loss such as vasoconstriction and increased secretion of the hormones aldosterone and vasopressin. Water can be a toxic agent when it produces an excessive dilution of extracellular fluids.

The mechanisms associated with water satiation and the blocking of drinking behavior are not well understood. Feedback signals from the hypothalamic nuclei are suspected, but the gradual cessation of peripheral cues that lead to the initial sensation of thirst are obviously important. Whether or not drinking is accompanied by eating is also important.

Water depletion is a powerful motivational state. Water is a reward routinely used by scientists who train animals for behavioral experiments involving learning. During the early sessions of operant conditioning (a form of learning to be reviewed in the next chapter), the successful execution of an act—eg, walking through an elevated alley—is rewarded by giving water. In the later phases of training, water availability can be conditioned to the execution of more complex acts.

A careful observation of thirst and drinking behavior is important for the understanding of metabolic, hormonal, kidney, and neuropsychological dysfunctions. A marked exacerbation of thirst is observed in pathological states such as bleeding, diabetes, and diseases of the pancreas. Thirst and drinking behavior have received little attention either from scientists working on basic mechanisms of neurotoxicity or from clinical neurotoxicologists. The literature amounts to isolated descriptions of case reports where thirst is described as a prominent symptom.

People undergoing lithium therapy often develop *polydipsia* (excessive water drinking). It has been suspected that lithium—an element of the same chemical group as sodium and potassium—may produce its therapeutic effect by modifying the ionic mechanisms of neurons.

Hunger

Eating behavior has also been suspected of being under the control of the hypothalamus. In the 1950s, the simple notion existed that hypothalamic nuclei contained centers that controlled the initiation and cessation of eating. It is now believed that the urge to eat is controlled by multiple signals including sensory information, arousal, alteration of hormonal balance, and the set point. The *set point*—a hypothetical physiological state—uses information from the body (its body weight, its nutritional status, etc), which in turn controls the intake of nutrients. Most laboratory animals regain the weight adequate for their age soon after prolonged periods of starvation or forced feeding.

But the feedback mechanism that seems to govern temperature control may not be similar to that governing eating. Temperature, for example, is remarkably constant within a single animal species, but there are large interindividual variations in body weight (more appropriately, the body weight that is expected for a given size). Among humans, the set point is known to be modified by numerous factors including environmental, cultural, and educational factors, exercise, emotional stress, depression, etc.

Children and, under certain pathological conditions, adults sometimes develop specific hungers, cravings for specific foods. The specific craving for salt—which is normal in parts of the world in which salt is not readily available—is well documented. For example, Brazilian Indians were said to have exchanged gold for salt from their Portugese conquerors.

It is commonly accepted that appetite disorders—most commonly present in the mild form of appetite loss or, in severe forms, as anorexia—are observed in many people exposed to neurotoxic agents.

Anorexia means lack of appetite. The essential features of *anorexia nervosa*—a complex disorder—are intense fear of becoming obese, disturbance of the body image, significant weight loss, refusal to maintain normal body weight, and amenorrhea (lack of menstruation). The term "anorexia" is recognized as a misnomer, since loss of appetite is usually rare until late in the illness.

Loss of appetite can be observed in conjunction with many other psychological disorders, particularly depression. Cultural factors and fads also need to be taken into consideration for the correct evaluation of appetite loss. Obesity is a health problem in the United States. However, in the early and middle 1980s, eating disorders associated with weight loss had achieved epidemic proportions in the United States; fads for achieving slimness and physical fitness are important factors accounting for these trends.

Many investigators suggest that eating disorders should be considered as a spectrum ranging from anorexia nervosa to *bulimia* (excessive eating) and compulsive overeating. Current research has been directed to the risk factors for bulimia. Bulimia is primarily a woman's problem; research suggests that 90% of bulimics are female. For a review of risk factors in adult bulimia, see Striegel-Moore and collaborators (1986).

Eating disorders found in infancy, childhood, and adolescence include anorexia nervosa, bulimia, pica, and rumination disorder. *Pica* is the persistent eating of nonnutritive substances. Infants affected by this eating disorder typically eat paint, plaster, strings, sand, insects, or pebbles. Pica is an important factor in lead poisoning in childhood—the child eats lead-containing paint chips frequently found in houses in decaying neighborhoods. *Rumination disorders* in infancy consist of repeated episodes of regurgitation—without nausea or associated gastrointestinal illness—lasting for at least a month following a period of normal functioning. Rumination disorder is predictably accompanied by weight loss or failure to make expected weight gain.

Sex

Sexual behavior seems to be controlled—more appropriately, "biased"—by hormonal events occurring at critical periods of fetal life. But this bias is neither immutable nor does it determine a person's sexual orientation.

From experimental animals and clinical observations it is possible to conclude that male and female behavior is largely determined and sustained by hormones throughout life. But the theory of sexual hormone specificity—the notion that all sexual behavior is determined by hormones—has largely been abandoned. The injection of male hormones into homosexual males, for example, will only increase the person's libido for homosexual encounters and the frequency of homosexual activity.

It has long been known that the neuroendocrine system is essentially dimorphic. (*Dimorphism* is the presence of physical or behavioral differences associated with gender.) The brain has also been found to be dimorphic. To a degree, the brain gender phenotype—the "gender" the brain appears to have—is determined by the amount and type of circulating steroid hormones present during critical periods of early fetal life. Thus, fetal exposure to male hormones in genetic females causes hermaphroditism—the presence of the sexual characteristics of both genders in the same individual.

In addition, the brain can be androgenized (masculinized) by several hormones (eg, testosterone, androstenedione), drugs (eg, barbiturates), and, of interest to us, by certain neurotoxic agents such as pesticides (eg, DDT).

There are important studies on the pharmacological basis of sexual behavior in laboratory animals. Clark and collaborators (1984) have postulated that α-adrenoreceptors are important modulators of sexual arousal in intact male rats. Yohimbine hydrochloride increases sexual motivation in male rats as evidenced by increased mounting performance in mating tests conducted after genital anesthetization. Moreover, yohimbine hydrochloride increases the percentage of male rats ejaculating in their first heterosexual encounter and induction of copulatory behavior in sexually inactive male rats. Similar experiments conducted in humans are inconclusive because of the difficulties in controlling for placebo effects. (A *placebo* is a preparation containing no medicine that, when given to unaware patients, sometimes produces therapeutic effects.)

Changes in sexual arousal and potency are common complaints in men who voluntarily ingest neurotoxic agents or workers occupationally exposed to certain neurotoxic agents such as lead and industrial solvents. In men, *sexual arousal* (ie, libido, sexual motivation) is distinguished from *potency* (ie, erectile and ejaculatory responses). (From the toxicological point of view, virtually nothing has been written on similar processes in women.) Questionnaires prepared to ascertain the effect of neurotoxic agents on neurological and psychological functions should ask for separate information on these two primary components of sexual behavior.

EMOTIONS

Emotion is a general term indicating both a series of responses toward the environment (the expression of emotions) and the subjective feelings that may or may not accompany these actions. Much has been achieved in our understanding of the neuroanatomic basis, electrophysiological events, and pharmacological mechanisms underlying some of the components involved in the production and expression of emotional behavior and subjective feelings. There have been many attempts to bring together all these facts in a comprehensive "theory of emotion." But, at present, there is no widely accepted theory that can explain all the components of this complex behavior.

Neural Basis

A brief review of the neural basis of emotion will concentrate on structures that most neuroscientists agree are involved in generating and expressing emotion: the hypothalamus and the limbic system.

In 1928, W. R. Hess, a Swiss neurologist continuing research work initiated in the 19th century, discovered that stimulation of the hypothalamus in the cat elicited attack behavior and expressions of fear and rage. Further research involving lesion and stimulation studies—or a combination of both—conducted in various areas of the world helped to establish the hypothalamus as an important integration site of autonomic nervous system functions and the expression of emotions. This is surprising in that the hypothalamus occupies no more than 1% of the entire volume of the brain, yet it controls a wide variety of functions including motivational states and emotional behavior.

Studies carried out in the 1960s helped to characterize aggressive displays and predatory behavior of laboratory animals such as the cat. Aggressive display and posturing—useful in establishing social dominance among members of the same species—is a highly emotional behavior. Interestingly, predatory behavior (killing) seems also to be mediated by the hypothalamus, but it is a "silent aggression" devoid of any emotional counterpart. For example, in the act of actually killing the mouse, the cat exhibits minimal emotional behavior.

The hypothalamus is not considered a center of emotions but as a "node" in a larger neural network controlling emotional behavior. (In the theory of networks, a "node" is where two or more lines converge.) The theory of emotion proposed by James Papez in 1937 aimed at naming all possible nodes of this network and at describing the flow of information from one node to another. It is pointless to review this brilliant theory—which was based on neurological observations in humans affected by tumors of the brain and some facts from comparative neuroanatomy—because it has never been proven in toto. However, the relationships of individual nodes taken two, three, and even four at a time can now be attempted.

Papez and his contemporaries, Klüver and Bucy, initiated interest in the experimental study of the amygdala and the role played by the hippocampus in learning. The amygdala is a spherical nucleus located inside the tip of the temporal lobes of the brain. In 1937, Henry Klüver and Paul Bucy in Chicago also performed a most significant piece of experimental work in the monkey. They demonstrated that after bilateral removal of the temporal lobe, monkeys became overattentive and restless and exhibited hyperorality (they compulsively examined objects by placing them in their mouths), "psychic blindness" (being unable to understand what they were seeing), sexual hyperactivity, and emotional changes (wild animals became tame after the operation). The syndrome is now known as the *Klüver–Bucy syndrome*.

In Papez's theory, the hippocampus was seen as part of the limbic system mediating emotions. However, the hippocampus is now seen as mediating learning and memory. The hippocampus may mediate motivation as well; learning is thought to be impossible in the absence of a motivating state.

Ekman and collaborators (1983) were able to demonstrate emotion-specific activity in the autonomic nervous system of humans by constructing facial prototypes of emotion, muscle by muscle, and by asking subjects to relive past emotional experiences. These investigators studied six target emotions (surprise, disgust, sadness, anger, fear, and happiness). In the facial prototypes, subjects were not asked to produce an emotional expression; instead, they were instructed which muscles to contract. In the relived-emotion task, subjects were asked to experience each of the six emotions by reliving a past emotional experience related to one of each target

emotions for 30 seconds. Measures of autonomic activity included heart rate, temperature of the left and right hand, skin resistance, and forearm tension. The autonomic activity produced distinguished not only between positive and negative emotions (eg, happiness versus disgust) but also negative emotions (eg, anger, fear, sadness, and disgust).

As we concluded in our discussion of motivational states, the study of the toxicity of environmental and occupational agents on human emotion, seen from an integrative point of view, has not received the attention it deserves. Most of the reports available are epidemiological studies or clinical observations with little emphasis on causation or possible pharmacological mechanisms of action. In contrast, the literature on the neurotoxicity of many therapeutic drugs affecting emotional states has been extensively studied (Goodman Gilman et al. 1980).

The Epidemiology of Panic Disorders

Panic disorder is a psychiatric condition characterized by recurrent, severe, and apparently spontaneous anxiety attacks accompanied by autonomic nervous system symptoms such as dyspnea (uneven breathing patterns), palpitations, dizziness, sweating, faintingness, and trembling (von Korff et al. 1985). Panic disorders are now recognized as a significant health problem. People affected by panic disorders develop phobic patterns of avoidance of situations during which such attacks have occurred in the past (eg, while traveling). Panic disorders may account for excess mortality from suicide and cardiovascular disease. An association has been reported between panic disorders and prolapse of the heart's mitral valve (Kantor et al 1980).

Simple panic attacks, severe and recurrent panic attacks, and panic disorders have been linked to occupational exposure to neurotoxic agents, notably solvents. However, the frequency of occurrence and the physiological, psychological, and social factors of panic attacks need to be known to rule out spurious associations between neurotoxic exposure and panic disorders. Von Korff and collaborators (1985) have performed an epidemiological study on panic attacks and panic disorders in three community surveys. What follows is a summary of this important research.

The study was conducted as part of the National Institute of Mental Health's Epidemiologic Catchment Area Program. Area probability samples (a form of sampling to avoid bias) were drawn from New Haven (Connecticut), eastern Baltimore (Maryland), and greater St. Louis (Missouri). In total, close to 10,000 people were interviewed. During the course of the epidemiological investigation, the screening question was: "Have you ever had a spell or attack when all of a sudden you felt frightened, anxious or very uneasy in a situation when most people wouldn't be afraid?" If the answer was affirmative, the interviewer asked whether or not a series of 12 autonomic symptoms were present in one of the worst of such attacks. They included breathing difficulty, heart pounding, dizziness, fingers and feet tingling, tightness or pain in the chest, a smothering sensation, feeling faint, sweating, trembling and shaking, hot and cold flashes, a sense of unreality, and fear of dying. In addition, the interviewer ascertained how frequently these attacks occurred, the age at which the first attack occurred, how recently the last attack occurred, whether the attacks occurred only in the presence of phobic stimuli, and asked three questions to assess severity (whether the attack prompted the subject to seek treatment or to use medicine and whether attacks interfered with life activities).

Among the most characteristic symptoms were heart pounding, trembling and shaking, sweating, hot or cold flashes, fear of dying, and difficulty in breathing. The age of onset was most often between 15 and 19 years of age. Females tended to report both simple and severe forms of panic attacks more frequently than men. Persons with less than high school education had higher prevalence rates.

Whites tended to have lower prevalence rates than people of other races, but the differences were small. Persons who were separated or divorced had substantially higher prevalence rates of panic than married persons. In a multivariate analysis, when all demographic variables were incorporated into a model, only gender and age were found to be significant.

One of the contributions of von Korff and his collaborators has been to show that there is a gradient from simple attacks through severe and recurrent attacks to panic disorder. They concluded that more attention needs to be paid to the utility of the diagnostic distinction between panic attacks and panic disorder. There was no unambiguous demarcation between panic disorder and severe and recurrent panic attacks in terms of expression of autonomic symptoms, age-at-onset distribution, or distribution by demographic factors. Rather, the distinction between simple panic attacks and more severe panic attacks appeared to be in the number of autonomic symptoms experienced.

MOODS

Moods (or *affects*) are persistent feelings and emotions that permeate every aspect of one's psychological makeup. Although there are many affective states that are moods, the term "moods" often refers to states of persistent depression, elation, or the cyclic presence of both.

Considerable efforts have been made in the past to clarify the psychological characteristics of mood states. Witness the attempts to define current guidelines for classification of affective disorders in the *Diagnostic and Statistical Manual of Mental Disorders,* third edition (DSM-III-R), of the American Psychiatric Association (1987). Since the primary objective of the DSM-III-R is the diagnosis of mental disorders, the possibility that some affective disorders may be caused by chronic, involuntary exposure to neurotoxic agents—such as those occurring during occupational exposures, for example—although hinted at in sections dealing with differential diagnoses, is not adequately covered. For example: "An Organic Affective Syndrome with depression may be due to substances such as reserpine, to infectious diseases such as influenza, or to hypothyroidism." Despite these shortcomings, a clinical neurotoxicologist needs to become familiar with the DSM-III-R nomenclature on the subclassification of affective disorders as major affective disorders, other specific affective disorders, and atypical affective disorders.

A major depressive disorder needs to be differentiated from a psychotic state. However, this differential sometimes is difficult to make because some psychotic disorders are accompanied by affective disorders, and some affective disorders are associated with clouding of cognitive functions. *Dysthymia* (mood alteration) is a less severe form of depression.

A simple depressive mood episode cannot be used to diagnose whether an individual has a major depressive disorder or dysthymia. Duration of symptoms—from a few weeks to a few months—must be established for a diagnosis of an affective disorder.

The Study of Moods

Moods can be assessed by observation of everyday behavior and by reliance on the subject's description of feelings. These two sources are complementary. Children may not be able to verbalize a state of depression, and therefore behavioral cues, such as those exhibited by playing, are important sources of information. There are numerous cultural groups and social circles in which the overt expression of individual emotions is not encouraged; symptoms of depression, therefore, need to be inferred through indirect methods such as, for example, the observation of ritualistic behavior.

Many efforts have been made to quantify moods, and these efforts are valuable if they are not taken as the sole source of information. In countries where there are marked

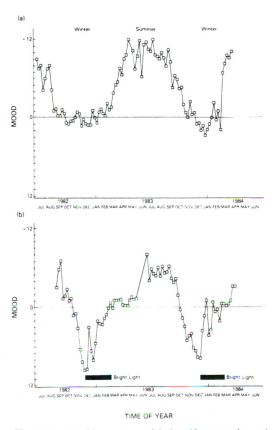

Fig. 28.1. Weekly averages of daily self-rating of mood over a 21-month period (shown for two different patients) showing the seasonal effect of light. (From Rosenthal 1987.)

seasonal changes, moods are influenced by ambient light (Fig. 28.1). Cultural factors and language always need to be taken into consideration, particularly in demographically heterogeneous communities.

A Profile of Mood States

The *Profile of Mood States* (POMS) is a questionnaire developed by McNier and collaborators (1971) to attempt to understand the psychology of emotions through information on subjective feelings, affect, and mood. The instructions call for checking on "how you have been feeling during the past week including today," using a rating scale ranging from 0 (indicating not at all) to 4 (extremely). The questionnaire is reported to measure six moods or affective states: tension–anxiety; depression–dejection; anger–hostility; vigor–activity; fatigue–inertia; and confusion–bewilderment.

The POMS has been applied for the evaluation of moods resulting from exposure to neurotoxic agents. In 1983, at a meeting of experts on the prevention of neurotoxic illness at the workplace, the POMS or a POMS-like questionnaire was recommended for the study of neurotoxin-induced changes in moods and feelings (Johnson 1987). The test may be either hand or computer scored.

There is considerable literature on the psychometric properties of the POMS. The internal consistency reliability scores between various items of the questionnaire (measured with coefficient alpha) is near 0.90 or above. Test–retest reliabilities for the six factors range from 0.61 to 0.69. There are numerous validity studies relating short-term psychotherapy and controlled outpatient drug trials. The POMS has only recently been used in community studies of blue-collar workers exposed to neurotoxic agents.

The POMS depends heavily on language (feelings and language are intimately related). Thus, it requires a good English language vocabulary and command of the language denoting feelings. For example, a subject who speaks English as a second language or who has had only a low level of education will probably have difficulty in understanding the words "peeved," "muddled," or "bushed."

Many other checklists and questionnaires on affects are of potential use in clinical neurotoxicology and neuroepidemiological research. One of the 10 "clinical scales" of the Minnesota Multiphasic Personality Inventory (MMPI-2) is depression (D) (Lachar 1983).

Anxiety Disorders

The DSM-III-R manual defines *anxiety disorders* as a group of disorders in which either anxiety is the predominant disturbance (as in the panic disorder or generalized anxiety disorder) or anxiety is experienced if the individual attempts to master the symptoms (as in confronting the dreaded object or situation in the phobic disorder or resisting obsessions or compulsions in the obsessive–compulsive disorder).

Importantly, a diagnosis of anxiety disorder is not made if the anxiety is caused by another disorder such as schizophrenia, affective disorder (discussed below), or an organic mental disorder. The DSM-III-R should be consulted for diagnostic criteria for *agoraphobia* (fear of open or public places), social phobia, simple phobia, panic disorder, generalized anxiety disorder, obsessive–compulsive disorder, and posttraumatic stress disorder.

Affective Disorders

The DSM-III-R defines *affective disorder* as a disturbance of mood, accompanied by a full or partial manic or depressive syndrome, that is not caused by any other physical or mental disorder.

The DSM-III-R diagnostic criteria for major depressive episodes include persistent mood alterations and symptoms, dysphoric mood, or loss of interest or pleasure in all or almost all usual activities and pasttimes. The *dysphoric* mood is characterized by symptoms such as depression, sadness, and feeling blue, hopeless, low, "down in the dumps," or irritable. The mood disturbance must be prominent and relatively persistent, but not necessarily the most dominant symptom, and does not include momentary shifts from one dysphoric mood to another (eg, anxiety to depression to anger) such as that seen in states of acute psychotic turmoil. (For children under six, dysphoric moods may have to be inferred from a persistent sad facial expression.)

Among the symptoms of *depression* are poor appetite, insomnia or hypersomnia, loss of interest or pleasure in one's usual activities, loss of energy or easy fatigability, feelings of worthlessness, self-reproach, excessive or inappropriate guilt, complaints, evidence of diminished ability to think, and recurrent thoughts of death, suicidal ideation, or actual suicide attempts.

Mania involves symptoms opposite to those of depression. The symptoms include hyperactivity, verborrhage (compulsion to speak), flight of ideas, inflated self-esteem, decreased need for sleep, and distractibility.

The *manic–depressive disorder* (*bipolar disorder*) is characterized by mood oscillations between manic and depressive states. Both the manic and depressive states are more frequent and of shorter duration than major depressive disorders. In rare cases there is a mood oscillation between manic and depressive states in the absence of any period of normal mood.

Affective Disorders and Alcoholism. Affective disorders and alcoholism are intimately related. Alcoholism can be a symptom of depression, and chronic ingestion of alcohol can produce a marked affective disorder. The neuropsychological correlates of alcoholism are the result of the direct influence of alcohol (ethyl alcohol), the effects of alcohol withdrawal, and malnutrition (Sterman and Schaumburg 1980).

The Epidemiology of Depression

Epidemiological studies have demonstrated that depression is one of the most frequent mental disorders (Weissman et al. 1978). Since the early 1980s, there have been many such studies on nationwide and regional samples of the United States population. One important study, by Eaton and Kessler (1981), has been performed in conjunction with the first Health and Nutritional Examination Survey (HANES) sponsored by the National Center for Health Statistics. Data were collected on 2867 respondents.

In the HANES study, depression was assessed by the Center of Epidemiologic Studies Depression Scale (CES-D). This is a 20-item scale asking for the frequency of a given symptom experienced during the previous week. The scale has been extensively used and validated (Comstock and Helsing 1976; Radloff 1977; Weissman et al. 1978). The data were analyzed by a statistical adjustment procedure that assesses the simultaneous impact of the major sociodemographic variables. The following are the major findings.

Females had more depressive symptoms than males; the trends did not change significantly as a result of controlling for other sociodemographic factors. Examination of single age trends was misleading because older persons are more likely than young people to be widowed, divorced, or separated and slightly more likely to have less education. All of these variables are associated with depression. When these confounding factors were controlled, younger people had more symptoms of depression than older ones. Blacks tended to have many more symptoms of depression than whites in univariate analyses. But when other sociodemographic factors were taken into account, race had little effect on measures of depression.

Multivariate procedures permit an insight into the strong interaction among race, other sociodemographic variables, and depression. Univariate studies (eg, studies on the prevalence of depression) are not designed to test these interactions. For example, the traditional contention that depression is more prevalent among the elderly is substantiated in prevalence studies using univariate statistics. But multivariate studies such as those described here seem to indicate an absence of age trends or even more depressive symptoms among the young.

Suicide. The frequency of suicide has been examined in epidemiological studies (Mac Mahon 1983). Suicide is more frequent on Mondays, and the frequency of occurrence declines during the week, being lowest on Saturdays (in the summer) or Sundays (in the winter). Suicides are more frequent around the fifth day of the month and least frequent in the last days of the month. These rates are important to take into consideration in large-scale studies such as epidemiological studies on the association between neurotoxic agents and depression.

The Biological Basis of Depression

There are numerous ethical considerations regarding biological research on depression in humans, and so the literature on the pharmacological basis of depression in humans is scant. Studies on the monoamine oxidase hypothesis of depression have used several research strategies (monoamine oxidase, or MAO, is an enzyme that is bound to the mitochondrial membrane of the neural cell; MAO can degrade cytoplasmic dopamine, a neurotransmitter):

- Measurement of indices of monoamine metabolism in accessible body fluids, such as blood, urine, or cerebrospinal fluid, of depressed patients.
- Postmortem studies of the brain of suicide victims.
- Analysis of the effects of drugs on central monoamine metabolism in patients with depression.
- Endocrine research on disturbances in the release of hormones of the pituitary gland.

Van Praag (1982) has reviewed the evidence linking alterations in neurotransmitters and depression. Interest in a possible correlation between monoamines and depression arose when it was discovered that antidepressant drugs enhance the availability of 5-hydroxytryptamine (5-HT) and norepinephrine at central (brain) receptors. For a review of pharmacological studies and hypotheses, see Goodman Gilman and collaborators (1980) and Feldman and Quenzer (1984).

Biological Markers of Depression. A biological indicator for depression has been long sought, since such a marker would help in the clinical identification of affective disorder and depressive states. The dexamethasone suppression test (DST) is a blood test to determine whether cortisol, a hormone secreted by the adrenal glands, is suppressed following injection of dexamethasone. In most normal people, dexamethasone temporarily suppresses cortisol, whereas in nearly half of depressed patients, the secretion is not suppressed. However, the test gives too many false positive results (it is also positive in people suffering from other ailments).

One of the most recent candidates for a biological marker is urinary phenyl acetate. The compound 2-phenylethylamine is an "endogenous amphetamine" that may modulate central adrenergic functions. 2-Phenylethylamine is mainly metabolized by monoamine oxidase to form phenyl acetate. Sabelli and collaborators (1983) measured 24-hour urinary excretion of phenyl acetate in healthy volunteers and depressed patients. Patients were diagnosed as depressed according to the diagnostic criteria of the DSM-III. Low urinary levels of phenyl acetate were observed among the depressive patients, and there were no significant differences between treated and untreated patients. The authors suggest that low urinary excretion of phenyl acetate may be a reliable marker for the diagnosis of unipolar major depressive disorder.

The Role of Affect on Cognitive and Motor Behavior

Neurotoxic agents may have a direct effect on cognitive and motor functions or an indirect effect through their influence on moods (affect). Depressed individuals may experience alterations in memory, attention, and concentration, lose interest in their immediate surroundings, and show profound cognitive deficits. A depressed individual may not have any interest in performing the task a neurologist or psychologist asks him/her to do. As a result, the individual may perform very poorly when a standard battery of neuropsychological testing is administered.

But depression may also be the result of neurotoxic exposure. The depressive picture associated with chronic alcoholism, for example, is well known and has been described in the classical neurotoxicological literature. Depression is a mood dominating the "crash" that follows smoking crack cocaine for several days. There are many studies showing that occupational exposure to neurotoxic agents, particularly industrial solvents, may create similar symptoms.

However, depression can be "reactive" (this is called *reactive depression*). A person may be depressed because of his/her reaction to a personal loss. In the case of major environmental accidents involving neurotoxic agents, reactive depression can be caused by many factors, such as financial loss, and thus needs to be separated from the true neurotoxic effects on affective behavior. To complicate matters further, someone experiencing an intellectual decline, as a result of neurotoxin exposure or for any other medical reason, may use excessive alcohol abuse as an escape. Clinical and experimental neurotoxicologists must be aware of these factors and sort out what is causing the depression. As we shall see, this is not an easy task.

MOOD ALTERATIONS PRODUCED BY ENVIRONMENTAL AND OCCUPATIONAL NEUROTOXIC AGENTS

Severe Depression Caused by Carbon Disulfide

Carbon disulfide is an inflammable and volatile liquid that, in the past, was an important solvent for sulfur in the rubber industry and a solvent for alkali-treated cellulose in the production of rayon and cellophane. In addition, it was used as a solvent for fats, lacquers, and camphor, for the extraction of oil from olives, and for the refining of paraffins and petroleum.

Carbon disulfide was discovered by W. A. Lampadius in 1796, and reports of its devastating neurotoxic properties—characterized by a generalized polyneuritis accompanied by personality changes and psychosis—began to be recognized in the middle of the 19th century (Delpeche 1856). However, carbon disulfide continued to be a widely unrecognized occupational neurotoxic agent until early in the 20th century, when Alice Hamilton, one of the founders of occupational medicine in the United States, reported cases of carbon-disulfide-induced psychosis that were largely misdiagnosed by neurologists and psychiatrists of her time (Hamilton 1925).

Reports on the behavioral effects of carbon disulfide continued to appear worldwide up through the 1970s with a publication by Hänninen (1971). Among the various effects of exposure to carbon disulfide are a severe form of depression leading to suicide. Up to now, there has been no comprehensive understanding of the neurological and neurochemical mechanisms of carbon disulfide poisoning. For a comprehensive discussion of the neurotoxic properties of carbon disulfide, see Seppäläinen and Haltia (1980).

Depression Caused by Organophosphate Pesticides

Organophosphate pesticides, also known as OP compounds, are a family of pesticides that are chemically similar in that all contain phosphorus. They are generally less persistent than the chlorinated hydrocarbon family, which they have replaced. Since they act by inhibiting the enzyme cholinesterase, they are also called anticholinesterase agents. The OP compounds are known to affect several areas of neuropsychological functioning including vigilance, information processing, motor processes, memory, and speech (Levin and Rodnitzky 1976).

Since the late 1960s, there have been numerous studies linking depression with exposure to these anticholinesterase agents, an interesting example of a link between occupational toxicology and pharmacology (Janowsky et al. 1972, 1974). There are numerous case reports linking OP exposure to depression and lethargy. Depression is the main psychiatric symptom in numerous cases of chronic OP toxicity. Associated symptoms of depression—such as sleep disturbances and decreases in libido—have also been reported. The link between OP exposure and anxiety and irritability, and even the induction of schizophrenia-like disorders, has not been established on an equal footing.

Studies on the neurotoxicity of OP compounds have greatly influenced the investigation of the pharmacological basis of depression and mania. Janowsky and collaborators (1972, 1974) postulated that affective disorders are caused by an imbalance between cholinergic and adrenergic systems of the central nervous system. Depression is considered to be an expression of cholinergic predominance and mania a result of adrenergic predominance.

Lithium: Industrial Uses and Use as a Therapeutic Agent Against Depression

Lithium is a metal that never occurs in pure form in nature, but rather exists in the form of salts. Lithium has industrial uses in alloys, as a catalytic agent, and as a lubricant. Because lithium hydride produces hydrogen on contact with water, it has been used in the manufacture of electronic equipment and ceramics. Except for lithium hydride, which produces skin and lung irritation because of its corrosive properties, none of the lithium salts are toxic.

Lithium has been found to be an effective pharmacological treatment for several affective disorders, particularly in the improvement of the manic phase in manic depression. When lithium is administered in an effective therapeutic dose to a healthy individual it has no adverse pharmacological effects, and when administered to people suffering from affec-

tive disorders it has the remarkable ability to prevent the occurrence of both mania and depression, although it does not have an established antidepressant action. Acute toxic effects resulting from overdose include vomiting, diarrhea, polydipsia (excessive water intake), ataxia, tremor, fatigue, coma, and seizures.

Lithium has a variety of biological effects on neuronal ionic mechanisms (suspected to cause its therapeutic effect), on the metabolism of carbohydrates, on the secretion of antidiuretic hormone, and on thyroid function.

Polybrominated Biphenyls and Depression

Polybrominated biphenyls (PBBs) are mixtures of brominated biphenyls, usually with four to eight bromine atoms per molecule, that have been useful as fire retardants in thermoplastic resins. One such mixture, Firemaster FF-1™, mainly hexobromobiphenyl, caused widespread contamination of livestock (dairy and beef cattle, poultry, and eggs) after an accidental introduction into feed in Michigan in early 1973. Before the cause and dimensions of the problem were fully appreciated, contamination of milk, beef, pork, eggs, and poultry had occurred, and ingestion of these foodstuffs resulted in PBB absorption by those who ate these products. At the time of the accident, no previous instance of human exposure to PBBs was known (Anderson et al. 1979; Valciukas et al. 1979).

By April 1976, the Michigan Department of Agriculture had characterized the extent of PBB contamination, involving 1039 farms. With this information, a cross-sectional clinical field study was carried out by the Environmental Sciences Laboratory of Mount Sinai Medical School in New York City, under the direction of Dr. Irving J. Selikoff, to assess the extent of the medical problems associated with PBB ingestion. The prevalence and incidence of neurological symptoms were analyzed in 626 adults from Michigan (the study group) and 153 from Wisconsin (the control group). Onset of neurological symptoms preceded that of all other symptoms in the Michigan group. The frequency of some of the symptoms, such as nausea and dizziness, increased slowly over months, whereas other symptoms, such as depression, nervousness, paresthesia, tiredness, sleepiness, and headaches, showed a more rapid increase in prevalence.

Depression was a prominent symptom of PBB intoxication. A time-course reconstruction of the onset of neurological symptoms revealed that depression was the first symptom to appear (Valciukas et al. 1979). However, to date, no conclusive link between symptoms and PBB levels has been established. Considerable pharmacological evidence exists that these symptoms are consistent with toxicological findings in clinical cases and animal experimentation (bromides were once used as hypnotics). However, depressive reactions associated with stress cannot be ruled out (Archibald and Tuddenham 1965; Stross et al. 1979).

The Evaluation of Moods in a Longitudinal Study of Lead Foundry Workers

The work by Hänninen and collaborators performed during the early 1970s and published in 1978 pinpointed the importance of assessing moods in studies of neurotoxicity. A questionnaire developed by Eysenck in England was used in these studies. [Unfortunately, the Eysenck factor (Cattell 1973) was called "neurotocism" (it implied that workers were "neurotic," thus being afflicted by a purely psychological illness). "Nervousness" would have been a more appropriate term.]

In 1985, Baker and collaborators utilized the Profile of Mood States (POMS) in the evaluation of the time course of improvement in 160 foundry workers who had been exposed to lead. When the subjects were no longer exposed, they showed improvements in levels of tension (20% reduction), anger

(18%), depression (26%), fatigue (27%), and confusion (13%). Multiregression analyses of moods versus six exposure indices showed significant correlations with some of the mood dimensions. Thus, the possible interpretation of reduction in mood measures as a purely psychological phenomenon seemed to be ruled out.

REFERENCES

American Psychiatric Association (1987) *Diagnostic and Statistical Manual,* 3rd ed, rev. Washington, DC: APA.

Anderson, HA, Wolff, MS, Lilis, R et al. (1979) Symptoms and clinical abnormalities following ingestion of polybrominated-biphenyl contaminated food products. *Ann NY Acad Sc,* 320:684–702.

Archibald, HC and Tuddenham, RD (1965) Persistent stress reaction after combat. *Arch Gen Psychiatry* 12(5):475–481.

Bernard C (1878–1879) *Leçons sur les phénomènes de la Vie Commus aux Animaux et aux Végétaux.* Paris: Baillière.

Cannon, W (1929) *Bodily Changes in Pain, Hunger, Fear and Rage,* 2nd ed. New York: Appleton.

Cannon, W (1939) *The Wisdom of the Body,* 2nd ed, New York: WW Norton.

Cattell, RB (1973) *Personality and Mood by Questionnaire: A Handbook of Interpretive Theory, Psychometrics, and Practical Procedures.* San Francisco: Jossey-Bass.

Clark, JT, Smith, E, and Davidson, JM (1984) Enhancement of sexual motivation in male rats by yohimbine. *Science* 225:847–849.

Comstock, GW and Helsing, KJ (1976) Symptoms of depression in two communities. *Psychosom Med* 6:551–563.

Delpeche, ALD (1856) Accidents produits dar l'inhalation du sulfure de carbone en vapeur: Expériences sur les animaux. *Gaz Hebd Med Chir* 3:384–385.

Eaton, WW and Kessler, LG (1981) Rates of symptoms of depression in a national sample. *Am J Epidemiol* 114:528–538.

Ekman, P, Levenson, RW, and Friesen, WV (1983) Autonomic nervous system activity distinguishes among emotions. *Science* 221:1208–1210.

Feldman, RS and Quenzer, LF (1984) *Fundamentals of Neuropsychopharmacology.* Sunderland, MA: Sinauer Associates.

Flower, RJ, Moncada, S and Vane, JR (1980) Analgesic-antipyretics and anti-inflammatory agents; drugs employed in the treatment of gout. In *Goodman and Gilman's The Pharmacological Basis of Therapeutics,* 6th ed, A Goodman Gilman, LS Goodman, and A Gilman (eds) p. 682. New York: Macmillan.

Goodman Gilman, A, Goodman, LS, and Gilman, A (eds) (1980) *Goodman and Gilman's The Pharmacological Basis of Therapeutics*, 6th ed. New York: Macmillan.

Hamilton, A (1925) *Industrial Poisons in the United States*. New York: Macmillan.

Hänninen, H (1971) Psychological picture of manifest and latent carbon disulphide poisoning. *Br J Ind Med* 28:374.

Hänninen, H, Hernberg, S, Mantere, P, et al. (1978) Psychological performance of subjects with low exposure to lead. *J. Occup Med* 20:683–689.

Janowsky, DS, Davis, JM, El-Yousef, M et al. (1972) A cholinergic–adrenergic hypothesis of mania and depression. *Lancet* 22:632.

Janowsky, DS, Davis, JM, El-Yousef, M et al. (1974) Acetylcholine and depression. *Psychosom Med* 36:248.

Johnson, FN (1987) *Depression and Mania: Modern Lithium Therapy*. Washington, DC: IRL Press.

Kantor, JS, Zitrin, CM and Seldis, SM (1980) Mitral valve prolapse syndrome in agoraphobic patients. *Am J Psychiatry* 137:467–469.

Klüver, H and Bucy, PC (1937) Psychic blindness and other symptoms following bilateral temporal lobectomy in Rhesus monkeys. *Am J Physiol* 119:352–353.

Lachar, D (1983) *The MMPI: Clinical Assessment and Automatic Interpretation*. Los Angeles: Western Psychological Services.

Levin, HS and Rodnitzky, RL (1976) Behavioral effects of organophosphates pesticides in man. *Clin Toxicol* 9(3):391–405.

MacMahon, K (1983) Short-term temporal cycles in the frequency of suicide, United States, 1972–1978. *Am J Epidemiol* 117:744–750.

McNier, DM, Lorr, M, and Droppelman, LF (1971) *Profile of Mood States*. San Diego: Educational and Industrial Testing Service.

Papez, JW (1937) A proposed mechanism of emotion. *Arch Neurol Psychiatry* 38:725–743.

Radloff, LS (1977) The CES-D Scale: A self-report depression scale for research in the general population. *J Appl Psychol Measure* 1:385–401.

Rosenthal et al. (1987) In *Encyclopedia of Neuroscience*, G Adelman (ed) p. 587. New York: Birkhäuser.

Sabelli, HC, Fawcett, J, Gusovsky, F, et al. (1983) Urinary phenyl acetate: A diagnostic test for depression? *Science* 220:1187–1188.

Seppäläinen, AM and Haltia, M (1980) Carbon disulfide. In *Experimental and Clinical Neuropathology*, PS Spencer and HH Schaumburg (eds) pp. 356–373. Baltimore: Williams & Wilkins.

Sterman, AB and Schaumburg, HH (1980) Neurotoxicity of selected drugs. In *Experimental and Clinical*

Neurotoxicology, PS Spencer and HH Schaumburg (eds) pp. 593–612. Baltimore: Williams & Wilkins.

Striegel-Moore, RH, Silberstein, LR, and Rodin, J (1986) Toward an understanding of risk factors for bulimia. *Am Psychol* 41:246–263.

Stross, JK, Bixon, RK, and Anderson, MD (1979) Neuropsychiatric findings in patients exposed to polybrominated biphenyls. *Ann NY Acad Sci* 320:368–372.

Valciukas, JA, Lilis, R, Anderson, HA, et al. (1979) The neurotoxicity of polybrominated biphenyls: Results of a medical field survey. *Ann NY Acad Sci* 320:337–367.

van Praag, HM (1982) Neurotransmitters and CNS disease: Depression. *Lancet* 2:1259–1264.

von Korff, M, Eaton, WW, and Keyl, PM (1985) The epidemiology of panic attacks and panic disorders: Results of three community surveys. *Am J Epidemiol* 122:970–981.

Weissman, MM, Myers, JK, and Harding, PS (1978) Psychiatric disorders in a US urban community 1975–1976. *Am J Psychiatry* 135:459–462.

Wolff, AV (1958) *Thirst: Physiology of the Urge to Drink and Problems of Water Lack*. Springfield, IL: Charles C Thomas.

SUGGESTED READINGS

Abramson, JH (1966) Emotional disorder, status inconsistency and migration: A health questionnaire survey in Jerusalem. *Milbank Mem Fund Q* 44:23–48.

Agras, S (1985) *Panic: Facing Fears, Phobias, and Anxiety*. New York: WH Freeman.

Andersen, AE (1983) Anorexia nervosa and bulimia: A spectrum of eating disorders. *J Adolesc Health Care* 4:15–21.

Aneshensel, C, Frerichs, R, and Clark, V (1981) Family roles and sex differences in depression. *J Health Soc Behav* 22:379–393.

Anthony, JC, Tien, AY, and Petronis, KR (1989) Epidemiologic evidence on cocaine use and panic attacks. *Am J Epidemiol* 129(3):543–549.

Attia, M and Engel, P (1980) A field study of thermal stress and recovery using thermoregulatory behavioral and physiological indicators. *Int Arch Occup Environ Health* 47:21–33.

Attia, M, Engel, P, and Hiddenbrandt, G (1980) Thermal comfort during work: A function of time of the day. *Int Arch Occup Environ Health* 45:205–215.

Attia, M, Khogali, M, El-Khatib, G, et al. (1983) Heat stroke: An upward shift of temperature regulation set point at an elevated body temperature. *Int Arch Occup Environ Health* 53:9–17.

Baker, EL, White, R, Pothier, LJ, et al. (1985) Occupational lead neurotoxicity: Improvement in behavioral effects after reduction of exposure. *Br J Ind Med* 42:507–516.

Barraclough, BM (1973) Differences between national suicide rates. *Br J Psychiatry* 122:95–96.

Bell, CR and Watts, AJ (1971) Thermal limits for industrial workers. *Br J Ind Med* 28:259–264.

Bell, DS and Treethowan, WH (1961) Amphethamine addiction and disturbed sexuality. *Arch Gen Psychiatry* 4:474–478.

Beller, AS (1977) *Fat and Thin: A Natural History of Obesity.* New York: Farrar, Straus & Giroux.

Berkman, LF, Berkman, CS, Kasl, S, et al. (1986) Depressive symptoms in relation to physical health and functioning in the elderly. *Am J Epidemiol* 124(3):372–388.

Blankfield, A (1982) Grief and alcohol. *Am J Drug Alcohol Abuse* 9:435–446.

Blumenthal, MD (1975) Measuring depressive symptomatology in a general population. *Arch Gen Psychiatry* 32:971–978.

Briddell, DW and Wilson, GT (1976) Effects of alcohol and expectancy set on male sex arousal. *J Abnorm Psychol* 85(2):225–234.

Bruch, H (1973) *Eating Disorders: Obesity, Anorexia Nervosa, and the Person Within.* New York: Basic Books.

Brumberg, JJ (1988) *Fasting Girls: The Emergence of Anorexia Nervosa as a Modern Disease.* Cambridge, MA: Harvard University Press.

Camhi, JM (1984) *Neuroethology: Nerve Cells and the Natural Behavior of Animals.* Sunderland, MA: Sinauer Associates.

Capurro, PU and Capurro, C (1979) Editorial: Solvent exposure and mental depression. *Clin Toxicol* 15(2):193–195.

Cooper, KE (1987) The neurobiology of fever: Thoughts on recent developments. *Annu Rev Neurosci* 10:297–324.

Crips, AH (1980) *Anorexia Nervosa: Let Me Be.* London: Academic Press.

Dally, PJ and Gomez, K (1979) *Anorexia Nervosa.* London: William Heinemann Medical Books.

Darwin, C (1872) *The Expression of the Emotions in Man and Animals.* London: Murray.

Dohrenwend, BS and Dohrenwend, BP (eds)(1981) *Stressful Life Events and Their Contexts.* New Brunswick, NJ: Rutgers University Press.

Douglas, J (1967) *The Social Meaning of Suicide.* Princeton, NJ: Princeton University Press.

Dublin, LI (1963) *Suicide: A Sociological and Statistical Study.* New York: Ronald Press.

Eibl-Eibesfeldt, I (1970) *Ethology: The Biology of Behavior.* New York: Holt, Rinehart and Winston.

Ekman, P, Sorenson, ER, and Friesen, WE (1969) Pan cultural elements in facial display of emotions. *Science* 164:86–88.

Epstein, AL, Kissileff, HR, and Stellar, E (1973) *The Neuropsychology of Thirst: New Findings, Advances, and Concepts.* New York:John Wiley & Sons.

Farmer, ME, Locke, BZ, Mosciki, EK, et al. (1989) Physical activity and depressive symptoms: The NHANES I epidemiologic follow-up study. *Am J Epidemiol* 128(6):1340–1351.

Fitzsimons, JT (1972) Thirst. *Physiol Rev* 52:468–561.

Franken, RE (1982) *Human Motivation.* Monterrey, CA: Brooks/Cole.

Freud, S (1940) *An Outline of Psychoanalysis.* New York: WW Norton.

Frohelich, A and Loewi, O (1908) Studies on the physiology and pharmacology of the autonomous nervous system: On the action of nitrite and atropine. *Arch Exp Pathol Pharmakol* 59:64.

Gale, CC (1973) Neuroendocrine aspects of thermoregulation. *Annu Rev Physiol* 35:391–430.

Garfinkel, PE and Garner, DM (1982) *Anorexia Nervosa: A Multidimensional Perspective.* New York: Bunner/Mazel.

Garner, DM and Garfinkel, PE (1979) The eating attitudes test: An index of the symptoms of anorexia nervosa. *Psychol Med* 9:273–279.

Garner, DM and Garfinkel, PE (1980) Sociocultural factors in the development of anorexia nervosa. *Psycho Med* 10:647–656.

Garner, DM, Garfinkel, PE, and O'Shaughnessy, M (1985) The validity of the distinction between bulimia with and without anorexia nervosa. *Am J Psychiatry* 142:581–587.

Gershon, S and Shaw, FH (1961) Psychiatric sequelae of chronic exposure to organophosphate insecticides. *Lancet* 1:1371.

Goldblatt, PB, Moore, ME, and Stunkard, AJ (1965) Social factors in obesity. *J AMA* 192:1039–1044.

Gould JL (1982) *Ethology: The Mechanisms and Evolution of Behavior.* New York: WW Norton.

Gove, WR (1972) Sex, marital status and suicide. *J Health Soc Behav* 13:204–213.

Halbreich, U (ed)(1988) *Hormones and Depression.* New York: Raven Press.

Hamilton, M (1961) A rating scale for depression. *J Neurol Neurosurg Psychiatry* 12:56–62.

Hess, WR (1954) *Diencephalon: Autonomic and Extrapyramidal Functions.* New York: Grune & Stratton.

Houston, JP (1985) *Motivation.* New York: Macmillan.

Iversen, LL, Iversen, DS, and Snyder, SH (eds)(1978) *Handbook of Psychopharmacology, Vol 14, Affective Disorders: Drug Actions in Animals and Man.* New York: Plenum Press.

Jung, J (1978) *Understanding Human Motivation: A Cognitive Approach.* New York: Macmillan.

Kagan, J, Reznick, JS, and Snidman, N (1988) Biological basis of childhood shyness. *Science* 240:167–171.

Kaplan, GA, Roberts, RE, Camacho, TC, et al. (1987)

Psychosocial predictors of depression: Prospective evidence from the human population laboratory studies. *Am J Epidemiol* 125:206–220.

Katchadourina, HA and Lunde, DT (1985) *Fundamentals of Human Sexuality,* 4th ed. New York: Holt, Rinehart & Winston.

Keyl, PM and Eaton, WW (1990) Risk factors for the onset of panic disorder and other panic attacks in a prospective population-base study. *Am J Epidemiol* 131(2):301–311.

Kliewer, EV and Ward, RH (1988) Convergence of immigrant suicide rates to those in the destination country. *Am J Epidemiol* 127(3):640–653.

Kolata, G (1987) Manic-depression gene tied to chromosome 11. *Science* 235:1139–1140.

Kupfermann, I (1985) Hypothalamus and limbic system I: Peptidergic neurons, homeostasis, and emotional behavior. In *Principles of Neural Science,* 2nd ed, ER Kandel and JS Schwartz (eds) pp. 611–625. New York: Elsevier.

Kupfermann, I (1985) Hypothalamus and limbic system II: Motivation. In *Principles of Neural Science,* 2nd ed, ER Kandel and JS Schwartz (eds) pp. 626–635. New York: Elsevier.

Lemere, F and Smith, J (1973) Alcohol-induced sexual impotence. *Am J Psychiatry* 130(2):212–213.

Lester, D (1972) *Why People Kill Themselves: A Summary of Research Findings on Suicidal Behavior.* Springfield, IL: Charles C Thomas.

Levin, HS, Rodnitzky, RL, and Mick DL (1976) Anxiety associated with exposure to organophosphate compounds. *Arch Gen Psychiatry* 33:225–228.

Lorenz, KZ (1950) The comparative method in studying innate behavior patterns. *Symp Soc Exp Biol* 4:221–268.

Mancuso, TF and Locke, BF (1972) Carbon disulfide as a cause of suicide. *J Occup Med* 14:595–606.

Mandler, G (1975) *Man and Emotion.* New York: John Wiley & Sons.

Marks, IM (1987) *Fears, Phobias and Rituals.* New York: Oxford University Press.

Marler, P and Hamilton, WJ (1966) *Mechanisms of Animal Behavior.* New York: John Wiley & Sons.

Master, WH, Johnson, VE, and Kolodny, RC (1985) *Human Sexuality,* 2nd ed. Boston: Little, Brown.

McAllister, TW (1981) Cognitive functioning in the affective disorders. *Comp Psychiatry* 22:572–586.

McCoby, EE and Jacklin, CN (1974) *The Psychology of Sex Differences.* Stanford, CA: Stanford University Press.

Metcalf, DR and Holmes, HH (1969) EEG, psychological, and neurological alterations in humans with organophosphorous exposure. *Ann NY Acad Sci* 160:357.

Miller, WR (1975) Psychological deficit in depression. *Psychol Bull* 82:238–260.

Money, J and Ehrhardt, AA (1972) *Man and Woman,* *Boy and Girl.* Baltimore: John Hopkins University Press.

Morgane, PJ (ed)(1969) Neural regulation of food and water intake. *Ann NY Acad Sci* 157:531–1216.

Morrison, J, Olton, D, Goldberg, A, et al. (1975) Alterations in consummatory behavior of mice produced by dietary exposure to inorganic lead. *Dev Psychobiol* 8:389–396.

Moscicki, EK, Locke, BZ, Rae, DS, et al. (1989) Depressive symptoms among Mexican Americans: The Hispanic health and nutrition examination study. *Am J Ind Med* 130(2):348–359.

Munjack, DJ (1979) Sex and drugs. *Clin Toxicol* 15(1):75–89.

Norman, DK and Herzog, DB (1983) Bulimia, anorexia nervosa, and anorexia nervosa with bulimia. *Int J Eating Disorders* 2:43–52.

Perlin, S (ed)(1975) *A Handbook for the Study of Suicide.* New York: Oxford University Press.

Quinn, MM, Wegman, DH, Greaves, IA et al. (1990) Investigation of reports of sexual dysfunction among male chemical workers manufacturing stilbene derivatives. *Am J Ind Med* 18:55–68.

Reich, T, Clayton, PJ, and Winokur, G (1969) Family history studies V: The genetics of mania. *Am J Psychiatry* 125:1358–1369.

Reiman, EM, Fusselman, MJ, Fox, PT, et al. (1989) Neuroanatomical correlates of anticipatory anxiety. *Science* 241:1071–1074.

Renshaw, DC (1975) Sexual problems of alcoholics. *Chicago Med* 78(10):433–435.

Rotton, J (1983) Affective and cognitive consequences of malodorous pollution. *Basic Appl Social Psychol* 4(2):171–191.

Sachar, EJ (1976) Neuroendocrine dysfunctions in depressive illness. *Annu Rev Med* 127:389–396.

Sachar, EJ (1985) Disorder or feeling: Affective diseases. In *Principles of Neural Science,* 2nd ed, ER Kandel and JS Schwartz (eds) pp. 717–725. New York: Elsevier.

Sachar, EJ and Baron, M (1979) The biology of affective disorders. *Annu Rev Neurosci* 2:505–518.

Satran, R and Dodson, VN (1963) Toluene habituation: Report of a case. *N Engl J Med* 268:719.

Schildkraut JJ (1965) The catecholamine hypothesis of affective disorders: A review of supporting evidence. *Am J Psychiatry* 122:509–522.

Schildkraut, JJ (1973) Pharmacology: The effects of lithium on biogenic amines. In *Lithium, Its Role in Psychiatric Research and Treatment,* S Gershon and B Shopsin (eds) pp. 51–74. New York: Plenum Press.

Schildkraut, JJ and Key, SS (1967) Biogenic amines and emotion. *Science* 156:21–30.

Schottenfeld, RS and Cullen MR (1984) Organic affective illness associated with lead intoxication. *Am J Psychiatry* 141(11):1423–1426.

Smith, WL (1986) The thirteen nerve: Sieben mit einem Streich. *Int J Clin Neuropsychol* 8(1):41–42.

Somervell, PD, Leaf, PJ, Weissman, MM, et al. (1989) The prevalence of major depression in black and white adults in five United States communities. *Am J Epidemiol* 130(4):725–735.

Spark, RF, White, RA, and Connolly, PB (1980) Impotence is not always psychogenic: Newer insights into hypothalamic-pituitary-gonadal dysfunction. *JAMA* 243:750–755.

Spioch, FM and Nowara, M (1980) Voluntary dehydration in men working in heat. *Int Arch Occup Environ Health* 46:233–239.

Steward, RD, Hake, CL, and Peterson, JE (1974) Degreasers flush. *Arch Environ Health* 29:1–5.

Story, NL (1974) Sexual dysfunctions resulting from drug side effects. *Sex Res* 10:132–149.

Strongren, LL (1977) The influence of depression on memory. *Acta Psychiatr Scand* 56:109–128.

Thayer, RE (1989) *The Biopsychology of Mood and Arousal.* New York: Oxford University Press.

Thomas, A and Chess, S (eds)(1977) *Temperament and Development.* New York: Brunner/Mazel.

Thorpe, WH (1956) *Learning and Instincts in Animals.* Cambridge, MA: Harvard University Press.

Tinbergen, N (1951) *The Study of Instinct.* Oxford: Clarendon Press.

Vernon, SW and Roberts, RE (1982) Prevalence of treated and untreated psychiatric disorders in three ethnic groups. *Soc Sci Med* 16:1575–1582.

Weisemberger, BL (1977) Toluene habituation. *J Occup Med* 19:569.

Whitlock, FA (1971) Migration and suicide. *Med J Aust* 2:840–848.

Wilson, GT and Lawson, DM (1976) The effects of alcohol on sexual arousal in women. *J Abnorm Psychol* 85:489–497.

Zaebst, DD, Tanaka, S, and Haring, M (1980) Occupational exposure to estrogens—problems and approaches. In *Estrogens in the Environment,* JA McLachlan (ed) pp. 377–388. New York: Elsevier.

Zuckerman, M (1960) The development of an affect adjective check list for the measurement of anxiety. *J Consult Psychol* 24:457–462.

29

Learning and Memory

As we go through life, each of us learns different things and acquires skills and stores of memories that ultimately modify our perception of the world (and of ourselves) and create our unique and relatively stable mode of behaving. (In Chapter 31, we will call this "personality.") Thus, to a great extent, learning and the storage of memory are the bases of our individuality.

Some definitions are necessary. *Learning* is the process of acquisition of skills and knowledge about the external environment and ourselves. *Memory* is the retention (storage) of that knowledge and skills and the possibility of their being recalled at will. *Short-term memory* is the ability to retain and recall information within short periods of time (ie, seconds, minutes, or hours). *Long-term memory* is the retention of that information for longer periods of time (weeks, months, and years).

This chapter is a review of the forms of learning, the neural basis of memory, and the behavioral techniques used for the assessment of memory, particularly in the adult. Some representative research on the effect of neurotoxic agents on memory functions is also reviewed.

LEARNING AND MEMORY AS PROCESSES

Perspectives of Learning and Memory

The human capacity to learn and to recall has been recognized since the Greeks. Aristotle (384–322 BC) himself wrote a small treatise on memory. His theory of association of ideas—a theory that explained sensory processes, memory, and thought—was so influential, its acceptance persisted into the early years of this century. In the 19th century, psychology became an independent discipline, and learning and memory were subjected to experimental analysis under laboratory conditions.

Many of us, professionals and laypeople alike, need to have a working knowledge of the process of learning and memory: for example, parents, psychologists, educators, linguists, neurologists, neurophysiologists, psychiatrists, biologists, ethologists, animal trainers, occupational therapists, and rehabilitation therapists. These specialists, of course, see the process of learning and memory from different points of view. Parents teach children how to speak using procedures that vary in different cultures. Some people need practical knowledge about the process of learning for rehabilitation following brain damage. Some others, conducting research with laboratory animals, look for an explanation of how learning occurs and for memory traces that are stored in the nervous system.

This chapter is limited to a review of three areas of research on learning and memory having significance for experimental and clinical neurotoxicity—namely, the views of neuroscience, neuropharmacology, and neuropsychology. A wider perspective of learning and memory is beyond the scope of this work.

Models of Learning and Memory

Historically, the search for understanding of how skills and memories are created and then remain a part of the behavioral repertoire has been inspired by models. A *model* is the physical or conceptual reproduction of the essential components of a functional organization or system. Models are almost invariably inspired by the technology of the times. The ancients, particularly Aristotle, used poetic images to describe memory and learning. Memory, they said, is like the mark imprinted on clay or wax. Man is a "tabula rasa" (a wax writing plate used by the Greeks in their daily business transactions), a blank surface, on which the events of one's personal world are imprinted. We now use computers to write, and computer scientists think of learning and memory in terms of computer components. Current models for memory storage include, for example, data storage and read-out mechanisms.

Very little is known about the effects of neurotoxic agents on learning and memory, primarily because we know very little about learning and memory. In addition, at least in our generation, with the enormous diversification of views, it has been close to impossible to suggest a coherent theory of learning and memory in which all the facts about these important psychological processes are brought together.

Anderson (1983) provides a good example of how a cognitive psychologist views "memory" as a scientific problem. Squire (1987) and Tulving (1985) report the current status of research on (primarily human) memory. This review of learning has been inspired by the enlightening chapters by Kupfermann ("Learning") and Kandel ("Cellular Mechanisms of Learning and the Biological Basis of Individuality") in *Principles of Neural Science* edited by Eric R. Kandel and James H. Schwartz (1985). The historical roots of the study of learning can be found in Boring (1950).

Forms of Learning

Two types of learning are recognized: nonassociative and associative learning. In *nonassociative learning*, learning occurs as a result of the repeated presentation of the stimulus. One form of nonassociative learning is *habituation*, in which one ceases to react to a stimulus that is neither threatening nor personally meaningful. For example, we ignore street noises until someone who visits our house for the first time notices them. Another form of nonassociative learning is *sensitization*, which is the increased reflex response to a large variety of stimuli after the elicitation of intense or threatening stimulation. For example, we may walk through a subway station in fear and suspicion of everyone if we have been victimized in that subway station or similar places. Sensitization may be involved in the intense emotional reactions some workers have to their workplace after a single exposure to a harmful physical or chemical agent, or even a distressing psychological situation. Other forms of nonassociative learning include some more complex forms of learning such as imitation; *imitation learning* makes learning of a language possible.

Two forms of *associative learning* are classical and operant conditioning. *Classical con-*

ditioning consists of the pairing of two stimuli, the conditioned stimulus (CS) and the unconditioned stimulus (US). The US can always produce a response (for example, salivation); the CS cannot produce such a response. But if a CS is systematically paired with a US so that the CS will always be present for a split second before the US, the CS by itself will be able to produce a response. Thus, classical conditioning is a way we learn to predict the relationships between events in our environment. *Operant conditioning* consists of the pairing of a response to the presence of a stimulus. If a hungry rat during its walks around the cage hits a lever that delivers a food pellet, the rat will learn to press the lever for food.

Once it was thought that classical and operant conditioning were fundamentally two different processes in which a behavior could be "shaped" (created). From a neural point of view, separate systems do not exist to accommodate these processes.

THE NEURAL BASIS OF LEARNING

Neuroscientists seek to understand how the neural trace for memory (the *engram*) is formed, how short-term and long-term memory are explained, and where and how in the nervous system these events take place.

A Model for Memory Storage and Retrieval

The model for a memory storage system can be described using computer terminology. Most investigators seem to agree on the existence of a short-term memory store, a long-term memory store, and a search and read-out system (Fig. 29.1). This model is supported by clinical observations of people who have suffered traumatic injuries of the brain. Many suffer selective injuries either of the short- or long-term memory store.

In *retrograde amnesia,* for example, the information or memory of events before the accident occurred is lost. This suggests an impairment either in the long-term memory store or in the search and read-out mechanism. Sufferers from traumatic retrograde amnesia usually recuperate gradually, and the memory of past events returns.

In *anterograde amnesia* people are unable to remember events that occurred after the accident. This suggests an impairment in the short-term memory store. Sufferers of this type of memory deficit never recuperate the information that is lost (it is thought that perhaps the information never registered). This is a type of memory deficit present in the aged or that results from an acute intoxication. The "blackout" that occurs during acute alcohol intoxication, for example, is probably caused by a failure in short-term memory storage.

Studies of people who receive shock therapy for treatment of severe depression seem to confirm the existence of a dual mechanism for short- and long-term memory storage. People who receive shock therapy momentarily lose the short-term memory, whereas long-term memory remains virtually unimpaired.

It has been suggested that short-term memory is kept momentarily in the brain via a reverberating circuit involving several neurons. In this view, recently incorporated information will travel around the reverberating circuit without leaving any physical mark of its presence. The fact that short-term memory is temporarily lost during deep anesthesia, by anoxia, and by cooling of the brain in experimental animals seems to support the existence of such circuits.

The Distributive Localization of Memory in the Brain

The key structures of the brain that seem to be implicated in the creation, retention, and retrieval of information have been identified primarily through three main sources: autopsies of the brains of people who, when alive, suffered from severe forms of amnesia;

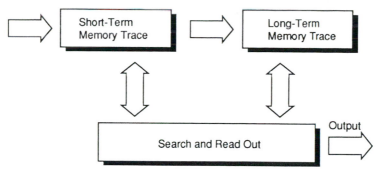

Fig. 29.1.   A diagrammatic model of memory storage.

studies of surgical (living) patients who suffered localized lesions of the brain in an attempt to control epileptic seizures; and stimulation, recording, and ablation studies (ie, selective removal of brain areas) in experimental animals.

Numerous cortical and subcortical centers of the brain are involved in the preservation of the memory trace. The medial temporal lobe and the diencephalon (in particular, the thalamus) are important. The limbic system—which, as we saw in the previous chapter, is related to the mechanism of emotions—reappears here as a key structure necessary for learning and memory. The hippocampus, which is a component of the limbic system, also seems to be a vital structure for the preservation of short-term memory.

Patients whose hippocampi have been surgically removed bilaterally display a total amnesia for recent events, amnesia that is not accompanied by perceptual or intellectual impairment. Long-term memory is also unimpaired. For example, such individuals can solve complex puzzles but, when probed, do not remember having worked with the puzzles after a few minutes have passed. Thus, bilateral hippocampal lesions produce not only specific and selective damage of memory functions but also impairment of short-term memory.

Neurotoxic agents and drugs do not usually produce a specific memory effect; they produce a generalized neuropsychological disturbance. Memory problems are often secondary to alterations in attention, arousal, or motivation. Only the severe amnestic syndrome associated with chronic alcoholism (to be described below) seems to be an exception, but this syndrome has a multiple causation, mostly from malnutrition. Thus, memory disturbances produced by chronic alcoholism cannot be used to model long-term effects of environmental or occupational neurotoxic agents.

The Basic Neurophysiological Processes of Learning and Memory

Research conducted on the neurophysiological basis of learning and memory has progressed from a molar and cellular to a molecular approach. Kandel and Schwartz (1982) have reviewed our current knowledge of behavioral, cell-physiological, ultrastructural, and molecular mechanisms in *Aplysia,* a marine snail.

Most of the cells involved in the gill- and siphon-withdrawal reflex of *Aplysia* are known, as are their interconnections. Unicellular recording of the electrical activity of neurons allows the understanding of the electrical and pharmacological status of one set of cells (eg, motor) when the cells are activated.

Several lines of work seem to indicate that serotonin is the neurotransmitter whose production is modulated while this organism is exhibiting behavioral signs of sensitization or habituation. Sensitization occurs as a strengthening of responses to a neutral stimulus (eg, a stream of water) after the snail has been exposed to a potentially threatening or noxious stimulus. Habituation occurs as a weakening of the response after the repetitive presentation of a neutral stimulus.

There is evidence that protein phosphorylation, which depends on cyclic adenosine monophosphate, can modulate synaptic action. Similar biochemical processes may be involved in the molecular mechanisms of long-term memory.

Additional studies have been conducted on the mollusk *Hermissenda* that are aimed at the ascertainment of the neural basis of a relatively higher-order level of learning, namely, associative learning (involving stimulus pairing in time). Learning behavior reminiscent of classical conditioning can be demonstrated in this organism. Postsynaptic membrane changes seem to account for the behavioral manifestations. Specific ionic currents in the neural tissue undergo transformations lasting days after associative training has taken place. During the acquisition phase of learning, intracellular calcium increases, and this increase is accompanied by specific potassium current reduction that lasts for days after conditioning. Alkon (1984), who has reviewed the experimental work with *Hermissenda,* concludes that the biophysical memory trace is a calcium-mediated reduction of ionic currents.

Thus, simple organisms that we do not normally think much about have provided valuable sources for our current understanding of the cellular and molecular mechanisms occurring during learning and memory.

The notion that memory traces are chemical has been reinforced by research on the neuropharmacological changes occurring in the hippocampus. Many scientists and clinical investigators now tend to agree that certain learning tasks may be mediated by subcortical structures such as the hippocampus, whereas others depend on cortical structures, a long-held view.

Lynch and Baudry (1986) have reviewed the experimental evidence supporting these

views and have proposed new and intriguing hypotheses. Briefly, high-frequency afferent stimulation produces postsynaptic changes in hippocampal neurons. The neurotransmitter involved seems to be either of the amino acids glutamate or aspartate, or both. The authors propose that a calcium proteinase receptor is involved in long-term potentiation (LTP) of monosynaptic hippocampal pathways. The LTPs and the associated chemical events that accompany their production seem to match fundamental features of memory in both lower and higher organisms.

Little is known about the neurophysiological basis of so-called "representational" memory—ie, memory involving images of the past. Studies that have been performed by clinical investigators are, in most cases, based on patients who need to be operated on because of brain pathological conditions such as epilepsy or tumors. Typically, the procedures are performed when the patient is awake (the stimulation of the brain is painless) and involve the electrical stimulation of brain areas suspected to be involved with memory. Since the middle 1950s, for example, it has been known that the stimulation of areas deep in the temporal lobe produce vivid memories of a patient's personal life. The discovery was made almost by accident.

The search for an animal model of the human amnestic syndrome—to be described below—has been frustrating because it is difficult to reproduce in animal species, such as the monkey, the tasks that are used for the diagnosis of human amnesia. Zola-Morgan and collaborators (1982) have utilized a technique described as "nonmatching-to-sample with trial-unique stimuli" that mimics tasks amnestic people are known to fail. Monkeys are trained in the Wisconsin General Testing Apparatus (WGTA) to displace an object placed over a central food well to obtain a raisin reward. After 8 seconds, they see two objects (the original one and a new one) and have to displace the new one in order to get the raisin reward. Twenty such trials are presented daily with an intertrial interval of 30 seconds. Each trial uses a new pair of objects, selected randomly from a collection of more than 300 junk objects. After reaching the learning criterion of 90 correct choices in 100 trials, monkeys are tested with longer delays between the sample and match trials.

Using the nonmatching-to-sample with trial-unique stimuli technique, these investigators were able to demonstrate that conjoint amygdala–hippocampal lesions produced a severe memory deficit. That the medial temporal region of the human brain, which includes the hippocampus, is a critical structure for memory has been known for some time (Milner 1966; Barbizet 1970).

Squire (1987) gives a comprehensive account of mechanisms of memory. John and collaborators (1986) provide a good review of recent attempts at localization of the engram. Olton et al. (1985) provide an integration of animal experimental and clinical perspectives. The neurology of learning and memory has been reviewed by Thompson (1986).

LEARNING AND MEMORY DISORDERS IN HUMANS

In humans, there are several important syndromes that are associated with learning and memory difficulties. Occasionally, these syndromes may be encountered in the occupational clinic, and a judgment needs to be made as to whether these conditions are linked to environmental or occupational factors.

Learning Disabilities

The ability to learn seems to be an innate capacity shared with most species of the animal kingdom. The notion that some individuals have learning difficulties or disabilities has long been proposed by educators. It is estimated that 10% of the American population is learning disabled (LD) (Byrne 1987).

Specific learning disabilities (SLD) is the name given to chronic conditions, assumed to be neurological in origin, which affect the development, integration, and/or demonstration of specific verbal or nonverbal abilities; SLD may be found in individuals who show no evidence of any other physical or mental handicap, are of average to superior intelligence, and have had adequate learning opportunities. The condition varies in its manifestation and in its degree of severity. Throughout life SLD can affect self-esteem, education, vocation, socialization, and/or daily living activities.

Current epidemiological studies have been directed at determining whether some forms of learning disabilities are associated with prenatal, perinatal, or early childhood exposure to neurotoxic agents. But large-scale epidemiological studies in which potential confounders have been controlled are rare. In Chapter 20 reference has been made to the difficulties in carrying out studies in which lead has been shown to be associated with a reduction in IQ among children.

Amnesia

Amnesia is a difficulty in learning new information or in remembering the past. The *Diagnostic and Statistical Manual of Mental Disorders* (DSM-III) published by the American Psychiatric Association (1980) offers three diagnostic criteria for amnestic syndrome:

1. An impairment in both short-term memory (characterized by the inability to learn new information) and long-term memory (inability to remember information known in the past).
2. Impairment of memory not explained by cloudiness of consciousness, as in delirium or intoxication, or general loss of major intellectual abilities, as in dementia.
3. Evidence from the history, physical examination, or laboratory tests of specific organic factors judged to be etiologically

related to the disturbance. (This is not always possible.)

Based on experimental studies in laboratory animals the etiological factors of the amnestic syndrome are thought to be caused by bilateral damage to the diencephalic and medial aspects of the temporal lobe including the amygdala and hippocampus. However, amnestic syndrome may be observed in the acute phase of brain trauma, surgical intervention, hypoxia, cerebral infarction, and herpes simplex encephalitis irrespective of its location. This relatively uncommon severe form of memory disorder has been linked to chronic alcoholism (see below) and also to chronic exposure to neurotoxic agents, particularly solvents, in the workplace.

Squire (1987) provides a good introduction to this neuropsychological problem and to how amnesia provides a window for the understanding of normal memory function in humans.

Alcohol Amnestic Syndrome. The most common form of amnestic syndrome is found in severe forms of chronic alcoholism. This thiamine-deficiency disorder is also known as *Korsakoff's disease.* The alcohol amnestic syndrome (AAS) often follows an acute episode of Wernicke's encephalopathy, a neurological disease characterized by confusion, ataxia, eye movement abnormalities, and other neurological signs.

Confabulation—nondeliberate fabrication of facts or events in response to questions about situations or events that are not recalled because of memory impairment—is often seen in alcohol amnestic syndrome. Clinical neuropsychologists may see these confabulations in the reproduction of test patterns during the administration of the Benton Visual Retention test and in tests requiring visual organization, such as the Embedded Figures test. In the former, the subject fills the gaps with patterns of his or her own invention just to avoid leaving the paper blank; in the latter, people may form new outlines out of fragments of outlines of other pictures. Testing procedures based on a menu of responses—which facilitate recall—may not unveil this significant sign of memory impairment.

ASSESSMENT OF HUMAN LEARNING AND MEMORY

There are four approaches to the assessment of human learning and memory.

The first approach originates in **experimental psychology** and can be traced to the pioneering work on pair-associates learning by Ebbinghaus, published in 1885 (Boring 1950). It is a cognitive approach aimed at the study of human memory capacities in normal individuals. The typical context of research is a laboratory of experimental psychology where college-age subjects are studied under controlled conditions. Studies on the human "channel capacity" and computer-based testing procedures for testing learning and memory can be considered part of this tradition.

Human learning is also studied by those interested in practical aspects of a **childhood education**, the second approach. It is traced to Binet in France and Terman in the United States (see Chapter 4 for their historical significance in psychometric testing). Pediatric neurotoxicologists, who study the effects of neurotoxic agents in the child, have profited from the wealth of assessment procedures in education.

The third approach is that originated by I. Pavlov (1849–1936) and B. F. Skinner (1904–1990), **classical behaviorists** who reject the concept of mind and instead study the objective manifestation of behavior. Learning and memory are described in terms of two basic paradigms: classical (Pavlovian) and operant conditioning. Skinner was a leading psychologist of his time, and his work and the work of his students have had a profound influence on psychologists' thinking in the United States and abroad. Experimental work in neurotoxicology in laboratory animals is dominated by this line of thought.

The last approach stems from **clinical neurology and neuropsychology**, with primary emphasis on the examination of qualitative aspects of memory dysfunctions in people affected by brain damage. Human research, performed in a clinical setting and primarily on the adult, is targeted to the accurate characterization of memory dysfunctions and the assessment of the degree of handicap and of the rehabilitation potential. The Wechsler's Memory Scale, the Benton Visual Retention test, and Memory Questionnaires (to be described below) originate within this background.

The Wechsler Scale for Memory

Wechsler's Memory Scale (WMS) has been in existence since the middle 1940s and was developed for the evaluation of people with severe neurological damage. Although the test is not challenging enough for workers examined for possible subclinical manifestations of neurotoxin-induced neuropsychological disorders, this test has often been very useful for clinical studies or health surveys. The classical questions "How old are you?" and "Who is the president of the United States?"—the first questions on the WMS—are likely to be resented by workers if the question is formulated devoid of an appropriate context. The scale is not truly a memory test but a probe of a variety of cognitive functions.

The WMS consists of seven subscales:

1. Personal and current information ("How old are you?" etc).
2. Orientation ("What year is this?" etc).
3. Mental control ("Count backwards from 20 to 1").
4. Logical memory (for example, recall of spoken stories—it is "logical" because the passage read to the examinee is best recalled if the relationships between characters and events are understood.)
5. Memory span (increasing numbers of digits that are repeated forwards or backwards, which are also part of intelligence tests).
6. Visual reproduction (reproduction of three cards with designs adapted from the Army Performance tests and the Binet scale).
7. Associated learning ("I am going to read to you a list of words, two at a time. Listen carefully because after I am through I shall expect you to remember the words that go together").

The Benton Visual Retention Test

This is a clinical and research instrument to assess visual perception and, in particular, visual memory. This specific test, or variations of it, has been recommended for the assessment of brain dysfunction caused by neurotoxic agents (Johnson 1987). The subject is shown 10 designs of increasing complexity, each for 10 seconds; this is followed by reproduction (from memory) of the designs by the subject either immediately or after a delay period. Both the number of correct reproductions and the error scores are used to assess the functional status of the subject's visual memory.

Some psychometric properties of both the WMS and the Benton Visual Retention test (BVRT) need to be emphasized. Although norms for certain populations are available in the literature, norms for blue-collar workers have yet to be developed. Information on the effect of age and education on the quantitative characteristics of the subject's response, characteristics that are important in the interpretation of the results, needs to be taken into consideration. The scoring procedure of both the WMS and BVRT is time consuming and quite elaborate. Commercially available sets give little information on validity and reliability studies. The report on standardization does not conform to modern psychometric thinking.

Most experts in the field of clinical neurotoxicology agree that a memory test suitable for the evaluation of acute or chronic neuropsychological effects of exposure to neurotoxic agents is still lacking. For a review of memory tests used in the evaluation of the brain-damaged, see Lezak (1976).

Assessment of Memory Problems by Means of Questionnaires

Wechsler's Memory Scale and the Benton Visual Retention test sometimes need to be supplemented with questionnaires aimed at the description of qualitative aspects of mem-

ory difficulties. Below is an example of the questionnaire used in clinical neurotoxicology at the Mount Sinai School of Medicine (developed by this author for the evaluation of common complaints of aging individuals).

Study of Human Memory under Laboratory Conditions

Experimental studies on the effects of neurotoxic agents on learning and recall have

---

Memory Questionnaire

To each question, the subject (or the person accompanying the patient) responds: never, occasionally, frequently, often, or all the time. The following is only a selection; questions include assessments of both short- and long-term memory.

1. Have you found yourself in the embarrassing situation of not knowing the name of the person you are talking to—a name you should know?
2. Are you bothered by your inability to remember names of people you came in contact with just a while ago?
3. When someone tells you his or her phone number or address, do you find yourself making mistakes in copying the numbers, particularly reversing or omitting numbers or letters?
4. Do you feel you need to make a list of the simplest things you are supposed to do because of fear of forgetting?
5. Do you need to tell your spouse (or partner) to remind you about things you ought to do?
6. Do you miss appointments because you just forget all about them?
7. Do you forget to do things you are supposed to do as a matter of routine?
8. Do you make mistakes so silly or so embarrassing that you tend not to talk about them to your spouse or close friend?
9. Have you ever found yourself needing to make up a story because you just cannot remember the circumstances under which something took place?
10. When you want to tell a story, do you find yourself needing to ask your spouse (partner, friend) for key details of the story such as names, places, etc?

11. Do you ever attempt to avoid people you think might notice a change in your behavior?
12. Have you found yourself in a place not really knowing what you were supposed to be doing there?
13. When you are suddenly interrupted while talking to someone, do you find it difficult to go back to the original topic of conversation?
14. Do you have difficulties handling a conversation with two or three people at the same time?
15. Do you miss the point of jokes told by people your own age?
16. Do you put things in places and then forget where you put them, requiring the help of your spouse (friend, partner) to find them?
17. Have you found yourself in the situation of not knowing how to return to a place you thought would be easy to find again?
18. Do you find yourself postponing tasks requiring a lot of mental effort (such as studying material on something you need to know) under the pretext you are not really interested in the task?
19. Do you find yourself thinking a lot about events of your childhood?
20. Is it easier for you to remember the details of events that took place a long time ago than the details of something that happened a few days ago?

been carried out on humans under controlled laboratory conditions. These are of two types: studies of acute and chronic effects. The acute studies are aimed at establishing the levels of environmental exposure to neurotoxic agents necessary to impair a learning task—for example, learning a series of numbers. The performance of these tasks is probably impaired because of the effects of neurotoxic agents on attention and concentration, which are intimately related to short-term memory. But acute effects on recall do not help in predicting the long-term effects of toxic agents or drugs on memory. For example, it is not known whether many such episodes over many years will eventually produce permanent damage of short- or long-term memory.

Because of ethical considerations, chronic studies are limited in scope and, as a rule, have not been designed to answer questions on the effects of neurotoxic agents on memory. However, profound memory disturbances have resulted from military experiments on volunteers and prisoners of war who were deliberately exposed to neurotoxic agents. (The possibility of emotional shock cannot be eliminated.) Sometimes, the purpose of these experiments has been for the development of incapacitating agents [eg, weapons such as LSD that would not kill but would temporarily disable the enemy, rendering him insane (see Chapter 35)].

CONCLUSIONS

Neurotoxic agents and drugs often produce a generalized acute or chronic neuropsychological impairment, and alterations in learning and memory are often a part of this generalized behavioral alteration. Few studies, however, have aimed at the effect of neurotoxic agents on specific learning or memory functions. This is to be expected because all brain functions—perception, attention, concentration, motor functions, motivation, emotions, etc—are intimately related, and only by abstracting these basic functions can they be conceived of as separate entities.

REFERENCES

Alkon, DL (1984) Calcium-mediated reduction of ionic currents: A biophysical memory trace. *Science* 226:1037–1045.

American Psychiatric Association (1980) *Diagnostic and Statistical Manual of Mental Disorders,* 3rd ed. Washington, DC: APA.

Anderson, JR (1983) Retrieval of information from long-term memory. *Science* 220:25–30.

Barbizet, J (1970) *Human Memory and Its Pathology.* San Francisco: WH Freeman.

Boring, EG (1950) *A History of Experimental Psychology.* New York: Appleton-Century-Crofts.

Byrne, WL (1987) Learning disabilities. In *Encyclopedia of Neuroscience, Vol I,* G Adelman (ed) pp. 580–582. Boston: Birkhäuser.

John, ER, Tang, Y, Brill, AB, et al. (1986) Double-labelled metabolic maps of memory. *Science* 233:1167–1175.

Johnson, BL (1987) *Prevention of Neurotoxic Illness in Working Populations.* New York: John Wiley & Sons.

Kandel, ER and Schwartz, JH (1982) Molecular biology of learning: Modulation of transmitter release. *Science* 218:433–443.

Kandel, ER and Schwartz, JH (eds) (1985) *Principles of Neural Science,* 2nd ed. New York: Elsevier.

Lezak, MD (1976) *Neuropsychological Assessment.* New York: Oxford University Press.

Lynch, G and Baudry, M (1986) The biochemistry of memory: A new and specific hypothesis. *Science* 224:1057–1063.

Milner, B (1966) Amnesia following operation on the temporal lobes. In *Amnesia,* CWM Whitty and OL Zangwill (eds) pp. 109–133. London: Butterworths.

Olton, DS, Gamzu, E, and Corkin, S (eds) (1985) Memory dysfunctions: An integration of animal and human research from preclinical and clinical perspectives. *Ann NY Acad Sci* Vol 44.

Squire, LR (1987) *Memory and the Brain.* New York: Oxford University Press.

Thompson, RF (1986) The neurobiology of learning and memory. *Science* 233:941–947.

Tulving, E (1985) How many memory systems are there? *Am Psychol* 40:385–398.

Zola-Morgan, S, Squire, LR, and Mishkin, M (1982) The neuroanatomy of amnesia: Amygdala–hippocampus versus temporal stem. *Science* 218:1337–1339.

SUGGESTED READINGS

Baddeley, AD (1976) *A Psychology of Memory.* New York: Basic Books.

Black, IB, Adler, JE, Dreyfus, CF, et al. (1987) Biochemistry of information storage in the nervous system. *Science* 236:1263–1268.

Bolla-Wilson, K, Wilson, RJ, and Bleecker, M (1988) Conditioning of physical symptoms after neurotoxic exposure. *J Occup Med* 30(9):684–686.

Bolles, RC (1979) *Learning Theory,* 2nd ed. New York: Holt, Rinehart and Winston.

Brady, K, Herrara, Y, and Zenick, H (1975) Influence of parental lead exposure on subsequent learning ability of offspring. *Pharmacol Biochem Behav* 3:561–565.

Brown, DR (1975) Neonatal lead exposure in the rat: Decreased learning as a function of age and blood lead concentration. *Toxicol Appl Pharmacol* 32:628–637.

Bushnell, PJ and Bowman, RE (1979) Reversal learning deficits in young monkeys exposed to lead. *Pharmacol Biochem Behav* 10:733–742.

Bushnell, PJ and Bowman, RE (1979) Persistence of impaired reversal learning in young monkeys exposed to low levels of dietary lead. *J Toxicol Environ Health* 5:1015–1023.

Butters, N and Cermak, LS (1980) *Alcoholic Korsakoff's Syndrome: An Information Processing Approach to Amnesia.* New York: Academic Press.

Catania, AC (1979) *Learning.* Englewood Cliffs, NJ: Prentice-Hall.

Cermak, LS (1972) *Human Memory: Research and Theory.* New York: Ronald Press.

Chalupa, B, Synková, J and Sevcík, M (1960) The assessment of electroencephalographic changes and memory disturbances in acute intoxications with industrial poisons. *Br J Ind Med* 17:238–241.

Crossen, JR and Wiens, AN (1988) Wechsler Memory Scale—Revised: Deficits in performance associated with neurotoxic solvent exposure. *Clin Neuropsychol* 2(2):181–187.

Del Ser, T, Espasandin, P, Cabetas, I, et al. (1986) Memory disturbances in the toxic oil syndrome [in Spanish]. *Arch Neurobiol* 49(1):19–39.

Del Ser, T (1985) Are there memory disturbances in toxic oil syndrome? A case-control study of one pair of twin girls [in Spanish]. *Arch Neurobiol* 48(3):124–132.

Donahue, JW and Wessels, MD (1980) *Learning, Language, and Memory.* New York: Harper & Row.

Dudai, Y (1989) *The Neurobiology of Memory: Concepts, Findings, Trends.* New York: Oxford University Press.

Erikson, RC and Scott, ML (1977) Clinical memory testing: A review. *Psychol Bull* 84:1130–1149.

Fox, JL (1983) Debate on learning theory is shifting. *Science* 222:1219–1222.

Hall, SS (1985) *Aplysia* and *Hermissenda. Science '85* May: 30–39.

Hebbs, DO (1949) *The Organization of Behavior.* New York: John Wiley & Sons.

Learner, J (ed) (1984) *Learning Disabilities: Theories,* *Diagnosis and Teaching,* 4th ed. Dallas: Houghton Mifflin.

Mackintosh, NJ (1983) *Conditioning and Associate Learning.* New York: Oxford University Press.

Maximilian, VA (1982) Regional cerebral flow and verbal memory after chronic exposure to organic solvents. *Brain Cognition* 1(2):196–205.

Mayes, AR (1986) Learning and memory disorders and their assessment. *Neuropsychologia* 24:25–39.

Mayron, LW (1978) Ecological effects in learning disabilities. *J Learning Dis* 11(8):495–505.

Mishkin, M and Appenzeller, T (1987) The anatomy of memory. *Sci Am* 256(6):80–89.

Neisser, U and Winograd, E (1988) *Remembering Reconsidered: Ecological and Traditional Approaches to the Study of Memory.* New York: Cambridge University Press.

Poon, LW (ed) (1986) *Handbook for Clinical Memory Assessment of Older Adults.* Washington, DC: American Psychological Association.

Prigatano, GP (1978) Wechsler Memory Scale: A selective review of the literature. *J Clin Psychol* 34(4):816–832.

Puff, CR (1982) *Handbook of Research Methods in Human Memory and Cognition.* New York: Academic Press.

Ross, ED (1982) Disorders of recent memory in humans. *Trends Neurosci* 6:170–173.

Schneider, W and Pressley, M (1988) *Memory Development between 2 and 20.* New York: Springer Verlag.

Smith, PJ and Langolf, GD (1981) The use of Sternberg's memory-scanning paradigm in assessing effects of chemical exposure. *Hum Factors* 23(6):701–708.

Smith, PJ, Langolf, GD, and Goldberg, J (1983) Effects of occupational exposure to elemental mercury on short-term memory. *Br J Ind Med* 40:413–419.

Sohler, A, Pfeiffer, CC, and Papaioannou, R (1981) Blood aluminum levels in a psychiatric outpatient population: High aluminum levels related to memory loss. *J Orthomol Psychiatry* 10(1):54–60.

Squire, LR (1982) Human memory: Neuropsychological and anatomical aspects. *Annu Rev Neurosci* 5:241–273.

Sternberg, S (1975) Memory scanning: New findings and current controversies. *QJ Exp Psychol* 27:1–32.

Stollery, BT and Flindt, ML (1988) Memory sequelae of solvent intoxication. *Scand J Work Environ Health* 14(1):45–48.

Störring, G (1936) *Gedächtnisverlust durch Gasvergiftung,* ein Mensch ohne Zeitgedächtnis. *Arch f. d. ges. Psychol* 95:436–511.

Thompson, RF and Spencer, WA (1966) Habituation: A model phenomenon for the study of neuronal substrates of behavior. *Psychol Rev* 173:16–43.

Wechsler, D (1945) A standardized memory scale for clinical use. *J Psychol* 19:87–95.

30

Cognition

"Cognition" is a construct—ie, a term designating an abstract entity; it replaces the old concept of "intelligence" with none of the difficulties in defining it. Cognition is a synthesis of many psychological functions, including spatial and time orientation, object recognition, skilled movements, the ability to elicit appropriate information from memory at the time needed, language comprehension, arithmetic calculation, reasoning, imagination, and problem solving.

Psychologists disagree among themselves about what functions should and should not be included in the definition of cognition. Although modern psychologists do not emphasize essential differences between sensory systems and cognitive functions as they did in the past, "achievement of meaning" is viewed as the quintessence of cognitive skills.

INTELLIGENCE

Hunt (1983) writes: "The study of intelligence has historically revolved around three questions: What does intelligence do, what causes it, and how should it be measured?" In recent years there has been a revival of the interest in a unified theory of cognition, such as the theory published by Anderson in 1983. Anderson established the fundamental distinction between *declarative knowledge*, the

knowledge that something is the case, and *procedural knowledge*, the knowledge of how to do something. In this theory, declarative knowledge is represented by a network in which nodes represent "cognitive units." Procedural knowledge is represented by "production rules," imperatives of the form "if a certain condition holds, then perform a certain action."

There is no single physical or neural basis for cognition. For generations, it was argued that intelligence was related to the size of the brain, development of the frontal lobes, the number of neural cells, etc. No scientific facts support these theories, which range from honest but biased observations to pure quackery. For an excellent review of theories of intelligence, see Sternberg (1985).

It is now possible to understand the neural basis of some localizable components of intelligence, such as perception, language, and memory. But the explanation for the neural basis of higher levels of cognitive functioning—such as the acquisition of knowledge, scientific understanding, ethical evaluation, etc—remains beyond our reach.

Tests of Intelligence

All tests of intelligence are based on views of human cognition. In certain cases a test is developed in connection with a particular theory of intelligence. One such test is the Raven Progressive Matrices test; the test consists of matrices (designs) from each of which a part has been removed. The examinee has to choose the missing insert from six or eight given alternatives. The items are grouped in a series of increasing difficulty. [Sometimes, even after the theory has been largely abandoned—as has the existence of the general intelligence factor g, which the Raven test was supposed to measure—such tests continue to remain in use.] Some other theories of intelligence, such as Piaget's, are not accompanied by formalized psychological tests.

LANGUAGE

In Chapter 25 the acoustic basis of speech intelligibility was discussed, and in Chapter 27 we addressed language as a motor activity. Language is mentioned once again here as the most important of the human cognitive functions.

Language has three different features: form, content, and use. The *form* of a language is the dictionary of words and the syntax that links words together in any language. The *content* of the language represents the ideas encoded in the spoken message. The *use* of a language is how people choose to respond to situations or contexts using verbal or nonverbal communication.

Certain neurological diseases can interfere with some or all three of these different features of language (see Chapter 27). Form, for example, can be affected by lesions of the cerebellum that alter the sequential programming of spoken words, causing dysarthria. Broca's aphasia is produced by lesions of the brain in the area of the cortex where language is, to a certain extent, localized. The slurred speech that is observed in acute alcoholic intoxication or acute solvent inhalation is also an alteration of language's form.

The content of language is disturbed by many neurological diseases that affect language and ideation. Alterations in content are observed, for example, in Wernicke's aphasia—a neurological condition characterized by a deficit in comprehension of language—and in schizophrenia. The content of the language can be modified by neurotoxic agents as well. Carbon disulfide poisoning, for example, is known to produce psychosis; many hallucinogenic drugs such as LSD produce alterations in the content of language.

Alterations in the use of language are seen in many psychiatric illnesses. In autism—a severe psychiatric disorder primarily affecting children—for example, the individual suffering the condition does not communicate. People affected by various psychiatric disorders employ body language or drawing as a means of expression. An important component of the training of psychologists is the identification of messages disturbed people convey in such different channels of human communication.

A good introduction to language and language disorders is the chapter by Mayeux and Kandel, "Natural Language, Disorders of Language, and Other Localizable Disorders of Cognitive Functioning," in Kandel and Schwartz (1985).

Language as Source of Information in Clinical Neurotoxicology

In the clinic, a wealth of information is obtained through the observation of spontaneous speech. As the examinee narrates the reason why he or she needs help, for example, the examiner pays attention to the form, content, and use of the language.

Through language, age, education, and sometimes cultural background are revealed. There is the language of the child, the teenager, the adult, and the aged. While in the clinic, and especially while talking to a professional, the examinee often uses his or her "best language"; different words might be used at home or at work. The richness of vocabulary, the choice of words, and the use of images and analogies reveal education (not necessarily achieved through schooling). Language is sometimes spoken with accents of foreign countries; geographic variations in speech and even local mannerisms can be detected.

There are normal but idiosyncratic uses of language. For example, some people consistently fail to refer to themselves. When A talks to B, A says "you would not like to be close to that place," meaning anybody including himself. In citing this example, we are introducing the use of language as a cue to the assessment of the individual's personality, the subject of the next chapter.

Surprisingly, there are only slight gender variations in some aspects of the language, such as the written form. In blind experiments, in which the identification of the author is not available, trained psychologists cannot tell the gender of the author of written stories when some key words indicative of gender are eliminated.

Language provides a measure of premorbid intelligence (the intelligence the subject had before a pathological condition affected the current level of brain functioning). Since language is acquired early in life, it is quite resistant to change such as that resulting from brain trauma.

In follow-up studies, the use and proficiency of language are found to be one of the few abilities that grows even past maturity. Language enrichment that occurs in normal aging is a fact consistently ignored in the description of the aging process, perhaps because it does not fit our stereotypes about aging.

Language conveys moods and emotions. The tone, the pauses, the sighs, the use of expletives to emphasize a point, are all important cues to the examinee's moods.

Because an important component of cognition is the understanding of spoken speech, the examiner's own speech and idiosyncratic use of language are also a factor in the evaluation of other people's cognitive abilities.

(The author, for example, speaks with an accent, a quality of speech almost unnoticeable in New York City but a relevant factor while conducting medical surveys in other areas of the country where exposure to foreign accents is unusual.)

Language as a Confounding Factor in Epidemiological Studies

Language, an important source of information in the clinic, needs to be either completely eliminated or accounted for in epidemiological studies on the effects of neurotoxic agents. During the course of a medical field survey, between 50 and 100 individuals need to be examined during 1 day, and the evaluation of each individual is carried out by several examiners. Failure to understand the instructions of a test that needs to be self-administered might be a reason for failing the test. Unexpected conditions that might or might not influence the results of psychometric testing need to be evaluated on the spot. In a random sample of the population of Michigan, for example, one subject came to the testing site carrying an electronic artificial larynx; his own larynx had been removed because of cancer years ago. The individual was tested after it was judged that the performance in our screening battery of tests would not be influenced by the use of the artificial larynx.

Language and Animal Models

The identification of an animal model of language has been largely unsatisfactory. No animal species, including the higher primates, have the capacity to learn language as we do. However, animal species can communicate. Monkeys can learn American Sign Language, the language of the American deaf. The largest number of sign-language words learned by a monkey is about 160, compared to 3000 learned by 4-year-old child.

Language and Speech Disorder in Children with Excessive Lead Absorption

Perino and Ernhart (1974) investigated the performance of children on verbal tasks from the McCarthy Scales of Children's Abilities (Kaufman 1973). The subjects of the study group were 80 black children residing in greater New York City. Thirty children—the study group—had elevated blood lead levels (40 to 60 μg/dL). The control group were 50 children whose blood lead levels ranged from 10 to 30 μg/dL. The elevated blood lead level group performed significantly worse than controls in the following tasks: (1) recalling names of pictures after a 10-second exposure; (2) naming picture objects; (3) vocabulary; (4) repeating words, sentences, and stories; (5) spontaneous naming of objects; and (6) naming opposites. The investigators concluded that children having subclinical levels of lead showed impairment similar to those exhibiting minimal brain damage.

ASSESSMENT OF COGNITION

Cognition is defined as a synthesis of many psychological functions including spatial and time orientation, object recognition, skilled movements, the ability to elicit appropriate information from memory at the time needed, language production and comprehension, arithmetic calculation, reasoning, and problem solving. It follows that each component tested to assess "lower order of functioning"—such as perception or memory—is also capable of furnishing information to a greater or lesser extent about the "high order of functioning" which we call cognition.

For example: the Embedded Figures test, consisting of the ability to detect outlines of figures intermingled with other outlines, has been (correctly) included as a test of visual perception, but the test can also be considered a test of cognitive functioning. The ability to distinguish figures from a background has long been considered a cognitive function par excellence.

A simple probe of motor function can also be a cognitive test. In the adult, the inability to tie shoes or button blouses might unveil apraxias. *Apraxia* is a disorder characterized by the failure to execute skilled purposive movements in the absence of significant motor weakness, incoordination, or sensory loss.

Drawings can reveal cognitive functioning. Among children, the Draw-a-Man test developed by Goodenough makes use of the observation that, with advancing age, children draw persons with increasing levels of complexity and attention to detail.

Arithmetic reasoning is widely used in the clinic as a cognitive probe. For example, "How many nickels are there in a dollar?"

The understanding of language—in particular, the abstract messages of proverbs—is also a cognitive function. For example, one may ask, "What does it mean that people in glass houses should not throw stones?"

A battery of tests of intelligence usually taps several of the abovementioned dimensions. To assess cognition, the examinee must be challenged. Experienced neuropsychologists develop a sense of the challenge that is adequate for various conditions—eg, a severe head trauma after an automobile accident, or a foundry worker who comes to the clinic because of concern about possible health effects related to neurotoxic metal exposure. In extreme situations, such as in the evaluation of accident victims, a physician or a paramedic needs to make a quick assessment of the cognitive functioning of an individual—the ability to talk, to state his or her name, to count forwards and then backwards, etc. In the clinic, there are a large variety of procedures that are available to evaluate the mental status of the patient.

Muriel D. Lezak's *Neuropsychological Assessment* (1976) is a comprehensive source of procedures, diagnostic issues, and interpretations of neuropsychological tests available for the evaluation of cognition that are normally used in the clinic. It should be stressed that, in the clinic, the neuropsychologist makes a professional judgment of the level and quality of cognitive functions in a descriptive manner. In epidemiological studies, on the other hand, in order to establish dose–response relationships between environmental or occupational levels of neurotoxic exposure (or biological indicators of absorption) and mental function, the level of cognitive functioning needs to be established in a quantitative manner. Thus, in neuroepidemiology, quantitative tools for neuropsychological assessment are essential.

The Intelligence Quotient

Alfred Binet (1857–1911), after losing faith in the theory that intelligence was correlated with children's head volume, decided in 1904 to adopt a psychological approach to the task of assessing intelligence. That year, France's Ministry of Public Education commissioned Binet to identify children who needed special education in the public school system. Binet's scale of intelligence, developed for that purpose, was the first psychometric technique for the evaluation of cognitive function and is the forerunner of modern IQ tests.

Binet's scale of intelligence consisted of a collection (a battery) of tasks that were judged essential in everyday life, such as counting coins. An age level was assigned to each task, specifically, the youngest age at which the task could be expected to be accomplished successfully. *Mental age* was defined as the age at which the task should be completed. After prolonged debate about how the relationship between mental age and chronological age (the actual age of the child) should be viewed, the German psychologist William Stern (1871–1938) proposed the concept of the *intelligence quotient,* most commonly known as IQ. The IQ is arrived at by dividing the mental age by the chronological age, multiplied by 100.

In Chapter 4 a brief history of psychometric methods including mental testing is

discussed. Chapter 20 contains a description of some intelligence scales for children.

Diagnostic Criteria for Mental Retardation in the Child

The DSM-III-R published by the American Psychiatric Association defines mental retardation as a subaverage general intellectual functioning (IQ less than 70) with concurrent deficits in adaptive behavior, taking the child's age into consideration, and with onset before the age of 18. Several subtypes of mental retardation are defined: mild (IQ between 50 and 70), moderate (35 to 49), severe (20 to 34), and profound (an IQ below 20).

DEMENTIA

Dementia is a sustained, multidimensional loss of cognitive functions resulting from central nervous system damage. Dementia is viewed as an "organic" dysfunction of the brain, such as, for example, that caused by chronic multiple brain trauma in boxing, metabolic conditions, or exposure to toxic agents. It needs to be emphasized that there is a lack of agreement about how dementia is defined.

Organic Mental Disorders in the Adult

The DSM-III establishes the distinction between organic brain syndromes and organic mental disorder. An *organic brain syndrome* is a constellation of psychological or behavioral signs or symptoms without reference to etiology (eg, delirium, dementia), whereas *organic mental disorder* refers to a particular organic brain syndrome in which the etiology is known or presumed (eg, alcohol withdrawal delirium, multiinfarct dementia). The DSM-III-R recommends that the word "organic" be replaced by the suspected causative agent when known. Thus, according to this recommendation, when carbon disulfide is highly suspected to be the causative factor for the organic brain syndrome, "organic hallucinosis" needs to be changed to "carbon disulfide hallucinosis".

Six categories of **organic brain syndromes** are described:

1. Delirium and dementia, characterized by global cognitive impairment.
2. Amnestic syndrome and organic hallucinosis, with selective cognitive impairment.
3. Organic delusional syndrome and organic affective syndrome, with features resembling schizophrenic or affective disorders.
4. Organic personality syndrome, in which personality is affected.
5. Intoxication and withdrawal, in which the disorder is associated with the ingestion or reduction in use of a toxic substance and does not meet any of the previous syndromes (intoxication and withdrawal are etiologically defined).
6. Atypical or mixed organic brain syndrome, a residual category for the classification of syndromes not falling into any of the above categories.

The following **organic mental disorders** are widely recognized, although a lively debate exists on the possible environmental and occupational causation of some of these disorders (see below):

1. Senile and presenile dementia
2. Substance-induced organic mental disorders
3. Alcoholic organic mental disorders
4. Barbiturate or similarly acting sedative or hypnotic organic mental disorders
5. Opioid organic mental disorders
6. Cocaine organic mental disorders
7. Amphetamine or similarly acting sympathomimetic mental disorders
8. Phencyclidine (PCP) or similarly acting organic mental disorders
9. Hallucinogen organic mental disorders
10. Cannabis organic mental disorders
11. Other or unspecified substance-induced organic mental disorders

Nomenclature for Dementia

There is wide professional, institutional, national, and international variation in naming a number of organic mental disorders, in characterizing clinical subtypes, and in summarizing the known pathological mechanisms of these disorders. Often, there are strong political forces supporting or rejecting a given classification system. Occupational (or industrial) physicians, neurologists, psychiatrists, clinical toxicologists, and clinical neuropsychologists use and contribute to the characterization of these terms. Inevitably, each profession is comfortable with its own particular language.

While studying the prevalence and incidence of neurotoxic illness, epidemiologists need to adhere to well-defined codes such as those of the DSM-III-R, although professionals do not have to adhere to these codes as strictly in the course of their professional practice.

One of the most important issues that has arisen in recent controversies is whether a new nomenclature should be proposed for organic mental disorders arising from chronic exposure to environmental or occupational neurotoxic agents or whether these disorders can be classified along the lines suggested, for example, by the DSM-III-R. Predictably, managers and labor organizations find themselves on opposite sides of this controversy. The adoption of a classification code that links dementia to an occupational toxic exposure, for example, has enormous implications for insurance and workers compensation policies. Environmental and occupational safety laws vary from country to country. In countries where such laws benefit workers, such as Denmark, there is a bitter controversy between those who wish to establish a link between organic mental disorders and neurotoxic exposures and those who do not. In the

United States, where such laws are not presently enforced, wide professional and public concern on probable occupational etiologies of dementia is still lacking.

The Distinction of Organic and Functional Neural Disorders May Not Be Warranted

At the conclusion of the monumental work *Principles of Neural Science* (Kandel and Schwartz 1985), Eric R. Kandel states:

> There is a tendency in medicine and psychiatry to think that biological determinants of behavior act on a different level of the mind than do social and functional determinants. For example, it is still customary to classify psychiatric illness into two major categories: organic and functional. Organic mental illness includes the dementias and the toxic psychoses, functional mental illnesses include the various depressive syndromes, the schizophrenia, and the neurotic illnesses. The distinction dates to the nineteenth century, when neuropathologists examined the brains of patients coming to autopsy and found gross and readily demonstrable disturbances in the architecture of the brain in some psychiatric diseases but not in others. Diseases that produced anatomical evidence of brain lesions were called organic; those lacking these features were called functional.
>
> [Experiments dealing with the cellular mechanisms of learning] show that this distinction is unwarranted. Everyday events—sensory stimulation, deprivation, and learning—have profound biological consequences, causing an effective disruption of synaptic connections under some circumstances, and a reactivation of connections under others. It therefore is incorrect to imply that certain diseases [organic diseases] affect mentation by producing biological changes in the brain, whereas other diseases [functional diseases] do not. All mental processes are biological, and any alteration in those processes is organic.
>
> Rather than making the distinction along biological and nonbiological lines, it is more appropriate to ask the following questions in each type of mental illness: To what degree is this biological process determined by genetic and developmental factors, to what degree is it determined by a toxic or an infectious agent, and to what degree is it environmentally or socially determined? Even in the most socially determined mental disturbances, the end result is biological, since it is the activity of the brain that is being modified (p. 831).

NEUROTOXIC AGENTS IN THE ENVIRONMENT AND THE WORKPLACE AS ETIOLOGICAL FACTORS FOR ORGANIC MENTAL DISORDERS

Effect of Mercury Absorption on Cognitive Functions in the Developing Child

In 1951, and again in 1960, Japan was hit hard with outbreaks of methylmercury poisoning occurring in Minamata Bay and the District of Niigata. In the Introduction to this book I refer to these episodes as important factors that increased awareness of the link between environment and public health around the world.

The source of exposure was methylmercury-contaminated fish. Profound mental retardation was reported among children born from intoxicated mothers. Animals such as cats, dogs, and birds that fed on some of the contaminated fish in the area also developed signs of poisoning. A new disease, Minamata disease, was named, associated with this tragedy. Until these episodes, methylmercury had not been recognized as an environmental health problem. Since then, vast literature has accumulated on the effects of methylmercury on the developing and adult brain.

In this case, the cause of mental retardation in the children was recognized as a failure to complete normal development of the brain and the cerebellum, caused by exposure to methylmercury in utero. The Minamata disease syndrome is accompanied by severe motor dysfunction such as muscular rigidity and exaggerated reflexes typical of the so-called "upper motor neuronal involvement." Cerebellar signs, such as ataxia, are also observed. Cerebral atrophy, particularly in the occipital lobes, can also be observed in the adult. These behavioral and neuropathological changes have been verified in experimental animals in which methylmercury was administered under controlled conditions.

Neurobehavioral Assessment of Mohawk Indians for Subclinical Indications of Methylmercury Neurotoxicity

The health consequences of the presence of methylmercury in waters, via consumption of fish, have been the object of concern since the tragic episode of mercury contamination in Japan described above. Methylmercury has also been found in fish and fish-eating mammals consumed by indigenous populations of North America. A study of Canadian Cree Indians with such a pattern of exposure was undertaken but failed to link neurological signs and symptoms with methylmercury absorption.

In connection with a larger study of health effects associated with toxic exposures among Mohawk Indians, Valciukas and collaborators (1986) performed a screening study to determine whether local residents in the St. Regis Reserve—an extended area at the convergence of Upper New York State, Ontario, and Quebec—were experiencing adverse health effects associated with undue absorption of methylmercury. The study was part of a comprehensive medical field study conducted by the Environmental Sciences Laboratory of the Mount Sinai School of Medicine in New York City, under the direction of Dr. Irving J. Selikoff, in the summer of 1981.

A total of 200 adult males and 200 females were examined by using a short battery of performance tests: the Block Design, Digit Symbol, and Embedded Figures test. Test selection was governed by two major considerations: time limitations inherent in clinical field studies, where the administration represents only one aspect of the medical examination, and the availability of data sets on control (nonexposed) groups.

The source of methylmercury was thought to be a chloralkali plant in the immediate vicinity of the reservation; however, contributions from other sources upstream in the St. Lawrence river had also been documented. The selection of subjects was based on "high" and "low" local fish consumption scores. Tests were administered in cooperation with specially trained local residents, and, whenever necessary, instructions were given in the Mohawk language.

No significant association between age-adjusted individual performance test scores and exposure was found. Males were found to eat more locally caught fish than females and had relatively higher methylmercury levels than females. It was concluded that, at the time of examination, St. Regis residents were exposed to almost "background" levels of methylmercury and did not exhibit either subclinical or clinical manifestations of methylmercury neurotoxicity.

The Link between Increased Lead in the Environment and Decreased IQ in Children

Several epidemiological studies in the late 1960s and early 1970s were aimed at determining the maximal allowable level of lead in children's blood.

The studies by Needleman and collaborators (1970, 1984) established a link between environmental lead levels and a decrement in IQ among children living in suburban Boston. The sample was drawn from 3229 children attending first and second grades in the period between 1975 and 1978 in Chelsea and Somerville, Massachusetts. Children were asked to submit their "baby" teeth to their teachers; the tooth dentine was then analyzed for lead content. A cumulative frequency distribution of dentine lead concentrations was drawn, and subjects were classified as having high or low blood lead levels, highest being defined as the highest 10th and lowest as the lowest 10th percentile, respectively. The final study group consisted of 58 children with high and 100 with low lead levels; 39 control variables entered in the analysis of covariance (a statistical procedure to control for possible confounding factors such the parents' IQ).

It was found that children with high lead levels in their dentine had significantly lower scores on the IQ test than those with low lead levels and that these children performed less well in various tests in addition to the IQ test. When the teacher's ratings were compared with the levels of lead in dentine, there was a remarkable dose–response relationship between dentine lead levels and negative rating of children's behavior (such as distractability, lack of persistence, dependency, etc).

As a result of these and numerous other investigations, maximal allowable exposure levels to lead have decreased. The level of 30 μg/dL of blood is the present recommended standard set by the US Department of Health, Education, and Welfare Center for Disease Control.

Effects of Lead Absorption on Cognitive Functions in the Adult

By the early 1970s in the United States the overt manifestations of lead poisoning were becoming increasingly rare in the adult, and the clinical picture of lead poisoning seemed to be well understood. Minimal allowable lead standards—expressed in maximal concentrations in blood—were set in many countries of the world. It was generally accepted that children suffered cognitive deficits. In adults, changes were restricted to a cluster of nonspecific symptoms and motor function alterations. Therefore, studies documenting cognitive dysfunctions in the adult—studies that were reported in the middle and late 1970s—were received with great interest.

In 1978 alone, three studies on the effect of occupational exposure to lead on cognition were published by Hänninen and collaborators, Valciukas and collaborators, and Grandjean and collaborators.

Hänninen et al. Study. In a study on the effects of low lead exposure on cognition—defined as "psychological performance," a term not widely accepted by U.S. psychologists—Hänninen and collaborators (1978) examined 49 exposed lead workers and 24 controls using a battery of tests. The examination consisted of a short interview, a neuropsychological test battery, and a personality inventory. The neuropsychological test battery comprised tasks representing a broad range of different functions. These included similarities, picture completion, block design, digit span, logical memory, visual reproduction, Bourdon–Wiersma (a test of vigilance), two scores in the Benton Visual Retention test (the time and the number of errors), the Santa Ana dexterity test, and simple and choice reaction time.

All the lead workers had been under regular surveillance, and only workers whose maximal blood lead concentration had never exceeded 70 μg/dL of blood were included in the study. At the time of the examination, the mean blood level was 32 μg/dL of blood. Comparisons were made both between exposed and nonexposed lead workers and within the exposed groups. In the exposed group, the maximal and the average blood lead concentrations and that taken closest to the moment of testing were used as measures of lead uptake. A time-weighted average (TWA) was calculated on the basis of the individual's historical blood lead values.

Significant negative correlations were observed between TWA blood lead levels and six test scores (the block design test, a test of visual reproduction, a test for verbal reproduction of digits, and dexterity tasks involving both hands, the preferred hand, and the nonpreferred hand). The TWA levels correlated best with these measures of neuropsychological functioning, whereas the blood lead level at the moment of testing was correlated the least. The block design tests and the visual reproduction tests correlated significantly with TWA levels only, and the digit span correlated significantly only with blood lead levels obtained closest to the moment of testing.

Hänninen, following the long tradition of factor analysis, attached names to the factors that neuropsychological tests are supposed to measure. Consistently, she and her collaborators in Finland interpreted these results as an indication of the effects of lead on "visual intelligence" and "visuomotor" functions, interpretations that sound somehow awkward for American neuropsychologists. The most important contribution of this study is that, even though no single blood lead level had ever exceeded 70 μg/dL of blood, at that time the Finnish standard for lead, her findings indicated the threshold for impairment to be far below that level.

Valciukas et al. Studies.   The association between lead absorption and performance in the adult at different levels of lead absorption was also studied by Valciukas and Lilis (1982). Four different occupational groups were studied: one reference group (control) and three groups with increasing levels of lead absorption (copper smelter workers, automobile production workers, and secondary lead smelter workers).

Blood lead levels ranged from 33 to 51 μg/dL of blood, whereas zinc protoporphyrin levels ranged from 37 μ/dL of blood in the nonexposed group to 193 μg/dL in secondary lead smelter workers.

The screening battery consisted of the Block Design, Digit Symbol, and Embedded Figures tests described in Chapter 10. It had been reported earlier (Valciukas et al. 1978) that secondary lead smelter workers had significantly lower performance test scores than did nonexposed controls, and the greater the lead absorption—as determined by blood lead levels and zinc protoporphyrin (ZPP) levels— the poorer the performance. The negative

correlation between indicators of lead absorption and performance were not related to age or education, since the effects of those confounding variables were controlled by appropriate statistical techniques. A significant association was found between deterioration of cognitive functions, as detected by performance tests, and increased levels of lead absorption. This association was most evident among secondary lead smelter workers, the occupational group with the highest level of lead exposure and absorption.

Grandjean et al. Study.   Grandjean and collaborators studied the effects of occupational exposure to lead on intelligence and on tests measuring motor performance and memory. The exposed group, consisting of 42 workers exposed to lead, comprised the study group. Thirty-four were employed at two enterprises manufacturing electric storage batteries, two individuals repaired automobile radiators, four were employed at a lead-rolling mill, and two worked in cable manufacturing. Twenty-two workers who processed edible oil and fatty acids in an oil mill comprised the reference group. Blood lead levels in the lead-exposed workers ranged from 12.6 to 88.2 μg/dL of blood (with a mean of 46.2 μg/dL). Hair lead and zinc protoporphyrin levels were also measured.

The psychological test battery consisted of the Wechsler Adult Intelligence Scale (described in Chapter 4) and the following additional tests: visual reproduction (to assess learning and reproduction of visually presented material), word pairs (to assess learning and reproduction of visual and auditory verbal material), graphic continuous performance test (to assess spatial orientation, attention, and maximal span), finger tapping (a measure of motor speed), repetition of a sentence (to assess short-term memory), story recall (to assess attention and short-term memory), and digit learning (to assess concentration and learning of meaningless material).

Significant differences in performance were

found between the two groups of workers, the exposed and the nonexposed group, especially in tests measuring memory, verbal and visuospatial abstraction, and motor speed. Decreased performance in these tests was in most cases associated with elevated levels of lead exposure. Blood lead levels and levels of zinc protoporphyrin correlated better than hair lead. Age and duration of lead exposure were not found to be significant confounding factors.

Longitudinal Studies of Neurotoxically Induced Cognitive Changes

The studies reviewed above are cross-sectional in design, all with the inherent limitations of cross-sectional studies—namely, that all neuropsychological testing was performed only once during the course of the study. More recently, more powerful longitudinal approaches have been directed to the study of the time course of lead neurotoxicity. Two studies illustrate this approach: the work by Mantere and collaborators in Finland and by Baker and collaborators in the United States.

Mantere and collaborators (1982) performed a prospective follow-up study on psychological effects on workers exposed to low levels of lead in a storage battery factory. The study was carried out between 1975 and 1981. Neuropsychological tests included tests of intelligence, memory, visuomotor functions, vigilance, and personality. Tests were administered after 1, 2, and 4 years of work. Of the initial 89 workers, 24 were available for the 1-year, 16 for the 2-year, and 11 for the 4-year reexaminations. The TWA ranged between 14 µg/dL and 46 µg/dL. A reference group was similarly followed. For some of the psychological tests, a learning effect occurred. The learning effect was more evident among the referents than among the lead workers during follow-up.

Among the lead workers, measures of "visual intelligence" and "visuomotor" functions were impaired significantly after 2 years of

follow-up. Although the impairment of the lead workers was rather slight, and the dispersion of the psychological changes wide, it was evident that cognitive functions were affected by lead levels above 30 µg/dL.

Baker and collaborators (1985) evaluated lead exposure and the reversibility of lead neurotoxicity on a group of 160 lead-exposed foundry workers. An unexposed reference group was also followed for 3 years. During this period, neuropsychological tests were administered, and several measures of lead exposure and absorption were obtained. Neuropsychological tests included tests of verbal ability (ie, vocabulary and similarities adapted from the Wechsler Scale of Adult Intelligence, WAIS), memory tests (digit span, digit symbol, paired-associate learning test, immediate and delayed visual reproduction), and visual and motor function test (including the Block Design test, continuous performance test, digit symbol substitute, and the Santa Ana dexterity test), and profile of mood states (POMS).

During the study period (1980–1982), the foundry was required by OSHA to lower blood lead levels progressively at the plant. To comply with this regulation, the company improved its ventilation system, developed a respirator program, monitored work practices, provided work clothing and worker education, and performed other activities to control occupational exposure to lead. As a result of all these activities, blood lead levels fell from a maximum of 80 µg/dL of blood in 1980 to blood lead concentrations no greater than 60 µg/dL of blood in 1981, and in 1982 the highest blood lead levels were 50 µg/dL.

As in the case of Hänninen's studies reviewed above, neuropsychological test scores correlated best with integrative indices of lead exposure. However, zinc protoporphyrin levels correlated less well with tests of cognitive function.

Hänninen (1982) has written an important review on the cognitive effects of occupational exposure to mercury and lead.

Cognitive Alteration and Chronic Occupational Exposure to Solvents

Clinical and epidemiological studies—to be reviewed below—support the view that chronic exposure to organic solvents is associated with a neurological picture called *toxic polyneuropathy,* which is a multiple-targeted neurological disorder in which the peripheral, central, and autonomic nervous systems are jointly or separately affected.

Much of the current knowledge on the clinical and subclinical manifestations of human solvent neurotoxicity has been gathered in Japan, Italy, Finland, Sweden, and, to a lesser extent, Denmark. This body of knowledge is usually—incorrectly—referred to as the "Scandinavian data" or the "Scandinavian experience." Comparatively, very little research on the human health effects of occupational exposure to solvents has been performed in the United States.

What is described below as "clinical observations" are, in most cases, studies of sick people who have been referred to or sought help in a medical unit. This grouping is contrasted with "epidemiological investigations," where public health workers study people at risk where they work, often while performing medical field surveys or health hazards evaluations. However, in many cases the justification for the two contexts is unwarranted. Epidemiological studies, for example, have been performed by inviting people at risk of solvent exposure—but not currently sick—for a thorough clinical evaluation in hospital units. On the other hand some advanced clinical cases are sometimes discovered as a result of a survey.

Solvent Poisoning.   The concept of solvent-induced polyneuropathy has been firmly established. This includes neurological signs and symptoms such as headaches, lightheadedness, lack of balance and coordination, paresthesia, memory problems, increased perspiration, euphoria, and sometimes tachycardia and hot flashes.

The acute effects of solvent exposure should be distinguished from its chronic effects. The acute effects of solvent exposure include short-lived symptoms such as dizziness, headaches, exhilaration, drowsiness, confusion, and disorientation that are time-linked to the presence of solvents in the environment. These symptoms disappear after the worker is removed from the exposure and do not appear during weekends or vacations.

The chronic effects of solvent exposure include persistent symptoms such as fatigue, sleep disturbances, irritability, lack of concentration, memory problems (recent memory), sleep disturbances, and sometimes changes in libido and potency.

The diagnosis of *chronic toxic encephalopathy* is made when:

1. Long-term, high-level organic solvent exposure can be demonstrated
2. A clinical neurological picture is present including one of the following:
   a. paresthesia
   b. impairment of memory
   c. impairment of concentration
   d. changes in mood or emotionality
3. Abnormal results are achieved in at least one of the following:
   a. psychometric tests specifically designed for the assessment of chronic toxic encephalopathies (most currently available batteries are not so designed)
   b. changes in nerve conduction velocities, particularly of lower limbs
4. Other obvious causes, such as chronic alcoholism, head trauma, vascular diseases, degenerative or metabolic conditions, are excluded

Note that there are no clinical chemistries (blood or urine) recommended for the diagnosis of chronic toxic encephalopathy.

Variation in Terminology.   There are large variations in the use of terms to designate the toxic-induced neuropsychological syndrome we have called "chronic toxic encephalopathy" here. In Sweden it is usually called "psychoorganic syndrome." Other authors refer to the syndrome as "toxic polyneuropathy." The term "painter's syndrome" has been proposed but is not generally accepted. For a good discussion of national variations of terminology (in Europe only), the WHO publication *Chronic Effects of Organic Solvents on the Central Nervous System and Diagnostic Criteria*, published in 1985, can be consulted.

In an international conference held in October 1985, the neurological effects of solvents on humans were classified into the following types (World Health Organization 1985):

- In *type I,* the patient complains of non-specific symptoms such as fatigue, poor memory, difficulties in concentration, and loss of initiative. These symptoms are thought to be reversible if exposure is discontinued.
- In *type IIa,* there is a marked and sustained change in personality as shown by fatigue, emotional lability, and lack of control of motivation and impulses.
- In *type IIb,* there are difficulties in concentration, memory impairment, and impairment in the capacity to learn. These symptoms, unlike those in type IIa, can be associated with measurable changes in psychometric tests. The complete reversibility of type IIb is questionable.
- *Type III* is characterized by dementia with pronounced global impairment in intellect and memory and is often accompanied by neurological signs.

Neuropsychological Changes among Shipyard Painters Exposed to Solvents. Valciukas and collaborators (1985) examined painters in three shipyards exposed to a wide variety of solvents. They administered a short battery of neuropsychological tests, a detailed occupational history, and a special questionnaire to assess acute (prenarcotic, transitory) and chronic (persistent) neurological symptoms. The results of their neuropsychological tests demonstrated decrements in central nervous system function in painters when compared with a control group matched for age, gender, race and education. The prevalence of reported acute neurological symptoms among painters was increased significantly compared to other occupational groups in the same shipyards, although for chronic, persistent symptoms the difference was not statistically significant. Neuropsychological test scores were significantly and negatively correlated with chronic symptoms but not with acute symptoms. No significant correlations between neuropsychological test scores and duration of solvent exposure or between symptoms and duration of solvent exposure were observed.

Occupational Exposure to Solvents as a Cause of Accelerated Aging. During the past decade, increasing concern has been expressed about whether occupational exposure to neurotoxic agents accelerates the normal aging of neuropsychological functions. Organic solvents have been placed on the top of the list of suspected causative agents of senile dementia. Chapter 32 is devoted to this topic.

MISINTERPRETATION OF FUNCTIONS AS COGNITIVE

Cognition is a catch-all term that, because of its overuse, is dangerously approaching the point of becoming meaningless. Contemporary research in neuropsychology recommends the diagnosis of "cognitive" dysfunction only when sensory and motor deficits and deficits caused by other factors are satisfactorily ruled out.

The literature of clinical neurotoxicology contains free use of the term "cognition," and in the vast majority of cases, the condition of existing sensory deficits is neither explored nor hinted at. Therefore, the task of reviewing the literature on cognitive effects of occupational and environmental neurotoxic agents is difficult. The fact that the key word "cognition" or "cognitive" is present in the title of a report is simply not enough reason to include it as such.

Dr. Morris B. Bender's major arguments against the use of the term "anomia" are illustrative of this situation. In classical neurology, anomia is described as a cognitive deficit characterized by the inability to "recognize" objects. Anomia has been defined as a percept—something that is perceived—devoid of its meaning. Because people with neurological deficits are unable to recognize fingers, faces, or other features of one's body or of one's immediate surroundings, anomias have been labeled based on the objects that are not recognized—eg, finger agnosia, face agnosia.

Bender used to claim that in his long years of clinical practice, he was unable to find a single person diagnosed as having anomia who did not also have slight and sometimes severe sensory deficits. To be able to bring these sensory dysfunctions to the surface, one obviously needs to know what to look for and to know a large variety of maneuvers, simple tests, or sophisticated ancillary procedures for sensory testing. The Embedded Figures test (described in Chapter 4) was born as a result of this challenge.

Curiously, even after a perceptual deficit such as a visual scotoma, elevated threshold for critical fusion frequency, or deficit in color perception has been thoroughly documented, clinically oriented professionals still use the label "anomia." We have important lessons to learn from the interpretation of anomia as a cognitive deficit. Are the deficits caused by acute or chronic exposure to lead "cognitive"? Yes, but only if primary sensory functions can be demonstrated to be unimpaired.

Often the use of the word cognition is a case of circular reasoning. "Cognitive tests" are those borrowed from IQ testing, such as the Block Design or Digit Symbol. If a person fails a test that claims to assess cognitive functions, then the deficit is "cognitive."

There are numerous reports in the human and animal research literature pointing to primary sensory deficits in vision and oculomotor behavior caused, for example, by lead. What if the person who exhibits a marked decrease in the ability to detect figures in the Embedded Figures test has a reduced ability to perform eye scanning with his or her eyes? Would we still use the term "cognitive" to describe these deficits? Certainly not. In this case, primary sensory deficits are the real explanation for the claimed cognitive deficits. In such cases, the word "cognition" accomplishes no purpose; it is superfluous, confusing, and misleading to describe a deficit this way.

Parsimony in the interpretation of clinical data has far-reaching consequences in rehabilitation programs for people suffering neuropsychological disturbances caused by acute or, most often, chronic neurotoxin exposure. There is an abundance of information on the devastating effects on cognition of early sensory deprivation in the child (eg, deafness resulting from ear infections). Should a primary sensory loss as a result of acute or chronic neurotoxin exposure be demonstrated, the primary objective of the rehabilitation program would be to enhance or compensate for the reduction or distortion of sensory information.

It has been indicated previously (Chapter 4) that there have been essentially two approaches giving psychometric techniques a solid foundation. The first, based on neurological grounds, attempts to give functions descriptive names and sometimes localizes functions in specific areas of the brain. Although this approach has been discredited for a number of years, we are experiencing a new wave of efforts to localize neuropsychological functions in specific sites of the brain. In the second approach, psychometric tests find their foundations in the statistical properties of test scores.

The second approach relies primarily on operational definitions. An operational definition is the specification of rules and procedures that have been used for the collection of data. A significant decrease in Block Design test scores can thus be interpreted as "a significant change in perceptual organization" or not be interpreted at all. Because in the majority of cases little is known about the biochemical and neurophysiological mechanisms underlying acute or toxic neurotoxin exposure, descriptive terms should be favored. The term "cognitive" throughout this chapter cannot be avoided but should be interpreted with caution in view of the above.

REFERENCES

Anderson, JR (1983) *The Architecture of Cognition.* Cambridge, MA: Harvard University Press.

Baker, EL, White, RF, Pothier, LJ, et al. (1985) Occupational lead neurotoxicity: Improvement in behavioural effects after reduction of exposure. *Br J Ind Med* 42:507–516.

Grandjean, P, Arnvig, E, and Beckmann, J (1978) Psychological dysfunctions in lead-exposed workers. *Scand J Work Health* 4:295–303.

Hänninen, H (1982) Behavioral effects of occupational exposure to mercury and lead. *Acta Neurol Scand* 66:167–175.

Hänninen, H, Hernberg, S, Mantere, P, et al. (1978) Psychological performance of subjects with low exposure to lead. *J Occup Med* 20(10):683–689.

Hunt, E (1983) On the nature of intelligence. *Science* 219:141–146.

Kandel, ER and Schwartz, JH (eds) (1985) *Principles of Neural Science,* 2nd ed. New York: Elsevier.

Kaufman AS (1973) Comparison of the WPPSI, Stanford–Binet, and McCarthy scales as predictors of first-grade achievement. *Percept Mot Skills* 36:67–73.

Lezak, MD (1976) *Neuropsychological Assessment.* New York: Oxford University Press.

Mantere, P, Hänninen, H, and Hernberg, S (1982) Subclinical neurotoxic lead effects: Two-year follow-up studies with psychologic test methods. *Neurobehav Toxicol Teratol* 4:725–727.

Mayeux, R and Kandel, ER (1985) Natural language, disorders of language and other localizable disorders of cognitive functioning. In *Principles of Neural Science,* 2nd ed, ER Kandel and JH Schwartz (eds) pp. 688–703. New York: Elsevier.

Needleman, HL, Gunnow, C, Leviton, A, et al. (1970) Deficits in psychologic and classroom performance in children with elevated lead levels. *N Engl J Med* 300(13):689–695.

Needleman, HL, Rabinowitz, M, Leviton, A, et al. (1984) The relationship between prenatal exposure to lead and congenital anomalies. *JAMA* 25(22):2956–2959.

Perino, J and Ernhart, CB (1974) The relation of subclinical lead level to cognitive sensorimotor impairment in black preschoolers. *J Learn Disabil* 7:616–620.

Sternberg, RJ (1985) Human intelligence: The model is the message. *Science* 230:1111–1118.

Valciukas, JA and Lilis, R (1982) A composite index of lead effects: Comparative study of four occupational groups with different levels of lead absorption. *Int J Occup Environ Health* 51:1–14.

Valciukas, JA, Levin, SM, Nicholson, WJ, et al. (1986) Neurobehavioral assessment of Mohawk Indians for subclinical indicators of methyl mercury neurotoxicity. *Arch Environ Health* 41(4):269–272.

Valciukas, JA, Lilis, R, Eisinger, J, et al. (1978) Behavioral indicators of lead neurotoxicity: Results of a clinical field survey. *Int Arch Occup Environ Health* 41:217–236.

Valciukas, JA, Lilis, R, Singer, RM, et al. (1985) Neurobehavioral changes among shipyard painters exposed to solvents. *Arch Environ Health* 40(1):47–52.

World Health Organization (1985) *Organic Solvents and the Central Nervous System.* Copenhagen: WHO.

SUGGESTED READINGS

Arlien-Søborg, P, Bruhn, P, Gyldensted, C, et al. (1979) Chronic painters' syndrome: Chronic toxic encephalopathy in house painters. *Acta Neurol Scand* 60:149–156.

Banks, HA and Stollery, BT (1988) The longitudinal evaluation of verbal reasoning in lead workers. *Sci Total Environ* 71(3):469–476.

Bender, MB (1952) *Disorders in Perception.* Springfield, IL: Charles C Thomas.

Block, NJ and Dworkin, G (eds) (1976) *The IQ Controversy.* New York: Pantheon.

Brim, OG, Glass, DC, Neulinger, J, et al. (1969) *American Beliefs and Attitudes about Intelligence.* New York: Russell Sage Foundation.

Brown, JW (1988) *Classics in Neuropsychology: Agnosia and Apraxia.* Hillsdale, NJ: Lawrence Erlbaum Associates.

Bruyer, R (1986) *The Neuropsychology of Face Perception and Facial Expression.* Hillsdale, NJ: Lawrence Erlbaum Associates.

Campion, J and Latto, R (1985) Apperception agnosia due to carbon monoxide poisoning: An interpretation based on critical band masking from disseminated lesions. *Behav Brain Res* 15(3):227–240.

Chastain, RL, Lehman, WEK, and Joe, GW (1986) Estimated intelligence and long-term outcomes of opioid addicts. *Am J Drug Alcohol Abuse* 12:331–340.

Churchland, PS and Sejnowski, TS (1988) Perspectives on cognitive neuroscience. *Science* 242:741.

Clarck, HH and Clarck, EV (1977) *Psychology and Language.* New York: Harcourt Brace Jovanovitch.

Coltheart, M, Job, R, and Sartori, G (1987) *The Cognitive Psychology of Language.* Hillsdale, NJ: Lawrence Erlbaum Associates.

Critchley, EMR (1987) *Language and Speech Disorders: A Neuropsychological Approach.* Hillsdale, NJ: Lawrence Erlbaum Associates.

Cronbach, LJ (1975) Five decades of public controversy over mental testing. *Am Psychol* 30:1–14.

Crystal, HA, Schaumburg, HH, Grober, E, et al. (1988) Cognitive impairment and sensory loss associated with chronic low-level ethylene oxide exposure. *Neurology (NY)* 38(4):567–569.

DeFranco, C, Tarbox, AR, and McLaughlin, EJ (1985) Cognitive deficits as a function of years of alcohol abuse. *Am J Drug Alcohol Abuse* 11:279–293.

DeVilliers, PA and DeVilliers, JG (1979) *Early Language.* Cambridge, MA: Harvard University Press.

Ellis, AW and Young, AW (1988) *Human Cognitive Neuropsychology.* Hillsdale, NJ: Lawrence Erlbaum Associates.

Feingold, A (1988) Cognitive gender differences are disappearing. *Am Psychol* 43:95–103.

Garth, TR and Smith, OD (1937) The performance of full-blooded Indians on language and non-language intelligence tests. *J Abnorm Soc Psychol* 34:376–381.

Goldberg, E (1989) *Contemporary Neuropsychology and the Legacy of Luria.* Hillsdale, NJ: Lawrence Erlbaum Associates.

Havighurst, RJ and Hilkevitch, RR (1944) The intelligence of Indian children as measured by a performance scale. *J Abnorm Soc Psychol* 39:419–433.

Herrick DJ (1921) A comparison of Brahman and Panchama children in South India with each other and with American children by means of the Goddard form board. *J Appl Psychol* 5:253–260.

Hilton, TL and Berglund, GW (1974) Sex differences in mathematics achievement: A longitudinal study. *J Educ Res* 67:231–237.

Keller, E and Gopnik, M (1987) *Motor and Sensory Processes of Language.* Hillsdale, NJ: Lawrence Erlbaum Associates.

Kineberg, O (1928) An experimental study of speed and other factors in "racial" differences. *Arch Psychol* 15(93):109.

Kyle, JH and Ghani, N (1982) Methylmercury in human hair: A study of a Papua New Guinean population exposed to methylmercury through fish consumption. *Arch Environ Health* 37:266–270.

Liebman, P (1984) *The Biology and Evolution of Language.* Cambridge, MA: Harvard University Press.

Loehlin, JC, Lindzey, G, and Spuhler, JN (1975) *Race Differences in Intelligence.* San Francisco, CA: Freeman.

Mann, CW (1939) A test of general ability in Fiji. *J Genet Psychol* 54:435–454.

McKeon-Eyseen, GE, Ruedy, J, and Neins, A (1983) Methylmercury exposure in northern Quebec. II. Neurologic findings in adults. *Am J Epidemiol* 118:461–469.

Moon, C, Marlowe, M, Stellern, J, et al. (1985) Main and interaction effects of metallic pollutants on cognitive functioning. *J Learn Dis* 18(4):217–221.

Nespoulous, J-L, Perron, P, and Lecaous, AR (1986) *Biological Foundations of Gestures.* Hillsdale, NJ: Lawrence Erlbaum Associates.

Nikki, P, Pfaffli, P, Ahlman, K, et al. (1972) Chronic exposure to anesthetic gases in the operating theatre and recovery room. *Ann Clin Res* 4:266.

Paradis, M (1987) *The Assessment of Bilingual Aphasia.* Hillsdale, NJ: Lawrence Erlbaum Associates.

Piaget, J (1952) *The Origins of Intelligence in Children.* New York: International Universities Press.

Plum, F (1988) *Language, Communication and the Brain.* New York: Raven Press.

Salvini, M, Binaschi, S, and Riva, M (1971) Evaluation of the psychophysiological functions in humans exposed to trichloroethylene. *Br J Ind Med* 28:293–295.

Selikoff, IJ, Hammond, EC, and Levin, SM (1984) *Environmental Contamination and the Health of the People of the St Regis Reserve, Vol II.* New York: Environmental Sciences Laboratory, Mount Sinai Medical School.

Seron, X and DeLoche, G (1989) *Cognitive Approaches in Neuropsychological Rehabilitation.* Hillsdale, NJ: Lawrence Erlbaum Associates.

Sherman, J (1978) *Sex-Related Cognitive Differences.* Springfield, IL: Charles C Thomas.

Smith, PJ (1985) Behavioral toxicology: Evaluating cognitive functions. *Neurobehav Toxicol Teratol* 7(4):345–350.

Snyderman, M and Rothman, S (1987) Survey of expert opinion on intelligence and aptitude testing. *Am Psychol* 42:137–144.

Steward RD, Dodd, HC, Gay, HH, et al. (1970) Experimental human exposure to trichloroethylene. *Arch Environ Health* 20:64–71.

Steward, RD, Fisher, TN, Hosko, MJ, et al. (1972) Experimental human exposure to methylene chloride. *Arch Environ Health* 25:342.

Stiles-Davis, J, Kritchesvsky, M, and Bellugi, U (1987) *Spacial Cognition: Brain Bases and Development.* Hillsdale, NJ: Lawrence Erlbaum Associates.

Takeuchi, T (1977) Neuropathology of Minamata disease in Kumamoto: Especially at the chronic stage. In *Neurotoxicology,* L Roizin, H Shiraki, and N Grevic (eds) pp. 235–246. New York: Raven Press.

Teuber, H-L, and Weinstein, S (1954) Performance on a formboard task after penetrating brain injury. *J Psychol* 38:177–190.

Vocate, DR (1986) *The Theory of Luria: Functions of Spoken Language in the Development of Higher Mental Processes.* Hillsdale, NJ: Lawrence Erlbaum Associates.

Wanner, E and Gleitman, L (1982) *Language and Acquisition: The State of the Art.* Cambridge (England): Cambridge University Press.

Wittig, M and Peterse, AC (eds) (1979) *Sex-Related Differences in Cognitive Functioning.* New York: Academic Press.

31

Personality

Personality is an individual's prevailing, fairly consistent mode of behavior. Personality results from the blending of: genetic and biological factors (our "temperament"); environmental influences resulting from our education and the culture in which we were born; the social pressures that have been and are presently being exerted on us; and our moral judgment of our own behavior and the behavior of others (our "character").

CATEGORIZATION OF PERSONALITY TYPES AND TRAITS

Insights into personality have been provided by literary writers, philosophers, psychologists, sociologists, and educators. As a result, it is difficult to propose a common framework into which all the relevant facets of a personality can be interwoven.

The most basic unit of analysis of personality is the *personality trait*. For clinical purposes, the recording of personality traits in narrative form is an acceptable—even recommended—procedure to describe a personality. However, over 3000 words are found in the English language dictionary that refer to personality characteristics (Allport 1937).

The description of a personality is heavily dependent on a knowledge of language and of a particular culture. Multilingual people often experience frustration in their inability to translate words that are descriptive of personality characteristics from one language to another. Thus, there is something to be gained by the development of universally used "labels" to describe personality or a personality classification system lumping these traits into more manageable and practical concepts. Our dependence upon language to describe aspects of personality makes the translation of most personality inventories and symptom questionnaires very difficult.

The definition of personality types is as old as humankind. The basic concept of "us" and "them" and the promulgation of racial personality stereotypes and personality stereotypes associated with red-haired people, short people, thin and tall people are well known. Don Quixote—the tall, thin man and the dreamer—and Sancho Panza—the short, fat man and the practical man—have been used as prototypes in many typologies emphasizing bodily and basic psychological makeup. Sad to say, historically such typologies have been more successful as a basis for discrimination and hate than as a scientific definition of personality.

Those interested in an historical account

of efforts to define "personality" and the various theories of personalities that have been proposed may consult Cattell (1965), Wiggins et al. (1971), and Gould (1981).

Sources of Information to Assess Personality

Cattell (1973) has argued that there are three sources of information about an individual's personality:

1. Responses to questionnaires in which the subject is at the same time both the observer and the describer of behaviors and feelings. The Minnesota Multiphasic Personality Inventory (MMPI, discussed in Chapter 4) is an example of such a questionnaire. These have been favored in clinical neurotoxicology.
2. The observation of the behavior of an individual in everyday life. An example of this is a student's class behavior evaluated by teachers (as in the study by Needleman on the association between lead in dentine and children's IQ, described in Chapter 20).
3. The observation of the individual's behavior in response to a challenge. An example of this is a situational test in which the subject's reactions are evaluated by placing him or her in a realistic situation—eg, a dinner with prospective professional colleagues. Situational tests are mainly used in the rehabilitation of individuals suffering from substance abuse.

Cattell proposed a classification of personality assessment data on the basis of their sources. Thus, Q-data are based on questionnaires; L-data are generated from the observation of subjects in everyday life; and T-data come from personality tests. This data classification has been extensively used by Cattell and collaborators in their work, but thus far this classification is not well known except by a relatively small circle of psychologists interested in personality research.

Questionnaires are by far the most widely used psychological methods for assessing personality changes produced by absorption of environmental and occupational neurotoxic agents.

Foundations of the Personality Questionnaire

As they apply to E & O neurotoxicology, personality questionnaires range from a collection of questions (eg, questionnaire items suggested by the clinical experience of the test administrator or the investigator) to widely accepted personality tests (eg, personality inventories such as the MMPI and MMPI-R).

Cattell and many personality theorists before him have argued in favor of a personality theory substantiating personality questionnaires. He was a strong advocate of conducting research on personality structure before constructing instruments to assess personality. Almost all the available literature on the effects of neurotoxic agents on personality are based on what Cattell considers the "itemetric approach," ie, personality assessed by a collection of individual personality traits.

However, a strict adherence to theories is not helpful in efforts to understand the effects of a large class of neurotoxic agents on moods and personality. Wiggins and collaborators (1971) have stated that "each of the . . . major viewpoints of personality study involves its own distinctive methods, procedures, and assumptions. It should also be apparent that each viewpoint imposes 'methodological blinders' on the study of man by purposely ignoring certain aspects of behavior and focussing on others."

In addition, it is not as yet clear whether personality changes observed as a result of neurotoxic action are statistical deviants of normal behavior or new disease processes.

The few investigators who have been attracted by the problems of environmental and occupational neurotoxic agents and personality have been overwhelmed by practical considerations regarding monitoring and prevention of neurotoxic illness at the workplace. As a rule, the field lacks documented speculation on the subject. Per force, analogies—not always valid—are drawn from experiences in psychopathology, neuropsychology, and the treatment of patients suffering from alcohol or drug abuse.

Use of Personality Inventories in Epidemiological Studies

Standardized and well-regarded personality inventories such as the MMPI or MMPI-R designed for use in the clinic are ill-suited for the documentation of personality disorders in an epidemiological/toxicological setting. Investigators rely on short inventories or symptoms questionnaires to document these changes.

It has been reported that the MMPI is included in the protocol of the study on the potential health effects associated with Agent Orange, a herbicide used during the Vietnam war; however, as of Fall 1990, no reports have become available to the public.

Need for Professional Training in the Interpretation of Personality Inventories or Symptoms Questionnaires. Data obtained from personality inventories and symptoms questionnaires need to be interpreted. The interpretation (literally, what the results mean) is a professional judgment requiring training and experience. The following examples illustrate the confounders encountered by professionals who are consulted on whether a link between paranoid behavior and chemical exposure may exist:

- A slight degree of paranoia is expected in people from neighborhoods close to a

chemical dump; a degree of concern is understandable.

- Paranoia is part of a personality disorder that may be induced by neurotoxic agents at the workplace (eg, carbon disulfide).
- Paranoia is a well-known personality trait that develops among abusers of cocaine, particularly the smokable form known as crack cocaine.
- Jealousy, very frequently found among paranoids, is known to occur in advanced stages of alcoholism and in other types of organic personality disorders.

The professional needs to make a judgment between alternatives such as: Is it a normal concern, caused by chemical exposure or drug abuse, an alcohol-related disorder, or the expression of a paranoid personality? Trained professionals are increasingly being called upon as witnesses to establish whether a link between patterns of occupational toxic exposure and neurobehavioral changes can be established with reasonable certainty. The section (later in this chapter) entitled "Psychotic Disorders and Personality Disorders" provides a brief review of the major neuropsychiatric disorders that neurologists, psychiatrists and psychologists must consider in establishing differential diagnoses of personality disorders.

Theories of Personality Derived from Clinical Observations

Early literature in personality has been dominated by clinical observations. The psychoanalytic theory has been the most influential. Its founders—Janet (1859–1947), Charcot (1825–1893), Freud (1856–1939), Jung (1875–1961), and McDougall (1871–1938)—were ". . . practicing physicians whose daily practice demanded a rationale and a set of procedures for coping with the psychological problems presented by their patients. The circumstances of 19th-century psychiatric practice gave rise to a kind of theorizing distinctively different from that of the academic psychology of the day" (Wiggins et al. 1971). The main thrust of psychoanalysis is the study of motivational forces that underlie behavior and as such it has had little influence on clinical neurotoxicology or neuroepidemiology research.

Among the most salient characteristics that distinguish clinically oriented personality theories from other psychological theories are the concerns with practical (medical) problems, concerns with causes of behavior, treatment of patients, and the integration of diverse findings (Hall and Lindzey 1970). These sets of theories have not been taken into serious consideration by investigators in the field of E & O neurotoxicology.

Factor-Analytical Theories of Personality

Research on personality theory has been dominated by factor analysis. The essentials of factor analysis are reviewed in Chapter 19. Thus far, the most significant work has been performed in Finland by Hänninen and Lindström. Briefly, these studies have aimed at demonstrating that control groups and groups occupationally exposed to neurotoxic agents have basic differences in personality. The point of these studies is that these differences are caused by neurotoxin exposure. This approach has not been favored in the United States.

It is important to observe that highly regarded instruments for personality assessment such as the MMPI-R are not based on any given personality theory or technique such as factor analysis, although factor-analytical studies have been extensively performed.

Wiggins and collaborators (1971) is an excellent, although dated, source for a detailed discussion of several personality theories. Edwards (1970) is a good source for the statistical concepts associated with the measurement of personality traits by scales and inventories.

Biological Determinants of Personality

In looking into the matter of how and to what extent personality is controlled by biological factors, there are profound contradictions that need to be confronted. On the one hand, the thought that personality—our individual or characteristic manner of behaving and thinking—is determined by biological factors is disconcerting. We think of ourselves as free individuals making free choices.

However, the thought that the way we behave might be determined by physical characteristics is embedded in many cultures. In looking into the possible truth of biological determinism (or scientific racism), scientists and scholars have many times "substantiated" the prejudices of their times—biological factors, for example, were named as explanations for the superiority of one race over others. The deep wounds that scientific racism created explain in part why scholars have stayed away from serious research into the matter of biological determinism.

The continuation of old research—such as the scientific study of identical twins reared apart—and the discovery of striking genetic characteristics of certain neurological diseases—such as Huntington's chorea, a disease affecting body movement—are creating a new interest in biological markers of personality. To us, these markers are important because they probably provide the link explaining why neurotoxic agents in the environment and the workplace produce changes in habitual modes of behavior.

Biological determinants of personality—determinants that are all interwoven—belong to four large groups: genetic, hormonal, neural, and pharmacological.

Genetic determinants shape our physique and also our behavior. The fact that one is born either male or female is an expression of a genetic process; many physical attributes are inherited following known laws of genetics, such the inheritance of eye color or the texture of our hair. Our physical attributes both potentiate and limit the range of our possible behavior at the same time. As seen in Chapter 20, chemical compounds can interfere with the genetic plan for organ formation and tissue development.

But behavior itself is determined in part by genetic factors. This is remarkably demonstrated in large-scale studies of psychological characteristics of identical twins reared apart. Identical twins develop from a single fertilized egg and are thus genetically identical. When identical twins are reared apart—sometimes in different cultures and speaking different languages—scientists have an unusual opportunity to study and separate the environmental from the genetic components of behavior. Studies of identical twins are remarkable in revealing psychological characteristics not usually thought of as genetic. For example, two identical twins who have never seen each other come to the first meeting wearing the same type of mustaches, wire-rimmed glasses, having the same taste in food, and enjoying an idiosyncratic sense of humor.

Our behavior is also created or modulated by **hormonal determinants**. Mental retardation can be created as a result of insufficient secretion of thyroid hormone in early childhood; hyperthyroidism can result in anxiety, tension, and hyperalertness.

The **neural determinants** of behavior can be recognized in affective and character traits that are anatomically localizable. Language, for example, involves motor, auditory, and emotionally expressive factors. Damage to the right temporal area causes disturbances in comprehension of the emotional aspects of the language, whereas damage to the left hemisphere leads to a deficit in expressing the emotional aspects of language. Kandel (1985) reviewed some examples of such localizations and discussed how and why the pendulum of scientific opinion has swing for and against these localizations.

Additional evidence for the neural determination of personality trait disorders comes from the study of epileptics and people who suffer panic attacks. Some people afflicted by a variety of epilepsy whose source is fairly well localized in the temporal lobe, for example, experience déjà vu (the sensation of having been in a place or situation before), transient visual and auditory hallucinations, feelings of depersonalization (seeing himself or herself as a separate individual), fear, anger, and sometimes paranoid ideation. Panic attacks can sometimes be traced to alterations in the temporal lobe. By using positron emission tomography (an imaging technique described in Chapter 6), it has been possible to demonstrate that some patients who have panic attacks also show a circumscribed abnormality in blood flow to the right parahippocampal gyrus.

The discovery of **pharmacological determinants** of behavior has revolutionized the manner in which certain mental disorders—thought to be "psychogenic" or "functional"—are viewed and treated. For example, the use (or abuse) of illicit drugs such as PCP ("angel dust") or hallucinogenic mushrooms has long been known to affect personality and even lead to temporary psychosis. The discovery of anxiolytic agents (literally meaning agents that "dissolve" anxiety) has stimulated research into the pharmacological basis of affects and other components thought to be characteristics of the personality of an individual. Some severe forms of depression can be treated by means of lithium therapy or other drugs.

PSYCHOTIC DISORDERS AND PERSONALITY DISORDERS

The *Diagnostic and Statistical Manual of Mental Disorders* (DSM-III-R) is published by the American Psychiatric Association (1987). The manual, developed and revised since 1952 by a group of advisory committees, provides a classification and coding system for mental disorders.

A group of professionals—psychiatrists, psychologists, psychiatric nurses, and forensic personnel—uses this document as a basis for diagnosis of major mental disorders and for the assessment of rehabilitation potential and treatment of affected individuals. A detailed review of this important source is beyond the scope of this chapter, but an examination of certain basic concepts for the assessment of mental disorders is essential. Unless otherwise noted, all definitions under this heading are from the DSM-III-R.

Mental Disorders, Neurosis, and Psychosis

A *mental disorder* is conceptualized as a clinically significant behavioral or psychological syndrome or pattern that occurs in an individual and that is typically associated with a painful symptom (distress) or impairment in one or more important areas of functioning (disability). In addition, there is an implication that there is a behavioral, psychological, or biological dysfunction and that this disturbance is not only in the relationship between the individual and society but also in the relationship of the individual with himself or herself. Organic mental disorders, schizophrenia, and paranoid disorders are all examples of mental disorders. (Note that the DSM-III-R does not accept the concept of mental "illness.")

A mental disorder does not classify an individual. For this reason, the manual recommends refraining from using such statements as "the schizophrenic" or "the alcoholic." In writing reports, health professionals are trained to use expressions such as "Mr. John Doe suffers from schizophrenia," or "he is afflicted by chronic alcoholism."

A *neurotic disorder* is a mental disorder in which the predominant disturbance is a symptom that is distressing to the individual and is recognized by him or her as unacceptable and alien, but reality testing (see below) is fairly intact. The disturbance may be enduring or recurrent, but there is no de-

monstrable organic etiology or factor. Examples of neurotic disorders are many psychosexual disorders and adjustment and personality disorders.

Psychosis is a term indicating a gross impairment in reality testing; ie, the individual incorrectly evaluates the accuracy of his or her perceptions and thoughts and makes incorrect inferences about external reality, even in the face of contrary evidence.

Psychotic Behavior in Chronic Alcoholism. People who suffer from chronic alcoholism may develop severe personality changes caused by the direct neurotoxic effects of alcohol, by effects of sudden alcohol withdrawal, or by malnutrition. For example, chronic alcoholism sufferers who suddenly stop drinking may develop visual and auditory hallucinations. Alcohol-related hallucinations usually start several hours after the onset of tremulousness, also characteristic of alcohol withdrawal. In certain cases of advanced alcoholism, the person may react appropriately to the hallucinations (eg, the individual may be terrorized by the crawling bugs on the wall and in bed and desperately try to kill them).

A paranoid personality may be established; paranoid behavior may persist even when the individual is not drinking. One of the most common emotions is jealousy. For example, while walking with one's spouse on the street, the sufferer of an alcohol-related mental disorder may interpret the spouse's most innocent acts—such as fixing his or her attire, combing his or her hair, or looking anyplace—as an attempt to establish contact with someone. These episodes of jealousy are sometimes increased by the sexual impotency that sufferers from chronic alcoholism sometimes suffer.

Schizophrenic Disorders

Schizophrenia is a term used for a group of disorders probably of different etiologies. The diagnostic criteria for schizophrenic disorders are:

1.   At least one of the following during a phase of the disorder:

a)   Bizarre delusions (content is patently absurd and has no possible basis in fact), such as delusions of being controlled, thought broadcasting (the idea that one's thoughts are heard by others through loudspeakers), thought insertion (the idea that people are inserting ideas in the affected individual's head), or thought withdrawal (the thought that ideas are being stolen away from the affected individual's head).

b)   Somatic, grandiose, religious, nihilistic, or other delusions without persecutory or jealous content.

c)   Delusions with persecutory or jealous content if accompanied by hallucinations of any type.

d)   Auditory hallucinations in which either a voice keeps a running commentary on the individual's behavior or thoughts or two or more voices converse with each other.

e)   Auditory hallucinations on several occasions with content of more than one or two words, having no apparent relation to depression or elation.

f)   Incoherence, making loose associations, markedly illogical thinking, or a marked poverty of contents of speech associated with at least one of the following: blunt, flat, or inappropriate affect; delusions or hallucinations; or catatonic or other grossly disorganized behavior. (Catatonic behavior is a marked motor anomaly frequently found among sufferers of psychotic disorders; in catatonic waxy flexibility, the person's limbs can be "molded" into any position, which is then maintained.)

2.   Deterioration from a previous level of functioning in such areas as work, social relations, and self-care.

3.   Continuous signs of the illness for at least six months at some time during the person's life, with some signs of illness at present.

The DSM-III-R cites additional criteria including prodromal (preclinical) and residual characteristics of this mental disorder.

Paranoid Disorders

The essential feature of *paranoid disorder* is a persistent persecutory delusion or delusional jealousy not caused by any mental disorder such as schizophrenia, affective disorder, or organic mental syndrome. A paranoid persecutory delusion is a false personal belief in which the affected person himself or herself is seen as being attacked, harassed, cheated, persecuted, or conspired against. A delusional jealousy is the belief that one's sexual partner is unfaithful. Interesting to us is the frequent belief that the "persecuting" person tries to poison water or food.

People affected by paranoid disorders have none of the incoherence of those affected by schizophrenia. Thus, environmental poisoning can be easily incorporated into a persecutory delusion; an intelligent individual can use sophisticated and persuasive language to describe the details of how the poisoning is being done.

The diagnostic criteria for paranoid disorder are:

1.   Persistent persecutory delusions or delusional jealousy.
2.   Emotions and behavior appropriate to the content of the delusional system.
3.   Duration of the illness for at least a week.
4.   None of the symptoms of criterion 1 that serve to identify schizophrenia, such as bizarre delusions, incoherence, or marked loosening of associations.
5.   No prominent hallucinations.

The DSM-III-R gives additional criteria and finer categories of paranoid disorders.

Personality Disorders

A *personality disorder* is the presence of inflexible or maladaptive personality traits that result in subjective distress or significant impairment of the afflicted individual in social or occupational functioning. A personality disorder is seen as a benign form of more serious mental disorders such as schizophrenia or paranoid disorders. A personality disorder can also be seen in the prodromal and residual phases of serious mental illness.

Numerous variations have been recognized. In children and adolescents, personality disorders include schizoid disorder of childhood or adolescence, avoidance disorder of childhood or adolescence, conduct disorder, oppositional disorder, and identity disorder. In the adult, personality disorders include schizoid or paranoid personality disorder, avoidance personality disorder, antisocial personality disorder, passive–aggressive personality disorder, and borderline personality disorder. The DSM-III-R contains diagnostic criteria for each of these disorders.

Adjustment Disorders

The main feature of *adjustment disorder* (AD) is a maladaptive reaction to a recognizable psychosocial stressor, such as death of a parent or spouse, occurring up to 3 months after the onset of the stressor. The maladaptive nature of the disorder is shown by an impairment in social or occupational functioning and by symptoms that are in excess of a normal and expected reaction to the stressor. Somatic symptoms such as headaches, fatigue, etc may be encountered as well. The disturbance does not meet the criteria for uncomplicated bereavement.

There are many types of adjustment disorders. Those recognized in the DSM-III-R include AD with depressive mood (sometimes called reactive depression), AD with anxious mood, AD with mixed emotional features, AD with disturbance of conduct, AD with work (or academic) inhibition, AD with withdrawal, and AD with atypical features.

Adjustment disorders also occur after catastrophic environmental events such as floods, earthquakes, explosions, plane accidents, random terrorist attacks, etc. Differential diagnosis between adjustment disorders and true neurotoxicological illness is particularly difficult in those instances when neuropsychological signs and symptoms occur after environmental disasters or occupational accidents—with or without loss of life—in which neurotoxic agents are involved. It is unfortunate that this important subject has not received the attention it deserves.

Adjustment disorders are observed following such negative life events as a death in the family (particularly death of a spouse), a mortgage foreclosure, death of a pet, or being fired from work and after positive life events such as a promotion at work or unexpected money gain. Current research on psychosocial stress indicates the importance of the degree of perceived control (ie, whether the individual can do anything to initiate or terminate the event) and various sources of support (ie, whether someone is available to console the sufferer) on the degree of stress. In the past two decades important literature has been accumulating on the role of psychosocial stress on immunologic changes. For a representative bibliography on stressful life events and their contexts, see Dohrenwend and Dohrenwend (1984).

EFFECTS OF NEUROTOXIC EXPOSURE ON PERSONALITY

Delayed Neurotoxicity and Personality Changes

Delayed neurotoxicity is the belated appearance of neurological and psychiatric symptoms after an acute episode of neurotoxic exposure, symptoms appearing 1 to 3 weeks after the exposure. Originally described in carbon monoxide poisoning, delayed neurotoxicity has now been described for other neurotoxic agents, notably organophosphate pesticides.

Many personality changes may be associated with the delayed appearance of symptoms. For example, for carbon monoxide poisoning, sudden disorientation, confusion, excitement, and restlessness or apathy may characterize the initial phases of the syndrome. In more advanced stages, profound alterations of behavior, including psychosis, might be observed.

Dose–Response Relationships between Lead Absorption and Subjective Symptoms

Differences in subjective symptoms between neurotoxin-exposed and control groups have been shown in various studies. Lilis et al. (1977a,b) reported that subjective symptoms such as headaches, irritability, and memory and sleep problems are prevalent among secondary lead smelter workers in proportion to lead dose.

Dose–response relationships between biological indicators of lead exposure and absorption and subjective symptoms have been reported. Hänninen et al. (1979), for example, found that when subjective symptoms of workers whose blood lead levels never exceeded 70 μg/dL of blood were compared to those of controls, there was an excess of almost all symptoms. When intergroup comparisons were made between a group having less than 50 μg/dL of blood lead and another having more than 50 μg/dL of blood lead, there was a dose–response relationship between biological levels of lead exposure and subjective symptoms.

More recently Fischbein et al. (1982) and Lilis et al. (1985) have shown that lead-related symptoms show higher correlations with zinc protoporphyrin (ZPP), a biological indicator of lead effects, than with blood lead levels.

Personality Changes and Occupational Solvent Exposure

There are very few clinical studies specifically designed to assess the effects of neurotoxic agents on personality. Linz et al. (1986) studied industrial painters for solvent-induced encephalopathy. Fifteen industrial painters underwent a complete medical examination and neuropsychological evaluation. The latter included the Revised Wechsler Adult Intelligence Scales (WAIS-R), measures of visual and memory functions, the Halstead–Reitan neuropsychology test battery, an aphasia-screening test, and the Minnesota Multiphasic Personality Inventory (MMPI). All these have been reviewed in Chapter 4 (dealing with psychometric techniques).

Painters as a group demonstrated clinically significant elevations (mean tests score greater than 70) on MMPI scales measuring somatization, depression, hysteria, anxiety, and schizoid tendencies. Psychiatric interviews failed to indicate a primary major psychiatric illness and supported the view that personality changes were caused by acute organic solvent intoxication. Psychiatric evaluations also emphasized the devastating effects of memory alterations and personality changes on the family and work life of painters, even when deficits were relatively mild or subtle. However, the authors do not tell whether test administrators and psychiatrists knew the occupational status of the workers exposed to solvents. In the best of circumstances, it is often difficult or impossible to avoid knowing the patient's occupational status during testing or interviews.

ISSUES RELATED TO PERSONALITY ASSESSMENT

Attitudes Toward the Environment

Sometimes, attitudes toward the local environment and the workplace and toward those who conduct health research testing cannot be easily separated from the effects of neurotoxic agents on basic personality traits. Attitudes should not be considered merely as prejudices of study subjects because it is not fully known whether or not absorption of neurotoxic agents is the cause of a change of attitude toward the environment.

Since the mid-1960s, there have been numerous studies of personal attitudes toward the environment inspired by environmental and ecological branches of psychology and human factor engineering (known in Europe as *ergonomics*). These studies are important if one is able to maintain the focus of research on the effects of neurotoxic agents on behavior. It was only in the mid-1980s that neurotoxicologists and social psychologists made an effort to join forces.

Anastasi (1982) provides a good introduction to the subject. In addition, a special issue of the journal *Environmental Research* (Bornschein and Rabinowitz 1985) contains various references to socioeconomic cofactors in neurotoxicology assessment. However, the research focuses on cognitive defects in children exposed to lead.

Malingering

We live in an increasingly litigious society. After environmental disasters and occupational accidents occur (by many, no longer considered acts of fate), people who are deemed responsible are sought and sometimes charged with criminal intent. In some cases, factory owners where workers have died or become disabled as a result of occupational exposure to toxic agents have been sent to prison for criminal behavior.

However, most commonly, rather than putting the blame on the employer, malingering is suspected among the victims of environmental and occupational hazards at a given site. Victims may attempt to seek compensation for resulting illness. Thus, when individuals are examined who might benefit from the presence of a sign, symptom, or

subaverage result in physiological and neuropsychological tests, malingering is often suspected. In addition, such individuals may, at times, try to manipulate the very decision process of ascertainment of toxic causation. In cases where a worker sues his or her employer, these signs, symptoms, test results, and the link between symptoms and exposure are vital to a successful legal case.

The *Diagnostic and Statistical Manual of Mental Disorders,* revised edition (DSM-III-R), defines *malingering* as the "intentional production of false or grossly exaggerated physical or psychological symptoms, motivated by external incentives such as . . . avoiding work, obtaining financial compensation, evading criminal prosecution, obtaining drugs, or securing better living conditions."

There are no clear rules for detecting and/or preventing malingering or minimizing its occurrence. Experienced forensic professionals follow procedures similar to those of scientists in not claiming an association between neuropsychological changes and neurotoxic exposure until this association is proven. (In legal terminology, a "preponderance of evidence" is needed in ruling civil cases; the criterion of "beyond reasonable doubt" prevails in criminal cases.) For the professional, the link needs to be demonstrated following detective work and in a logical manner. However, with so little known in the field of clinical neurotoxicology of occupational and environmental toxic agents, a rigid scientific attitude toward people being examined for suspected exposure is not recommended.

Malingering needs to be differentiated from many other conditions (such as hysteria) that can produce an impression that signs and symptoms are under the subject's control. In Chapter 34 the topic of working conditions leading to mass illness will be examined.

Malingering is hard to detect even by the most experienced professionals. The DSM-III-R states that malingering should be strongly suspected if any combination of the following is noted:

- Signs and symptoms of disorders are presented in a medicolegal context; eg, the afflicted person is being referred by his or her attorney.
- There is a marked discrepancy between the person's claimed distress and disability and the result of objective methods (eg, psychometric, electrophysiological testing).
- There is a lack of cooperation during the diagnostic evaluation and lack of complying with prescribed treatments if any.
- Antisocial personality disorder (a diagnostic category in the DSM-III-R) is present.

Many professionals who work in forensic disciplines allied to the occupational and environmental health sciences—forensic psychiatry, forensic psychology—have proposed their own detection methods. The following is an expansion of one developed by Resnick (1984) in the context of forensic psychiatry in which the defendant has something to gain if found "mentally incompetent." A brief critique of such attempts follows.

The person who is malingering often shows an overreaction to being "mentally sick." By subtle or sometimes not-so-subtle means, often very early in the evaluation, the defendant tries to make sure that it is understood that he or she is a "very sick person."

The person suspected of malingering often shows eagerness to call attention to his or her illness. If one tries to follow a questionnaire in which questions are scheduled to be asked in order, one often finds that the individual soon manages to tell a lot of what he or she wants to relate but is unable to follow the planned order of questions.

He or she often shows inconsistencies in responses and behavior. There are personality tests, such as the MMPI-2, that contain specially designed scales to show when the subject is inconsistent. Some of these inconsistencies are best detected by several different people in different contexts. An individual may volunteer cocaine/crack abuse at the time of the environmental incidents to a "sympathetic" interviewer and later vehemently deny its use to someone who appears threatening. The inconsistencies are detected when all the information from several individuals collecting the data, independently of one another, is put together.

He or she may be able to imitate the content but not the form of a mental disorder. Trained professionals pay attention not only to the things defendants say but the manner in which the ideas are communicated. An alert clinician may be able to detect that a 15-year-old has suffered a stroke even if he or she has never suspected that he has suffered a cerebrovascular accident. (As a rule, a stroke is unlikely to be clinically linked to an environmental and occupational exposure except in the case of chronic toxin-induced elevation of blood pressure.)

Symptoms often do not fit a known diagnostic entity, or fit "too well." Occasionally, people who are examined in an occupational health clinic or who are involved in environmental disasters bring newspaper clippings—and even papers published in the scientific literature—with descriptions of signs or symptoms derived from exposure to given neurotoxic compounds (eg, solvents, pesticides, dioxins). The afflicted individual brings the information, sometimes with the totally honest belief that the examining professional may not be aware of the symptoms of the disease, in order to show that he or she perfectly fits what is described in the literature.

Unless the subject is a trained health professional himself or herself—which is very possible, for instance, in the evaluation of occupational exposure to anesthetic gases among surgeons and other professionals in hospitals—defendants often are not aware of, or pay little attention to, the clinical significance of the time course of signs and symptoms. Sudden onset of illness is a common complaint among people who malinger, whereas experts know that the complaints are known to take several weeks, months, or even years to develop.

Inconsistency may exist between mental symptoms (what they say they feel) and behavior (what they do). However, sometimes this inconsistency is not a sign of malingering—workers sometimes need to suppress their signs and symptoms of illness in order to keep their jobs.

People who malinger may tell far-fetched stories to fit their needs. In addition, they may show contradictions in accounts of their stories; this is the reason why the evaluative session of individuals suspected of being malingerers needs to be especially long— "exhaustive" and "exhausting"—to allow the interviewer to recognize these contradictions and self-serving versions of environmental and occupational toxic exposures.

The net implication is that the malingerer is blameless within the framework of the feigned illness; often "others" are responsible for "symptoms" of disease; alternatives—often very plausible alternatives— are selectively ignored.

Malingerers often engage in delaying tactics to buy time to think of the "right answer" to the question. Sometimes, people who malinger give vague answers to specific questions, repeat the question just asked, and delay the answers to some questions. After giving answers of low informational content, the malingerer would carefully study the reporter's minute reactions and then selectively add additional comments, also of very low information content.

At times, an individual appears to attempt to "please" the interviewer or to create a favorable impression of himself or herself. At other times, the defendant will try to express interest about the professional background of the interviewer (eg, "If you would just listen to what I am telling you, you may be on the threshold of making the most remarkable discovery of this decade").

Malingering should be suspected in a criminal defendant's pleading mental disorder if a partner (or a large group of individuals) is involved in the litigation (this topic is further developed in Chapter 34).

Malingerers are likely to have nonpsychotic alternative motives for their behavior; in contrast, signs and symptoms without motive may add credence to the presence of mental illness (as in the case of someone who is called to testify but who did not originally complain or file suit against a company).

Signs and symptoms that individuals who malinger **do not** show should also be suspected:

It is rare for malingerers to show signs of perseveration, a sign one often encounters in mental and neuropsychological impairment.

Malingerers are unlikely to show "negative symptoms" of a serious mental illness, such as blunted affect or total indifference to the surroundings. On the contrary, signs and symptoms of anxiety are prevalent among malingerers.

It is rare for malingerers to complain of hallucinations, possibly on grounds that if one experiences them one is "crazy" to start with. Hallucinations, when they occur, are often reported by relatives and friends based on a subject's odd behavior. However, when convenient, malingerers who have suffered hallucinations in the past may malinger hallucinations.

Malingerers almost never describe themselves as "delusional"; people and events are "really" after them. (From the clinical point of view, the belief that someone or something is poisoning them is common among people affected by delusions. A sufferer from a delusional disorder is sometimes able to convince a number of people that his complaints have substance.)

Malingerers often have studied, or have close relatives or friends who have studied, psychology, psychiatry, or mental or environmental health. They are often the children, spouses, companions, or close friends of psychologists, psychiatrists, or journalists. (The dangers of such "profiling" are discussed below.)

There has been little research on the subject of malingering as applied to the occupational and environmental health sciences. Some opinions as to when a subject is likely to be malingering are based on the technique called *profiling*. For example, statistics may show that minorities who drive beat-up cars are likely to carry drugs through the Lincoln Tunnel into New York City. It would thus appear to "make sense" to search for drugs among minorities driving beat-up cars. Similarly, experience shows that mass psychogenic illness often involves young women— particularly young girls—who show a close bond amongst themselves and who share the collective perception of a common source of threat. Thus, it would appear "logical" that a reported health hazard among young women is most likely caused by mass psychogenic illness.

But "common sense" and "logic" are often the substrate for stereotyping and prejudice. Unfortunately, we know that prejudice often exists among the best-informed people. Thus, it is unwarranted to conclude that people who show what expert professionals say are signs and symptoms of malingering are in fact malingerers. Stereotyping and profiling, no matter how scientifically founded, may in many cases be just plain wrong and in some others may violate individuals' rights.

Subjective Responses as Scientific Data

Introspection is the "looking into oneself." In human health studies on the effects of neurotoxic agents on personality, the wealth and quality of the clinical or epidemiological information rest on the individual's capacity to introspect. When the professional asks the interviewee "How would you say you have been feeling for the past month?", the subject has to direct his or her attention to a reservoir of memories and experiences and respond "in a nutshell" (eg, "In good spirits, most of the time").

Subjective symptoms are still poorly regarded in E & O neurotoxicology. "Subjective" data are often equated with "unreliable," and are thus something that cannot be trusted in any serious study on the prevalence or causes of illness.

Sometimes the interviewer attempts to circumvent the very person he or she is trying to examine in search of the truth. Psychoanalysis, for example, analyzes dreams, looking for unfulfilled needs; polygraphy relies on the questionable premise that neurophysiological processes, such as changes in the electrical conductance of the skin, blood flow, heart rate, and breathing rate reveal what the individual does not want to tell.

However, subjective phenomena have had a fairly good standing in many scientific disciplines intimately related to E & O neurotoxicology, such as pharmacology and the social sciences. For example, quantitative study of pain—a subjective phenomenon—is essential in the development of pain killers. Beecher (1959), summarizing work on pain performed since the middle 1940s, concluded that subjective responses and symptoms could be expressed in quantitative forms through the use of rating scales.

As seen in Chapter 25 while discussing psychophysical methods, S. S. Stevens was able to develop laws linking subjective phenomena—such as the perception of loudness, brightness, roughness, viscosity, etc—with physical properties of sensory stimuli. Stevens' power law describes in quantitative terms the relationships between the intensity of stimulus and the magnitude of our impressions.

These findings are significant for prevention because reports of subjective symptoms often serve as warnings (or "sentinel events") of real neurotoxic effects. Should lead-related symptoms and elevated ZPP be found to be increased in a group exposed to lead, symptoms cannot be dismissed as "soft" data or data that could be easily tampered with. Workers cannot create a dose–response relationship. Those trends are discovered by investigators in laboratories where symptoms are compared with biological indicators of neurotoxic absorption.

Group differences in subjective symptoms reported by workers exposed to solvents are a consistent finding in the literature (Cherry and Waldron 1983; Valciukas et al. 1985). However, the vast majority of studies fail to demonstrate a dose–response relationship between exposures and symptoms. Since the questionnaires used to study the effects of lead toxicity are very similar to those in the study of solvents, it cannot be concluded that the questionnaires used are inadequate tools, or that the use of subjective symptom descriptions is too unreliable. Most human studies on the chronic effects of long-term, low-level exposure to solvents have failed because of the great difficulties in quantifying exposures rather than in quantifying subjective changes.

Studies of the Effects of Neurotoxic Agents on Personality Are Often Mislabeled

If one is to follow the criterion that one should label a study as a "personality study" only when a standardized personality inventory is used, most clinical studies containing the key word "personality" in the title would be mislabeled. In most cases, a neurological or psychiatric questionnaire of signs and symptoms has been used. Sometimes a semistructured psychiatric interview is added to the research protocol.

Following this criterion, up to the present time there have been no large-scale epidemiological studies on the effects of neurotoxic agents on personality. A long-advertised study on the effect of Agent Orange on thousands of Vietnam veterans, which is said to contain the MMPI in the research protocol mentioned above, is yet to be published.

REFERENCES

Allport, GW (1937) *Personality: A Psychological Interpretation.* New York: Holt, Rinehart, and Winston.

American Psychiatry Association (1987) *Diagnostic and Statistical Manual of Mental Disorders,* 3rd ed, revised. Washington, DC: APA.

Anastasi, A (1982) *Psychological Testing,* 5th ed. New York: Macmillan.

Beecher, HK (1959) *Measuring of Subjective Responses: Quantitative Effects of Drugs.* New York: New York University Press.

Bornschein, RL and Rabinowitz, MB (1985) The Second International Conference on Prospectives Studies of Lead, Cincinnati, Ohio April 9–14, 1984. *Environ Res* 38(1):1–210.

Cattell, RB (1965) *The Scientific Analysis of Personality.* Chicago: Aldine Publishing Co.

Cattell, RB (1973) *Personality and Mood Questionnaire: A Handbook of Interpretative Theory, Psychometrics, and Practical Procedures.* San Francisco: Jossey–Bass.

Cherry, N and Waldron, HA (1983) *The Neuropsychological Effects of Solvent Exposure.* Havant: Colt Foundation.

Dohrenwend, BS and Dohrenwend, BP (1984) *Stressful Life Events and Their Contexts.* New Brunswick, NJ: Rutgers University Press.

Edwards, AL (1970) *The Measurement of Personality Traits by Scales and Inventories.* New York: Holt, Rinehart, and Winston.

Fischbein, A, Thornton, JC, Sarkosi, L, et al. (1982) Subjective symptoms in workers with low level exposure to lead. *J Appl Toxicol* 2(6):289–293.

Gould, SJ (1981) *The Mismeasure of Man,* New York: WW Norton.

Hall, CS and Lindzey, G (1970) *Theories of Personality,* 2nd ed. New York: John Wiley & Sons.

Hänninen, H, Mantere, P, Hernberg, S, et al. (1979) Subjective symptoms in low-level exposure to lead. *Neurotoxicology* 1:333–347.

Kandel, ER (1985) Brain and behavior. In *Principles of Neural Science,* 2nd ed, ER Kandel and JH Schwartz (eds) pp. 3–12. New York: Elsevier.

Lilis, R, Fischbein, A, Diamond, S, et al. (1977a) Lead effects among secondary lead smelter workers with blood lead levels below 80 μg/100 mL. *Arch Environ Health* 32:256–266.

Lilis, R, Fischbein, A, Eisinger, J, et al. (1977b) Prevalence of lead diseases among secondary lead smelter workers and biological indicators of exposure. *Environ Res* 14:255–285.

Lilis, R, Valciukas, JA, Malkin, J, et al. (1985) Effects of low-level lead and arsenic exposure on copper smelter workers. *Arch Environ Health* 40(1):38–47.

Linz, DH, De Garmo, P, Morton, WE, et al. (1986)

Organic solvent-induced encephalopathy. *J Occup Med* 28(2):119–129.

Resnick, PJ (1984) The detection of malingered mental illness. *Behav Sci Law* 2(1):21–38.

Valciukas, JA, Lilis, R, Singer, RM, et al. (1985) Neurobehavioral changes among shipyard painters exposed to solvents. *Arch Environ Health* 40(1):47–52.

Wiggins, JS, Renner, KE, Clore, GL, et al. (1971) *The Psychology of Personality*. Reading, MA: Addison-Wesley.

SUGGESTED READINGS

Anderson, SC (1981) Alcoholic women: Personality traits during adolescence. *Am J Drug Alcohol Abuse* 8:239–247.

Angleitner, A and Wiggins, JS (1986) *Personality Assessment Via Questionnaire: Current Issues in Theory and Measurement*. New York: Springer-Verlag.

Axelson, O, Hane, M, and Hogsteadt, C (1976) A case-referent study on neuropsychiatric disorders among workers exposed to solvents. *Scand J Work Environ Health* 2:14–20.

Baelum, J, Andersen, I, and Mølhave, L (1982) Acute and subacute symptoms among workers in the printing industry. *Br J Ind Med* 39:70–75.

Barnes, JM (1961) Psychiatric sequelae of chronic exposure to organophosphorus insecticides. *Lancet* 2:102.

Biking, MS and Bieber, I (1949) DDT poisoning—a new syndrome with neuropsychiatric manifestations. *Am J Psychother* 3:261.

Biskind, M and Mobbs, RF (1972) Psychiatric manifestations from insecticide exposure. *JAMA* 220:1248.

Bistrup, PL (1961) Psychiatric sequelae of chronic exposure to organophosphorus insecticides. *Lancet* 2:103.

Braceland, FJ (1942) Mental symptoms following carbon disulfide absorption and intoxication. *Ann Intern Med* 16:246–261.

Brieger, H (1972) Chronic carbon disulfide poisoning. *J Occup Med* 14:123–124.

Broad, W (1981) Sir Isaac Newton: Mad as a hatter. *Science* 213:1341–1344.

Brown, GG and Nixon, RK (1979) Exposure to polybrominated biphenyls: Some effects on personality and cognitive functioning. *JAMA* 242:423–526.

Butcher, JN and Tellegen, A (1978) Common methodological problems in MMPI research. *J Consult Clin Psychol* 46:620–628.

Chandra, SV (1983) Psychiatric illness due to manganese poisoning. *Acta Psychiatr Scand* 67:49–54.

Cherry, N, Hutching, H, and Waldron, HA (1985) Neurobehavioral effects of repeated occupational exposure to toluene and paint solvents. *Br J Ind Med* 42:291–300.

Dager, SR, Holland, JP, Cowley, DS, et al. (1987) Panic disorder precipitated by exposure to organic solvents in the work place. *Am J Psychiatry* 144(8):1056–1058.

Dohrenwend, BP and Dohrenwend, BS (1969) *Social Status and Psychological Disorder: A Causal Inquiry*. New York: John Wiley & Sons.

Eløfsson, S-A, Gamberale, F, Hindmarsh, T, et al. (1980) Exposure to organic solvents: A cross-sectional epidemiological investigation on occupationally exposed car and industrial spray painters with special reference to the nervous system. *Scand J Work Environ Health* 6:239–273.

Eysenck, HJ (1982) *Personality, Genetics and Behavior*. New York: Praeger.

Eysenck, H and Eysenck, S (1964) *Manual of the Eysenck Personality Inventory*. London: University of London Press.

Feshbach, S and Weiner, B (1986) *Personality*, 2nd ed. Lexington, MA: Health.

Forzi, M, Cassito, MG, Gilioli, R, et al. (1976) Persönlichkeitsfehlentwicklungen in Arbeitern bei der elektrolytischen Chlor-Alkali-Gewinnung. In *Proceedings of the 2nd Industrial and Environmental Neurology Congress*, E Klimkova-Deutschova and E Lukás (eds) pp. 79–82. Prague: Universita Karlova.

Gershon, S and Shaw, FB (1961) Psychiatric sequelae of chronic exposure to organophosphorus insecticides. *Lancet* 1:1371.

Giannini, AJ and Castellani, S (1982) A manic-like psychosis due to khat (*Catha edulis Forsk*). *J Toxicol* 19(5):455–459.

Goldbloom, D and Chouinard, G (1985) Schizophrenic psychosis associated with chronic industrial toluene exposure: Case report. *J Clin Psychiatry* 46(8):350–351.

Green, LM (1987) Suicide and exposure to phenoxy acid herbicides. *Scand J Work Environ Health* 13(5):460.

Guildford, JP (1954) *Psychometric Methods*. New York: McGraw-Hill.

Hall, CS and Lindzey, G (1985) *Introduction to Theories of Personality*. New York: John Wiley & Sons.

Hall, W and MacPhee, D (1985) Do Vietnam veterans suffer from toxic neurasthenia? *Aust NZ J Psychiatry* 19(1):19–29.

Hänninen, H (1971) Psychological picture of manifest and latent carbon disulphide poisoning. *Br J Int Med* 28:374–381.

Harkönen, H (1977) Relationships of symptoms to occupational styrene exposure and to the findings of electroencephalographic and psychological examinations. *Int Arch Occup Environ Health* 40:231–239.

Harvey, PD and Walker, E (1987) *Positive and Negative*

Symptoms in Psychosis: Description, Research and Future Directions. Hillsdale, NJ: Lawrence Erlbaum Associates.

Hogstedt, C, Hane, M, Agrell, A, et al. (1983) Neuropsychological test results and symptoms among workers with well-defined long-term exposure to lead. Br J Ind Med 40:99–105.

Holden, C (1986) Researchers grapple with problems of updating classic psychologic test. Science 233:1249–1251.

Husman, K (1980) Symptoms of car painters with long-term exposure to a mixture of organic solvents. Scand J Work Env Health 6:33–39.

Iregren, A (1986) Subjective and objective signs of organic solvent toxicity among occupationally exposed workers. Scand J Work Environ Health 12(5):469–475.

Kirby, H, Nielson, CJ, Nielson, VK, et al. (1983) Subjective symptoms after long-term exposure in secondary lead smelting workers. Br J Ind Med 4:314–317.

Lachar, D (1983) The MMPI: Clinical Assessment and Automatic Interpretation. Los Angeles: Western Psychological Services.

Lanyon, RU and Goodstein, LD (1982) Personality Assessment, 2nd ed. New York: John Wiley & Sons.

Levenson, H, Glenn, N, and Hirschfeld, ML (1988) Duration of chronic pain and the Minnesota Multiphasic Personality Inventory: Profiles of industrially injured workers. J Occup Med 30(1):809–812.

Levin, HS (1976) Anxiety associated with exposure to organophosphorus compounds. Arch Gen Psychiatry 33:225–228.

Levy, CJ (1988) Agent Orange exposure and posttraumatic stress disorder. J Nerv Ment Dis 176(4):242–245.

Lewey, FH (1941) Neurological, medical, and biochemical signs and symptoms indicating industrial carbon disulfide absorption. Ann Intern Med 15:869–883.

Lieben, J and Williams, RA (1974) Five years of experience with carbon disulfide. In Behavorial Toxicology: Early Detection of Occupational Hazards, C Xintaras, BL Johnson, and I DeGroot (eds) pp. 60–63. Washington DC: US Department of Health, Education and Welfare, Public Health Service, Centers for Disease Control, NIOSH.

Lilis, E (1974) Behavioral effects of occupational carbon disulfide exposure. In Behavioral Toxicology: Early Detection of Occupational Hazards, C Xintaras, BL Johnson, and I DeGroot (eds) pp. 51–59. Washington DC: US Department of Health, Education and Welfare, Public Health Service, Centers for Disease Control, NIOSH.

Lindström, K, Harkonen, H, and Hernberg, S (1976) Disturbances in psychological functions of workers occupationally exposed to styrene. Scand J Work Environ Health 3:129–139.

López-Ibor, JJ (1987) Social reinsertation after catastrophes: The toxic oil syndrome experience. Eur J Psychiatry 1(1):12–19.

López-Ibor, JJ, Soria, J, Cañas, F, et al. (1985) Psychopathological aspects of the toxic oil syndrome catastrophe. Br J Psychiatry 147:352–365.

Maddi, R (1989) Personality Theories: A Comparative Analysis, Pacific Grove, CA: Brooks/Cole.

Olsens, J and Sabroe, S (1980) A case-referent study of neuropsychiatric disorders among workers exposed to solvents in the Danish wood and furniture industry. Scand J Soc Med [Supp] 16:44–49.

Ørbæk, P and Nise, G (1989) Neurasthenic complaints and psychometric function of toluene-exposed rotogravure printers. Am J Ind Med 16:67–77.

Ryckman, RM (1985) Theories of Personality, 3rd ed. Monterey, CA: Brooks/Cole.

Sakurai, H, Sugita, M, and Tsuchiya, K (1974) Biological response and subjective symptoms in low level lead exposure. Arch Environ Health 29:157–163.

Savage, EP, Keefe, TJ, Mounce, LM, et al. (1988) Chronic neurological sequelae of acute organophosphate pesticide poisoning. Arch Environ Health 43(1):38–45.

Spigelberg, U (1961) Psychopathologisch-neurologische Schaden nach Einwirkung synthetischer Giftem Wehdients und Gesundheit, Vol III. Darmastaedt: Wehr und Wissen Verlagsgesellshaft.

Stevens, SS (1975) Psychophysics: Introduction to its Perceptual, Neural and Social Prospects. New York: John Wiley & Sons.

Stoller, A, Krupinski, J, Christophers, AJ, et al. (1965) Organophosphorus insecticides and major mental illness. Lancet 1:1387.

Tola, S and Norman, CH (1977) Failure to find excessive symptoms in the general population and in workers exposed to lead. Int Arch Occup Environ Health 40:153–162.

Turner, CF and Martin, E (1984) Surveying Subjective Phenomena, Vols 1 and 2. New York: Russel Sage Foundation.

Vigliani, EC (1954) Carbon disulfide poisoning in viscose rayon factories. Br J Ind Med 11:235–244.

Vigliani, EC (1961) Erkrangungen durch schwefelkohlenstoff. In Handbuch der gesamten Arbeitmedizin, EW Baader (ed) II pp. 313–325. Berlin: Urban and Scharzenberg.

Warheit, GH, Holzer, CF, and Arey, SA (1975) Race and mental illness: An epidemiologic update. J Health Soc Behav 16:243–256.

Part VI

Confounders and Current Issues

32

The Question of Senile Dementia

In the late 1970s, a growing number of reports—particularly from Finland, Sweden, and Denmark—indicated that workers occupationally exposed to organic solvents were at risk of developing polyneuropathy. By the middle 1980s, some investigators proposed that occupational exposure to solvents may also induce senile dementia (WHO 1985). However, Americans who deal with problems of aging have defined senile dementia as a condition in which other etiological factors, such as exposure to toxic agents, are ruled out. A heated debate has resulted. This chapter reviews the highlights of this ongoing controversy.

DEFINITIONS OF AGING

We need to differentiate between chronological age (ie, the age the calendar says we are) and functional age (ie, the age indicated by the appearance and performance of our various physiological systems). Chronological age is not a predictor of functional age. Indeed, not everyone ages at the same rate or in the same manner: at age 30, and even younger, some people have white hair; some people lose motor coordination in their forties but remain intellectually active; some people are

bed-ridden in nursing homes while still in their sixties; some musicians, such as Pablo Casals or Arthur Rubinstein, kept busy performance schedules well into advanced age; a lady in her nineties jogs in Central Park in New York City.

The examples above illustrate a key question in gerontological research: Why is there a mismatch between chronological and functional age, and which one is the best indicator of aging? Functional indicators of aging that have been proposed in large epidemiological studies include changes in the genetic composition of cells, the capacity of the immune system to fight diseases, sensory loss, and decreasing levels of performance and capacity to adapt to social change. Taking these measures one at a time or in composite indices—ie, combining several promising measures at one time—one may question how good these measures are for predicting chronological age. Despite the immense effort to identify markers of aging, the results of large epidemiological studies are frustrating. Some suggest that when supposed objective markers are pitted against chronological age, by far the most practical measure is chronological age (Costa and McCrae 1980).

The argument in favor of the use of chronological age as a marker is compelling.

Granted, nobody should be forced to retire because he or she is 65. But how fair is it to take graying of the hair or the breadth of the ear lobe as a criterion of functional age? In addition, not all jobs require identical skills: our swimming abilities reach their peak in the late teens and go downhill after that, but our verbal abilities remain unchanged and, depending on our criteria, may even improve throughout life.

What has thwarted many scientific efforts in the search for objective indicators of aging is the preconceived idea that aging is a single process. Yet we know it is not. Efforts to create some magic index similar to IQ (itself under fire) between chronological and functional age have failed time and again.

BIOLOGICAL MECHANISMS OF AGING

Is aging an inexorable biological process, or are there factors that contribute to early aging? If so, what are the important factors? The search for possible mechanisms to explain aging has been accelerated in recent years for two main reasons: (1) because of improved health care, the population of the United States is getting older and "by the year 2020, the percentage of people over 65 is expected to nearly double from 11% to 20%" (Mount Sinai Medical Center 1985); and (2) dementia, particularly Alzheimer's disease, has reached epidemic proportions.

Why should one discuss Alzheimer's disease in the context of biological mechanisms of aging? It is not yet clear whether dementia is an exacerbated condition of an essentially normal mechanism—ie, the manifestation of a built-in biological clock—or is caused by external factors such as the food we eat, the exercises we perform, or a slow-acting virus.

Possible Etiological Factors for Aging

Scientists have proposed several conceptual models for aging and dementia: genetic, ab-

normal protein generation, abnormal blood flow, changes in the biochemical properties of neurotransmittors in the brain, infectious agents, toxic agents, and other theories abound. A brief review of some of these models is appropriate before considering the possibility that dementia may be caused by chronic environmental or occupational exposure to neurotoxic agents.

Genetic Causation.   Certain families have a very high rate of longevity with little mental deterioration, whereas in others the incidence of Alzheimer's disease is disproportionately high. The possibility that what is labeled "genetic" is in fact the sharing of common environmental factors—eg, rural living or nutritional habits—cannot be ruled out, however. Abnormalities in the genetic material in the cells of the aged are highly suspected. Inability of DNA to code for normal proteins, which in turn may affect neurotransmission between neurons, has been reported. Chromosomal aberrations have been proposed as cytogenetic markers of aging.

Abnormal Protein Generation.   When Alzheimer first described the disease that now bears his name in 1907, he observed that the neural tissue exhibited a characteristic neurofibrillar appearance. He also observed that a substance—later known to be a protein—wrapped around cerebral blood vessels, replacing degenerating nerve terminals. The hypothesis is that this abnormal generation of proteins leads to the formation of neural plaques, which in turns causes severe intellectual impairment. This hypothesis seems to be supported by the common observation that in postmortem examination of the brains of affected individuals, the more numerous the neural plaques, the more profound the mental deterioration while the individual was alive.

Poor Blood Circulation.   "Bad circulation" and "hardening of arteries" have been popular explanations of why mental capacity declines with age. It has been postulated that people suffering from Alzheimer's disease suffer from a marked reduction in blood flow. Thus, the brain may lose its ability to receive adequate oxygen and glucose from blood, both of which are vital to normal brain functioning. Today, the hypothesis of brain atherosclerosis has few supporters. But it is possible that numerous subclinical strokes may lead to dementia, for example, in those who are occupationally exposed to head trauma, such as boxers.

The Biochemical Hypothesis. Spontaneous or environmentally induced biochemical disturbances in neural transmission have been thought to be very plausible causative factors in senile dementia. The hippocampus and the cerebral cortex of patients suffering from Alzheimer's disease show markedly reduced levels of the enzyme choline acetyltransferase (CAT). It is speculated that some of the profound memory disturbances and cognitive deficits seen in this disease are the results of biochemical alterations in acetylcholine-mediated neurotransmission.

Slow-Acting Viruses. Viruses are known to be causative agents in many progressively debilitating and fatal diseases such as Creutz-feld-Jakob's and AIDS (acquired immune deficiency syndrome). It has been found that 25% of all AIDS cases develop neurological problems including dementia. Certain degenerative diseases such as Creutzfeld-Jakob's may be caused by *prions,* infectious agents that lack RNA or DNA (unlike viruses, which usually contain either RNA or DNA).

Alterations in the Immune System. Some investigators have proposed changes in cells generated by the thymus gland (T cells) and bone-marrow-generated cells (B cells) as biological markers of aging. The viral and the immunologic hypotheses may be related, since the AIDS virus, for example, may cause dementia and destroys the body's immunologic system.

Lathyrism. Excessive consumption of chick pea or vetch (*Lathyrus sativus*) and related

species is associated with a nonprogressive, irreversible neurological disease called *lathyrism.* Paralysis of the lower limbs occurs in both genders and at all ages, but it seems more prevalent among young males. It is one of the oldest neurotoxic diseases known to humans and once was prevalent in Europe, northern Africa, the Middle East, and parts of the Far East. Now it is restricted to India, Bangladesh, and Ethiopia. The disease tends to develop in times of flood or drought when other crops are ruined or become unavailable; at those times, the hearty plant *Lathyrus* becomes the major dietary staple. The causative agent is suspected to be β-(N)-oxalyl-amino-L-alanine (BOAA). Spencer and Schaumburg (1983) have written a comprehensive article on the subject.

Aging As an Example of Abiotrophic Processes

In the mid 1980s comprehensive hypotheses were proposed for common mechanisms underlying several neurodegenerative diseases. Calne et al. (1986), for example, has proposed the hypothesis that "... Alzheimer's disease, Parkinson's disease, and motorneuron disease are (all) due to environmental damage to specific regions of the central nervous system. ... The damage remains subclinical for several decades and makes those affected specially prone to the consequences of age-related neuronal attrition."

The authors of this hypothesis argue that several neurodegenerative diseases may be initiated by environmental factors: for example, parkinsonism, poliovirus infection, and postpolyomyelitic syndrome by the presence of methylphenyltetrahydropyrine; lathyrism by chick pea ingestion; and pugilist's encephalopathy by physical trauma. Each of these neurodegenerative diseases may be an expression of *abiotrophy,* a selective, premature decay of a functionally related population of neurons. It is speculated that abiotrophic disorders were not recognized earlier because before the 20th century few people reached 50 years of age.

THE HYPOTHESIS THAT AGING MAY BE TOXICALLY INDUCED

The Difficulty of Testing Neurotoxic Hypotheses of Accelerated Aging

The hypothesis that occupational neurotoxic agents may accelerate aging is hardly new. Dr. Alice Hamilton observed early in this century that lead workers looked twice their age. Dr. Irving J. Selikoff, one of the leaders of occupational medicine in our time, made a similar observation in describing patients who were occupationally exposed to solvents. Thus far, the hypothesis that chronic, low-level occupational or environmental exposure to neurotoxic agents may accelerate functional aging has never been postulated in a manner that could be adequately tested in epidemiological studies. However, the idea has been postulated time and time again. There are many methodological problems that make it difficult to design an appropriate study— namely, adequate epidemiological design, the availability of cohorts, the quantitative definition of long-term exposure and absorption of neurotoxic agents, and matters of statistical analysis of data.

Decline in neuropsychological functioning with normal aging may be an artifact of epidemiological study design. Aging of psychological functioning—the backbone of the definition of senile dementia—is very much in question. Most of us have been led to believe that our mental abilities diminish as we grow older. However, scientific observations do not seem to support this contention. When data are obtained in cross-sectional studies, older individuals will tend to have been less educated than younger ones. "Age differences in education are inevitable if a test standardization sample is to be truly representative of the population of [a given] country at the time the norms are established" (Anastasi

1982). The apparent decline of psychological functions in cross-sectional studies may then be a methodological artifact: cultural and experiential effects are confounded with aging.

Longitudinal studies in which individuals are tested at regular time intervals for many years and therefore act as their own controls tell a much different story. Fundamental psychological functions such as "understanding of verbal meaning" actually show an increase with chronological age in longitudinal studies. Identical functions when tested in cross-sectional studies show a decline. Anastasi (1982) concludes that ". . . the results of the better-designed studies of adult intelligence strongly suggest that the ability decrement formerly attributed to aging is predominantly due to intergeneration or intercohort differences, probably associated with cultural changes in our society. Genuine ability decrements are not likely to be manifested until well over the age of 60." Anastasi, an authority in the field of psychological testing, believes that what counts are the changes in performance that occur with age. Many people, of course, do experience a decline in intellectual abilities and performance with age. But in proportions that are still unknown, some others show no changes. These facts do not fit our prejudices.

All the reports claiming an association between environmental or occupational exposure and early aging to this date have been cross-sectional studies. For a prospective study, a cohort that is occupationally exposed to neurotoxic agents and can be observed for a number of years needs to be identified and examined. The identification of people who are exposed to neurotoxic agents such as solvents at the workplace is difficult because such exposures are not likely to be known outside the premises in which they occur. In addition, chronic exposure to neurotoxic agents often occurs in small shops with a rapid turnover rate. Affected individuals may leave their jobs, and the subjects who are available for study might not be the most appropriate to study.

In order to claim that an occupational neurotoxic agent is the causative factor of dementia, long-term exposure to such an agent needs to be thoroughly documented. For example, quantitative assessment of environmental exposure to solvents in every job where painters are exposed to solvents in paints is a formidable task. In the United States, the cooperation of management in such assessment is the exception more than the rule. Sometimes, in order to define "personal dose," diaries documenting paint use need to be kept; from these diaries, industrial hygienists need to identify the chemical composition of paints used in every case. In Chapter 16 additional factors of solvent exposures that need to be accounted for—such as methods of paint application (eg, brushing, rolling, or spraying), and use of protective equipment—were reviewed.

There are aspects of statistical analysis of data that need to be considered. The analysis of data claiming an association between solvent dose and chronic neuropsychological function is performed with a "repeated-measures design," a data-analytical technique in which each subject is his or her own control. Some of the models require complete availability of all measures for all subjects at all points in time in which subjects were studied, requirements that are sometimes difficult to meet. In certain branches of the social sciences, rules regarding the "filling in" of missing values are accepted, whereas in occupational health research they are frowned on.

Judging from the few examples reviewed below, it is clear that most of these important considerations in study design and data analysis have not been applied in well-known studies.

Chronic Toxic Encephalopathies in Solvent-Exposed Workers

Several case reports and epidemiological studies seem to indicate that professional painters with long-term occupational exposure to solvents may develop toxic encephalopathy characterized by headaches, dizziness, memory impairment, fatigue, and personality changes. Some of these studies have stimulated heated debates between defenders and detractors at meetings devoted to the review of the neurotoxicology of solvents. The following are examples of the studies that have often been quoted to support the notion that occupational exposure to solvents may cause senile dementia.

The Chronic Painter's Syndrome. Arlien-Søborg et al. (1979) published a study of 70 house painters referred to a clinic because organic solvent intoxication or dementia was suspected. In 50 of these cases, no competitive etiological factors to the cerebral symptoms other than exposure to organic solvents could be ascertained. In neuropsychological examinations, 39 patients showed signs of intellectual impairment. Neuroradiological examination by fractional pneumoencephalography (PEG) and cranial computerized tomography (CT) demonstrated the presence of cerebral atrophy in 31 patients. Further, 38 patients studied with CT were compared to an age-matched control group with regard to the width of cerebral foldings, and a significant difference was found.

The conclusion of this study was that long-term exposure to turpentine substitutes—often accompanied by a period of acute symptoms of intoxication—may gradually lead to the development of a chronic brain syndrome, which the authors call "chronic painter's syndrome." The existence of such a syndrome has been widely debated in the literature.

Occupational Exposure to Solvents in Recipients of Pension Funds. The contention that chronic occupational exposure to solvents, particularly among painters, leads to premature signs of aging, has been made in several epidemiological studies in Sweden, Denmark, Finland, and Great Britain. The study designs are similar. Cases and referents (controls) were selected from employment pension funds providing disability pensions.

Lindström (1981, 1982) for example, sought to answer the question of whether there was a positive history of solvent exposure among all male construction workers in Finland who had been granted a disability pension because of certain neuropsychiatric disorders during the period 1978 to 1980. The principal psychiatric diagnoses excluded were "primary debility," schizophrenia, and mental diseases caused by extraneous factors such as encephalitis, traumatic disorders, etc. Diseases were classified according to the eighth revision of the *International Classification of Diseases* (ICD-VIII). The cases and the referents were matched in pairs with regard to the time of pensioning and age at the time of the study within a range of 2 years. The mean age of all subjects was 49.1 years. The study showed that solvent exposure increased the risk of being prematurely pensioned due to toxic encephalopathy.

In 1976, Axelson and collaborators performed a case–referent study of data from a regional Swedish pension fund register. They found a risk ratio of 1.8 for nonspecific neuropsychiatric disorders among workers such as painters, varnishers, and carpetlayers who were exposed to solvents as compared with workers not so exposed. Moreover, a dose–response relationship was noted between exposure, defined as years of occupational exposure to solvents, and eligibility for disability pensions.

Rasmussen and collaborators (1985) published a report on the risk of encephalopathy among retired solvent-exposed workers who applied for nursing home accommodations in Denmark. The study was carried out in the city of Odense (population 170,000), located on the island of Funen. In this city, about 1800 persons a year apply for supportive facilities in addition to the ones provided by health care centers. This additional support is provided—among others—in the form of home helpers or home nurses. All persons applying are admitted to the local geriatric hospital ward, where the allocation of nursing homes is made. The investigation was conducted as a case–control study among all males less than 81 years of age who were admitted to this geriatric ward to obtain these additional supportive facilities from 1981 through 1983.

The study group included 767 males, of whom 229 had a diagnosis of dementia or other kinds of encephalopathy. Control subjects were selected from the remaining group. The main diagnoses for controls were ischemic heart disease, chronic bronchitis, and lung cancer. Questionnaire and telephone interviews sought information about the longest-held occupation, about occupations with known risk of solvent exposure held for more than 5 years, and about alcohol consumption.

In the words of the authors:

> [The] results of this study are neither conclusively positive nor negative. The workers formerly exposed to solvents have an increased risk ratio [of developing encephalopathy later in life] which is on the borderline of being statistically significant. . . . However, the authors believe that the findings do, to some degree, support the hypothesis that exposure to organic solvents increases the risk of chronic encephalopathy. They think the study strengthens the evidence of a link between solvent exposure and permanent brain disorders. (Rasmussen et al. 1985)

Cherry and Waldron (1984) failed to replicate these findings in their study performed in Great Britain. They used data originally collected between 1970 and 1976 as part of a morbidity study in general practice. They estimated the prevalence of minor neuropsychiatric illness among workers exposed to organic solvents. No differences were found between the rates of consultations for mental illness in any solvent-exposed group, either male of female. Nor was any difference found in the prevalence of mental illness between workers exposed to solvents and nonexposed referents when data from two smaller studies were examined.

Aluminum as a Possible Etiological Factor of Aging

Aluminum has also been suspected to be a causative agent for senile dementia. People who require aluminum-rich dialysis for kidney ailments have been shown to have elevated aluminum levels in the brain, followed by senile dementia. But the explanation for these findings is not clear. The presence of aluminum in the brain may be an artifact. Once the neurofibrils characteristic of Alzheimer's disease are formed, they may have an affinity for aluminum. It has also been stated that aluminum by itself may not be the cause of the disease but may facilitate the effects of other causative factors. Today, the toxic hypothesis applied to aluminum has few supporters. The hypothesis itself suffers from a common aberration in science: the theory has been stated and rejected with very little experimentation.

CONCLUSIONS

The hypothesis of a possible role of environmental or occupational neurotoxic agents in producing senile dementia is presently clouded by an unproductive controversy over diagnostic terminology and interpretation. Is a documented reduction in cognitive function and performance (ie, dementia) produced by an exogenous factor such as solvents? How much of a reduction must one observe to be able to use the term? Are neurotoxically induced dementia and senile dementia two expressions of a common underlying phenomenon or not?

It is the sentiment of many that the United States is at least a decade behind other developed countries—particularly the Scandinavian nations—in the study of changes in cognitive functions and performance caused by chronic low-level exposure to neurotoxic agents at the workplace. But the "facts" that have been brought up as "proof" that occupational exposure to toxic agents may cause a permanent impairment in neuropsychological functions are both insufficient and inadequate.

REFERENCES

Alzheimer, A (1907) Über eine eigenartige Erkrankung der Hirninde. *Allg Z Psychiatrie* 64:146–148.

Anastasi, A (1982) *Psychological Testing,* 5th ed. New York: Macmillan.

Arlien-Søborg, P, Bruhn, P, Gyldensted, C, et al. (1979) Chronic painter's syndrome: Chronic toxic encephalopathy in house painters. *Acta Neurol Scand* 60:149–156.

Axelson, O, Hane, M, and Hogstedt, C (1976) A case-referent study on neuropsychiatric disorders amongst workers exposed to solvents. *Scand J Work Environ Health* 2:14–20.

Calne, DB, Geer, EM, Eisen, A, et al. (1986) Hypothesis Alzheimer's disease, Parkinson's disease, and motoneurone disease: Abiotropic interaction between ageing and environment? *Lancet* 2:1067–1070.

Cherry, N and Waldron, HA (1984) The prevalence of psychiatric morbidity in solvent workers in Britain. *Int J Epidemiol* 13(2):197–200.

Costa, PT and McCrae, RR (1980) Functional age: A conceptual and empirical critique. In *Proceedings of the 2nd Conference on the Epidemiology of Aging,* SG Haynes and M Feinleib (eds) pp. 23–50. Washington, DC: US Department of Health and Human Sciences, NIH Publication No. 80-969.

Lindström, K (1981) Behavioral changes after long-term exposure to organic solvents and their mixtures. *Scand J Work Environ Health* 7(Supp 4):48–53.

Lindström, K (1982) Behavioral effects of long-term exposure to organic solvents. *Acta Neurol Scand* 92:131–141.

Mount Sinai Medical Center (1985) *Newsletter of the Gerald and Mary Ellen Riter Department of Geriatrics and Adult Development, Vol 2, No. 3.* New York: Mount Sinai Medical Center.

Rasmussen, H, Olsen, J, and Lauritsen, J (1985) Risk of encephalopathia among retired solvent-exposed workers: A case-control study among males applying for nursing home accommodation or other types of social support facilities. *J Occup Med* 27:561–566.

Spencer, PS and Schaumburg, HH (1983) Lathyrism: A neurotoxic disease. *Neurobehav Toxicol Teratol* 5:625–629.

World Health Organization (1985) *Organic Solvents and the Central Nervous System.* Copenhagen: WHO.

SUGGESTED READINGS

Baker, SR and Rogul, M (1985) *Environmental Toxicity and the Aging Process.* New York: Alan R Liss.

Bayley, N and Oden, M (1955) The maintenance of intellectual ability in gifted adults. *J Gerontol* 10:91–107.

Birren, JE and Schaie, KW (eds) (1985) *Handbook of the Psychology of Aging.* New York: Van Nostrand Reinhold.

Blessed, G, Tomlinson, BE, and Roth, M (1968) The association between quantitative measurements of dementia and of senile changes in the cerebral gray matter of elderly subjects. *Br J Psychiatry* 114:797–811.

Bollerup, TR (1985) Prevalence of mental illness among 70-year olds domiciled in nine Copenhagen suburbs: The Glostrup survey. *Acta Psychiatr Scand* 51:327–339.

Bolton, N, Britton, PG, and Savage, RD (1966) Some normative data on the WAIS and its indices in an aged population. *J Clin Psychol* 22:184–188.

Botwinick, J and Storandt, M (1974) *Memory, Related Functions and Age.* Springfield, IL: Charles C Thomas.

Brody, JA (1982) An epidemiologist views senile dementia: Facts and fragments. *Am J Epidemiol* 115(2):155–162.

Brody, JA and Kurland, LT (1973) Amyotrophic lateral sclerosis and Parkinsonism–dementia in Guam. In *Tropical Neurology,* J Spillane (ed) pp. 355–375. London: Oxford University Press.

Brooks, Br, Jubett, B, Swartz, JR, et al. (1979) Slow viral infections. *Annu Rev Neurosci* 2:309–340.

Brown, P, Cathala, F, and Gaddusek, DC (1979) Creutzfeldt–Jakob disease in France: III. Epidemiological study of 170 patients dying during the decade 1968–1977. *Ann Neurol* 6:438–446.

Butler, RN (1975) *Why Survive? Being Old in America.* New York: Harper & Row.

Chokroverty, S, Breutman, ME, Berger, V, et al. (1976) Progressive dialytic dementia. *J Neurol Neurosurg Psychiatry* 39:411–419.

Chong, JP, Turpie, I, Haines, T, et al. (1989) Concordance of occupational and environmental exposure information elicited from patients with Alzheimer's disease and surrogate respondents. *Am J Ind Med* 15:73–89.

Clarfield (1988) The reversible dementias: Do they reverse? *Ann Intern Med* 109:476–486.

Cliff, J, Martelli, A, Molin, A, et al. (1984) Mantakassa: An epidemic of spastic paraparesis associated with chronic cyanide intoxication in a cassave staple area of Mozambique. I. Epidemiology and clinical and laboratory findings in patients. *Bull WHO* 62:477–484.

Cohn, NB, Dustman, RE, and Bradford, DC (1984) Age-related decrements in Stroop Color Test performance. *J Clin Psychol* 40:1244–1250.

Corsellis, J (1962) *Mental Illness and the Ageing Brain.* London: Oxford University Press.

Crapper, DR, Krishnan, SS, and Quittkat, S (1976) Aluminum, neurofibrillary degeneration and Alzheimer's disease. *Brain* 88:67–80.

Crook, TH and Miller, NE (1985) The challenge of Alzheimer's disease. *Am Psychol* 40:1245–1250.

Daniels, N (1988) *Am I My Parents' Keeper?* New York: Oxford University Press.

Dirken, JM (1972) *Functional Age of Industrial Workers.* Groningen, The Netherlands: Wolters-Noordhoff.

Dolezal, J, Perkins, ES, and Wallace, RB (1989) Sunlight, skin sensitivity and senile cataract. *Am J Epidemiol* 129(3):559–568.

Eaton, WW and Kessler, LG (1981) Rates of symptoms of depression in a national sample. *Am J Epidemiol* 114(4):528–638.

Fillerbaum, G, Heyman, A, Williams, B, et al. (1990) Sensitivity and specificity of standardized screens of cognitive impairment and dementia among elderly black and white community residents. *J Clin Epidemiol* 43(7):651–660.

Finch, CE and Schneider, EL (eds) (1985) *Handbook of the Biology of Aging,* 2nd ed. New York: Van Nostrand Reinhold.

Foster, HD (1988) The geography of schizophrenia: Possible links with selenium and calcium deficiencies, inadequate exposure to sunlight and industrialization. *J Orthomol Med* 3(3):135–140.

French, LR, Schuman, LM, Mortiner, JA, et al. (1985) A case-control study of dementia of the Alzheimer type. *Am J Epidemiol* 121(3):414–421.

Gajdusek, DC (1977) Unconventional viruses and the origin and disappearance of kuru. *Science* 197:943–960.

Gajdusek, DC and Zigas, V (1957) Degenerative disease of the central nervous system in New Guinea: The endemic occurrence of "kuru" in the native population. *N Engl J Med* 257:974–978.

Goldman, R (1978) The social impact of the organic dementias of the aged. In *Senile Dementia: A Biomedical Approach,* K Nandy (ed) pp. 3–17. New York: Elsevier.

Goodwin-Austen, R and Bendall, J (1990) *The Neurobiology of the Elderly.* New York: Springer-Verlag.

Haynes, SG and Feinlieb, M (eds) (1980) *Second Conference on the Epidemiology of Aging.* Washington, DC: US Department of Health and Human Services, Public Health Service, NIH Publication No 80-969.

Heckler, MM (1985) The fight against Alzheimer's disease. *Am Psychol* 40:1240–1244.

Henderson, VW (1986) Non-genetic factors in Alzheimer's disease pathogenesis. *Neurobiol Aging* 7(6):585–587.

Holden, U (ed) (1989) *Neuropsychology and Aging.* New York: New York University Press.

Holland, AJ (1986) Down's syndrome and Alzheimer's disease: A review. *Psychol Med* 16:307–322.

Horne, RD (1987) Age of onset of Alzheimer's disease: Clue to the relative importance of etiologic factors? *Am J Epidemiol* 126(3):409–414.

Hurd, MD (1989) The economic status of the elderly. *Science* 244:659–663.

Inglis, J (1957) An experimental study of learning and memory function in elderly psychiatric patients. *J Ment Sci* 103:796–803.

Inglis, J (1959) Learning, retention and conceptual use in elderly patients with memory disorder. *J Abnorm Soc Psychol* 59:210–215.

Jacoby, RJ and Levy, R (1980) Computed tomography in the elderly: 2. Senile dementia: Diagnosis and functional impairment. *Br J Psychiatry* 136:256–269.

Jarvik, LF, Ruth, V, and Mastsuyama, SS (1980) Organic brain syndrome and aging: A six-year follow up of surviving twins. *Arch Gen Psychiatry* 37:280–286.

Jorm, A (1987) *A Guide to the Understanding of Alzheimer's Disease and Related Disorders.* New York: New York University Press.

Kendrick, DC and Post, F (1967) Differences in cognitive status between healthy, psychiatrically ill, and diffusely brain damaged elderly subjects. *Br J Psychiatry* 11:75–81.

Khachaturian, ZS (1985) Progress of research on Alzheimer's disease: Research opportunities for behavioral scientists. *Am Psychol* 40:1251–1255.

Kiloh, LG (1961) Pseudo-dementia. *Acta Psychiatr Scand* 37:336–351.

Liu, IY and Anthony, JC (1989) Using the "mini-mental state" examination to predict elderly subjects's completion of a follow-up interview. *Am J Epidemiol* 130(2):416–422.

Marx, JL (1989) Brain protein yields clues to Alzheimer's disease. *Science* 243:1664–1666.

Marx, R (1988) Evidence uncovered for second Alzheimer's gene. *Science* 241:1432–1433.

Mikkelsen, S (1980) A cohort study of disability pension and death among painters with special references to disabling presenile dementia as an occupational disease. *Scand J Soc Med* 16:34–43.

Miller, BL (1986) Aluminum in Alzheimer's disease: A testable hypothesis. *Neurobiol Aging* 7(6):570–571.

Miller, E (1973) Short- and long-term memory in presenile dementia (Alzheimer's disease). *Psychol Med* 3:221–224.

Nappi, G, Homyliewicz, O, Fariello, RG, et al. (eds) (1988) *Neurodegenerative Disorders: The Role Played by Endotoxins and Xenobiotics.* New York: Raven Press.

O'Flynn, RR (1988) Do organic solvents "cause" dementia? *Int J Geriatric Psychiatry* 3(1):5–15.

Olsen, J and Sabroe, S (1980) A case-referent study of neuropsychiatric disorders among workers exposed to solvents in the Danish wood and furniture industry. *Scand J Soc Med* 16:44–49.

Osuntokun, BO (1981) Cassava, diet, chronic cyanide intoxication and Nigerian Africans. *World Rev Nutr Diet* 26:141–173.

Pfeffer, RI, Kurosaki, TT, Harrah, CH, et al. (1981) A survey diagnostic tool for senile dementia. *Am J Epidemiol* 114(4):515–527.

Pfeffer, RI, Afifi, AA, and Chance, JM (1987) Prevalence of Alzheimer's disease in a retirement community. *Am J Epidemiol* 125:420–436.

Podlisny, MB, Lee, G, and Selkoe, DJ (1987) Gene dosage of the amyloid beta precursor protein in Alzheimer's disease. *Science* 238:669–671.

Post, F (1965) *The Clinical Psychiatry of Late Life.* Oxford: Pergamon Press.

Price, DL (1986) New perspectives on Alzheimers' disease. *Annu Rev Neurosci* 9:489–512.

Prusiner, SB and McKinley, MP (eds) (1987) *Prions: Novel Infectious Pathogens Causing Scrapie and Creutzfeld–Jacob Disease.* New York: Academic Press.

Roberts, E (1986) Alzheimer's disease may begin in the nose and may be caused by aluminosilicates. *Neurobiol Aging* 7(6):561–567.

Rosenberg, GS (1970) *The Worker Grows Old.* San Francisco: Jossey-Bass.

Roth, M and Hopkins, B (1953) Psychological test performance in patients over 60: I. Senile psychosis and the affective disorders of old age. *J Ment Sci* 99:439–538.

Rothschield, H (1984) *Risk Factors for Senility.* New York: Oxford University Press.

Rowe, JW and Kahn, RL (1987) Human aging: Usual and successful. *Science* 237:143–149.

St George-Hyslop, P, Tanzi, RE, Polinsky, RJ, et al. (1987) Absence of duplication of chromosome 21 genes in familial and sporadic Alzheimer's disease. *Science* 238:664–666.

Salthouse, TA (1978) The role of memory in the age decline in digit symbol substitution performance. *J Gerontol* 33:232–238.

Scheibel, AB and Wechsler, AF (eds) (1986) *The Biological Substrates of Alzheimer's Disease.* New York: Academic Press.

Schellenberg, GD, Bird, TD, Wijsman, EM, et al. (1988) Absence of linkage of chromosome 21q21 markers to familial Alzheimer's disease. *Science* 241:1507–1510.

Scherr, PA, Albert, MS, Funkenstein, HH, et al. (1988) Correlated or cognitive function in an elderly community population. *Am J Epidemiol* 128(5):1084–1101.

Schneidman, E (1989) The indian summer of life: A

preliminary study of septuagenerians. *Am Psychol* 44:684–694.

Selkoe, DJ (1990) Deciphering Alzheimer's disease: The amyloid precursor protein yields new clues. *Science* 248:1058–1060.

Shalat, SL, Seltzer, B, Pidcock, C, et al. (1987) Risk factors for Alzheimer's disease: A case-control study. *Neurology (NY)* 37(10):1630–1633.

Snyder, SH and D'Amato, RJ (1986) MPTP: A neurotoxin relevant to the pathophysiology of Parkinson's disease. *Neurology (NY)* 36:250–258.

Spencer, PS, Ludolph, A, Dwivedi, MP, et al. (1986) Lathyrism: Evidence for role of the neuroexcitatory aminoacid BOAA. *Lancet* 2:1066–1067.

Strong, R, Wood, G, and Burke, WJ (1988) *Central Nervous System Disorder of Aging.* New York: Raven Press.

Tanzi, RE, Bird, ED, Lati, SA, et al. (1987) The amyloid beta protein is not duplicated in brains from pa-

tients with Alzheimer's disease. *Science* 238:666–669.

Terry, RD (ed) (1988) *Aging and the Brain.* New York: Raven Press.

Terry, RD and Davies, P (1980) Dementia of the Alzheimer type. *Annu Rev Neurosci* 3:77–95.

White, RF (1987) Differential diagnosis of probable Alzheimer's disease and solvent encephalopathy in older workers. *Clin Neuropsychol* 1(2):153–160.

Woodruff, DS and Birren, JE (1983) *Aging: Scientific Perspectives and Social Issues,* 2nd ed. Monterey, CA: Books/Cole.

Woodruff-Pak, DS (1988) *Psychology and Aging.* Englewood Cliffs, NJ: Prentice-Hall.

Yankner, BA, Dawes, LR, Fisher, S, et al. (1989) Neurotoxicity of a fragment of the amyloid precursor associated with Alzheimer's disease. *Science* 245:417–420.

33

Alcoholism, Smoking, and
Other Substance Abuse

Sometimes, in epidemiological studies of large groups and in the clinical evaluation of single individuals, the link between neuropsychological findings and neurotoxic exposures is difficult to establish because of the presence of alcoholism and other substance abuse.

It is also true that alcoholism—and, more recently, drug abuse—has often been wrongfully blamed for workers' subjective complaints and neurological signs. It has been said that ignorance and bad faith share the same symptoms; sometimes such misdiagnosis is the result of a conscious effort to deflect an occupational health problem so that the problem looks as if it were the worker's personal problem.

From the outset, it must be emphasized that without the full cooperation of affected individuals a differential diagnosis separating occupational illnesses and substance abuse is very difficult if not impossible to establish. The problem is compounded by the fact that substance abuse can itself be an occupational disease—eg, alcoholism associated with the inability to cope with stress. In other instances both problems are present at the same time: occupational neurotoxic exposure and alcoholism. Some research workers (eg, Hänninen in Finland) argue that solvent exposure

and alcoholism may be related as a cross-addiction, citing the case of alcohol abuse and toluene addiction as an example.

Professionals dealing with individuals and investigators studying the health consequences of environmental and occupational exposure to neurotoxic agents are familiar with the clinical manifestations of alcoholism and drug abuse and the misuse of these observations. Alice Hamilton (1943) reports in her remarkable biography that, in numerous instances, managers and even physicians often attribute signs and symptoms of neurotoxic illness—notably occupational exposure to solvents—to an employee's chronic alcohol problems.

ALCOHOLISM

Acute Alcoholic Intoxication and Chronic Alcoholism

The acute picture of ethyl alcohol (or ethanol) intoxication includes general disinhibition, slurred speech, dizziness, nausea, unsteady gait, coma, and death through respiratory depression. However, the acute picture varies markedly in inexperienced drinkers and chronic alcoholics. The latter rarely experience "hangovers." Chronic alcoholics learn to manipulate food intake and pace drinks to avoid any unpleasant toxic side effects.

Psychologists who administer neuropsychological tests in the clinic or during the course of medical field surveys often encounter individuals in various phases of acute alcohol intoxication or the "morning after" syndrome. Instructions for participants in medical surveys sometimes contain a reminder to refrain from drinking alcoholic beverages at least 24 hours prior to testing. The fact that some individuals do not comply with these instructions may itself be indicative of a drinking problem. Sometimes it is possible to smell the aroma of beer, wine, whiskey, gin, brandy, or liquors on the breath of an individual. But experienced drinkers may drink vodka, which is comparatively— but not totally—odorless.

Neuropsychologists should be alerted to the possibility that an individual who is examined in the context of litigation with his or her employer may purposely drink large quantities of alcohol for several days before testing to alter the result of the tests. There are no guidelines as to what test results may be more susceptible to this type of malingering. Most of the psychometric test results that are recommended for inclusion in a core battery of neurotoxicological assessment can be significantly altered in this manner. Certain electrophysiological tests— such as the determination of nerve conduction velocity of peripheral nerves—are unlikely to be influenced by a single instance of excessive alcohol intake. But the results of other electrophysiological procedures such as nystagmography are extremely sensitive to even minute amounts of alcohol intake. Examination of the eye movements of people suspected to be intoxicated by alcohol (the "gaze test") is a common practice in many states.

The neuropsychological picture of chronic alcoholism is important to bear in mind in either clinical neurotoxicology or epidemiological studies of neurotoxic illness. Chronic alcoholism has a profound effect on mood, cognitive functioning, personality, and social behavior; in advanced stages of alcoholism, neurological signs such as peripheral neuropathies and cerebellar disorders may be present.

Chronic alcohol abuse may create mood lability, that is, quick shifts from exhilaration to depression. Inappropriate sentimentality is sometimes apparent in people suffering from chronic alcoholism. The afflicted person may cry listening to music or a story having a particular sentimental bent, or recalling sad—or even happy—episodes of his or her childhood. Alcohol is described as anxiolytic (having the capacity to reduce anxiety), and its intake in moderate amounts can have beneficial health effects. Aggressive behavior, too, can be unleashed during episodes of alcohol consumption. Criminal acts such as spouse and child abuse, rape, and murder are often committed under the influence of alcohol.

People who suffer from chronic alcoholism cannot drink in moderation. A reevaluation of the hypothesis that chronic alcoholics can control their drinking instead of abstaining totally has failed to support early contentions (Pendery et al. 1982). A history of alcohol consumption can have devastating effects. Some experts refuse to use the expression "ex-alcoholic" in the classification of people who have ceased to drink, pointing to the lifelong vigilance on drinking behavior such individuals must exert.

Symptoms of *alcohol withdrawal* include tremulousness ("morning shakes"), malaise, irritability, and gastrointestinal and autonomic symptoms. Hallucinations and seizures may also occur. These symptoms may be alleviated by the intake of alcohol. *Delirium tremens* (DT) is the most severe manifestation of alcohol withdrawal. It includes extreme agitation, confusion, tremors of the face, tongue and extremities, and sometimes hallucinations.

Malnutrition often accompanies excessive alcohol consumption. Korsakoff's psychosis (a disease characterized by confusion and severe memory deficits) and alterations of peripheral nervous system functions—including paresthesia and sometimes paralysis—are now understood to be caused by nutritional factors and not the alcohol per se. Malnutrition may be voluntary, as in the cases of women who drink to avoid eating in order to stay thin—the "three martini diet."

Persons at High Risk of Alcoholism

A conservative estimate is that about 10% of the population who drink develop the psychological and physiological dependence on alcohol that characterizes alcoholism. On the basis of epidemiological and sociological data, the National Council on Alcoholism has pinpointed the following factors for the development of alcoholism. There is no complete agreement on the extent of the risk for each factor.

- A family history of alcoholism, including parents, siblings, grandparents, uncles, and aunts.
- A history of teetotalism in the family, particularly where strong moral overtones were present and, most particularly, where the social environment of the patient has changed to associations in which drinking is encouraged or required.
- A history of alcoholism or teetotalism in the spouse or the family of the spouse.
- Coming from a broken home or one with much parental discord, particularly where the father was absent or rejecting but not punitive.
- Being the last child in a large family.
- Heavy drinking is often associated with heavy smoking, although the opposite need not be true.
- Membership in certain cultural groups that are recognized as being more associated with drinking than others (Polish, Scandinavian, etc versus Chinese, for example). However, alcoholism can be encountered in any culture.

Diagnostic Criteria for Alcoholism

The DSM-III-R published by the American Psychiatric Association (1987) suggests the following diagnostic criteria:

1. Pattern of pathological use of alcoholic beverages. Need for daily use of alcohol for adequate functioning; inability to cut down or stop drinking; repeated efforts to control or reduce excess drinking by "going on the wagon"—periods of temporary abstinence—or restricting drinking to certain times of the day; binges (remaining intoxicated throughout the day for at least 2 days); occasional consumption of a fifth of spirits (or its equivalent in wine or beer); amnestic periods for events occurring while intoxicated (blackouts); continuation of drinking despite a serious physical disorder that the individual knows is exacerbated by alcohol use; drinking of nonbeverage alcohol.

2. Impairment in social or occupational functioning as a result of alcohol use. Violence while intoxicated; absence from work; loss of job; legal and financial difficulties (eg, arrest for intoxicated behavior, traffic accidents while intoxicated); arguments or difficulties with family or friends because of excessive alcohol use.

3. Duration of disturbance of at least a month. Signs and symptoms need not be present continuously during this period.

The DSM-III-R establishes the distinction between alcohol abuse and alcohol dependence. *Alcohol dependence* is characterized by all the symptoms of alcohol use plus the pathological characteristic of daily need of alcohol ingestion for adequate functioning. Tolerance or withdrawal must be present. *Alcohol tolerance* is defined as the need for marked increases in amounts of alcohol to achieve the desired effects, or markedly diminished effects with regular use of alcohol.

Difficulty in Obtaining Reliable Data on Alcohol Consumption

Reliable data on patterns of alcohol consumption are difficult to obtain. The toxicological approach to data gathering is to estimate the amount and frequency of drinks, equating a can of beer to a glass of wine or a shot of hard liquor (either by itself or in highballs). This approach is used in most epidemiological studies of work-related neurotoxic illness.

The behavioral approach used by expert groups such as the National Council on Alcoholism or the DSM-III-R is to ascertain the degree to which an individual's behavior is patterned around alcohol intake. The behavioral approach is followed by most professionals who deal with alcoholics and alcoholism.

Toxicological Assessment of Ethanol Dose

The following is an example of a basic questionnaire to assess drinking habits.

Data are abstracted and transformed into several indices of alcohol intake on the basis that beer contains 4.5%, table wine 12%, and whiskey 45% ethyl alcohol (ethanol). Body weight must be taken into consideration, since the same amount of alcohol creates an effective dose of alcohol in a 120-lb person that is almost double that in a 200-lb person. Some investigators define alcoholism on the basis of dose alone. A heavy drinker is thus defined as one who drinks between 70 g of alcohol per day (low figure) and 100 g per day (high figure).

Although in epidemiological research there have been many attempts to improve the data acquisition portion of this questionnaire, it

---

Drinking Habits Questionnaire

1. Have you drunk as many as 20 alcoholic beverages in your entire life?
   IF NO, terminate questionnaire on alcohol intake.
2. Do you now drink alcoholic beverages?
   IF NO, how old were you when you gave up drinking?
   IF NO, answer question 3 and continue with question 10.
3. How old were you when you first started drinking?
4. About how often do you drink some kind of alcoholic beverage?
   1 = almost every day
   2 = three or four times a week
   3 = once or twice a week
   4 = once or twice a month
   5 = less than once a month
   6 = don't know/not applicable
5. When you drink beer, about how many cans or bottles do you usually drink?
6. When you drink wine, about how many glasses of wine do you usually drink?
7. When you drink highballs, mixed drinks, or other kinds of liquor, about how many drinks do you usually have?
8. Have your drinking habits changed over time?
9. If you have ever reduced your alcohol intake, indicate the year.
10. In the past, about how often did you drink some kind of alcoholic beverage?
    1 = almost every day
    2 = three or four times a week
    3 = once or twice a week
    4 = once or twice a month
    5 = less than once a month
    6 = don't know/not applicable
11. When you drank beer, about how many cans or bottles did you usually drink.
12. When you drank wine, about how many glasses did you usually drink?
13. When you drank highballs, mixed drinks, or other kinds of liquor, about how many drinks did you usually have?

has major flaws: people have poor recall of their alcoholic intake—most underestimate their alcoholic consumption; some drinkers follow a consistent pattern of alcohol intake, whereas others do not—for example, some people drink wine with their meals every day, and others engage in alcoholic binges lasting several days; in certain areas of the country where there are marked seasonal changes, drinking intake varies markedly in summer and in winter, being more common in winter; behavioral aspects of drinking (the need to drink just when one rises in the morning, typical of chronic alcoholics) are lost in this type of questionnaire.

Despite their toxicological aura, questionnaires of this type are difficult to code and have questionable validity when measured against behavioral indicators of alcoholism. It is as if one were to attempt to tell whether a person is alcoholic from his or her intake rather than by directly asking the subject about the significance alcohol plays in his or her life. In addition, in a medical field survey, an attempt to include all possible patterns of alcohol intake would make the questionnaire unusually long, thus taking a valuable segment of the total time slot intended for the medical and neuropsychological evaluation of a single subject and the collection of laboratory specimens.

Behavioral Signs and Symptoms of Alcoholism

On the following page is a questionnaire on symptoms of alcoholism prepared by the National Council on Alcoholism (NCA). The NCA questionnaire is self-administered and takes only a few minutes to complete.

Epidemiological Studies on Alcohol Use and Cognitive Functioning

There have been numerous studies on the possible effects on cognitive functioning of alcohol use at levels that are considered "slight" or "moderate." Some of these have been conducted on large numbers of people,

paying attention to important issues of study design. But because of time limitations inherent in these large-scale epidemiological studies, the task of assessing "cognition" is hardly comparable to that used by neuropsychologists in the course of their clinical evaluation.

The study by Parker and collaborators (1983) is an example. This report is based on a representative sample of 1367 employed men and women. The respondents were drawn from employed people in the three-county central core of metropolitan Detroit consisting of Wayne, Oakland, and McComb counties. Respondents were asked about their alcohol consumption during the month before the interviews and about periods of heavier or lighter drinking, in terms of quantity and frequency, throughout the course of their lives.

The questions were open-ended, and the interviewers were trained to probe for types, numbers, and sizes of drinks usually consumed. Reported types, numbers, and sizes of drinks were used to determine total ounces of specific beverages consumed. The analysis was confined to the most frequently consumed beverage of each respondent because of the errors inherent in reports of occasional drink consumption.

Cognitive functioning was measured by the Shipley Institute of Living Scale (SILS), which was completed by respondents at the end of the interview. The SILS is a self-administered paper-and-pencil test comprised of two parts: 40 multiple-choice questions about word meaning (vocabulary) and 20 questions that require the subject to complete sequential patterns. The influence of reported alcohol consumption on cognition was then analyzed using multiple-regression procedures. In this model, abstraction score was the dependent variable, and vocabulary scores, quantity of alcohol consumed per drinking occasion, frequency of consumption, age, education level, and race were the independent (predictor) variables. Abstraction, tested while respondents were sober, decreased significantly as the reported quantity of alcohol usually consumed per drinking occasion increased.

Questionnaire on The Symptoms of Alcoholism

1. Do you occasionally drink heavily after a disappointment, a quarrel, or when the boss gives you a hard time?
2. When you have trouble or feel under pressure, do you always drink more heavily than usual?
3. Have you noticed that you are able to handle more liquor than you did when you were first drinking?
4. Did you ever wake up on the "morning after" and discover that you could not remember part of the evening before, even though your friends tell you that you did not "pass out"?
5. When drinking with other people, do you try to have a few extra drinks when others will not know it?
6. Are there certain occasions when you feel uncomfortable if alcohol is not available?
7. Have you recently noticed that when you begin drinking you are in more of a hurry to get the first drink than you used to be?
8. Do you sometimes feel a little guilty about your drinking?
9. Are you secretly irritated when your family or friends discuss your drinking?
10. Have your recently noticed an increase in the frequency of your memory "blackout"?
11. Do you often find that you wish to continue drinking after your friends say they have had enough?
12. Do you usually have a reason for the occasions when you drink heavily?
13. When you are sober, do you often regret things you have done or said while drinking?
14. Have you tried switching brands or following different plans for controlling your drinking?
15. Have you often failed to keep the promises you have made to yourself about controlling or cutting down on your drinking?
16. Have you ever tried to control your drinking by making a change in jobs, or moving to a new location?
17. Do you try to avoid family or close friends while you are drinking?
18. Are you having an increasing number of financial and work problems?
19. Do more people seem to be treating you unfairly without good reason?
20. Do you eat very little or irregularly when you are drinking?
21. Do you sometimes have the "shakes" in the morning and find that it helps to have a little drink?
22. Have you recently noticed that you cannot drink as much as you once did?
23. Do you sometimes stay drunk for several days at a time?
24. Do you sometimes feel very depressed and wonder whether life is worth living?
25. Sometimes after periods of drinking, do you see or hear things that aren't there?
26. Do you get terribly frightened after you have been drinking heavily?

Adapted from "What Are the Signs of Alcoholism?" © 1987 National Council on Alcoholism Inc. Reproduced with permission of the National Council on Alcoholism Inc.

Alcohol and the Child

Clinical neurotoxicologists performing individual evaluation of children and epidemiologists carrying out large-scale studies on the influence of alcohol on children's behavior distinguish three major problem areas:

1. The fetal alcohol syndrome—ie, neuropsychological deficits in the child caused by the mother's excessive drinking during pregnancy (reviewed in Chapter 20).
2. The fact that alcoholism tends to be present in successive generations of a family (people who drink sometimes have a family history of alcohol abuse).
3. The extent of alcoholism as a problem among children and adolescents, which is unknown but suspected to be high.

Is the Study of Alcohol Abuse Paradigmatic?

There is no other single neurotoxic agent that has been more extensively studied than alcohol, either from the clinical, experimental, or epidemiological point of view. Literature on the pharmacological, physiological, and psychological effects of alcohol abuse in humans and animal models amounts to hundreds of publications a year around the world. Several dozen of periodic publications are specifically devoted to alcoholism. Alcoholism is a major community and occupational health problem around the world, and the amount of research reflects in part the effort to control the magnitude of the problem and reduce human suffering.

But alcohol, like lead, has often been claimed to be "paradigmatic" of all other research in environmental and occupational toxicology. Some investigators claim that since alcohol is a solvent, the study of the chronic effects of occupational exposure to solvents should be modeled after the extensive research performed on alcoholics. This strategy is reinforced by the fact that because of the relative novelty of the discipline, environmental and occupational neurotoxicology still lacks well-established research canons. It therefore seems reassuring to build new research on existing methodologies and techniques created for other purposes and in a different context. There are, however, important differences.

On one hand, alcoholism is a complex disease that begins (arguably) as a choice and—in a number of individuals—ends with catastrophic consequences. It is (again, arguably) a voluntary intake of a powerful mood modifier. People seek alcohol as a reinforcer to produce a complex array of individual psychological changes.

Neurotoxic agents in the environment or in the workplace, on the other hand, are not the choice of individuals. They are often unrecognized by the people of a community or workers at the worksite, who have no control over the exposure. In addition, people do not voluntarily seek to be exposed to neurotoxic agents—although exposure to certain solvents is known to produce addictions as a sequel to occupational exposure.

In conclusion, the basic information on the clinical picture of alcoholism—the epidemiological trends, the predisposing factors, the techniques and statistical methodology—all need to be known by the professional who works in any of the several contexts of environmental and occupational neurotoxicology. But he or she should be cautious in assessing the influence of alcohol-related problems in the evaluation of the health status of individuals, work groups, or of a given community.

CIGARETTE SMOKING AND NICOTINE

The Prevalence of Smoking

Cigarette smoking is one of the most common forms of drug dependence. The prevalence of smoking varies widely—between 7% and 70%—in different countries and cultural groups. Much is known about the prevalence of smoking because of its role in causing cancer as well as many other adverse health effects. The Surgeon General's report contains a periodic update of smoking habits and health problems associated with smoking in the United States.

Cigarette smoking depends on the effects of several demographic factors. Although men used to be the heaviest smokers, women are now smoking in increasing numbers. Less-educated people smoke in larger numbers than more-educated people. The differential effects of ethnic background are difficult to ascertain because of confounding factors such as education and income.

In epidemiological studies, smoking habits can be ascertained by the use of questionnaires such as that shown on the following page. This questionnaire is aimed at establishing the individual "dose" of cigarette smoking.

Smoking Habits Questionnaire

1. Do you now smoke cigarettes?
   IF YES, go to question 4.
2. Have you ever smoked cigarettes regularly in the past?
   (Count as YES anyone who has smoked more than 1 cigarette per day for more than 6 months.)
   IF NO, go on to question 7.
3. In what year did you stop smoking?
4. In what year did you start smoking?
5. How many do/did you smoke per day on the average?
   (number of cigarettes, not packs)
6. What do/did you mostly smoke? Type: 1 = filter; 2 = non-filter
7. Do you smoke a pipe?
   IF YES, go on to question 9.
8. Have you ever smoked a pipe?
   (Count as YES more than 1/day for more than 6 months.)
   IF NO, go on to question 10.
9. How many pipefuls per day do/did you smoke?
   (Code = number of pipefuls per day.)
10. Do you smoke cigars?
    IF YES, go on to question 12.
11. Have you ever smoked cigars?
    (Count as YES more than 1/day for more than 6 months. IF NO, terminate the questionnaire.)
12. How many cigars per day do/did you smoke?
    (Code = number of cigars per day.)

Active Ingredients in Tobacco and Cigarette Smoking

Over 90% of tobacco is used in the form of cigarettes. Although cigars, pipes, chewing tobacco, and snuff also contain tobacco, their numbers are minor compared to cigarettes. The primary neurotoxic agent in tobacco is nicotine, but carbon monoxide is also important.

Nicotine is a naturally occurring alkaloid found in the tobacco plant, *Nicotiana*. Although the tobacco plant is the primary source of nicotine, many other plants produce nicotine in lesser concentrations. Nicotine appears to have evolved as the plant's natural protection against predators; in fact, it is still used as an effective insecticide. Nicotine is very toxic to humans—ingesting as little as 60 mg can be fatal to an adult. An ordinary cigar contains at least two lethal (if ingested) doses of nicotine.

Cigarette smoking may be the unsuspected source of other neurotoxic agents. While smoking at the workplace with dirty hands, for example, the worker may increase his or her intake of toxic agents in the environment

severalfold: the worker touches the cigarette and deposits toxins on the cigarette paper which he or she later inhales. Such routes have been documented for lead and cadmium.

The Pharmacological Effects of Tobacco

The pharmacokinesis of nicotine has been extensively studied. Nicotine is readily absorbed from several parts of the body, mainly through mucous membranes, the epithelium of the respiratory track, and skin; nicotine is not absorbed in the stomach, but it is absorbed by the small intestine.

Nicotine receptors are one of the two types of receptors that respond to acetylcholine (the others are muscarinic receptors). As discussed in Chapter 2, nicotinic receptors are associated with rapid conduction across the synapse, that is, for rapid transmission of information such as that necessary at the neuromuscular junction.

Nicotine stimulates both the autonomic ganglia of the peripheral nervous system and centers located in the central nervous system;

it also has a wide variety of other physiological effects. Some of these effects are complex. For example, nicotine can directly increase the heart rate by stimulation of the sympathetic ganglia or by release of epinephrine from the stimulated adrenal gland.

Acute nicotine poisoning is possible through accidental ingestion of insecticides containing nicotine. Children can sometimes develop signs of acute nicotine poisoning from swallowing cigarettes. But such an ingestion is rarely fatal because the slow absorption through the stomach and the low levels of nicotine stimulate the chemical trigger zone (vomiting center) in the area postrema of the medulla, causing vomiting.

The Smoking Habit

Although many factors contribute to initiating and maintaining the smoking habit, it has been fairly well established that the smoking habit is an expression of nicotine-seeking behavior. Smokers will often compensate for changes in the availability of nicotine in order to maintain an optimum blood level. The prevailing view today is that tobacco smoking creates a physical rather than a psychological dependence on nicotine.

Nonsmokers often find tobacco smoking aversive. Along with the desirable features of euphoria, beginners often experience nausea, vomiting, pallor, abdominal pain, headache, dizziness, and weakness.

The smoking habit is maintained by several reinforcing effects of cigarette smoke, which are most likely produced by nicotine. These reinforcers are arousal, improved attention, diminution of aggression and irritability, and inhibition of appetite with a consequent weight reduction.

Tobacco Withdrawal

The *Diagnostic and Statistical Manual of Mental Disorders* (DSM-III-R) defines tobacco withdrawal as "a characteristic withdrawal syndrome due to recent cessation or reduction in tobacco use that has been at least moderate in duration and amount." The syndrome includes a craving for tobacco, irritability, anxiety, difficulty in concentrating, restlessness, headache, drowsiness, and gastrointestinal disturbances. The associated features of tobacco withdrawal include increased slow rhythms on the electroencephalogram, decreased heart rate and blood pressure, weight gain, and impairment in performance of tasks requiring vigilance.

The course of symptoms begins within 24 hours of cessation or reduction in tobacco use and decreases in intensity over a period of a few days to several weeks. The diagnostic criteria for tobacco withdrawal are use of tobacco for at least several weeks at a level equivalent to more than 10 cigarettes per day, with each cigarette containing at least 0.5 mg of nicotine, and subsequent abrupt cessation or reduction in tobacco use, followed within 24 hours by at least one of the symptoms listed above.

Tobacco Dependence

The DSM-III-R defines tobacco dependence as "continuous use of tobacco for at least one month" with either (1) unsuccessful attempts to stop or significantly reduce the amount of tobacco use on a permanent basis, (2) the development of tobacco withdrawal upon attempting to stop or reduce tobacco use, or (3) continuation of tobacco use despite the presence of a serious physical disorder (eg, respiratory or cardiovascular disease) that the individual knows is exacerbated by tobacco use.

In the middle 1980s, smoking was reported to be on the decline in the United States in part because of the Surgeon General's (1985) report on smoking and health. In attempts to reduce smoking and particularly to avoid the inhalation route, an unrecorded number of individuals have resorted to the use of nicotine-containing chewing gum. The rationale for the use of the gum is to reduce the withdrawal pangs and allow the smoker to reduce dependence gradually. The literature on adverse neuropsychological effects associated with long-term use of chewing gum is scant.

Teratological Effects of Cigarette Smoking

Cigarette smoking is a known neuroteratogen (affecting the development of the nervous system). Although nicotine addiction in the unborn cannot be ruled out, the primary suspect is carbon monoxide generated while smoking. Exposure to carbon monoxide in the unborn is suspected to cause mental retardation by inhibiting the normal development of the brain.

COFFEE, TEA, AND HERBAL TEAS

The consumption of coffee, teas, and other products containing substances that affect the nervous system is pervasive in the United States and other parts of the world. Caffeine, for example, is found not only in coffee but in numerous other beverages such as soft drinks and over-the-counter drugs. Caffeine is sometimes added to certain drugs to counteract drowsiness created by some of their other components.

Caffeine Intoxication

According to the *Diagnostic and Statistical Manual of Mental Disorders* (DSM-III-R),

> The essential features [of caffeine intoxication] are restlessness, nervousness, excitement, insomnia, flushed face, diuresis, and gastrointestinal complaints. These symptoms appear in some individuals following intake of as little as 250 mg of caffeine per day, whereas others require much larger doses. At levels of more than 1 g/day there may be muscle twitching, periods of inexhaustibility, psychomotor agi-

tation, rambling flow of thought and speech, and cardiac arrhythmia. Mild sensory disturbances such as ringing in the ears and flashes of light have been reported at higher doses.

The diagnostic criteria for caffeine intoxication includes the recent consumption of caffeine, usually in excess of 250 mg, and the presence of at least five of the symptoms named above. Caffeine intoxication and certain mental disorders—such as anxiety disorders—can present similar symptoms.

Toxic Effects of Herbal Teas

Common tea (*Camellia sinensis*) is neurotoxic because of its caffeine content. Consumption in large amounts may lead to irritability, tremor, premature ventricular beat, and acute hypertension.

Ridker (1987) reviewed the toxic effects of some herbal teas consumed by individuals attempting to reduce their caffeine intake. Several herbal teas contain the anticholinergic compounds atropine, scopolamine, and hyoscyamine. These include mandrake (*Mandragon officianurum*), thornapple (*Datura* sp.), lobelia (*Lobelia inflata*), and burdock root (*Arctium lappa*). Burdock roots have been associated with the acute anticholinergic symptoms of blurred vision, dry mouth, dilated pupils, distended bladder, disorientation, and delirium. Adrenergic complications have not been reported, although Mormon tea is known to contain ephedrine. Tea prepared from yihimbe bark (*Corynanthe yohimbe*) contains yohimbine, a presynaptic α_2 blocking agent. In northern Argentina, Bolivia, and other Andean countries, the leaves of the coca plant—a powerful stimulant which is the basis of cocaine—are brewed in tea; in the early 1900s coca was part of the formula for the now popular beverage *Coca-Cola*.

Some herbal teas might contain neurotoxic contaminants. There are case reports of arsenic poisoning resulting from consumption of herbal teas.

Forensic Substance Abuse Questionnaire

The defendant began to use drugs at the age of _____.

At one time or another the defendant used the following (Yes/No):

Marijuana	Cocaine + heroin (smoked)
Cocaine (snorted)	Cocaine + heroin (injected)
Cocaine (injected)	LSD
Crack cocaine	"Uppers" (amphetamines)
(smoked)	"Downers" (Valium)
Heroin (snorted)	"Angel dust" (PCP)
Heroin (injected)	

Others ("poppers," designer drugs, mushroom, peyote, pain killers, etc.)

The defendant used the following *on a regular basis* (Yes/No):

Marijuana	Cocaine + heroin (smoked)
Cocaine (snorted)	Cocaine + heroin (injected)
Cocaine (injected)	LSD
Crack cocaine	"Uppers" (amphetamines)
(smoked)	"Downers" (Valium)
Heroin (snorted)	"Angel dust" (PCP)
Heroin (injected)	

Defendant abused drugs for _____ hours at a time.
Defendant abused drugs for _____ days at a time.
On a single day the defendant spent as much as $_____ on drugs.

The defendant uses drugs to counteract withdrawal symptoms or "crashes." (Yes/No)
Events leading to the charges occurred when the defendant was on drugs, needed drugs, or needed money to buy drugs. (Yes/No)
Many times the defendant would mix drugs and alcohol. (Yes/No)

OTHER SUBSTANCE ABUSE

The DSM-III-R recognizes several classes of substance abuse: alcohol (described above), barbiturates or similarly acting sedatives or hypnotics, opiates, amphetamines or similarly acting sympathomimetics, cannabis, tobacco, caffeine, and other mixed or difficult-to-classify substances such as amyl nitrite, mushrooms, peyote, etc.

Most people use, are dependent on, or are addicted to a combination of neurotoxic agents (eg, alcohol, cigarettes, and coffee; drugs and alcohol; etc). Above is a questionnaire in use at the Forensic Psychiatry Clinic for the Criminal and Supreme Courts of New York State, for the assessment of substance abuse in criminal defendants.

An important difference between drug abuse and alcohol abuse is the relative risk of addiction. It takes the consumption of large quantities over long periods of time to become an alcoholic, but the risk of addiction to illegal drugs is considerably higher. Some experts claim that the addiction to crack cocaine is almost immediate for some individuals.

Inhalants

The National Institute of Drug Abuse has published literature for the lay public on inhalants, their general effects, the extent of the problem, and the danger. The following information is abstracted from these publications.

Inhalants are a diverse group of chemical compounds that produce profound psychological effects, particularly alterations in mood. Many addicts describe the action of some inhalants ". . . as a suffusion of pleasant warmth, a feeling of disengagement and relaxation and slowly approaching peaceful sleep" (Alapin 1973). Sometimes inhalants are not recognized as drugs because they were never meant to be used that way. Thus, the presence of dried paint or spray on clothes and body, empty spray cans, or tubes of glue in a teenager's room are not suspected as a source of problems by a parent. Inhalants may be products used as cleaners, beauty agents (eg, acetone used as a nail polish remover), glues (as used in model airplane making), or fuel for commercial vehicles (eg, there are reports on addiction to gasoline).

Inhalants fall into three major categories: aerosol sprays, solvents (eg, toluene, n-hexane, trichloroethylene), and anesthesics. They all produce effects similar to anesthesics. At low doses, users may feel slight stimulation; at higher amounts, they may feel less inhibited; at high doses, loss of consciousness and death can occur. The effects of inhalants are immediate and can last from 15 to 45 minutes. Drowsiness usually follows, and headache and nausea can also occur. Sniffing of inhalants for even brief periods of time can produce alterations in vision and cognition, and can reduce muscle and reflex control.

In the middle 1980s the National Institute of Drug Abuse estimated that about seven million Americans had experimented with inhalants. Most of the people who experiment with inhalants are under 20 years old, many as young as seven or eight. They usually start sniffing when they see friends, brothers and sisters, or other neighborhood people doing it. Sometimes the child will experiment with some household products and discover their psychoactive properties by accident. Repeated sniffing over a period of a number of years can produce permanent, irreversible damage to the nervous system. Sniffing high concentrations of aerosols can produce heart failure and death. Others produce death by acting on the respiratory centers of the brainstem. Deliberate inhaling from plastic bags carries the added risk of death by suffocation.

The first case of trichloroethylene addiction was reported about 60 years ago. At first, most addicts "stumbled on its narcotic action by accident and subsequently become addicts" (Alapin 1973). Since the 1970s it has been a problem confined mostly to young adults with a history of psychological disturbance (which is exacerbated even further by the addiction).

Since the early 1960s, there have been numerous case reports on the devastating neurological effects of glue sniffing. In some of them, occupational exposure to these solvents may have been the trigger for the addiction. Shirabe and collaborators (1974), for example, reported two patients with polyneuropathy following glue sniffing. The cases involved a 20- and a 19-year-old painter who worked in the same workshop and who each developed a subacute, predominantly motor polyneuropathy after sniffing vapor for 2.5 and 3 years, respectively. The polyneuropathy progressed for 3 months even after the exposure ceased. As a result of chromatographic analysis, the glue was proven to contain both n-hexane and toluene as volatile substances. Although n-hexane seems likely to have been the major cause, toluene may have been a contributing factor in the onset of the polyneuropathy. As a result of light and electron microscopy, it was concluded that both solvents, but primarily n-hexane, acted on the axon cylinders of the peripheral nerves, resulting in axonal degeneration, thus producing a predominantly motor polyneuropathy with marked neurogenic muscular atrophy.

Sometimes the source of inhalants can be unusual. Sahenk and collaborators (1978) reported a generalized toxic polyneuropathy in a 23-year-old woman after excessive intentional inhalation of compressed nitrous oxide delivered from cartridges through a whipped-cream dispenser. Chromatographic analysis of the cartridges revealed an exposure to nitrous oxide and 26 other compounds including trichloroethylene, toluene, and phenol, all known neurotoxic agents.

DRUG DEPENDENCY

The World Health Organization defines drug dependence as

> A state, psychic and sometimes also physical, resulting from the interaction between a living organism and a drug, characterized by behavioral and [other] responses that always include a compulsion to take the drug on a continuous or periodic basis in order to experience its psychic effects, and sometimes to avoid the discomfort of its absence. Tolerance may or may not be present. A person may be dependent on more than one drug. (Falk et al. 1982)

Until recently, substance abuse was considered to be primarily an "urban problem." However, there have been many accounts of the rapid extension of this severe health problem to suburban and rural communities.

At the time of this writing the use of cocaine in the United States has reached epidemic proportions. In the early 1980s, the drug was still a status symbol, but by the middle 1980s its use was prevalent in every social segment of the (primarily) urban population.

Assessing Substance Abuse through Questionnaires

Because of the sensitive nature of the questions and the illegality of drug use, inquiry into a subject's history of drug use is confined to clinical settings only. But even during the course of a clinical examination, an examiner cannot be sure he/she is obtaining a reliable history of drug abuse. Attempts to obtain data on drug use during the course of medical field surveys are generally avoided lest they discourage subject participation.

Studies on the use of recreational drugs (eg, marijuana, cocaine) among blue-collar workers are scant.

Long-Term Use of Cannabis

Few neurotoxic drugs have received more attention than marijuana and other cannabis products. When smoked or ingested, these substances produce changes in perception, performance, cognitive functioning, and moods. As Mason and McBay (1985) have stated,

> [There] has been a great concern that the psychoactive response experienced by marijuana users has a detrimental effect on the performance of complex coordinate psychomotor skills. Naturally, the impairment of performance would be of greatest concern in those individuals whose impaired actions could potentially be dangerous to themselves or to others near them. Motor vehicle operators, pilots, air traffic controllers, law enforcement or emergency aid personnel, military personnel, and industrial workers are all good examples of people whose impaired performance could potentially be dangerous.

These authors made an extensive review of 123 studies and concluded that the "data base for interpretation of the relationship between cannobinoid concentration and effects is woefully inadequate." This is primarily based on retrograde temporal extrapolation, or "back calculations" on concentrations of any cannobinoid in any human physiological fluid or tissue. This method is not supportable by pharmacological experiments, and thus interpretations of effects based on back-calculated concentrations are not scientifically defensible.

MPTP

In 1983 there was a report of four persons who developed marked parkinsonism-like symptoms after injection of 1-methyl-4-phenyl-1,2,5,6-tetrahydropyridine (MPTP) sold as "synthetic heroine" (Langston et al. 1983). On the basis of the striking parkinsonian features observed in these patients and additional pathological data from similar cases, it has been proposed that the substantia nigra—a diencephalic nucleus—is the target of MPTP.

CULTURAL AND COMMUNITY STANDARDS AND THE ASSESSMENT OF SUBSTANCE ABUSE

Workers share the standards of the communities in which they live. Study protocols aimed at determining the effect of neurotoxic occupational exposure need to include questions regarding substance abuse. Sometimes this is difficult, and the questioning alone may jeopardize the overall efforts of a medical field survey.

There are many cultural and community standards by which substance abuse needs to be evaluated, and community standards may vary over time. Until recently, for instance, alcohol consumption and cigarette smoking were considered part of the American social fabric. New attitudes toward physical fitness and health have dramatically changed the patterns of alcohol and cigarette use, leading to their progressive decline. The cultural context of psychological approaches to alcoholism has been examined by Peele (1984).

CONCLUSIONS

Professionals who wish to assess the health consequences of environmental and/or occupational exposure to neurotoxic agents need to be aware of the behavioral and psychological effects of important confounders, such as alcoholism, cigarette smoking, drinking of coffee and herbal teas, and other substance abuse.

Those who perform epidemiological studies among workers recognize that workers share the standards of the community in which they live. One should be careful not to under- or overestimate the impact of substance-abuse-related problems in the evaluation of individuals, work groups, or the health status of a given community. The "occupational link" fallacy (see Chapter 12) should also be recognized.

REFERENCES

Alapin, B (1973) Trichloroethylene addiction and its effects. Br J Addict 68:331–335.

American Psychiatric Association (1987) Diagnostic and Statistical Manual of Mental Disorders, 3rd ed, revised. Washington, DC: APA.

Falk, JL, Schster, CR, Bigelow, GE, et al. (1982) Progress and needs in the experimental analysis of drug and alcohol dependence. Am Psychol 37:1124–1127.

Hamilton, A (1943) Exploring the Dangerous Trades. Boston: Little, Brown.

Langston, JW, Tetrud, JW, and Irwin, I (1983) Chronic parkinsonism in humans due to a product of meperidin-analog synthesis. Science 219:979–980.

Mason, AP and McBay (1985) Cannabis: Pharmacology and interpretation of effects. J Forensic Sci 30(3):615–631.

National Council on Alcoholism Inc. (1987) "What Are The Signs of Alcoholism?" (brochure) New York: National Council on Alcoholism Inc.

Parker, DA, Parker, ES, Brody, JB, et al. (1983) Alcohol use and cognitive loss among men and women. Am J Pub Health 73:521–526.

Peele, S (1984) The cultural context of psychological approaches to alcoholism: Can we control the effects of alcohol? Am Psychol 12:1337–1351.

Pendery, ML, Malzman, IM, and West, LJ (1982) Controlled drinking for alcoholics? New findings and a reevaluation of a major affirmative study. Science 217:169–175.

Ridker, PM (1987) Toxic effects of herbal teas. Arch Env Health 42(2):133–136.

Sahenk, Z, Mendell, JR, Couri, D, et al. (1978) Polyneuropathy from inhalation of N_2O cartridges through a whipped-cream dispenser. Neurology (Minneap.) 28:485–487.

Shirabe, T, Tsuda, T, Terao, A, et al. (1984) Toxic polyneuropathy due to glue sniffing: Report of two cases with a light and electron-microscopic study of the peripheral nerves and muscles. J Neurol Sci 21:101–113.

Surgeon General (1985) The Health Consequences of

Smoking; Cancer and Chronic Lung Disease in the Workplace. Rockville, MD: US Department of Health and Human Services, Public Health Service, Office of Smoking and Health.

SUGGESTED READINGS

Anderson, FJ (1977) *An Illustrated History of the Herbals.* New York: Columbia University Press.

Anderson, SC (1981) Alcoholic women: Personality traits during adolescence. *Am J Drug Alcohol Abuse* 8:239–247.

Arnold, WN (1989) Absinthe. *Sci Am* 260(6):112–117.

Bandroft, J (1977) People who deliberately poison or injure themselves: Their problems and their contacts with helping agencies. *Psychol Med* 7(2):289–303.

Bauman, KE, Koch, GG, Bryan, ES, et al. (1989) On the measurement of tobacco use by adolescents: Validity of self-reports of smokeless tobacco use and validity of cotinine as an indicator of cigarette smoking. *Am J Epidemiol* 130(2):327–336.

Blair, A and Steenland, K (eds) (1988) Smoking and occupations in epidemiologic studies. *Am J Ind Med* (special issue) 13(1).

Blankfield, A (1982) Grief and alcohol. *Am J Drug Alcohol Abuse* 9:435–446.

Bollinger, L (1972) Alcoholism and drug abuse. *Chem Eng* 79(25):139–142.

Boyd, G and associates (1987) Use of smokeless tobacco among children and adolescents in the United States. *Prev Med* 16:402–421.

Bruckner, JV and Peterson, RG (1981) Evaluation of toluene and acetone inhalant abuse. I. Pharmacology and pharmacodynamics. *Toxicol Appl Pharmacol* 61:27–38.

Carney, J (1969) Some realities of a joint management–labor alcoholism program. *Rehab Health* 7(1):31.

Carone, P and Krinsky, L (eds) (1973) *Drug Abuse in Industry.* Springfield, IL: Charles C Thomas.

Chambers, C and Heckman, R (1972) *Employee Drug Abuse: A Manager's Guide for Action.* Boston: Cahners Books.

Chassin, L, Presson, C, Sherman, SJ, et al. (1985) Psychological correlates of adolescent smokeless tobacco use. *Addict Behav* 10:431–435.

Chastian, RL, Lehman, WEK, and Joe, GW (1986) Estimated intelligence and long-term outcomes of opioid addicts. *Am J Drug Alcohol Abuse* 12:331–340.

Cho, AK (1990) Ice: A new dosage form of an old drug. *Science* 249:631–634.

Cole, C (1976) Drugs in the workplace. *Clin Toxicol* 9(2):185–197.

Committee on Passive Smoking, Board of Environmental Studies and Toxicology, National Research Council (1986) *Environmental Tobacco Smoke: Measuring Exposures and Assessing Health Effects.* Washington, DC: National Academy Press.

Corry, JM and Cimbolic, P (1985) *Drugs: Facts, Alternatives, Decisions.* Belmont, CA: Wadsworth Publishing.

Criteria Committee, National Council on Alcoholism (1972) Criteria for the diagnosis of alcoholism. *Am J Psychiatry* 120(2):127–135.

DeFranco, C, Tarbox, AR, and McLaughlin, EJ (1985) Cognitive deficits as a function of years of alcohol abuse. *Am J Drug Alcohol Abuse* 11:279–293.

Feeney, DM (1976) The marijuana window: A theory of cannabis use. *Behav Biol* 18:455–471.

Fisher, S, Raskin, A, and Uhlenhuth, EH (eds) (1987) *Cocaine: Clinical and Biobehavioral Aspects.* New York: Oxford University Press.

Fitzgerald, JH and Mulford, HA (1979) Rural vs urban problem drinker clients. *Am J Alcohol Abuse* 6:235–343.

Gawin, FH and Ellinwood, EH (1988) Cocaine and other stimulants: Actions, abuse and treatment. *N Engl J Med* 318:1173–1182.

Gay, GR, Ianba, DS, Sheppard, CW, et al. (1975) Cocaine: History, epidemiology, human pharmacology and treatment. A perspective of a new debut for an old girl. *Clin Toxicol* 8(2):149–178.

Glasser, H and Massengale, O (1962) Glue sniffing in children: Deliberate inhalation of vaporized plastic cements. *JAMA* 181:300–303.

Goldenberg, I (1972) *Employment and Addiction: Perspective on Existing Business and Treatment Practices.* Springfield, VA: National Technical Information Service.

Grabski, DA (1962) Toluene sniffing producing cerebellar degeneration. *Am J Psychiatry* 118:461–462.

Greathouse, P (1969) The union and the problem drinker. *Rehab Health* 7(1):27.

Green, M and Suffet, F (1981) The neonatal narcotic withdrawal index: A device for the improvement of care in the abstinence syndrome. *Am J Drug Alcohol Abuse* 8:203–213.

Hänninen, H, Antti-Poika, M, and Savolainen, P (1987) Psychological performance, toluene exposure and alcohol consumption in rotogravure printers. *Int Arch Occup Environ Health* 59:475–483.

Hart, JB and Wallace, J (1975) The adverse effects of amphetamines. *Clin Toxicol* 8(2):179–190.

Hunter, SM, Croft, JB, Burke, GL, et al. (1986) Longitudinal patterns of cigarette smoking and smokeless tobacco use in youth. *Am J Publ Health* 76:193–195.

Jackson, GW (ed) (1986) Substance abuse. *Semin Occup Med* (special issue) 1(4).

Johnson, S and Garzon, SR (1978) Alcohol and women. *Am J Drug Alcohol Abuse* 5:107–122.

Johnson, SF, McCarter, RJ, and Ferencz, C (1987) Changes in alcohol, cigarette and recreation drug use during pregnancy: Implications for intervension. *Am J Epidemiol* 126:695–702.

Jones, BM (1971) Verbal and spatial intelligence in short and long term alcoholics. *J Nerv Ment Dis* 153:292–297.

Juntunen, J (1982) Alcoholism in occupational neurology: Diagnostic difficulties with special reference to the neurological syndromes caused by exposure to organic solvents. *Acta Neurol Scand* 66 (Supp 92):89–108.

Kaufman E (1982) The relationship of alcoholism abuse to the abuse of other drugs. *Am J Drug Alcohol Abuse* 9:1–17.

Kelinknecht, RA, and Golstein, SG (1972) Neuropsychological deficits associated with alcoholism: A review and discussion. *Q J Stud Alcohol* 33:999–1019.

Kerr, P (1988) Crime study finds recent drug use in most arrested. *The New York Times* Jan, 22.

Kloc, JC, Boerner, U, and Becker, CE (1975) Coma, hyperthermia and bleeding associated with massive LSD overdose: A report of eight cases. *Clin Toxicol* 8(2):191–203.

Knox, JW, and Nelson, JR (1966) Permanent encephalopathy from toluene inhalation. *N Engl J Med* 275:1494–1486.

Kopin, IJ (1987) MPTP: An industrial chemical and contaminant of illicit narcotics stimulates a new era in research on Parkinson's disease. *Environ Health Perspect* 75:45–61.

Korobkin, R, Ashbury, AK, Summer, AJ, et al. (1975) Glue-sniffing neuropathy. *Arch Neurol* 32:158–162.

Kosten, TR, Gawin, FH, Rousaville, BJ, et al. (1986) Cocaine abusers among opioid addicts: Demographic and diagnostic factors in treatment. *Am J Drug Alcohol Abuse* 12:1–16.

Lachar, D, Berman, W, Grisel, JL, et al. (1976) The MacAndrew alcoholism scale as a general measure of substance misuse. *J Stud Alcohol* 37:1609–1615.

Learner, SE (1976) PCP revisited. *Clin Toxicol* 9(2):339–348.

Lings, S, Jensen, J, Christense, S, et al. (1984) Occupational accidents and alcohol. *Int Arch Occup Environ Health* 53:321–329.

Mackinnon, GL and Parker, WA (1982) Benzodiasepine withdrawal syndrome: A literature review and evaluation. *Am J Drug Alcohol Abuse* 9:19–33.

Marchiafava, E (1933) The degeneration of the brain in chronic alcoholism. *Proc R Soc Med* 26:1151.

Markey, SP, Castagnoli, N, Trevor, AJ, et al. (eds) (1986) *MPTP: A Neurotoxic Producing a Parkinsonian Syndrome.* New York: Academic Press.

Martin, TR and Bracken, MB (1987) The association between low birth weight and caffeine consumption during pregnancy. *Am J Epidemiol* 126:813–821.

Mason, P (1973) Drug users and job. *Manpower* 5(4):3.

Massengale, O and Glasser, H (1963) Physical and psychological factors in glue sniffing. *N Engl J Med* 269:1340–1344.

Matsumura, M, Inoue, N, Onishi, A, et al. (1972) Toxic polyneuropathy due to glue-sniffing. *Clin Neurol* 12:290–296.

Merry, J and Zachariadis, N (1962) Addiction to glue sniffing. *Br Med J* 2:1448.

Miller, WR (1976) Alcoholism scales and objective assessment methods: A review. *Psychol Bull* 83:649–674.

National Council on Alcoholism (1974) *A Cooperative Labor–Management Approach to Employee Alcoholism Programs.* New York: NCA.

National Institute on Alcohol Abuse and Alcoholism (1982) *Occupational Alcoholism, Monograph 8.* Washington, DC: US Government Printing Office.

National Institute of Drug Abuse. *Inhalants* [brochure]. Washington, DC: NIDA.

Parker, ES and Noble, EP (1977) Alcohol consumption and cognitive functioning in social drinkers. *J Stud Alcohol* 38:1224–1232.

Parker, WA (1982) Alcohol-containing pharmaceuticals. *Am J Drug Alcohol Abuse* 9:195–209.

Parsons, OA (1977) Neuropsychologic deficits in alcoholics: Facts and fancies. *Alcoholism* 1:51–56.

Primavera, LH and Pascal, R (1986) A comparison of male users and non-users of marijuana on the perceived harmfulness of drugs. *Am J Drug Alcohol Abuse* 12:71–77.

Rankin, JG (ed) (1975) *Alcohol, Drugs, and Brain Damage.* Toronto: Addiction Research Foundation of Ontario.

Redda, KK, Walker, CA, and Barnett, G (1989) *Cocaine, Marijuana, Designer Drugs: Chemistry, Pharmacology, and Behavior.* Boca Raton, FL: CRC Press.

Reid, LD (ed) (1988) *Opioids, Bulimia, and Alcohol Abuse and Alcoholism.* New York: Springer-Verlag.

Roads, PM, Tong, TG, Banner, W, et al. (1984) Anticholinesterase poisonings associated with commercial burdock root tea. *J Toxicol* 22:581–584.

Romano, J, Michael, M Jr, and Merritt, HH (1940) Alcoholic cerebellar degeneration. *Arch Neurol Psychiatry* 44:1230.

Rosett, HL and Weiner, L (1984) *Alcohol and the Fetus: A Clinical Perspective.* New York: Oxford University Press.

Ryall, RW (1974) Nicotine. In *Neuropoisons: Their Pathophysiological Actions, Vol 2, Poisons of Plant Origin,* LL Simpson and DR Curtis (eds) pp. 61–97. New York: Plenum Press.

Ryen, C and Butters, N (1980) Learning and memory impairments in young and old alcoholics: Evidence for the premature-aging hypothesis. *Alcoholism* 4:288–293.

Satran, R and Dodson, VN (1963) Toluene habituation: Report of a case. *N Engl J Med* 268:719–721.

Spears, RA (1986) *The Slang and Jargon of Drugs and Drinks.* Metuchen, NJ: Scarecrow Press.

Stewart, M (1987) The validity of an interview to assess a patient's drug taking. *Am J Prev Med* 3(2):95–100.

Susuki, T, Shimbo, S, Nishitani, H, et al. (1974) Muscular atrophy due to glue sniffing. *Int Arch Arbeitmed* 33:115–123.

Takenaka, S, Tawara, S, Ideta, T, et al (1972) A case with polyneuropathy due to glue sniffing. *Clin Neurol* 12:747.

Tartar, RE (1975) Psychological deficit in chronic alcoholics: A review. *Int J Addict* 10:327–368.

Taylor, P (1988) It's time to put warnings on alcohol. *The New York Times* March 20.

Taylor, S (1988) VA's denial of benefits to alcoholics is upheld. *The New York Times* April 21.

Trice, HM and Roman, PM (1979) *Spirits and Demons at Work: Alcohol and Other Drugs on the Job.* Ithaca, NY: ILR Press, Cornell University.

Wallace, L, Pellizzari, E, Hartwell, TD, et al. (1987) Exposures to benzene and other volatile compounds from active and passive smoking. *Arch Environ Health* 42(5):272–279.

Watson, RR (ed) (1989) *Diagnosis of Alcohol Abuse.* Boca Raton, FL: CRC Press.

Weingarter, H, Faillance, LA, and Markley, HG (1971) Verbal information retention in alcoholics. *QJ Stud Alcohol* 32:293–303.

Wilkinson, A (ed) (1982) *Cerebral Deficits in Alcoholism.* Toronto: Addiction Research Foundation.

Wyse, DG (1973) Deliberate inhalation of volatile hydrocarbons: A review. *CMA J* 108:71–74.

Yamada, S (1964) An occurrence of polyneuritis by *n*-hexane in polyethene laminating plants. *Jpn J Ind Health* 6:192–194.

Yamamura, Y (1969) *n*-Hexane polyneuropathy. *Fol Psychiatr Neurol Jpn* 23:45–57.

34

Mass Psychogenic Illness

A differential diagnosis sometimes needs to be made between widespread neurotoxic illness and mass psychogenic illness, a strange sociological phenomenon with which health professionals, investigators, labor leaders, and managers often have to deal. Without doubt, mass psychogenic illness is one of the most spectacular—in the literal sense—of all social behaviors. Should the reader have reservations about the reality of group behavior, the Jonestown tragedy in Guyana on November 19, 1978 (where 913 people committed suicide following a leader's command) may serve as a grim reminder.

Mass psychogenic illness tends to occur in situations where a number of people find themselves exposed to sources of strain from which no fully acceptable means of escape is available (Kerckhoff 1982). The term "psychogenic" emphasizes the psychological—more precisely, psychosociological—basis of the illness. It is labeled as such after other possible causative factors such as medical conditions, true epidemics, etc have been ruled out.

Mass psychogenic illness is an important sociological phenomenon that should be taken seriously in evaluating the possible effects of neurotoxic agents in a group. But extreme caution should be exercised. The illness is diagnosed by default when no environmental toxic conditions or other causative factors are found. As we shall soon see, such conditions may not be known at the time the phenomenon occurs.

Mass psychogenic illness has occurred throughout history, and outbreaks continue to be reported from time to time. The purpose of this chapter is to summarize present knowledge of the phenomenon and discuss current thoughts regarding the nature of the phenomenon, to review the heated controversy surrounding its very consideration as a cofactor in the onset of illness, and to show conditions favoring mass psychogenic illness at the workplace.

CONCEPTS OF HYSTERIA

Mass psychogenic illness is thought to be closely related to hysteria. Indeed, *mass hysteria* is a term commonly used to characterize outbreaks of emotionality, anxiety, excitability, sensory and motor disturbances, and vocalization occurring in groups of people. What makes hysteria unique and what has intrigued generations of scholars is somatization. *Somatization* is the accompaniment of physical conditions such as blindness, paralysis, and rashes along with the hysteria syndrome. Somatization can sometimes be produced at will, in the absence of medical explanations.

The fact that no medical conditions can be established does not mean that somatization does not have a physiological basis. Serious investigators have often avoided the scientific study of hysteria for fear of ridicule. But as we learn more about the physiology of the autonomic nervous system and brain neurotransmitters, hysteria no longer needs a physiology of its own.

"Hysteria" is a term first introduced by Hippocrates in about 400 BC. A variety of symptoms such as convulsions, twitching, shouting, muscle spasms, and paralysis were explained by sexual abstinence in unmarried women. The unsatisfied womb ("hystera" means "womb" in Greek) was thought to wander throughout the body in search of sexual satisfaction, producing the symptoms.

Modern scholars are divided in their interpretation of episodes of the Saint Vitus Dance epidemics that affected Europe in the 15th and 16th centuries as examples of mass psychogenic illness (Colligan et al. 1982). The story that supposedly explains these episodes is interesting. It tells of a curse imposed by a parish priest on peasants who were loudly celebrating Christmas, disturbing church services. They were condemned to dance without rest for a full year. Outbreaks of Saint Vitus Dance epidemics appeared in Europe in the middle ages on several occasions and were always explained as supernatural phenomena. The "medieval mind" had the irrepressible tendency to attach symbolism to anything that happened.

In the 13th century, a form of Saint Vitus Dance involving shouting and uncontrollable movements was thought to be produced by the bite of the tarantula spider. This is the origin of the name of the traditional Italian dance, the "tarantella."

Many reports still refer to outbreaks of hysteria as purely psychosocial phenomena. However, it has been known for quite some time that many episodes of Saint Vitus Dance epidemics and wild forms of behavior often

interpreted as witchcraft were actually caused by ergot poisoning. *Ergot* is a toxic substance derived from a fungus often found in rye. Some other episodes may have been caused by avitaminosis, since malnutrition has been, and still is, endemic in many regions of the world.

The concept of hysteria took an interesting turn back to its original Greek definition when Freud resurrected the concept that the illness was caused by unfulfilled sexual desires. Freud published extensively on the subject; many contemporary psychiatrists and professional psychotherapists still adhere to this interpretation.

Many hysterics are easily hypnotized; while under this state symptoms and psychological traits can be created and made to disappear with ease. The concept of *suggestibility* is of paramount importance in linking hysteria—as applied to a given individual—to social phenomena such as mass psychogenic illness. Individual susceptibility and psychological explanations of contagion are at the top of the modern interpretation of mass psychogenic illness.

Modern sociobiology has produced some information that may be relevant to the explanation of mass psychogenic illness. For instance, it seems that social animals, including humans, have never lost the capacity to relate to each other through behavioral patterns, visual cues, and even chemical signals. Lorenz and Tinbergen spent their lifetimes observing how animals use these cues to regulate their behavior (Gould 1982). Members of an ant nest, for example, emit chemical signals that serve to trigger behaviors in other members of their social community.

Mass psychogenic illness has been the domain of philosophers, theologians, physicians, biologists, sociologists, psychologists, and mass media analysts. It has only on rare occasions received the emotionally neutral treatment that other life phenomena have received. It has suffered from both excessive attention and oblivion, yet it is unfailingly rediscovered in every generation. In spite of this, it is fair to say that a convincing explanation of mass psychogenic illness is lacking. Even reputable scholars accept that theories of mass psychogenic illness are ex post facto explanations of fleeting, confusing, and difficult-to-study real events.

CURRENT PERSPECTIVES ON MASS PSYCHOGENIC ILLNESS

Background and Causative Factors

There are circumstances and promoting conditions that have been described in the relatively few good publications on mass psychogenic illness. The following has been abstracted from a variety of sources and review articles but is not intended as a checklist.

Mass psychogenic illness involves:

- Large numbers of people
- Generally, young females in their early teens and 20s
- Individuals who are linked by bonds of friendship or work-related associations
- Workers of low economic status and poor job satisfaction
- Conditions of stress, particularly where limiting rules for acceptable behavior are imposed
- A sudden onset, appearing with little or no warning
- At times, a stimulus or circumscribed event (real or imaginary)
- A high degree of "infection": it spreads very quickly within facilities or in neighboring facilities where similar circumstances exist
- A high rate of repeats
- Subsidence within a week or two
- An additive factor of local customs or folklore
- Psychological measures, such as firm authoritative stands taken by management, that are not very effective (indeed, they sometimes aggravate the situation)
- A triggering agent that is a real or ima-

ginary presence of a physical or biological agent; attempts to interpret the situation as a purely psychological phenomenon are quickly dismissed as scientifically unsound

Modes of Presentation

The prevailing modes of presentation are hysterical seizures, nausea, dizziness, fainting, trance states, and spells of fright. Table 34.1 is a brief summary of episodes interpreted by various authors as indicative of mass psychogenic illness.

Contributing Factors

Colligan and Murphy (1982) define mass psychogenic illness as a "collective occurrence of physical symptoms and related beliefs among two or more persons in the absence of an identifiable pathogen." The explanation for its occurrence varies from relatively straightforward observations of job characteristics to elaborate sociological or biological theories (to be reviewed below). Explanations based on job conditions are noteworthy.

Job stress is a recurrent factor. Colligan and Murphy (1982) state that mass psychogenic illness tends to be present in situations where the job is boring and repetitive with little opportunity for advancement. To this they add work pressure, physical stress, unresolved problems in labor–management relationships, and lack of communication between workers and management. The illness tends to appear where the psychological environment is "... formally structured involving well-defined roles and regimentations." Finally, the affected tend to have a history of absenteeism.

The psychosocial explanations of mass psychogenic illness are intriguing. It is thought to be a form of **crowd response**, "... some sort of emotional identification with others in the same settings" so that one person's experience becomes meaningful to others (Kerckhoff 1982). The contagion is thought

Table 34.1. Some Examples of Mass Psychogenic Illness

Source	Setting	Symptoms	Trigger
Chew 1978	Television assembly plant in Singapore	Screaming, fainting, fear, anxiety, trance state, violent acts	No apparent trigger ("spirit possession")
Chew 1978	Dry cuttlefish factory in Singapore	Screaming, crying, violent acts	Visions of black man with hairy arms trying to frighten people
Chew 1978	Camera manufacturing plant in Singapore	Headaches, screaming, fainting, crying, violent acts	No apparent trigger
Chew 1978	Telecommunication facility in Singapore	Fainting, screaming, violent acts	No apparent trigger
Chew 1978	Ballbearing plant in Singapore	Dizziness, nausea, fainting, watery eyes	Acidic odor
Kerckhoff and Back 1968	Dressmaking plant in southern USA	Nausea, skin rash, fainting, headaches, weakness	Bug bite
Maguire 1978	Ceramics factory in northern England	Skin rash on face, neck and forearms	Ceramics
Maguire 1978	Large textile plant in northern England	Eye and skin irritation	Dyes used in nylon fabric
McEvedy 1966	Textile plant in Midlands (England)	Dizziness, blurred vision, stomach complaints	No apparent trigger
NIOSH HHE 78-116-557	Garment storage warehouse in eastern USA	Headache, lightheadedness, dry mouth, sleepiness, dizziness	Foul odor
NIOSH-HHE 77-27-437	Lawn furniture assembly plant in midwestern USA	Headache, bad taste in mouth, dizziness, lightheadedness	Strange odor
Sheppart and Kroes, 1975	Garment manufacturing plant in southwestern USA	Respiratory irritation, headaches, muscle weakness, nausea	Strange odor
Stahl and Lebedum, 1974	University data processing center in midwestern USA	Nausea, vomiting, dizziness, fainting	Strange odor

Adapted from Colligan and Murphy (1982).

563

to be ". . . the spread of affect or behavior from group member to member, one person serving as [the] stimulus for the imitative act of another" (Colligan and Murphy 1982). Thus, many sociologists and psychologists postulate that mass psychogenic illness is a normal sociological phenomenon of a normal population under conditions of physical or psychological stress.

Theories of Contagion of Mass Psychogenic Illness.   Since the late 19th century, several theories have been proposed to explain why large groups of people display "crowding behavior" (ie, act as a unit rather than as individuals). The core of these theories is the explanation of the *contagion:* the mechanisms and the conditions under which crowding behavior occurs. Most of the theories have been proposed by sociologists and social psychologists trained in traditional schools. What follows is based on a lucid review article by Freedman (1982).

The term contagion was proposed by LeBon in 1895 to explain "why in a mob, all the people tend to feel and behave the same way." LeBon argued that ". . . the emotions and actions of one person spread through the group." He is also credited with the observation that ". . . in a mob people behave in ways they would not have if they were alone." These thoughts gave rise to the development of social psychology as we know it today.

Early sociology was founded on biology, particularly on the observations of the behavior of social animals. These foundations were dismissed by many generations of American sociologists who preferred to interpret social phenomena in human terms. Sociobiologists, inspired by ethology, a branch of biology created by Lorenz and Tinbergen, put sociology back among the natural sciences (Gould 1982). In both cases—the biological and sociological interpretations— scientists contend that the proper unit of analysis is not the individual's behavior but that of the group to which he/she belongs.

According to Friedman (1967), contagion is a term closely related to social conformity and emergent norms. *Conformity* describes a situation in which a person tends to do what other members of the group do. The underlying mechanism is social pressure. *Emergent norms* is the tendency of a group to behave in a similar manner: the social norm. The group establishes a particular form of behavior as both acceptable and desirable.

Freud (1940) explained that the group releases primitive impulses by suppressing the individual's restraints. These thoughts have been invoked to explain why a group is likely to engage in aggressive or other forms of antisocial behavior.

Another important concept is that of *anonymity of behavior,* the idea than anonymity frees people to worry less about the consequences of their actions.

Friedman has proposed an important theoretical approach that, although based on pure sociological theory, is not likely to be dismissed by sociobiologists: the concept of *critical crowd density.* "Increased density (ie, less space available per person) tends to intensify people's reactions to one another. . . . As density increases, other people become a salient aspect of the environment. The actions of others are likely to be noticed and to impinge on the individual, and therefore reactions are magnified" (Friedman 1967).

THE EPIDEMIOLOGY OF MASS PSYCHOGENIC ILLNESS

Mass Psychogenic Illness in Classical Occupational Medicine

In Alice Hamilton's autobiography, an interesting account is given of both a real neurotoxic disease of epidemic proportions and mass psychogenic illness that occurred in Russia at the beginning of this century.

I was reminded of an interesting incident in a rubber factory during the Czarist days which was related by a Russian doctor, Dworetsky, in 1914 in a German medical journal, since he was forbidden to publish it in Russia. He tells of a mysterious outbreak of illness among women working with rubber solution in a large factory in St. Petersburg. A new solvent had been introduced, and, soon after, many of the women began to complain of headache, dizziness, nervousness, some were greatly excited, some fainted, others had epileptoid convulsions. The foremen evidently did nothing sensible about it, and by the end of four days 231 had been affected. The tale spread and with it the rumor that the employers were starting a wholesale murder of the workers, so then the sickness spread to the women in chocolate and tobacco factories. The employers lost their tempers and declared a lockout, whereupon the Duma voted an emergency fund for the thousands thus turned out in the depth of the winter. Naturally the doctors were much interested and eager to discover whether this was really an instance of intoxication by a volatile solvent or only mass hysteria, but they were not allowed to find out, for the chief of police stepped in, declared that it was all the work of radical agitators, forbade any discussion of the subject by a group larger than three, and refused to let the Duma distribute any relief. The factories were reopened after the workers had been brought to a proper state of meekness, and the incident was closed. About the same time a similar situation developed in rubber works in Moscow and in Riga, where a quiet investigation revealed the illness to be acute benzol intoxication, for the new cement had been made with almost pure benzol. The illness in the chocolate and tobacco factories was undoubtedly hysterical (Hamilton 1943, pp. 333–334.)

Sick Building Syndrome

The term "sick building syndrome" is used to describe symptoms associated with the occupation of sealed buildings—that is, those that depend on air conditioning for normal ventilation. Symptoms that have been related to this syndrome include blocked and runny nose, dry and itchy eyes, dryness of the throat, lethargy, headache, and sometimes wheezing and breathlessness.

Sick building syndrome and mass psychogenic illness are sometimes related. Episodes of mass psychogenic illness can occur in large, impersonal, and confined office buildings.

In recent years, there have been attempts to characterize the sick building syndrome. Burgue and collaborators (1987) performed a study involving 4373 office workers—one of the largest ever reported in the literature. They found that the mean number of work-related symptoms was significantly greater in females than males (3.66 versus 2.75 symptoms out of a possible 10 symptoms). Furthermore, symptoms were greatest in clerical and secretarial workers (3.65), followed by technical or professional workers (2.85) and managers (2.50). Overall, buildings with ventilation from local or central air conditioning had more work-related symptoms per worker than buildings that relied on natural or mechanical ventilation. The most common work-related symptom was lethargy (57%), closely followed by blocked nose (47%), dry throat (46%), and headache (46%). The authors of this study argue that symptoms of building sickness are widespread and not necessarily related to a few problem buildings. As has been shown by many previous studies, the design characteristics of buildings and plants are associated with substantial differences in the reported frequencies of symptoms in those working in those buildings.

Significance of Group Phenomena in the Study of Neurotoxic Effects

Mass psychogenic illness is difficult to study scientifically. It is unfortunate that epidemiologists, sociologists, and biologists do not meet more frequently to appreciate each other's potential contributions to the understanding of this phenomenon. Epidemiologists take the individual as the primary datum of information and reconstruct the group by a process of aggregation.

Anyone with a basic knowledge of the history of behavioral sciences recognizes the background against which Gestalt psychology was established: a reaction against the atomism of early psychologists inspired by the physical sciences. There is, in fact, ample documentation today to establish that the group is an adequate unit of analysis. The source of this truism is not only sociological research but also top-rated biological observations. **Mass psychogenic illness should not be ruled out as a causative agent even if a neurotoxic agent is found in the environment or the workplace.**

Health scientists and investigators are painfully aware of the consequences of wrong judgments when dealing with mass psychogenic illness. Is it a neurotoxic disease or a case of mass psychogenic illness? The consequences of confusing the two are serious. Consider these scenarios: a group of health scientists loses credibility if an epidemic thought to be a case of mass psychogenic illness is found later to be caused by an unknown virus or a new chemical substance; a group of workers and labor leaders may find themselves in a very embarrassing situation before the mass media if, after months of militant demands that a toxic agent be studied, the "toxic agent" is found to be a classic case of "agent X" sometimes associated with mass psychogenic illness.

Statistically speaking, it is commonly agreed among experts that mass psychogenic illness is the exception rather than the rule as an explanation of human behavior in the workplace. But its potential to be used as a rationale for not acting on a neurotoxic threat is always present. This is possibly why it took so long for behavioral toxicology to be accepted as a serious discipline in the United States: often, neurotoxic effects are dismissed as sociological phenomena. Populations affected by serious stressful conditions find an escape in real or imaginary neurotoxic agents. "Neither employees nor management . . . (to which I add scientists and health officers) . . . are currently equipped to deal with mass psychogenic illness" (Colligan and Murphy 1982).

REFERENCES

Burgue, S, Hedge, A, Wilson, S, et al. (1987) Sick building syndrome: A study of 4,373 office workers. *Ann Occup Hyg* 31:493–504.

Colligan, MJ and Murphy, LR (1982) A review of mass psychogenic illness in work settings. In *Mass Psychogenic Illness: A Social Psychological Analysis*, MJ Colligan, JW Pennebaker, and LR Murphy (eds) pp. 33–52. Hillsdale, NJ: Lawrence Erlbaum Associates.

Colligan, MJ, Pennebaker, JW, and Murphy, LR (eds)(1982) *Mass Psychogenic Illness: A Social Psychological Analysis*. Hillsdale, NJ: Lawrence Erlbaum Associates.

Freedman, JL (1982) Theories of contagion as they relate to mass psychogenic illness. In *Mass Psychogenic Illness: A Social Psychological Analysis*, MJ Colligan, JW Pennebaker, and LR Murphy (eds) pp. 199–215. Hillsdale, NJ: Lawrence Erlbaum Associates.

Freud, S (1940) *An Outline of Psychoanalysis*. New York: WW Norton.

Friedman, TI (1967) Methodological considerations and research needs in the study of epidemic hysteria. *Am J Publ Health* 57:2009–2011.

Gould, JL (1982) *Ethology: The Mechanisms and Evolution of Behavior*. New York: WW Norton.

Hamilton, A (1943) *Exploring the Dangerous Trades*. Boston: Little, Brown.

Kerckhoff, AC (1982) A social psychological view of mass psychogenic illness. In *Mass Psychogenic Illness: A Social Psychological Analysis*, MJ Colligan, JW Pennebaker, and LR Murphy (eds) pp. 199–215. Hillsdale, NJ: Lawrence Erlbaum Associates.

SUGGESTED READINGS

Ackerman, SE and Lee, RLM (1978) Mass hysteria and spirit possession in urban Malaysia: A case study. *J Sociol Psychol* 1:24–35.

Araki, S and Honma, T (1986) Mass psychogenic system illness in school children in relation to the Tokyo photochemical smog. *Arch Environ Health* 41:159–162.

Barger, G (1931) *Ergot and Ergotism*. London: Gurney and Jackson.

Bove, FJ (1970) *The Story of Ergot*. Basel: S Karger.

Chang, M and Kee, WC (1983) Epidemic hysteria: A study of high risk factors. *Occup Health Safety* 52:550–564.

Chan, OY, Zee, KO, and Wong, CK (1979) High risk factors in Singapore factory workers. *Occup Health Safety* 48:58–60.

Colligan MJ and Murphy, LR (1979) Mass psychogenic illness in organizations: An overview. *J Occup Psychol* 52:77–90.

Colligan, MJ and Smith, MJ (1978) A methodological approach for evaluating outbreaks of mass psychogenic illness in industry. *J Occup Med* 20:401–402.

Donnell, HD, Bagby, JR, Harmon, RG, et al. (1989) Report of an illness outbreak at the Harry S Truman state building. *Am J Epidemiol* 129(3):550–558.

Faust, HS and Brilliant, LB (1981) Is the diagnosis of "mass hysteria" an excuse for incomplete investigation of low-level environmental contamination? *J Occup Med* 23:22–26.

Finnegan, MJ, Pickering, CAC, and Burge, PS (1984) Sick building syndrome: Prevalence studies. *Br Med J* 289:1573–1575.

Friedman, AP (1979) Ergotism. In *Handbook of Clinical Neurology, Vol 22: Intoxications of the Nervous System*. Amsterdam: North Holland.

Galanter, M (1989) *Cults: Faith, Healing and Coercion*. New York: Oxford University Press.

Grant, IWB (1985) The sick building syndrome. *Br Med J* 290:321.

Kerckhoff, AC and Back, KW (1968) *The June Bug: A Story of Hysterical Contagion*. New York: Appleton-Century-Crofts.

Kiesler, S and Finholt, T (1988) The mystery of RSI. *Am Psychol* 43(12):1004–1015.

Landrigan, PJ and Miller, B (1983) The Arjenyattah epidemic: Home interview data and toxicological aspects. *Lancet* 2:1474–1476.

Lieber, EG (1970) On contaminated cereals as a cause of epidemics. *Bull Hist Med* 44:332–345.

Mackay, C (undated) *Extraordinary Popular Delusions and the Madness of Crowds*. New York: Barnes and Noble.

Markusch, RE (1973) Mental epidemics; A review of the old to prepare for the new. *Publ Health Rev* 2:353–442.

McLeod, WR (1975) Merphos poisoning or mass panic? *Aust NA J Psychiatry* 9(4):225–229.

Modan, R, Swartz, TA, Tirosh, M et al. (1983) The Arjenyattah epidemic: Spread and triggering factors. *Lancet* 2:1472–1474.

Murphy, LR and Colligan, MJ (1979) Mass psychogenic illness in a shoe factory: A case report. *Int Arch Occup Environ Health* 44:133–138.

Nitzkin, JL (1976) Epidemic transient situational disturbance in an elementary school. *J Florida Med Assoc* 63:357–359.

Small, GW and Borus, JF (1983) Outbreak of illness in a school chorus: Toxic poisoning or mass hysteria. *N Engl J Med* 308:623–635.

Stahl, SM and Lebedum, M (1974) Mystery gas: An analysis of mass hysteria. *J Health Soc Behav* 15:44–50.

Tan, ES (1963) Epidemic hysteria. *Med J Malaya* 43:72–76.

Veith, I (1965) *Hysteria: The History of a Disease*. Chicago: University of Chicago Press.

Woon, TH (1976) Epidemic hysteria in a Malaysian Chinese extended family. *Med J Malaysia* 31:108–112.

35

Neurotoxic Agents in Chemical Warfare

The use of neurotoxic agents and naturally occurring neurotoxins as weapons represents one of the most frightening chapters of modern history, and yet this topic is rarely mentioned in professional toxicological literature. It is hard to know the reason for this, but some potential explanations are that: the story of chemical and biological warfare has been covered in mass media, and therefore the subject matter is perceived as unfit for serious treatment in scientific and technical publications; the use of chemical and biological weapons has been shrouded in mystery—one is apt to err trying to cover material about which so little is known (in fact, many of the documents on this subject are likely to be classified, and many sources of information are known to have been destroyed); there may be some who adhere to the illusion that morality and scientific knowledge are intimately related. For many of us, it is unthinkable that top scientists have devoted their talents (and still do) to the destruction of human lives under any type of euphemism, including war deterrence.

THE RISE OF CHEMICAL WEAPONS

A U.S. Government document published in 1985 described how chemical weapons de-liver agents that react with human tissue, chemically changing it in a way that injures or kills. Like the radiation effect of nuclear weapons—as opposed to the heat and blast associated with the nuclear explosion—chemical weapons attack the physiology rather than the external anatomy of the body.

Chemical and bacteriological warfare has a long history, but the first use of chemicals and other biological agents to kill thousands still lies in the memory of some. Chemical warfare was born precisely on the 22nd of April in 1915 in the village of Langemarck, near Ypres, Belgium (Harris and Paxman 1982) (Fig. 35.1). After a long-lasting confrontation with the German army, thousands of Allied soldiers (French reservists and Algerians from French former colonies) were killed by chlorine gas. The gas, delivered by opening the valves of 6000 cylinders, spread along a 4-mile front. The new "experiment" with chemical weapons resulted in 5000 men dead and 10,000 wounded.

Chlorine gas was used many times during World War I by both the Germans and the Allies. Soon enough ". . . a pattern was established which was to persist to the end of the war: The Germans would initiate the use of a new gas to try to break through; it would fail, be copied by the Allies, and the cycle would repeat itself" (Harris and Paxman

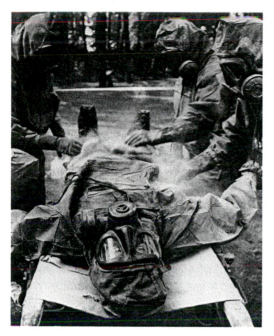

Fig. 35.1. Decontaminating a casualty during British exercises in Germany during World War I. (From Harris and Paxman 1982)

1982). Gas readiness was an integral part of training in both military and civilian programs on both sides.

Types of Chemical Weapons

According to the most recent sources on the subject (U.S. Government 1985), chemical weapons can be classified according to the way they are dispersed, the way they attack the body, and the length of time they remain able to attack the body. Although the term "poison gas" continues to be used in the literature, not all chemical weapons are gases. The term poison gas is a grim reminder of gases (eg, chlorine, mustard, phosgene) that were used during World War I. Other chemical weapons include liquids, sprays, and vapors.

There are essentially three types of chemical weapons: *blister agents* (eg, mustard gas, Lewisite) burn body surfaces and kill through secondary effects of blistering on the respiratory system; *blood agents* (eg, hydrogen cyanide, cyanogen chloride) attack blood cells, preventing the normal uptake of oxygen; and *nerve agents* (eg, Tabun, Sarin, Soman, V agents) attack the chemical process of neurotransmission, particularly on the autonomic nervous system. Nerve agents developed in the 1930s and 1940s acted through the respiratory system, whereas those created in the 1950s act by absorption through the skin.

In scientific and technical literature, nerve agents are known as acetylcholinesterase agents (of which organophosphorus compound pesticides are one family) because the first nerve agents bound to acetylcholinesterase, the enzyme that breaks down the neurotransmitter acetylcholine after its release; however, other nerve agents developed after World War II probably involve other mechanisms and neurotransmitters and other neurobiological principles.

During World War I many of these substances were often known by code names. (Chemical weapons were ready for use but were not actually delivered in World War II.) Code names continue to be attached to these and other weapons. For example, persistent nerve agents developed in the mid-1950s that are absorbed through the skin are known as "V agents."

Another class of neurotoxic weapons are the *bacteriological weapons* (also known as biological or toxin weapons). These are living organisms that are used to cause death or incapacitation [eg, anthrax, botulism, plague, mycotoxins (toxins produced by fungi)].

In recent years, it has been suggested that human research on volunteers was carried out with many other neurotoxic agents including strychnine, arsenicals, and LSD. The rest of this chapter is devoted to a discussion of nerve agents only. The well-researched book by Harris and Paxman (1982) contains a comprehensive treatment of chemical and bacteriological warfare and the prospects of genetic engineering for a new family of chemical weapons.

NEUROTOXIC AGENTS USED IN CHEMICAL WARFARE

The vast majority of nerve agents are based on the pharmacological action of anticholinesterase. Acetylcholinesterase inhibitors increase the duration of the effects of endogenous acetylcholine at the cholinergic receptor sites by blocking its removal by hydrolysis. Nerve agents were discovered while trying to develop more powerful insecticides.

Deployment

Nerve agents can be delivered by any usual munition: bombs, artillery and mortar shells, mines, rockets, missiles, and spray tanks. The concept of *binary weapons* was developed during World War II. Briefly, these weapons consist of two nonlethal chemical components stored in separate compartments. The chemical compound contained in each compartment becomes lethal when the two are combined on impact. Binary weapons are a practical solution to many problems originally associated with the manufacture, transportation, and deployment of neurotoxic weapons. By using nonlethal components, the danger to nonintended victims is minimized.

Chemical poisoning is an ancient art. There are many well-documented episodes in spy confrontations in which neurotoxic agents have been delivered to individuals in a manner that serves as inspiration for mystery novels and television programs.

Protection

Protection against nerve agents is difficult. Chemical weapons, depending on conditions such as wind direction, affect victims and aggressors on an equal basis. Mask protection is known to be adequate for nerve agents in gas form. Whole-body protection is required for the V family of nerve agents, since the neurotoxic agent can be absorbed through the skin. The use of such cumbersome equipment makes simple operations such as carrying gear extremely difficult.

CURRENT DEBATES AND MORAL ISSUES

The use of poison gas was specifically outlawed by the The Hague Declaration of 1899, where it was agreed that certain methods of combat where outside the scope of "civilized" warfare. As stated above, the use of chemical weapons began in 1915. The reaction against their use at that time was universal; since then there have been many meetings attempting to ban their use. The Geneva Protocol of 1925 was signed by 38 powers, and this document supposedly is still in effect. The conference leading to the Geneva Protocol was led by the United States in hope of reducing the "barbarity of modern warfare" (Harris and Paxman 1982). In 1969, under the Nixon administration, the United States unilaterally ceased the production of chemical weapons.

At the moment of this writing debate continues as to whether the United States should continue the manufacture and stockpiling of nerve agents as a deterrent against a similar buildup in other countries. The progress of this debate is likely to be followed in the mass media.

Chemical weapons were once considered to be a humane form of killing. In fact, the title of a superb book by Harris and Paxman is *A Higher Form of Killing,* a phrase supposedly used by Professor Fritz Haber, pioneer of gas warfare, while receiving the Nobel Prize for Chemistry in 1919.

More recently, the use of chemical and biological agents in warfare has been called "public health in reverse." It is important that the story of the use of chemical weapons in the past 70 years be retold time and again and the gruesome physiological effects of chemical weapons be known by scientists and laypersons alike. Educated decisions on the offensive use of chemical weapons and the need to have deterrents need to be made by people of all nations.

REFERENCES

Harris, R and Paxman, J (1982) *A Higher Form of Killing: The Secret Story of Chemical and Biological Warfare*. New York: Hill and Wang.

US Government (1985) *Report of the Chemical Warfare Review Commission, June 1985*. Washington, DC: US Government Printing Office.

SUGGESTED READINGS

Bodansky, O (1945) Contributions of medical research in chemical warfare to medicine. *Science* 102:517.

Blum, A (1984) Chemical weapons: A question of morality. *NY State J Med* 84(3, part 2):104–105.

Brooks, FR, Ebner, DG, Xenakis, SN, et al. (1983) Psychological reactions during chemical warfare training. *Milit Med* 148(3):232–235.

Cecil, PF (1986) *Herbicidal Warfare: The Ranch Hand Project in Vietnam*. New York: Praeger.

Dickson, D (1986) Approval seen for new US chemical weapons. *Science* 232:567–568.

Dickson, D (1988) Hopes recede for early ban on chemical arms. *Science* 240:22–23.

Directorate for Scientific and Technical Intelligence of the Defense Intelligence Agency (1985) *Soviet Chemical Weapons Threat, DST-1620F-051-85*. Washington, DC: Defense Intelligence Agency.

Douglass, JD and Livingstone, NC (1987) *America the Vulnerable: The Threat of Chemical and Biological Warfare*. Lexington, MA: Lexington (Heath).

Grob, D (1956) The manifestation and treatment of poisoning due to nerve gas and other organic phosphate anticholinesterase compounds. *AMA Arch Intern Med* 98:221–239.

Grob, D and Harvey, AM (1953) The effects and treatment of nerve gas poisoning. *Am J Med* 14:52–63.

Grob, D and Harvey, AM (1958) Effects in man of the anticholinesterase compound sarin (isopropyl methyl phosphonofluoridate). *J Clin Invest* 37:350–368.

Haber, LF (1986) *The Poisonous Cloud: Chemical Warfare in the First World War*. New York: Oxford University Press.

Heller, CE (1985) *Chemical Warfare in World War I: The American Experience 1917–1918*. Fort Leavenworth, KS: Combat Studies Institute.

Hooper, RR (1983) The covert use of chemical and biological use against United States Strategic Forces. *Milit Med* 148(12):901–902.

Horgan, J (1988) Poisoning the air: The US resumes production of lethal nerve-gas weapons. *Sci Am* 258(3):17–18.

Keller, B (1989) Soviets report use of toxic gas in putting down strife in Georgia. *The New York Times* April 20.

Lubasch, AH (1987) $700,000 award is made in '53 secret test death: The patient was not told he was used in a chemical warfare experiment. *The New York Times* May 6, p. B3.

McDonald, A (1985) Ethics and editors: When should unethical research be published? *Canad Med Assoc J* 133:803–805.

Meselson, M and Robinson JP (1980) Chemical warfare and chemical disarmament. *Sci Am* 242(4):38–47.

Rothshield, JH (1964) *Tomorrow's Weapons*. New York: McGraw-Hill.

SIPRI (Stockholm International Peace Research Institute) *Delayed Toxic Effects of Chemical Warfare Agents*. New York: Almquist and Wiksell.

Spiers, EM (1986) *Chemical Warfare*. Urbana, IL: University of Illinois Press.

Sun, M (1988) EPA bars use of Nazi data. *Science* 240:21.

36

Environmental and Occupational Neurotoxicology and the Changing Concept of "Quality of Life"

Behavioral toxicology is defined as the study of the effects of toxic agents on behavior and the use of behavioral methods for the monitoring of toxic substances in the environment and the workplace. This discipline seems to have existed in Europe without a name as early as 1930. In the Introduction to this book I argued that one can view the birth of behavioral toxicology merely as a novel approach in toxicological evaluation or as an expression of social changes—particularly changes in views about occupational health. Although this book is devoted to reviewing the scientific basis of environmental and occupational neurotoxicology as a novel toxicological approach, it would be incomplete if the social (and even moral) context of this discipline were not mentioned.

From the sociological point of view, behavioral toxicology was born when, as a result of more than 200 years of social turmoil, some dating back to the Industrial Revolution, the concept of the "quality of life" changed. Standards of quality of life changed from a fatalistic, unchallenged, even accepted view that death may result from one's job to the successful plea that dangerous workplace conditions—including psychological factors—should be seriously considered.

Abbott (1988), in *The Systems of Professions: An Essay on the Division of Labor,* wrote:

In the mid- to late-nineteenth-century America, there was no general conception of problems of living. Nor were angst and maladjustment subjectively real categories of experience. To the extent that such things were experienced at all, they were construed within a vague cultural category of everyday life problems. People might have family or marital quarrels, career difficulties, financial problems, "disappointed affections," chronic minor illness, or even be generally unhappy. But these were seen as diverse exigencies of life, not as forces shaping the quality of life or as encroachments preventing individuals reaching some highest levels of personal functioning, as they do today. A notion of careers, career success, and career contingencies had coalesced at this time, but the ideas of personal adjustment and self-realization had not emerged, under any label.

QUALITY OF LIFE

Societal Perception of Quality of Life and Prevention of Neurotoxic Illnesses

Quality of life and health are intimately related. It is difficult to conceive of the "good" life along with poor health. Neurotoxic agents are particularly pernicious; they may even hamper our ability to make intelligent decisions about our lives by affecting our brains.

In many societies, though, human beings are still a commodity that can be spared. And when we need to count bodies, who cares about changes in motor dexterity, cognition, and feelings resulting from neurotoxic agents in the environment and the workplace that we sometimes cannot even see? Quality of life and health depends on societal goals, and these goals have changed throughout time; prevention of neurotoxic illness in the environment and the workplace seems to be a higher form of prophylaxis. It looks as if this sort of luxury is a valid societal (or health) goal only where other preventable and curable deadly diseases have been eradicated or are almost absent. Thus, it is possible to argue that in underdeveloped countries—which, parenthetically, comprise the vast majority of the world's countries—prevention of neurotoxic illness has a low priority at best.

We thus have to conclude that it is probably not possible to develop a discipline that has an immediate global significance. Curiously, at international meetings, the very subject that has not been discussed is how behavioral toxicology—and later E & O neurotoxicology—fills societal goals. For example, a local health officer fighting for the eradication of malaria or AIDS in a given country might resent, to say the least, implementation of research programs on behavioral toxicology; similarly, a physician fighting endemic plumbism among children may find it frivolous to test their IQs.

Prevention of neurotoxic illness in the environment and the workplace can thus be conceived as representing the highest stage of an evolution in our thinking about disease prevention. The sad conclusion is that not many countries around the world can afford such a luxury.

The Dollar Value of One's Life

Even in countries such as the United States, where the plea for a healthy environment is understood, things in the environment and the workplace that affect our minds and behavior have a lower priority than, say, things that affect our heart or lungs. We can attach a dollar value to life (as insurers do); but how can we attach a dollar value to an externally caused diminution of our intellect, the quality of our performance, or the narrowing range of our feelings?

Although we may view the mere question of determining the dollar value of life with disdain, since ancient times societies have created systems of compensation for injuries and deaths. The Babylonian Code of Hammurabi and other ancient and medieval laws, for example, contained such a system. On the American continent, the Aztecs had a similar system. Greer (1985) has written a short and enlightening review of the different methods used by societies, insurance agents, economists, legal experts, scientists, and agency administrators to assign monetary values according to different formulas.

One well-known method of calculating the value of a life is by evaluating the chemical elements a human being contains—carbon, hydrogen, oxygen, nitrogen, calcium, phosphorus, potassium, sulfur, sodium, magnesium, and some traces of iron, copper, and iodine. In 1990 on a chemical basis, the body is worth about $10. Another method is to estimate the street value of human life, namely, the amount of money paid in a contract murder. The price is variously quoted at $50 to $5000 or more.

In a more serious vein, life insurance calculations must determine what people would have earned had they lived, that is, the economic value of an individual. This is usually determined by considering the individual's earning power over the course of his or her working life. Airplane victims' families are compensated by this method and can recover between $300,000 and $500,000 with isolated cases in the millions of dollars. In 1985, the Federal Aviation Administration estimated human life at about $650,000 for compensation purposes. For a given individual, the Environmental Protection Agency chooses a number between $400,000 and $7 million, whereas the Occupational Safety and Health Administration scale ranges from $2 million to $5 million.

Other formulas are based on the perceived risks of different occupations. For example, in high-risk industries such as mining and oil-rig drilling, human life has a price tag of about $600,000. Interestingly, though—and for reasons that are not always clear—white-collar workers in what is generally considered the relative safety of city offices may get between $7 million to $10 million.

Environmental exposures, disasters, and occupational accidents involving neurotoxic agents have created new challenges. The issues related to compensation for cancer and death associated with exposure to chemicals or agents such as asbestos in the environment and the workplace are at present an active source of debate (Kimbrough and Simonds 1986).

Monetary Compensation for Neuropsychological Impairment

How long will it take to develop compensation policies dealing with permanent neuropsychological damage? What would be adequate compensation to a young victim of a long-lasting behavioral or psychological impairment, such as mental retardation, associated with methylmercury poisoning in the womb (such as that caused in Minamata disease)? What if chronic, low-level exposures to solvents are proved to accelerate neuropsychological impairment and cause dementia in middle-aged workers?

It is hoped that these topics will someday also be a source of active debate.

REFERENCES

Abbott, A (1988) The Systems of Professions: An Essay on the Division of Labor. Chicago: University of Chicago Press.

Greer, WR (1985) Value of one life? From $837 to $10 million. The New York Times June 26.

Kimbrough, RD and Simonds, M (1986) Compensation of victims exposed to environmental pollutants. Arch Environ Health 41(3):185–189.

SUGGESTED READINGS

Bloom, BR (1988) A new threat to world health. Science 239:9.

Daniel, TC (1990) Measuring the quality of natural environment. Am Psychol 45(5):633–637.

Demick, J and Wapner, S (1990) Role of psychological science in promoting environmental quality. Am Psychol 45(5):631–632.

Emshwiller, JR (1988) California ushers in environmental law placing warning levels [sic] on 29 substances. The Wall Street Journal February 23.

Hardison, NM and Vanier DJ (1976) Environment and quality of life: Attitudinal measurement and analysis. Psychol Rep 39(3, Part 1):959–965.

Howe, HL (1988) A comparison of actual and perceived residential proximity to toxic waste sites. Arch Environ Health 43(6):415–419.

Jacobs, S, Evans, GW, Catalano, R, et al. (1984) Air pollution and depressive symptomatology: Exploratory analysis of intervening psychosocial factors. Popul Environ Behav Soc Issues 7(4):260–272.

Levenson, H (1973) Perception of environmental modifiability and involvement in antipollution activities. J Psychol 84(2):237–239.

Nelkin, D (1983) Workers at risk. Science 222:125.

New York Times (1988) "The Environment: US and Soviet Groups Joining for Quality of Life." December 12.

Peck, DL (ed) (1989) Psychosocial Effects of Hazardous Toxic Waste Disposal on Communities. Springfield, IL: Charles C Thomas.

Samuels, SW (1986) *The Environment of the Workplace and Human Values*. New York: Alan R Liss.

Selikoff, IJ (1984) Twenty lessions from asbestos: A bitter harvest of scientific information. *EPA* 10(4):21–24.

Weir, D (1986) *The Bhopal Syndrome: Pesticide Manufacturing and the Third World*. Penang, Malaysia: International Organization of Consumers Unions. (1981)

Weir, D and Schapiro, M (1981) *Circle of Poison: Pesticides and People in a Hungry World*. San Francisco, CA: Institute for Food and Development Policy.

EPILOGUE

Environmental & Occupational Neurotoxicology as a Profession

Neurotoxicology is a discipline that studies the effects of chemical compounds on the nervous system. Its two major objectives are (1) the evaluation, diagnosis, treatment, and prevention of neurological dysfunctions caused by toxic agents in humans, and (2) the study of how neurotoxic compounds cause their effects.

Over the years, several overlapping specialties within the field of neurotoxicology have emerged. There are professionals who deal with the clinical evaluation of single individuals affected by neurotoxic agents (clinical neurotoxicology); the evaluation of health effects caused by toxic agents among large human groups (neuroepidemiology); the evaluation of the environment where people live and work (industrial hygiene); the study of the effects of neurotoxic agents in ecological systems (environmental toxicology); the experimental study of neurotoxic agents in laboratory animals (experimental animal neurotoxicology); the experimental study of neurotoxic agents in human volunteers (experimental human neurotoxicology); and, finally, the compilation of existing knowledge for legislation and law enforcement (meta-analysis research).

Each of these areas attracts different professionals with different training, professionals who tackle a large array of problems, who use varied research tools, who apply a large variety of different procedures, and who view the field from different perspectives. Below is a matrix identifying the manner in which different professionals contribute to the field.

THE CLINICAL EVALUATION

The clinical evaluation of individual workers affected by exposure to neurotoxic agents in the workplace is performed by specially trained physicians with the aid of other personnel including neuropsychologists, analytical chemists, and radiologists. Although the term "environmental and occupational (E & O) medicine" has long been in existence, a joint specialization in these two intimately related fields has only recently emerged.

Environmental and Occupational Medicine

Environmental and occupational physicians evaluate, diagnose, and treat people affected by exposure to toxic substances in the envi-

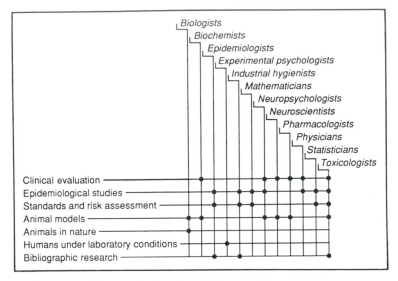

E & O neurotoxicology professionals and their areas of
involvement.

ronment and the workplace. The term "occupational neurology" was first proposed in
the early 1980s as a medical discipline that
deals with people affected by neurotoxic agents
at the workplace. An E & O physician observes the sick, asks questions relative to his
or her health history, takes a detailed account
of the person's present job(s), performs a
physical examination, requests the performance of tests when indicated, consults experts or available literature when in doubt,
ponders the contribution of various other
medical or psychological confounding factors, and—on the best evidence—arrives at a
professional opinion on the causes of illness.

Environmental and occupational physicians are familiar with a large body of knowledge, including not only medicine but also
the large number of toxic agents, their targets, techniques that are appropriate to detect
their presence in the environment or worksite, and the manner in which chemical compounds or their metabolites may be detected
in the human body.

The clinical examination may take place
in many different places, including private
offices, private and publicly owned hospitals,
occupational clinics in major hospitals, medical facilities attached to industrial com-
plexes, forensic clinics, and under field conditions. In Europe—where occupational
medicine has a long tradition, particularly in
England, Germany, France, Russia, Yugo-
slavia, Romania, Czechoslovakia, Finland,
Sweden, Denmark, and Italy—there are special institutes of occupational health devoted
to the diagnosis, treatment and rehabilitation
of people affected by occupational diseases.
In Japan, there are entire universities devoted
to the study of industrial hygiene and industrial medicine as well as specialized centers
such as the National Institute for Minamata
Disease (for the long-term evaluation of victims of the contamination by methylmercury
that took place in the Minamata Bay in the
1950s and 1960s).

Environmental and occupational physicians are sometimes the first to detect an environmental or occupational health problem.
The examination of an individual patient affected by a work-related disease may lead to
the examination of other people working under similar conditions in the same facilities.
A medical field survey can result after an oc-

cupational physician detects a cluster of illnesses among workers.

Forensic Toxicology

Crisso (1987) has defined the term "forensic" as "... any information that is appropriate for a legal forum." A "... forensic psychologist refers to any psychologist, experimental or clinical, who specializes in producing or communicating psychological research of assessment information intended for application to legal issues." A forensic neurotoxicologist is a professional who can advise the courts on matters of the effects of neurotoxic agents in humans.

Forensic toxicologists are physicians with special training in pathology and toxicology; sometimes they are trained in pharmacology and chemistry. They are called upon when the medicolegal aspects of harmful chemicals arise, especially when death or serious injury results from chemical exposure. Forensic toxicologists are often required to appear in court during the course of such proceedings and explain their findings in language that a jury of laypeople can understand.

Until recently, assessments performed by psychologists in courts were limited to areas such as criminal responsibility, competence to stand trial, child custody in cases of divorce or abuse, injury, etc. More recently, research and clinical psychologists have been called on to advise or to act as expert witnesses in matters of regulation and control of toxic agents in the environment and the workplace.

Because of the nature of their work—and its legal implications—forensic toxicologists have an encyclopedic knowledge of the harmful effects of chemicals that may be involved in accidental poisoning, their criminal use, and drug addiction. To accommodate this information explosion, an increasing number of universities offer programs in forensic toxicology at the graduate—and even at the undergraduate—level.

Clinical Neurotoxicology

The link between clinical neurotoxicology and environmental and health problems occurred in the early 1980s. Until then, the term "neurotoxicology" was almost invariably associated with drug abuse or experimental animal research. The field of clinical neurotoxicology is shared by occupational physicians, clinical neuropsychologists, neurologists, psychiatrists, and pediatricians. What clinical neurotoxicology "is" and what clinical neurotoxicologists do vary from institution to institution and from country to country. In Western Europe, for example, psychologists who work in clinical neurotoxicology rely on psychometric tests as the primary source for diagnosis. In Russia, electrophysiological procedures are favored. In the United States, neuropsychologists are trained in both psychometric, psychophysical, and electrophysiological procedures. As a result, in this country it is not uncommon for a neuropsychologist to issue a clinical report in which electrophysiological methods—such as nerve conduction velocity determinations—are used.

Clinical neuropsychologists in the United States participate in the assessment and diagnosis of environmental and occupational neurological disease. To be able to examine patients and to provide a professional judgment on the psychological picture of a patient, psychologists are required to have state licenses. It is only recently that psychologists are being trained to recognize that certain neuropsychological disorders may be caused by exposure to environmental and occupational toxic agents.

Neuropathological Perspectives

Neuropathological observations at the gross morphological, cellular, and molecular levels for determining possible toxic causation are one of the pillars of modern E & O neurotoxicology. In the past decade, several sources have become available on this topic. Stata Norton's chapter "Toxic Responses of the Central Nervous System" in *Casarett and Doull's Toxicology,* edited by C. D. Klaasen, M. O. Amdur, and J. Doull (1986), is an outstanding example. A chapter on "Nervous System Injury" by C. M. Shaw and E. C. Alvord in a book awkwardly titled *Environmental Pathology,* edited by N. K. Mottet (1985), is also an example of this approach.

Some neuropathologists seem to have only recently appreciated the shortcomings of exclusive reliance on morphological evidence as a possible indication of toxic causation. Although in the past decade there have been many efforts to impose this as the primary source of evidence for regulation and control of neurotoxic agents in the environment and the workplace—as in *Principles and Methods for the Assessment of Neurotoxicity with Exposure to Chemicals,* published by the World Health Organization in 1986—there are two important problems with this approach.

First, structural changes in the nervous system caused by exposure to toxic chemicals may occur at a later stage, long after neurochemical changes (eg, alterations in the pharmacokinesis of neurotransmission) have occurred. Historically, the morphological view of toxic causation was valuable at a time when little was known about the neurochemical processes that could be used as biological indicators of toxic exposure. In environmental health research, the neuropathological perspective of toxic causation occupies a relatively less prominent place because of these advances. Morphological alterations may be indicative of a very advanced stage of chemical effect and thus cannot be used for either prevention, monitoring, or control of neurotoxicologic exposure in the environment.

In forensic toxicology, however, particularly applied to the assessment of individual cases, the preeminence of the neuropathologist's testimony has never been questioned.

THE EVALUATION OF HEALTH EFFECTS ON LARGE HUMAN GROUPS

Two important study situations—short-term and long-term—are encountered when observing the health consequences of toxic exposure in large groups of people. The association between human neurotoxic exposures and diseases may be ascertained as a result of a well-planned epidemiological study that lasts several years. More frequently, however, these links are discovered as a result of environmental disasters or occupational accidents that happen in a matter of hours or days. For this reason, these two important contexts are reviewed separately.

Clinical Epidemiology

Epidemiology is the "study of the distribution and determinants of health-related states and events in populations, and the application of this study to the control of health problems" (Last 1983). An epidemiologist is "an investigator who studies the occurrence of disease or other health-related problems or events in defined populations." The **control** of disease in populations is also often considered a task for the epidemiologist, especially in speaking of certain specialized fields such as malaria epidemiology. In addition, epidemiologists may sometimes study disease in populations of animals and plants.

For many years the field of epidemiology was dominated by the study of diseases caused by biological vectors, particularly infectious diseases. In spite of the fact that epidemiology as a scientific discipline can be traced to the 17th century, epidemiologists have only recently became interested in morbidity studies of environmental and occupational origin where chemical agents are the vectors. (Epidemiologists have long been involved in mortality studies of workers and are responsible for the current concern regarding the possible occupational etiology of cancer.) The primary contributions of epidemiology are methodological, such as the improvement of study design, the adequate control of bias, and the perfecting of techniques for conducting surveys.

Broadly speaking, a survey is the systematic observation of a large number of people. A survey is both the context within which the study is performed and the instrument with which such research is performed, such as a questionnaire, a telephone interview, or a mail probe. An important difference exists between a health survey and a medical survey. In the former, interviewers ask questions about people's health. A questionnaire is the most common way this information is obtained. In a medical survey, various licensed professionals collect information that leads to the ascertainment of the people's current health status. For example, a physician performs a medical examination; a neuropsychologist administers a performance test; a nurse draws blood, etc.

There are many areas of overlap between statisticians and epidemiologists. Traditionally, epidemiologists were viewed as professionals who would have something to say about how the data are **collected**, whereas statisticians would have a similar claim on how the data are **analyzed**. But these differences are becoming blurred as the result of increasing collaboration among epidemiologists, statisticians, social scientists, econometricians, and many other professionals. Issues on study design, sampling, bias, the power of inferences, matters regarding techniques of test validation, statistical treatment of exposure data, and analysis of dose–response relationships are common to a large number of professionals.

Schoenberg (1978) has proposed the term "neuroepidemiology" to describe a discipline that studies the prevalence, incidence, and mechanisms of human neurotoxic diseases in populations. But the term has not been generally adopted by epidemiologists and other health scientists. The major problem with the term is that it emphasizes superspecialization at a time when many disciplines are discovering the advantages of the opposite trend, toward multidisciplinary research.

Environmental Disasters and Occupational Accidents

During environmental disasters or occupational accidents, emergency health surveys are performed by environmental response teams to determine the extent and the magnitude of health problems. Emergency surveys are reviewed in detail because, as stated above, they have given rise to vital information in E & O neurotoxicology. House-to-house inspections during devastating epidemics and industrial surveys performed in the middle of the 19th century in England, France, and Germany to cope with accidents produced by the then new chemical industry were antecedents of modern medical surveys.

In a medical field survey, the research team goes to the actual site where the problem has occurred. Thus, there are important differences in study conditions between institution-based surveys and field surveys. In the laboratory-based medical survey, all resources of a well-equipped research facility are available to scientists and professionals, and workers may be examined for several consecutive days. In a medical field survey the scope is much more limited because of time and equipment constraints.

It must be recognized that a battery of tests given under field conditions is never a substitute for the comprehensive evaluation performed in a medical center. This is clearly explained to participants before they give their informed consent.

SETTING STANDARDS AND ASSESSING RISKS

Industrial hygiene began in Europe in the middle of the 19th century to combat the excesses brought about by the Industrial Revolution and the innumerable—and unanticipated—health problems associated with the birth of industry. The first industrial standards were issued in the late 1880s. Setting standards and assessing risks is essentially a social and humanitarian issue. In the United States a safe environment and a healthy workplace are considered a human right.

There are many disciplines that contribute to the characterization of the chemical environment; this information is essential for the regulation and control of neurotoxic substances and law enforcement. Four are reviewed here: chemistry, toxicology, industrial hygiene, and risk assessment.

Chemistry

Chemists work in close association with toxicologists, epidemiologists, statisticians, physicians, neuropsychologists, and others when dose–response relationships between chemical exposures and effects need to be known. Chemical analysts determine not only the presence of indicators of environmental exposure—eg, lead at the worksite—but also biological indicators of exposure—ie, chemical substances, such as lead, present unchanged in biological specimens such as hair, nails, blood, urine, or dentine. They sometimes develop techniques for the assessment of biological indicators of effect. [The zinc protoporphyrin test used for the monitoring of lead poisoning was developed by physicists at Bell Laboratories, professionals that had another interest, that of the fluorescent patterns of biological materials (Blumberg et al. 1977).]

Analytical chemists analyze samples of chemicals present in the environment or the workplace in order to identify the substance(s) that may be harmful. For this purpose they use essentially three methods:

1. Classical chemical methods—eg, whether the substance is primarily an acid or base, gravimetric analysis, and solid–liquid, liquid–liquid, or solid–gas extractions.

2. Instrumental methods of analysis—eg, the selective absorption of visible, infrared, or ultraviolet light or X-rays, X-ray diffraction patterns and fluorescence, emission spectrophotometry, and a large variety of electrochemical procedures.

3. Physicochemical procedures such as the flame emission and emission spectrography used for qualitative and quantitative determination of chemical substances; for certain substances, such as metals, new imaging techniques allow the evaluation of whole-body contents of these substances.

The world of chemistry has been reviewed in an excellent book published in 1985 aimed at the general public: *Opportunities in Chemistry* by the Committee to Survey Opportunities in the Chemical Sciences.

Toxicology

Various branches of toxicology provide information leading to the setting of standards and the evaluation of human risks; these include descriptive, environmental, economic, and regulatory toxicology.

Descriptive Toxicology. The early studies on toxic effects in animals or humans are almost always descriptive. In animal experimentation, descriptive toxicologists trained in pharmacology and toxicology ascertain the lethal dose of chemical compounds with the assumption that this may provide information on the risks posed to humans.

Environmental Toxicology. The spread and effects of chemical pollutants in soil, water, and air, particularly those chemicals present around a known source of toxic materials, are studied by biologists and ecologists, who make important contributions to this branch of toxicology. This discipline is also called ecotoxicology. A specific branch of environmental toxicology is industrial and occupational toxicology, which studies the harmful effects of chemicals in the working environment.

Economic Toxicology. This discipline deals with chemicals used as drugs, food additives, cosmetics, pesticides, and veterinary drugs having an economic value for society. Economists study such problems as the financial consequences of implementing alternative methods to protect individuals or reduce or eliminate a toxic substance from the environment, and the projected medical costs of dealing with disease and death resulting from toxic agents in the environment and worksites.

Regulatory Toxicology. The federal government of the United States has several regulatory agencies dealing with the safety of drugs and toxic agents in the environment and the workplace—eg, the Food and Drug Administration (FDA), the Environmental Protection Agency (EPA), the Occupational Safety and Health Administration (OSHA), and the National Institute of Occupational Safety and Health (NIOSH). Regulatory toxicologists have the important responsibility of evaluating the existing data for a given drug or product, the intended mode of application for its use as a drug, its release into the environment, or its presence in the workplace. The American Conference of Governmental Industrial Hygienists (ACGIH), for example, periodically publishes and updates information on permissible levels of a large number of industrial toxic agents.

Industrial Hygiene

According to Clayton (1973), "industrial hygiene is both a science and an art. It covers the total realm of control, including recognition and evaluation of those factors of the environment emanating from the place of work which may cause illness, lack of well-being or discomfort either among workers or among the community as a whole." The industrial hygienist is someone educated in engineering, chemistry, physics, medicine or a related biological science. His or her abilities may encompass three major areas: recognition of the interrelation of environment and industry, evaluation of the impairment of health and well-being by work and work operations, and formulation of recommendations for alleviation of such problems.

Industrial hygienists participate—with the help of other health professionals, particularly occupational physicians—in periodic monitoring of the quality of the environment and the workplace through sampling of soil, water, and air using a variety of sampling devices. They may also design and develop protective devices or systems with the aid of environmental engineers. Their role in training, education, and prevention is important because they have intimate contact with workers and the health problems they experience. Industrial hygienists also play a major role in the training of workers in the use of protective equipment and hygiene practices.

Risk Assessment

Risk assessment, or risk analysis, is a discipline that deals with the quantitative analysis of risk factors. A risk factor is a background condition, physical attribute, or exposure that increases the probability of disease or some other outcome. Mathematical and statistical models allow one to make such predictions. Many risk assessments are performed to predict future outcomes in order to design preventive measures, and thus are intimately associated with economic toxicology, described above.

Within the framework of E & O neurotoxicology, risk analysis is one of the youngest disciplines. Very little theoretical or empirical work has been done in the field except in pediatric neurotoxicology. Recent work has been directed to the contribution of social and economic factors in the elevation of blood lead levels in children, levels that may in turn adversely affect intelligence.

PERFORMING TOXICOLOGICAL EXPERIMENTS ON LABORATORY ANIMALS

Industrial chemical compounds and drugs are tested in animals under controlled conditions to ascertain their toxic properties. In drug manufacture, toxicity testing is performed first; laboratory animals sometimes are tested after an outbreak of neurotoxic E & O illness has occurred.

What "toxicity" means has changed in the past 40 years. For example, since the tragic episode of thalidomide—a hypnotic drug used by mothers during pregnancy that caused limb deformities in the unborn—all new drugs are required to be tested for teratogenic effects. The notion that—in addition to toxicological and teratogenic evaluation—behavioral tests should also be performed before chemical compounds are released to the market is still in the process of being implemented.

Animal experimentation is sometimes performed after neurotoxic effects have already been observed in humans. For example, occupational exposure to n-hexane—an industrial solvent—causes severe peripheral neuropathy in humans; animal experimentation proved n-hexane to be the causative agent. The mechanism of action of n-hexane neurotoxicity is now understood because of extensive animal experimentation.

Research on absorption, distribution, and excretion of neurotoxic agents, their receptor sites, mechanisms of toxicity, pharmacological actions of neurotoxic agents, side effects, and dose–response relationships in experimental animals are performed by scientists who have different backgrounds, such as neuropharmacology/toxicology, psychopharmacology, and behavioral toxicology.

Neuropharmacology/Toxicology

Neuropharmacology is a discipline dealing with the chemical and therapeutic properties of drugs and agents that have the nervous system as a target. The term is used very loosely, and it sometimes implies the discipline in which experiments are performed in vitro (meaning in a laboratory dish), such as the study of isolated cells, or in vivo (the study of whole organisms), such as the observation of behavior after injection of a toxic substance into a rat. Neuropharmacology is an outgrowth of the sciences of pharmacology and biochemistry.

Neuropharmacology is concerned with the understanding of the physicochemical, pharmacological, neurophysiological, and behavioral (or psychological) mechanisms by which neurotoxic agents exert their effects on the nervous system. That is why neuropharmacology and mechanistic toxicology—a term that now has largely been abandoned—have no clear boundaries. The understanding of such mechanisms is essential for the development of therapeutic drugs. Whether this knowledge is also essential for regulation and control of E & O neurotoxic agents is arguable. As the mode of action of the vast numbers of chemicals in the human environment is still being studied, offenders in the meantime have no legal barriers to continuing chemical pollution.

Psychopharmacology

"Psychopharmacology" is a term that first appeared in scientific literature in the middle 1950s in connection with the development of "wonder drugs" (chlorpromazine and diazepam or Valium™). A new breed of investigator surfaced: psychologists with classical training in animal laboratory research and, at the same time, neuroanatomy, neurophysiology, biochemistry, and pharmacology.

The term "psychoneuropharmacology" is a relatively new specialization within pharmacology and indicates the territory psychopharmacology covers. The qualifier "psycho" is intended to incorporate the realm of subjective phenomena, which is largely ignored by behaviorists working with animal models. However, the term is unlikely to catch on in scientific circles. In 1984 Robert S. Feldman and Linda F. Quenzer published an excellent textbook titled *Fundamentals of Neuropsychopharmacology,* an equally unwieldy term.

Behavioral Toxicology

The term "behavioral toxicology" has been widely used in the scientific literature since the late 1960s to characterize a discipline that studies the effects of toxic chemicals on behavior and uses behavioral methods for the monitoring and control of exposure to neurotoxic agents in the environment and the workplace. It was coined by experimental and clinical psychologists who work either with experimental animals or—less frequently—people exposed to neurotoxic agents in the workplace. The term "behavioral toxicology" is essentially incorrect: a drug or toxic agent cannot act directly on behavior but only through its action on the nervous system. The term, which appeared in many reports between the 1960s and the early 1980s, is gradually being replaced by "neurotoxicology."

OBSERVATIONS OF NONHUMAN SPECIES IN THEIR NATURAL HABITATS

Changes in the normal patterns of behavior have often served as clues of impending environmental disasters. Rachel Carson's (1962) book *Silent Spring* describing observations of the devastating effects of pesticides on wildlife is the best illustration. There are many others. In Michigan, for example, observation of abnormal physical and behavioral changes in farm animals intoxicated by polybrominated biphenyls (PBBs) preceded the appearance of neurological symptoms in people.

Environmental research is closely identified with the study of the effects of toxic agents on living organisms in their natural habitats. Research is conducted by different professionals trained in the natural sciences, including several specialties of biology such as insect physiology, marine biology, lake fishery, agricultural sciences, forestry, zoology, and veterinary medicine. (However, many environmental problems involving neurotoxic agents—such as mass deaths—have been spotted first not by scientists but by people who work outdoors or enjoy outdoor activities, such as park managers, farmers, fishermen, and sportspeople.)

The observation of animals in the wild has had a long and uninterrupted tradition. But it is *ethology* that has the most relevance to our field. Ethology deals with the observation of animals in their natural environment, and gained prominence as a result of the studies of Nikolaas Tinbergen, Konrad Lorenz, and Karl von Frisch, who in 1973 won the Nobel prize for their studies on ethology and the biological basis of animal behavior (Gould 1982).

Ethologists have been the most acerbic critics of investigators who perform animal research under laboratory conditions, for the following reasons: (1) animals are not likely to display their full repertoire of behavioral patterns under laboratory conditions; (2) many behavioral toxicologists coming from highly automated, technician-run laboratories have little or no contact—much less familiarity—with the animals whose behavior they claim to study; and (3) "The selection of a behavior pattern for assessing the effects of a given neurotoxin would dictate which experimental methods and measuring techniques are appropriate, rather than the methodology determining which form of behavior might be examined" (Davis 1982).

Ethologists, ecologists, and many biologists working in environmental research have made important conceptual contributions to the field of environmental neurotoxicology by emphasizing the need to see problems beyond the tools used for the study of these problems. Yet, the contribution of ethology to the field is mainly programmatic. Except for rare articles, such as Davis (1982), ethological approaches in neurotoxicology have been underrepresented in the body of neurotoxicological literature.

PERFORMING HUMAN STUDIES UNDER LABORATORY CONDITIONS

Human studies under laboratory conditions have a long tradition in experimental psychology (Boring 1950). The use of instrumentation for the objective study of a variety of psychological functions such as attention, concentration, reaction time, sensory processes, memory function, cognition, etc made the birth of psychology possible as an independent discipline. The oldest laboratories of experimental psychology in the United States were founded soon after they were created in Germany in the middle of the 19th century.

A serious effort to bring together the tools of the trade of toxicology and experimental psychology occurred in many countries around the late 1960s. Human studies under laboratory conditions seemed to be the only true counterpart to toxicological research carried out in animals under controlled conditions. However, these experiments were short-lived.

The goals of human experimentation under laboratory conditions were: (1) to study permissible levels of environmental and occupational exposures—ie, measurable levels that just produce observable behavioral alterations; (2) in the majority of cases, to monitor the absorption and excretion of neurotoxic agents, particularly in the case of solvents, at the same time psychological tests are administered; and (3) to ascertain dose–effect relationships between concentrations of neurotoxic exposure and psychological functions or between exhaled or excreted metabolites and psychological function.

Because of ethical considerations, human experimentation needed to be restricted to acute exposure, although studies of effects of chronic exposure in volunteer subjects are also reported from time to time in the literature. The manner by which these cumulative effects of acute episodes are transformed into chronic effects—an important question in human neurotoxicology—cannot be effectively studied in volunteers.

We should not lament the progressive disappearance of this type of research. In the United States, human studies involving exposure to neurotoxic agents under laboratory conditions have been seriously curtailed because of ethical considerations. Clearance by ethical committees at institutional levels, informed consent, freedom to withdraw from the experiment without fear of penalty, and the prohibition of use of deception have now become standard requirements in human laboratory experimentation (Adair et al. 1985). The concensus is that utilization of data—or even their citation in any form—derived from human experiments performed in concentration camps or among people who have been experimented upon against their will violates similar ethical principles.

Experimental neurotoxicology, however, made an important contribution to the field: the use of laboratory instrumentation for the measurement of basic psychological functions and the use of computer-based testing procedures.

SUMMING UP RESEARCH RESULTS

The results of research eventually need to be distilled, and the significance of the major findings communicated. Summing up such literature—sometimes called "meta-analysis" by social scientists—is also an important research activity. For example, lead is known to be neurotoxic because of the hundreds of published observations and studies that have been performed in humans as well as in laboratory animals. In general, in order to understand how a neurotoxic agent or drug affects nervous system function and behavior, the results of both animal and human experiments need to be summarized.

Summing up scientific literature is accomplished by specially trained people. In the early 1980s several excellent books appeared with recommendations on how the science of reviewing other people's research ought to be performed (Glass et al. 1981; Hunter et al. 1982; Light and Pillemer 1984).

A review of the scientific literature is essential for other scientists, for educated people who want to be informed on matters concerning them, and for legislation. A review of literature is sometimes a form of research in that a hypothesis is supported or discounted as a result of such a search. New research is often necessary to resolve conflicting research findings.

The art and science of summing up is the direct result of the information explosion. When one cannot read all the facts, a summary of the facts published by a reputable reviewer is essential. In 1980 TOXLINE, a valuable computer-based reference databank in toxicology, became available; its information is derived from 14,000 journals listed at least once (Kissman 1980). Read-only disks designed for personal computers—CD-ROM—have also been increasingly available. The information explosion has generated the need for professionals to understand the available primary bibliographic sources and to review major findings following strict statistical principles.

The information explosion has also given rise to the phenomenon of reviewing reviews—a feature of the journal *Annual Review of Pharmacology and Toxicology*—thus distancing the information obtained from the original conclusions reached by the investigators themselves. Current recommended standards for toxic agents are preceded by such exhaustive bibliographic research. The conclusions obtained from conducting bibliographic research are very important and play a powerful role when legislation is at stake.

It is often the case that people who participate in influencing legislation—particularly lawyers, professional lobbyists, managers, leaders of labor organizations—do not have the background or time to read the scientific literature or the details of significant documents supporting either side of a controversy. (The background documents associated with the new lead standard provide an example of this.)

Documents circulating in Washington, DC are usually accompanied by an *executive abstract* intended to be read in a few seconds. Until recently, no scholarly rules for abstracting the information existed; the conclusions reached were those of the person who performed the bibliographic search and wrote the abstract. Without rigorous methodology, it is almost unavoidable that those writing such abstracts impose their own bias, thus eliminating the very essence of what scientists try to provide.

Meta-Analysis

Meta-analysis is the use of statistical methods for the investigation of results obtained from a series of separate experimental or observational studies. In practice, meta-analytical work involves the use of summary statistics (most commonly dimensionless quantities to facilitate comparisons), correlation coefficients, and probability values that events may have occurred by chance alone.

Meta-analysis is a branch of statistics and is not to be confused with literature review. In reviewing past published results, strict adherence to statistical thinking is maintained. An example of meta-analysis is the document published in 1984 entitled *Toxicity Testing: Strategies to Determine Needs and Priorities*, published as a joint effort by the Steering Committee on Identification of Toxic and Potentially Toxic Chemicals for Consideration by the National Toxicology Program, and the Board on Toxicology and Environmental Health Hazards, the Commission on Life Sciences, and the National Research Council. In this document, a "select universe" of 65,725 substances that are of possible concern to the National Toxicology Program (NTP) because of their potential for human exposure were identified. Of these, a random sample of 675 substances covering seven major intended-use categories were further selected. From this sample, a subsample of 100 substances was selected by screening for the presence of at least some toxicity information. In the great majority of cases, data considered to be essential for conducting a health assessment are lacking. This document contains an appendix (Appendix I) discussing the need for guidelines or reference protocols for neurobehavioral toxicity tests in animals.

CONCLUSIONS

In all scientific disciplines the context of research is dictated by research objectives. Environmental and occupational neurotoxicology is a discipline that originated in medicine, with the examination of individuals affected by agents that had the nervous system as a primary target of toxicity. It acquired momentum and achieved a generally recognized social significance when unsuspected victims, because of occupational exposures or environmental accidents, became ill and even died as a result of these exposures. It is closely related to the work performed by those who measure levels of neurotoxic exposure and who recommend maximum allowable exposures at the workplace.

But the discipline also legitimately covers the efforts of those who perform neurotoxicological experiments in laboratory animals under controlled conditions, looking for basic mechanisms of neurotoxic action; those who examine marked changes in the behavior of wildlife with signs of environmental neurotoxic contamination; and those who perform human studies under controlled laboratory conditions. Finally, it also encompasses the work of those who summarize the wealth of knowledge, efforts that ultimately are reflected in national, state, and local laws and recommendations essential for enforcement, leading to a safe environment and a healthy workplace.

Context of research refers to where the research takes place, by whom, and why the research is performed. The context, thus defined, determines the specific professional training necessary to perform the study, dictates a language that professionals use among themselves, brings to focus a specific set of problems, influences the choice of tools and procedures to study selected problems, and ultimately affects the fate of the practical uses of the information obtained.

Unfortunately, the context of a study is often unrecognized by those who work and think from a perspective other than that used in the study. Characteristically, for some there is a sense of pride in viewing problems from a given angle; not uncommonly other perspectives are respectfully ignored—less frequently, they are even secretly derided. The end result is that valid research often does not receive the attention it deserves and potentially important information remains unrecognized.

Environmental and occupational neurotoxicology is applied research. It is intimately linked to the objective of effective monitoring of the quality of our environment, the safety of our workplace, and, ultimately, the improvement of the quality of our lives.

REFERENCES

Adair, JG, Dushenko, TW, and Lindsay, RCL (1985) Ethical regulations and their impact on research practice. *Am Psychol* 40:59–72.

Blumberg, WE, Eisinger, J. Lamola, AA et al. (1977) The hematofluorometer. *Clin Chem* 23:270–274.

Boring, EG (1950) *A History of Experimental Psychology.* New York: Appleton-Century-Crofts.

Carson, R (1962) *Silent Spring.* Greenwich, CT: Fawcett.

Clayton, GD (1973) Introduction. In *The Industrial Environment—Its Evaluation and Control.* Washington, DC: US Department of Health Education and Welfare, Public Health Service, NIOSH.

Committee to Survey Opportunities in the Chemical Sciences, Board on Chemical Sciences and Technology,

Commission on Physical Sciences, Mathematics, and Resources and National Research Council (1985) *Opportunities in Chemistry.* Washington, DC: National Academy of Sciences.

Crisso, T (1987) The economic and scientific future of forensic psychological assessment. *Am Psychol* 42:831–838.

Davis, JM (1982) Ethological approaches to behavioral toxicology. In *Nervous System Toxicity,* CL Mitchell (ed) pp. 29–44. New York: Raven Press.

Feldman, RS and Quenzer, LF (1984) *Fundamentals of Neuropsychopharmacology.* Sunderland, MA: Sinauer Associates.

Glass, GV, McGaw, B, and Smith, ML (1981) *Meta-Analysis of Social Research.* Beverly Hills, CA: Sage.

Gould JL (1982) *Ethology: The Mechanisms and Evolution of Behavior.* New York: WW Norton.

Hunter, JE, Schmidt, FL, and Jackson, GB (1982) *Meta-Analysis: Cumulating Research Findings Across Studies.* Beverly Hills, CA: Sage.

Kissman, HM (1980) Information retrieval in toxicology. *Annu Rev Pharmacol Toxicol* 20:285–305.

Last, JM (ed)(1983) *A Dictionary of Epidemiology.* New York: Oxford University Press.

Light, RJ and Pillemer, DB (1984) *Summing Up: The Science of Reviewing Research.* Cambridge, MA: Harvard University Press.

Norton, S (1986) Toxic responses of the central nervous system. In *Casarett and Doull's Toxicology: The Basic Science of Poisons,* 3rd ed. CD Klaasen, MO Amdur, and J Doull (eds) pp. 359–386. New York: Macmillan.

Schoenberg, BS (1978) *Advances in Neurology, Vol 19.* New York: Raven Press.

Shaw, CM and Alvord, EC (1985) Nervous system injury. In *Environmental Pathology,* NK Mottet (ed) pp. 368–453. New York: Oxford University Press.

Steering Committee on Identification of Toxic and Potentially Toxic Chemicals for Consideration by the National Toxicology Program, the Board on Toxicology and Environmental Health Hazards, the Commission on Life Sciences, and the National Research Council (1984) *Toxicity Testing: Strategies to Determine Needs and Priorities.* Washington, DC: National Academy Press.

World Health Organization (1986) *Principles and Methods for the Assessment of Neurotoxicity Associated with Exposure to Chemicals,* Environmental Health Criteria 60. Geneva: WHO.

SUGGESTED READINGS

Ad Hoc Committee, American Industrial Hygiene Association (1959) Industrial hygiene: Definitions, scope, function and organization. *Am Ind Hyg Assoc J* 20:428–430.

American Conference of Governmental and Industrial Hygienists. *TLVs*™: Threshold Limit Values and Biological Indices for 1985–1986.

American Psychological Association (1973) *Ethical Principles in the Conduct of Research with Human Participants.* Washington, DC: APA.

Arezzo, JC and Schaumburg, HH (1989) Office and field diagnosis of neurotoxic disease. *J Am Coll Toxicol* 8(2):311–319.

Ashford, NA and Bingham, E (1989) *Environmental and Occupational Health Training.* Princeton, NJ: Princeton Scientific Publications.

Barners, DM (1989) Neurotoxicity creates regulatory dilemma. *Science* 243:29–30.

Capurro, PU (1966) The clinical pathologist as hospital toxicologist. *Bull Pathol* 132.

Castleman, B and Ziem, G (1988) The corporate influence on threshold limit values. *Am J Ind Med* 13:531–559.

Checkoway, H, Dement, JM, Fowler, DP, et al. (1987) Industrial hygiene involvement in occupational epidemiology. *Am Ind Hyg Assoc J* 48(6):515–523.

Cochran, WG (1937) Problems arising in the analysis of a series of similar experiments. *J R Stat Soc (Suppl)* 4:102–118.

Comstock, EG (1979) The practice of medical toxicology. *Clin Toxicol* 15(1):1–11.

Cook, TD and Leviton, LC (1980) Reviewing the literature: A comparison of traditional methods with meta-analysis. *Person* 48:449–472.

Cook, RS and Trainer, DO (1966) Experimental lead poisoning of Canada geese. *J Wildlife Manage* 30:1–8.

Cools, A, Salle, HJA, Verberk, MM, et al. (1976) Biochemical response of male volunteers ingesting inorganic lead for 49 days. *Int Arch Env Occup Health* 38:129–139.

Cooper, HM (1982) Scientific guidelines for conducting integrative research reviews. *Rev Educ Res* 52:291–302.

Cooper, HM and Rosenthal, R (1980) Statistical versus traditional procedures for summarizing research findings. *Psychol Bull* 87:442–449.

Forssman, S (1967) Occupational health institutes: An international survey. *Am Ind Hyg J* 28:197–203.

Friedman, SM, Dunwoody, S, and Rogers, CL (1986) *Scientists and Journalists: Reporting Science as News.* New York: The Free Press.

Gad, SC (1989) Screens in neurotoxicity: Objectives, design and analysis with the functional battery as a case example. *J Am Coll Toxicol* 8(2):287–301.

Gehring, PJ (1979) Clinical toxicology viewed from an industrial setting. *Clin Toxicol* 15(4):401–404.

Glass, GV (1976) Primary, secondary and meta-analysis of research. *Educ Res* 5:3–8.

Glass, GV, McGaw, B, and Smith, ML (1981) *Meta-Analysis of Social Research.* Beverly Hills, CA: Sage.

Goldberg, L (1980) Broader aspects of clinical toxicology. *Clin Toxicol* 16(3):365–370.

Hedges, LV and Olkin, I (1980) Vote-counting methods in research synthesis. *Psychol Bull* 88:359–369.

Hedges, LV and Olkin, I (1985) *Statistical Methods for Meta-Analysis.* New York: Academic Press.

Jackson, GB (1980) Methods for integrating reviews. *Rev Educ Res* 50:438–460.

Johnson, BL (ed) (1987) *Prevention of Neurotoxic Illness in Working Populations.* New York: John Wiley & Sons.

Johnson, BL, Anger, K, Durao, A, et al. (eds) (1990) *Advances in Neurobehavioral Toxicology: Applications in Environmental and Occupational Health.* Boca Raton, FL: Lewis.

Kehoe, RA (1961) Experimental studies on the inhalation of lead by human subjects. *Pure Appl Chem* 3:129–144.

Kehoe, RA (1962) Cummings memorial lecture: Education and training in industrial hygiene. *Am Ind Hyg Assoc J* 23:175–180.

Laties, VG (1982) Contributions of operant conditioning to behavioral toxicology. In *Nervous System Toxicology,* CL Mitchell (ed) pp. 67–79. New York: Raven Press.

Levine, RJ, McLaren, RM, Barthel, WF, et al. (1976) Occupational lead poisoning, animal deaths, and environmental contamination at a scrap smelter. *Am J Publ Health* 66:548–552.

Light, RJ and Pillemer, DB (1982) Numbers and narrative: Combining their strengths in research reviews. *Harvard Educ Rev* 52:1–26.

Mackay, CJ, Campbell, L, Samuel, AM, et al. (1987) Behavioral changes during exposure to 1,1,1-trichloroethane: Time course and relationship to blood solvent levels. *Am J Ind Med* 11:223–239.

Mann, C (1990) Meta-analysis in the breech. *Science* 249:476–480.

Mattison, JL, Albee, RR, and Eisenbrandt, DL (1989) Neurological approach to neurotoxicological evaluation of laboratory animals. *J Am Coll Toxicol* 8(2):271–286.

Meltzer, HY (1987) *Psychopharmacology: The Third Generation of Progress.* New York: Raven Press.

Miller, NE (1985) The value of behavioral research on animals. *Am Psychol* 423–440.

O'Connor, M, (1979) *The Scientist as Editor: Guidelines for Editors of Books and Journals.* New York: John Wiley & Sons.

Perrow, C (1984) *Normal Accidents: Living with High-Risk Technologies.* New York: Basic Books.

Pillemer, DB and Light, RJ (1980) Synthesizing outcomes: How to use research evidence from many studies. *Harvard Educ Rev* 50:176–195.

Poling, A, Cleary, J, and Monaghan, M (1980) The use of human observers in psychopharmacological research. *Pharmacol Biochem Behav* 13:243–246.

Putz, VR, Johnson, BL, and Setzer, JV (1979) A comparative study of the effects of carbon monoxide and methylene chloride on human performance. *J Environ Pathol Toxicol* 2:97–112.

Rosenthal, R (1979) The "file drawer problem" and tolerance for null results. *Psychol Bull* 86:638–461.

Russell, RW (1981) Behavioral toxicology: Development of a science and a profession. *Acad Psychol* 3(2):177–189.

Seaman, J (ed)(1984) *Epidemiology of Natural Disasters.* Basel: S Karger.

Sharp, CW and Carroll, LT (eds)(1978) *Voluntary Inhalation of Industrial Solvents.* Washington, DC: US Department of Health, Education and Welfare.

Smith, HF (1963) Industrial hygiene in retrospect and prospect. *Toxicol Aspects* 24:222–226.

Steward, RD, Baretta, ED, and Dodd, HC (1970) Experimental human exposure to tetrachloroethylene. *Arch Environ Health* 20:224–229.

Steward, RD, Dodd, HC, Milwaukee, AB, et al. (1970) Experimental human exposure to trichloroethylene. *Arch Environ Health* 20:64–71.

Steward, RD, Fisher, TN, Hosko, MJ, et al. (1972) Experimental human exposure to methylene chloride. *Arch Environ Health* 25:342–348.

Trainer, DO and Hunt, RA (1965) Lead poisoning of waterfowl in Wisconsin. *J Wildlife Manage* 29:95–103.

US Congress, Office of Technology Assessment (1990) *Neurotoxicity: Identifying and Controlling Poisons of the Nervous System.* OTA-BA-436. Washington, DC: Government Printing Office.

Verberk, MM (1976) Motor-nerve conduction velocity in volunteers ingesting inorganic lead for 49 days (technical note). *Int J Occup* 38(2):141–143.

Weiss, B (1983) Intersections of psychiatry and toxicology. *Int J Mental Health* 14(3):7–25.

Weiss, B (1983) Behavioral toxicology and environmental health science: Opportunities and challenge for psychology. *Am Psychol* 38(11): 1174–1187.

Wilson, JT (1980) Concepts to facilitate a combined program of clinical pharmacology and clinical toxicology. *Clin Toxicol* 16(3):371–376.

Winneke, G (1974) Behavioral effects of methylene chloride and carbon monoxide as assessed by sensory and psychomotor performance. In *Behavioral Toxicology, Early Detection of Occupational Hazards,* C Xintaras, BL Johnson, and I DeGroot (eds) pp. 130–144. Washington, DC: US Department of Health, Education and Welfare, Public Health Center for Disease Control, National Institute for Occupational Safety and Health.

Name Index

Subject Index

2,4,5-T, *see* 2,4,5-Trichlorophenoxyacetic acid
2,4-D, *see* 2,4-Dichlorophenoxyacetic acid
AAS, *see* Alcohol amnestic syndrome
Abdominal pain, caused by nicotine
    intoxication, 551
Abiotrophic process, and aging, 535
Abiotrophy, definition of, 535
Ablasion studies, providing information about
    mechanisms of memory, 491
Abnormal walk, 61
Absorption of neurotoxic agents, 175–179
Acaricides, 161
Acceleration, as a stimulus for vibration, 386
Accelerometer, vestibular system as an, 395,
    396
Accidents (chemical)
    epidemiological study of, 207–208
    as national problems, 2
Acetylcholine, 54, 55
Acetylcholinesterase agents, used in chemical
    warfare, 569
ACGIH, *see* American Conference of
    Government and Industrial Hygienists
Achievement of meaning, as quintessence of
    cognitive skills, 499
Achromatopsia, 430
Acoustic basis of speech intelligibility, 419
Acoustic imaging, 148
Acoustic nerve, 416
Acrylamide, 11
  as a cause of motor tremor, 65
Actin, 446
Action potential, 50, 51
Active transport, 179
Acute effects, toxicological definition of, 191
Acute neurological symptoms, in shipyard
    painters exposed to solvents, 311

Acute symptoms, definition for data analysis,
    288
Acute toxic effects, definition of, 72
Acute toxic encephalopathy, as an example of
    clinical syndrome, 72
Adaptation to external environment, 469
Addiction risks, in alcohol and drug abuse, 553
Additive effects of chemicals, 192
Adjustment disorder(s)
  caused by environmental accidents, 522
  definition, 522
Advance notice, in the organization of a medical
    field survey, 236
Adverse effects, of teratogens, 342
Aerosol(s)
  inhalation of, 176
  sprays used as inhalants, 554
  types, 176
Affect
  definition of, 68
  range of, 69
Affective disorders
  and alcoholism, 479
  types, 478–480
Afferent system, 444
Age trends
  ascertained in cross-sectional studies, 536
  correction in group data, 303–305
  disruptions created by computer-simulated
    "impairments," 295
  in psychometric test scores, 293
  in electrophysiological data, 304–305
  selective effects of toxic agents on, 294
Age
  and depression, 479
  as a factor in onset of panic disorder, 476
  and language, 500